Pulmonary Differential Diagnosis

Commissioning Editor: Serena Bureau
Production Manager: Mark Sanderson

Pulmonary Differential Diagnosis

Harold Zackon MD
Associate Professor of Medicine,
Clinical Director, Respiratory Division,
St. Mary's Hospital,
McGill University Health Centre,
Montreal, Quebec
Canada

WB Saunders
London • Edinburgh • New York • Philadelphia • Toronto •
St Louis • Sydney • Tokyo

WB Saunders
An imprint of Harcourt Publishers Limited

First published 2000

ISBN 0-7020-2577-1

British Library Cataloguing in Publication Data
A catalogue record for this book is available from the British Library

Library of Congress Cataloging in Publication Data
A catalog record for this book is available from the Library of Congress

Note
Medical knowledge is constantly changing. As new information becomes available, changes in treatment, procedures, equipment and the use of drugs become necessary. The editors/authors/contributors and the publishers have, as far as it is possible, taken care to ensure that the information given in this text is accurate and up to date. However, readers are strongly advised to confirm that the information, especially with regard to drug usage, complies with the latest legislation and standards of practice.

Printed in China

The
Publisher's
policy is to use
paper manufactured
from sustainable forests

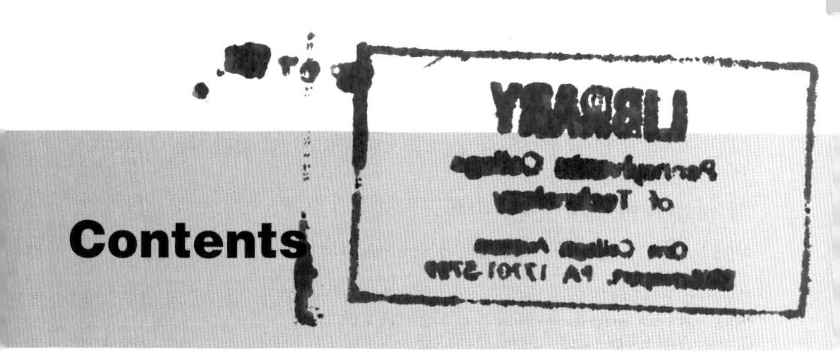

Contents

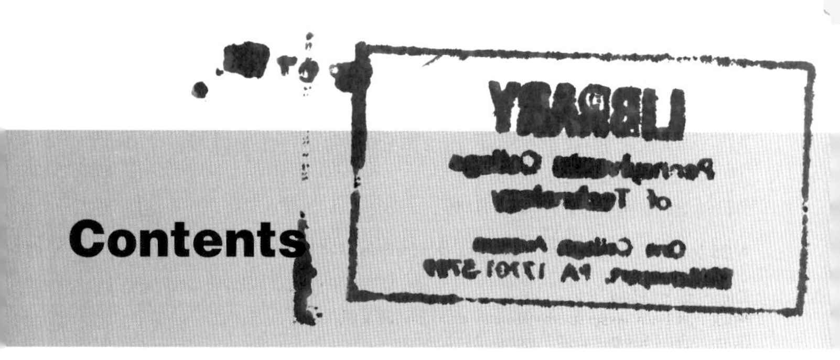

Contents

Contributors

Pierre Ernst, MD, MSc, FRCPC
Professor of Medicine,
McGill University
Montreal, Quebec
Canada

Guy Fradet, MD, MSc, FRCSC, FACS
Associate Professor, Department of Surgery
University of British Columbia
Vancouver, British Columbia
Canada

R. John Kimoff, MD, FRCPC
Associate Professor of Medicine
Director, MUHC Sleep Laboratory
McGill University
Montreal, Quebec
Canada

Robert D. Levy, MD, FRCPC
Associate Professor of Medicine
Vancouver General Hospital
University of British Columbia
Medical Director, Lung Transplant Program
British Columbia Transplant Society
Vancouver, British Columbia
Canada

Michael Libman, MD, FRCPC
Microbiologist-in-Chief
Montreal General Hospital
McGill University Montreal, Quebec
Canada

E. Matouk, MD ChB, FRCPC
Associate Professor of Medicine
McGill University
Director, Adult Cystic Fibrosis Clinic
Montreal Chest Institute, Royal Victoria Hospital
Montreal, Quebec
Canada

James Gerard Martin, MD
Professor of Medicine
Director, Meakins-Christie Laboratories
McGill University
Montreal, Quebec
Canada

Dick Menzies, MD, MSc
Associate Professor of Medicine, Epidemiology
and Biostatistics
McGill University
Montreal, Quebec
Canada

Kevin Schwartzman, MD, MPH, FRCPC
Assistant Professor of Medicine, Epidemiology
and Biostatistics
McGill University
Montreal, Quebec
Canada

Harold Zackon MD
Associate Professor of Medicine
Clinical Director, Respiratory Division

St Mary's Hospital
McGill University Health Centre
Montreal, Quebec
Canada

Preface

The symptoms and signs of pulmonary disease are often non-specific as the lungs can react to numerous insults in a limited number of ways. Similarly, radiologic imaging, our most important diagnostic tool, is frequently non-pathognomonic in its manifestations, but often compatible with a large group of disorders.

In spite of spending much time teaching pulmonary medicine, it is impossible to remember all the pertinent diagnostic features of the common and uncommon diseases increasingly described to involve the lungs. As the pulmonary literature has expanded annually, so have the size and volume of our textbooks. We cannot practically carry four volumes with us. In addition, the above texts cover physiology, pathology, pathogenesis, epidemiology, molecular biology, immunology, anatomy and treatment – all of which do not directly affect our initial differential diagnoses. The wealth of information available in present textbooks often results in difficulty extracting the pertinent diagnostic information. It is thc consideration of the wide range of diagnostic possibilities that will expedite investigations and lead to a prompt and correct diagnosis.

Statement of Purpose

My purpose is to develop a **portable practical handbook** that can be used by physicians at the bedside, in the Radiology Department, in the office, in the clinic setting as well as in preparation for teaching rounds with house staff. This portability is required as there is simply too much information to keep in our heads. This book is not a condensation of standard texts but rather those facts a consultant would like at his or her fingertips. I have tried to extract clinically relevant diagnostic information and organize it in an easily accessible alphabetic manner. This book will, hopefully, form a diagnostic framework for clinicians.

The subjects covered by the book are clinical problems or questions we have personally faced as pulmonary consultants:

- in office practice;
- in hospital practice at primary, secondary and tertiary care hospitals;
- as an emergency room consultant;
- teaching (and learning from) medical and respiratory residents;
- attending and organizing rounds at the McGill University Teaching Hospitals;
- attending pulmonary meetings e.g. ATS.

Users' Guide

Having identified the problems, i.e. radiologic abnormalities, pulmonary signs or symptoms, abnormal lab findings, I have tried to develop:

- a 'bottom-up' approach, e.g. airspace disease, where the range of diagnostic possibilities is listed and clues provided;
- a 'top-down' approach when the underlying pulmonary disease, e.g. alveolar proteinosis, or extrapulmonary disease, e.g. systemic lupus, is known but the pulmonary manifestations are described.

Target Audience

The target audience includes pulmonary physicians, pulmonary residents or fellows in training, internists, and internal medicine residents. It is, therefore, intended for those individuals with a background knowledge of pulmonary anatomy, physiology, pathology, radiology and clinical medicine.

'IF YOU BECOME A TEACHER, BY YOUR PUPILS YOU'LL BE TAUGHT'
Rodgers and Hammerstein – *The King and I*

Practicing pulmonary medicine for 20 years makes diagnosis almost 'second nature'. Through my encounters with students, interns and residents, I have had to articulate knowledge, transforming tacit knowledge into explicit knowledge. It has allowed me to identify clinical problems and develop a diagnostic approach to them that I hope will be useful to my readers.

H. Zackon
2000

Acknowledgements

This book is based on years of clinical experience and knowledge gleaned from my teachers, colleagues and students at the McGill University Health Center. The clinico-radiologic-pathologic approach to pulmonary medicine was emphasized by my outstanding physician-teachers including Drs. J.A. Peter Pare, P.D. Pare, Robert G. Fraser and Richard S. Fraser. A special thanks to Dr. Manuel Cosio who, as Director of the Respiratory Division, MUHC, gave me encouragement, support, clinical and common sense advice in writing this book. The manuscript could not have been completed without the tireless efforts of Sylvie DesRosiers and Barbara Robson. Finally, I would like to dedicate this book to my loving wife Janet and daughter Alysha.

Regards, Harold.

1 A, B, Cs of Radiologic Evaluation

CHEST X-RAY – WHAT TO LOOK FOR

Technical factors

- Name and age of patient
- Date of the film
- Right–left markers
- Properly centred and penetrated
- Adequate inspiration, i.e. at least 9 posterior ribs are seen above the diaphragm

Airways

1 Tracheal air column on PA film
  - Deviation
  - Narrowing: N > 10 mm female, >13 mm male
  - Dilatation:
    N < 21 mm coronal, < 23 mm sagittal } female; < 25 mm coronal, < 27 mm sagittal } male
  - Loss of distinct air–tissue border
  - Well-defined opacity within the air column

2 Carinal angle usually ~60° and <90°
3 Air in the main stem bronchi
4 Visualization of the tracheal air column as well as the right and the left upper lobe bronchi on lateral film

Parenchyma

5 Size
6 Symmetry
7 Abnormal opacities or lucencies

Pleura

8 Examine the lung circumference (including the costophrenic and cardiophrenic angles) as well as the fissures looking for nodularity, irregularity, mass lesions, loculated fluid, calcifications

Hilum and vasculature

9 Hilar regions for their size, shape, density, angle, relative heights and any change from previous films
10 Abnormal tapering or cut-off of the hilar vessels
11 Peripheral vasculature for increase, decrease or discrepancy between the two lungs

Chest wall (ABCD)

12 Asymmetric breast shadows
13 Bones, including the clavicles, ribs, scapula and spine on PA as well as the sternum and spine on lateral
14 Chest wall, neck and abdominal soft tissues for air, surgical clips, calcifications
15 Diaphragm height and contour

Mediastinum and heart

16 Paratracheal, para-aortic, aortopulmonary, pulmonary outflow tract, subcarinal and paraspinal areas on the PA film for a mass lesion and/or adenopathy
17 Retrosternal and retrotracheal areas as well as the posterior mediastinum on the lateral film for evidence of a mass lesion and/or adenopathy
18 Cardiac silhouette re size, sharp borders, apex, configuration (LV or RV), chamber enlargement, calcifications
19 Major arteries and veins

Expiratory film is useful for detection of

1 Pneumothorax
2 Localized air trapping
   - Results from the obstruction to air leaving the lung and may be secondary to partial obstruction (endobronchial, peribronchial) or complete obstruction and collateral air drift
   - Manifest by hyperlucency and oligemia but may not

be appreciated on films exposed at TLC where the involved area of lung can be of normal, increased or decreased volume

- An obstructing endobronchial lesion almost always results in reduced volume of the obstructed area of lung at TLC whereas hyperinflation is seen with (a) congenital atresia of the apico-posterior segments of the LUL and (b) neonatal lobar emphysema
- Findings on an expiratory film include
  - Maintenance of volume in the region of air trapping (segmental, lobar, entire lung) *vs.* decreasing lung volume in normal areas
  - Little alteration in density of the abnormal area *vs.* a diffuse increase in density of normal lung, accentuating the differences
  - Contralateral mediastinal shift
  - Failure of elevation of the ipsilateral hemidiaphragm

Oblique film is useful for distinguishing the opacity of overlapping bronchovascular markings from a parenchymal or rib lesion

- Ordered less often today as it has been replaced by CT scan

AP portable film limitations

- Magnification of the heart, mediastinum and hilar vasculature
- Difficult identification of abnormalities in the posterior costophrenic angles, mediastinum or areas adjacent to the spine
- Impaired assessment of pleural effusions or pneumothorax (when supine)
- Pulmonary redistribution to the upper lobes (when supine)
- Diaphragmatic elevation with compressive atelectasis of the lower lobes, resembling an expiratory film and mimicking heart failure or basilar pneumonia (when supine)

OTHER RADIOLOGIC STUDIES

Chest Fluoroscopy – Indications

1. Assessment of diaphragmatic movement, e.g. paralysis
2. Lesion localization for TTNA or transbronchial biopsy

HRCT Scan – Features (vs regular CT)

- Vessels are sharper defined and more nodular in appearance
- Better airway visualization
- Improved visualization of pleural fissures
- Better definition of parenchymal disease including interstitial, airspace and cystic disorders
- Artifactual increased density of the dependent lung zones

HRCT scan – indications

1. Detection of disease not apparent on chest X-ray in patients presenting with undiagnosed
   - Hemoptysis, e.g. bronchiectasis, central endobronchial lesion
   - Dyspnea, e.g. early interstitial disease (sarcoid, UIP, allergic alveolitis, miliary TB, asbestosis)
     e.g. emphysema
     e.g. accentuated pattern of mosaic attenuation on expiratory HRCT with bronchiolitis obliterans
   - Cough, e.g. ILD, airway lesion
   - Fever in an immunocompromised host, e.g. pneumonia
   - Abnormal PFTs, e.g. ILD
2. Limit the differential diagnosis, strongly suggest or diagnose specific diseases when X-rays are abnormal
   - Airways, e.g. bronchiolitis, bronchiectasis, Boop
   - Airspaces, e.g. alveolar proteinosis, non-resolving pneumonia secondary to airway narrowing or cavitation in an area of consolidation
   - Interstitial, e.g. IPF, sarcoid, lymphangitic cancer

- Cystic, e.g. LAM, histiocytosis-x, IPF, centrilobular emphysema (can simulate cystic disease)

3 Exclude or confirm the presence of diffuse interstitial lung disease (accuracy ~95%) when chest X-rays reveal 'increased markings'
4 Assess 'activity' of ILD by the presence of 'ground glass' opacities
5 Guide biopsy site

MRI

Advantages and uses

1 No radiation exposure
2 Iodine-allergic patient
3 Renal patients who cannot tolerate contrast
4 Imaging in the sagittal and coronal planes with improved visualization of
   - Lung apex, e.g. superior sulcus tumors
   - Diaphragm, e.g. hernias
   - Chest wall invasion, e.g. neoplasms, infections
   - Vertebral column and spinal cord invasion
5 Vascular imaging without contrast for
   - Systemic vessels, e.g. SVC, aorta
   - Pulmonary arteries and veins
   - Pericardium
6 Mediastinal masses
7 Specific mediastinal lesions
   - Radiation fibrosis *vs.* active lymphoma
   - Thymic hyperplasia (*vs.* tumor recurrence) following cessation of chemotherapy for lymphoma

V/Q Scan

1 Diagnosis of thrombo-embolic disease
2 Differential lung function as part of the pre-op assessment for lobectomy or pneumonectomy
3 Documentation of right-to-left shunts by measuring the radioactivity trapped in the lung *vs.* that in the brain or kidneys

Gallium Scan

In the presence of disease on chest X-ray, gallium uptake is seen in the lung parenchyma and/or lymph nodes in a variety of infectious, inflammatory and neoplastic disorders

Gallium uptake with normal chest X-rays

1 Inflammatory
   - Usual interstitial pneumonitis (UIP)
   - Asbestosis
   - p.o. drugs, e.g. amiodarone, bleomycin
   - i.v. injections, e.g. i.v. drug abusers, post-lymphangiography
   - sarcoid
2 Infections
   - Pneumocystis or MAI in AIDS patients
3 Neoplasms
   - Lymphangitic cancer
4 Radiation pneumonitis

Angiography

1 **Pulmonary angiography**
   - Gold standard for the diagnosis of pulmonary emboli, acute or chronic (?replaced by spiral CT angio)
   - Evaluation of arteriovenous malformations where diagnosis is not confirmed on CT scan
2 **Bronchial arteriography**
   - Diagnosis and therapeutic embolization in severe hemoptysis
3 **Aortography**
   - For suspected dissection, traumatic injury or aneurysm

SIGNS AND FINDINGS

Positive Bronchus Sign (PBS)

Definition: The CT finding of a tubular area of hypoattenuation, representing an air-filled bronchus, that leads to, +/– into, a peripheral lung nodule

- The PBS does not distinguish benign from malignant lesions as the sign is described with peripheral carcinomas as well as infarcts, tuberculosis and other inflammatory lesions
- Significance of the sign lies in the higher yield of diagnosis of malignancy by bronchoscopy and transbronchial biopsy when the PBS is present
- Absence of the sign might suggest a TTNA as the initial biopsy procedure of choice

Meniscus Sign

Definition: A fixed or mobile mass within a cavity

The air surrounding the mass varies from a rim of air at the periphery of the mass to a small mass in a large cavity

Etiologies include

1. Fungus ball or mycetoma – usually aspergillosis, rarely mucormycosis, candida
2. Invasive aspergillosis
3. Blood clot
4. Hydatid cyst
5. Rasmussen aneurysm in an old tuberculous cavity
6. Cavernolith
7. Cavitary carcinoma
8. Bronchogenic cancer in a bulla
9. Pulmonary gangrene
10. Septic emboli

'Extrapleural' Sign

Definition: An opacity with a sharply defined convex contour facing the lung, accompanied by superior and inferior margins which are tapered and may be concave toward the lung

- Metastatic rib tumor is the commonest cause of this sign and therefore rib films are essential (bony destruction, periostitis)

1. **Rib or sternal lesion** with adjacent soft tissue mass
    - Vascular, e.g. extramedullary hematopoiesis, fracture with hematoma

- Infections, e.g. tuberculosis, actinomycosis, nocardia, blastomycosis
- Inflammatory, e.g. eosinophilic granuloma
- Neoplastic
  - Benign, e.g. *enchondroma, *fibrous dysplasia, hemangioma
  - Primary malignancy, e.g. chondrosarcoma, *plasmacytoma, lymphoma, sarcoma
  - Local metastatic spread, e.g. Pancoast's, mesothelioma, breast cancer, mediastinal tumors
  - Hematogenous metastases, e.g. GU, thyroid, colon, lung, others

2 **Soft tissue neoplasm** – benign, e.g. lipoma
– malignant, e.g. fibrosarcoma

3 **Neurogenic tumor** – e.g. neurofibroma (rib notching)

4 **Vessels**
- Neoplastic lesion
- AV malformation

5 **Pleura**
- Pleural plaque
- Loculated effusion
- Mesothelial cyst
- Round atelectasis
- Neoplasms – benign, e.g. lipoma
  – malignant, e.g. liposarcoma, localized fibrous tumor, mesothelioma, metastases
- Plombage, e.g. oleothorax

6 **Diaphragm**
- Rupture
- Hernias
- Neoplasms
  - Benign, e.g. lipoma
  - Malignant, e.g. fibrosarcoma, metastatic disease

7 **Mediastinum** – e.g. 'mass' lesion

Silhouette Sign

Definition: Loss of the border of a structure which is normally seen on chest X-ray

Loss of right heart border

1 Right middle lobe atelectasis or airspace consolidation
2 Pleural disease
3 Mediastinal disease
4 Pectus excavatum
5 Scimitar syndrome

Loss of aortic knob

1 Left upper lobe disease
2 Mediastinal disease
3 Pleural disease

Loss of left heart border

1 Lingular collapse or airspace consolidation
2 Pleural disease
3 Mediastinal disease
4 Pericardial fat

Loss of hemidiaphragm

1 Lower lobe disease
2 Pleural disease

'Ground Glass' Opacities

Definition: Hazy increase in lung density without loss of vascular definition

- Anatomically may be due to disorders affecting the **airspaces** and/or **interstitium** and pathologically may reflect **inflammation** and/or **fibrosis**

The following disorders result in 'ground glass' opacities on HRCT, with or without associated airspace consolidation

1 Interstitial pneumonitides, including
    - Non-specific interstitial pneumonitis (NSIP)
    - Acute interstitial pneumonitis (AIP)
    - Desquamative interstitial pneumonitis (DIP)
    - Usual interstitial pneumonitis (UIP)
    - Lymphoid interstitial pneumonitis (LIP)
    - Respiratory bronchiolitis – interstitial lung disease (RB-ILD)
2 BOOP
3 Alveolar proteinosis
4 Pulmonary edema
5 Pulmonary hemorrhage

6 Pneumonias – pneumocystis, CMV, others
7 Eosinophilic pneumonia
8 Sarcoid
9 Allergic alveolitis
10 Any cause of airspace disease in its early stages, e.g. alveolar cell carcinoma

'Ground glass' opacities on CT scan with normal chest X-rays

1 Pneumocystis
2 Sarcoid
3 Allergic alveolitis
4 Interstitial pneumonitides, including: DIP, UIP, RB-ILD, NSIP

Clinically, when 'ground glass' opacification is present in isolation or with minimal signs of fibrosis, e.g. DIP, NSIP, it predicts a positive response to steroids and a good prognosis

- When present with findings of fibrosis, i.e. architectural distortion, traction bronchiectasis, honeycombing, it predicts a poor response to steroids with serial films showing the areas of 'ground glass' evolving into areas of progressive fibrosis

Diagnostic pitfalls **radiologically** include difficulty

1 Recognizing 'ground glass' opacification if it is bilateral and diffuse *vs.* patchy in distribution
2 Distinguishing from mosaic perfusion (see below) reflecting perfusion differences in the lungs

Mosaic Perfusion

Definition: Attenuation differences seen on HRCT reflecting areas with reduced lung perfusion, which can be secondary to

1 Pulmonary vascular obstruction, e.g. pulmonary emboli
   - Vessels in the lucent areas are smaller than those seen in the denser normal areas unlike 'ground glass' opacities
2 Airways disease, e.g. bronchiolitis, with secondary vasoconstriction and hyperinflation where hyperlucent

areas are interspersed with areas of increased attenuation

- Bronchial wall thickening
- Hyperlucent areas on inspiration show little attenuation increase or even a reduced attenuation on expiratory CT, whereas increased attenuation is seen with
  - Normal lungs
  - 'Ground glass' opacities
  - Mosaic perfusion secondary to vascular disease

Fraser R.S., Muller N.L., Colman N., Paré P.D. (1999) Diagnosis of Diseases of the Chest 4th Edn., WB Saunders.

Naidich, D.P., Zerhouni, E.A., Siegelman, S.S. *Computed Tomography and Magnetic Resonance of the Thorax*, 2nd edn. New York: Raven Press.

Moss, Gamsu, Genant, Thorax and neck. In: *Computed Tomography of the Body with Magnetic Resonance Imaging*, 2nd edn, vol. 1.: W.B. Saunders.

Reed, J.C. (1997) *Chest Radiology. Plain Film Patterns and Differential Diagnoses*, 4th edn.: Mosby.

Felson, B. (1973) *Chest Roentgenology*.: W.B. Saunders.

2 Abscess of Lung

Definition: Pathologically defined by a localized area of necrosis and suppuration within the lung parenchyma and may be solitary or multiple

- Usually develops as a complication of bacterial pneumonia and less often from hematogenous spread, although may be the initial manifestation of disease

Etiologies include

1. *Anaerobes (often more than 3 species), including *Fusobacterium nucleatum*, *Bacteroides melaninogenicus*, peptostreptococci, others
2. *Anaerobes and aerobes, e.g. aerobic and microaerophilic streptococci
3. Aerobes only, e.g. *Staph. aureus*, gram negatives, legionella
4. 'Chronic' bacteria, e.g. tuberculosis, atypicals, nocardia, actinomycosis
5. Fungi
6. Parasites, e.g. amebiasis

Clinically, the presentation can vary from insidious to acute with non-specific respiratory and systemic symptoms, predisposing conditions including

- Risk factors for aspiration and anaerobic infection
  - Altered sensorium (structural or functional), e.g. CVA, alcoholism
  - Dysphagia (mechanical or neuromuscular), e.g. carcinoma, myasthenia
  - Anaerobic upper respiratory infection, e.g. poor dentition, abscess
- Bronchial obstruction, e.g. neoplasm
- Bronchiectasis
- Cardiac or systemic septic focus

Complications

1 Parapneumonic effusion
2 Empyema
3 Hemoptysis (can be massive)
4 Tracheobronchial spread of infected material with new areas of pneumonitis from a bronchopulmonary fistula
5 Sepsis
6 Brain abscess
7 Amyloid (chronic abscess)

Differential diagnosis of a simple lung abscess

1 Necrotic tumor
2 Post-obstructive pneumonitis with cavitation
3 Necrotizing pneumonia (pneumonia with air–fluid levels) caused by multiple organisms including gram negatives, staphylococcus, others
4 Infected bulla or cyst (air–fluid level in a pre-existing bulla with little infiltrate in the surrounding parenchyma)
5 Tuberculosis
6 Fungal or parasitic infection
7 Empyema
8 Septic emboli (look for a primary infective focus)
9 Rheumatoid nodule (cavitated)
10 Amyloid
11 Wegener's granulomatosis
12 Churg-Strauss
13 Bronchopulmonary sequestration

Non-responsiveness of a simple abscess to antibiotic therapy is manifest by

- Failure to resolve radiologically
- Continued spread to the other areas of lung
- Significant hemoptysis
- Persistent sepsis

Radiology

Chest X-ray findings

1 Single or multiple opacities, spherical or oval in shape

2 Prior to communication with the bronchial tree it presents as a solid opacity
3 Air–fluid levels are common with the width of equal length on PA and lateral films
4 Does not conform to the shape of the chest wall but forms an acute angle with it
5 Anaerobic abscesses are usually in an 'aspiration' segment, i.e. posterior segment of upper lobe, superior segment of lower lobe, basal segment of lower lobe
6 Associated atelectasis, foreign body or a mass lesion suggests a post-obstructive process
7 Radiologic resolution depends on the cavity size and may take 2–3 months for cavity closure and complete disappearance, whereas non-resolution should suggest
   - Unsuspected organisms, e.g. TB, fungi, parasite
   - Organisms resistant to antibiotics chosen
   - Inadequate antibiotic dosing
   - Obstructed bronchus, e.g. tumor or foreign body
   - Misdiagnosis, e.g. necrotic tumor

CT with infusion

1 An abscess typically forms in an area of consolidated lung and appears as a sharply defined, smooth walled lesion
2 After communication with the bronchial tree or pleural space there is a central lucency while the wall is thick, irregular and shaggy, seldom compressing adjacent lung tissue
3 A complicating mycetoma may be present
4 Lung gangrene rarely develops (fragments of necrotic lung within an abscess cavity)
5 May demonstrate associated bronchial obstruction if present, e.g. foreign body, endobronchial lesion
6 Suggest malignancy by the presence of mediastinal lymphadenopathy (although inflammatory adenopathy may occur)
7 May distinguish the thin walls of infected bullae versus the thick walls of a primary lung abscess

Investigations

1 Sputum gram stain typically shows a mixed flora with multiple species in anaerobic infections but is neither sensitive nor specific
   - A single species seen on a good specimen suggests an aerobe, e.g. *Staph. aureus*
   - Sputum culture is of no value for anaerobic abscess
   - Smears and cultures for tuberculosis and fungi should be done when clinically suspected
2 Blood cultures will be positive with hematogenous seeding or may be positive with a primary pulmonary infection
3 Pleural fluid should be tapped if present
4 TTNA with a fine needle may yield an uncontaminated sample
5 Bronchoscopy should be performed if
   - Neoplasm is suspected, e.g. smoker without risk factors for aspiration, edentulous subject
   - Samples are required for tuberculosis or fungi but sputum is unavailable
   - History is suggestive of foreign body aspiration
   - Poor response to antibiotics

Fraser R.S., Muller N.L., Colman N., Paré P.D. (1999) Diagnosis of Diseases of the Chest 4th Edn., WB Saunders.

Naidich, D.P., Zerhouni, E.A., Siegelman, S.S. *Computed Tomography and Magnetic Resonance of the Thorax*, 2nd edn. New York: Raven Press.

Moss, Gamsu, Genant, Thorax and neck. In: *Computed Tomography of the Body with Magnetic Resonance Imaging*, 2nd edn, vol. 1.: W.B. Saunders.

Thurlbeck, W., Churg, A. (eds) (1995) *Pathology of the Lung*, 2nd edn.: Thieme Medical Publishers.

Reed, J.C. (1997) *Chest Radiology. Plain Film Patterns and Differential Diagnoses*, 4th edn.: Mosby.

3 Acid – base Disorders – Respiratory

RESPIRATORY ACIDOSIS

Acute respiratory acidosis

- Each 10 mmHg ↑ in PCO_2 → 1 MEq ↑ in HCO_3 and 0.08 reduction in pH
- Serum HCO_3 above approximately 32 indicates a complicating metabolic alkalosis
- Serum HCO_3 below normal reflects a complicating metabolic acidosis

Chronic respiratory acidosis

- Each 10 mmHg ↑ in PCO_2 → 3.5 MEq ↑ HCO_3 and 0.03 reduction in pH
- The resultant secondary metabolic alkalosis should be distinguished from other causes which include
  - Sodium restriction
  - Diuretics
  - Steroids
- Complications of metabolic alkalosis include
  - Respiratory center depression and ↑ PCO_2
  - Hypokalemia and muscle weakness with ↑ PCO_2

Pulmonary Etiologies

1 **Airways obstruction**
  - Upper acute, e.g. edema, abscess, hemorrhage, foreign body
  - Upper chronic, e.g. *OSA, macroglossia, micrognathia,

vocal cord paralysis, neoplasms, post-intubation, tonsillar hypertrophy
- Lower acute, e.g. bronchiolitis, asthma, pulmonary edema
- Lower chronic, e.g. bronchiolitis, bronchiectasis, *COPD

2 **Parenchymal disease**
- e.g. *Emphysema, severe pneumonia or pulmonary edema

3 **Pleural disease (uncommon)**
- e.g. Tension pneumothorax, bilateral fibrothoraces

Extrapulmonary Etiologies

1 **Brain**
- e.g. Narcotic overdose, status epilepticus, trauma, ischemia, bulbar polio, myxedema, obesity-hypoventilation, idiopathic hypoventilation

2 **Spinal cord**
- e.g. Trauma, tumors, transverse myelitis, disc disease, ALS

3 **Anterior horn cells**
- e.g. Polio, ALS

4 **Peripheral nerves**
- e.g. Guillain-Barré, vasculitis

5 **Myoneural junction**
- e.g. Myasthenia gravis or myasthenia-like syndromes, botulism

6 **Chest wall**
- e.g. Kyphoscoliosis, thoracoplasty, flail chest, obesity

7 **Myopathy**
- Inherited, e.g. congenital nemaline rod, acid maltase deficiency, mitochondrial myopathies, muscular dystrophies, periodic paralysis
- Acquired, e.g. SLE, poly/dermatomyositis, steroids,

hypo/hyperthyroid, ↓ K, ↓ PO_4, rhabdomyolysis, nutritional

RESPIRATORY ALKALOSIS

Acute respiratory alkalosis

- Each 10mmHg ↓ PCO_2 → 2MEq ↓ HCO_3 and 0.08 increase in pH

Chronic respiratory alkalosis

- Each 10mmHg ↓ PCO_2 → 5MEq ↓ HCO_3 and 0.01 increase in pH

Pulmonary/Extrapulmonary Etiologies

1. Hypoxemia
2. Pulmonary receptor activation in the airways, parenchyma, pleura, vasculature, chest wall
3. Psychogenic
4. CHF, e.g. Cheyne-Stokes
5. Drugs, e.g. ASA, progesterone, catecholamines, theophylline
6. CNS disorders, e.g. subarachnoid hemorrhage, CVA, tumor, infection
7. Cirrhosis
8. Pregnancy
9. Fever
10. Sepsis
11. Hyperthyroidism

Fraser R.S., Muller N.L., Colman N., Paré P.D. (1999) Diagnosis of Diseases of the Chest 4th Edn., WB Saunders.

Narins, R., Emmet, M. (1980) Simple and mixed acid-base disorders: a practical approach. *Medicine* **59**: 161–185.

4 Airspace Disease

ETIOLOGIES

Definition: Lung disease primarily affecting the alveoli and respiratory bronchioles, classic radiologic signs being:

- **Air bronchogram**, i.e. airless alveoli outlining air-filled bronchi
- **Air alveologram**, i.e. normal radiolucent areas of lung interspersed between opacified acini

Seen with a wide range of disorders which pathologically can originate not only within the lung **parenchyma**, but also in the **airways** or **vasculature**, and present as airspace disease

Primary Parenchymal Diseases

1 *Aspiration
  - Near-drowning
  - Oropharyngeal/gastric/small bowel secretions
  - Mouth flora
  - Lipid (lipoid pneumonia)
  - Vegetable material (miliary granulomatosis)

2 *Inhalation
  - Inorganic dusts, e.g. acute silico-proteinosis, acute berylliosis, progressive massive fibrosis
  - Organic dusts, e.g. allergic alveolitis
  - Gases, e.g. smoke inhalation, chlorine, ammonia, nitrogen dioxide

3 *Ingestions, e.g. drug reactions

4 *Edema
  - Transudative, e.g. cardiac, pulmonary venous obstruction
  - Pneumonias: bacterial, mycoplasma, viral, fungal, parasitic, rickettsial, chlamydial origin
  - ARDS: multiple causes
5 *Neoplasms, e.g. peripheral bronchogenic, alveolar cell, lymphoma, leukemia,
6 Sarcoid
7 Alveolar proteinosis
8 Alveolar microlithiasis
9 Acute interstitial pneumonitis (Hamman-Rich)
10 Desquamative interstitial pneumonitis
11 Lymphoid interstitial pneumonitis
12 Pseudolymphoma
13 Inflammatory pseudotumor (organizing pneumonia)
14 Radiation pneumonitis
15 Amyloid
16 Metastatic calcification

Primary Airways Diseases

1 Complications of allergic bronchopulmonary aspergillosis, bronchopulmonary sequestration, pseudosequestration
2 Bronchocentric granulomatosis
3 BOOP

Primary Vascular Diseases

1 Whole blood – any cause of alveolar hemorrhage
2 Vasculitides/collagen vascular diseases
3 Eosinophilic lung diseases
4 Vascular tumors, e.g. pulmonary capillary hemangiomatosis
5 Blood-borne, e.g. embolic disease, sepsis

RADIOLOGIC CLUES TO DIAGNOSIS (CHEST X-RAY/CT)

1 Pattern of disease
  - 'Ground glass' opacity (see p. 9)

- Airspace consolidation-homogeneous or non-homogeneous, defined as an increased lung opacity resulting in obscuration of vessels plus air bronchograms, e.g. bacterial pneumonia
- Airspace ('acinar') nodules, e.g. bronchogenic spread of tuberculosis
- Masses and conglomerate masses, e.g. progressive massive fibrosis of silicosis, talcosis or coal workers' pneumoconiosis

2 Density features
- Fat, e.g. lipoid pneumonia
- High iodine content, e.g. amiodarone
- Calcifications, e.g. metastatic calcinosis, microlithiasis

3 Cystic/cavitary disease (see p. 178)

4 Distribution characteristics
- Central, e.g. alveolar proteinosis
- Peripheral, e.g. eosinophilic pneumonia, sarcoid, drug reaction, BOOP, UIP, DIP
- Upper lobe, e.g. tuberculosis *vs.* lower, e.g. cardiac edema
- Segmental, e.g. mycoplasma *vs.* non-segmental, e.g. *Strep. pneumoniae*
- Peribronchial, e.g. sarcoid
- Sharp borders, e.g. radiation pneumonitis
- Unifocal, e.g. *Strep. pneumoniae vs.* multifocal, e.g. alveolar proteinosis

5 Associated abnormalities on chest X-ray or CT involving the airways (e.g. endobronchial obstruction), pleura (e.g. effusion, nodularity), vasculature (e.g. Kerly B lines), chest wall (e.g. metastatic rib lesion), hilum (e.g. adenopathy) or mediastinum (e.g. cardiomegaly, esophageal lesion)

6 Duration of the radiologic process
- Acute, e.g. pneumonia
- Subacute, e.g. alveolar cell carcinoma
- Chronic, e.g. lipoid pneumonia

7 Changing pattern of airspace disease with recurrent infiltrates in different areas of lung (see p. 357)

RAPIDLY PROGRESSIVE AIRSPACE DISEASE – COMMUNITY-ACQUIRED

Clinically, patients present with
- Acute onset of non-specific respiratory symptoms, i.e. dyspnea, cough, fever, chest pains
- Rapidly progressive disease radiologically with severe hypoxemia, occasionally requiring ICU admission and intubation
- No obvious predisposing cause to explain the disease process after the history, physical and routine labs have been obtained

Differential diagnosis

1 ***Infections** (see CAP Requiring ICU Admission, p. 598)
   - *Streptococcus pneumonia or other bacteria including hemophilus, anaerobes, *Staph. aureus*, gram negatives, moraxella, tuberculosis
   - *Viral, e.g. influenza, parainfluenza, adeno, respiratory syncitial, hanta
   - *Atypicals, e.g. mycoplasma, legionella, *Chlamydia pneumoniae*
   - Uncommon atypicals, e.g. *F. tularensis* (tularemia), *Chlamydia psittaci*, *Coxiella burnetti*
   - Fungal, e.g. pneumocystis, coccidioides, histoplasma
   - Parasitic

2 **Acute interstitial pneumonia – Hamman-Rich**

3 **Alveolar hemorrhage syndromes**, e.g. Goodpasture's

4 **Vasculitis/collagen vascular diseases**, e.g. Wegener's, systemic lupus

5 **Acute eosinophilic pneumonia**

6 **ARDS**, characterized pathologically by diffuse alveolar damage (DAD), with disruption of the alveolo-capillary barrier and resultant protein-rich edema, inflammation with neutrophil accumulation, alveolar hemorrhage
   - Sequelae vary from resolution within days to an intense proliferative response with fibrosis and death

   Clinical correlates of the above include

a. Acute onset of respiratory failure lasting days to weeks
b. Hypoxemia
c. Bilateral diffuse pulmonary infiltrates
d. Wedge pressure < 18 mmHg
e. Identification of a precipitating risk factor:

Primary Pulmonary	Extrapulmonary
• Gastric aspiration	• Sepsis
• Near-drowning	• Trauma
• Inhalation injury	• Pancreatitis
• Contusion	• Hypotension
• Infections	• Anaphylaxis
• Fat emboli	
• Drugs	

Table 4.1

7 **Allergic alveolitis**
8 **Pulmonary edema**, e.g. cardiac, pulmonary venous obstruction
9 **BOOP**
10 **Drug reactions**, e.g. amiodarone
11 **Neoplastic disease**, e.g. lymphoma, alveolar cell cancer, lymphangitic carcinomatosis
12 multiple pulmonary infarcts

AIRSPACE DISEASE – MULTIFOCAL (>4 WKS)

Intervening areas of **uninvolved lung** are present, distinguishing these disorders from **diffuse** lung disease

- Presentation varies from asymptomatic to non-specific respiratory symptoms
- The following **differential diagnosis** and **diagnostic clues** apply for multifocal airspace disease in the absence of cavitation, lymphadenopathy and pleural effusion

1 **Chronic infection** with tuberculosis, atypicals, nocardia, fungi or opportunistic infection, e.g. pneumocystis

- Immunologic status of the patient
- Endemicity of infection
- Sputum and BAL studies

2 **Atypical pulmonary edema**
- Evidence of cardiac disease with signs of pulmonary venous hypertension
- Extracardiac pulmonary vein obstruction

3 **Alveolar cell carcinoma**
- Bronchorrhea

4 **Sarcoid**

5 **BOOP**

6 **Drug reaction**
- Drug history
- Accompanying peripheral eosinophilia

7 **Alveolar hemorrhage or aspiration of blood**
- Hemoptysis
- Falling hemoglobin
- Elevated diffusing capacity
- Hemosiderin-laden macrophages on BAL

8 **Lipoid pneumonia**
- History of mineral oil ingestion or use of oily nose drops
- Lipid-laden macrophages on BAL
- Fat density on CT scan

9 **Chronic eosinophilic pneumonia**
- Peripheral distribution of airspace disease
- Blood and BAL eosinophilia

10 **Lymphoproliferative disorders**
- LIP
- Lymphoma
  - Rare without concurrent lymphadenopathy or evidence of extrathoracic disease
- Lymphomatoid granulomatosis
  - Systemic symptoms
  - Concurrent disease of skin and nervous system

11 **Wegener's granulomatosis**
- Hemoptysis
- Upper and/or lower respiratory symptoms

- Sinus, renal and often other systemic disease
- ⊕ cANCA

12 **Churg-Strauss**
- History of asthma
- Peripheral eosinophilia
- ⊕ pANCA

13 **Amyloid**

14 **Microscopic polyarteritis**
- Hemoptysis
- Glomerulonephritis
- ⊕ pANCA

15 **Alveolar proteinosis**
- CT appearance of 'crazy-paving'
- PAS ⊕ material from BAL

16 **Allergic bronchopulmonary aspergillosis**
- History of asthma
- Eosinophilia, ↑ IgE
- Serum precipitins

17 **Bronchocentric granulomatosis**
- One third of patients are asthmatic with peripheral eosinophilia

Fraser R.S., Muller N.L., Colman N., Paré P.D. (1999) Diagnosis of Diseases of the Chest 4th Edn., WB Saunders.
Reed, J.C. (1997) *Chest Radiology. Plain Film Patterns and Differential Diagnoses*, 4th edn.: Mosby.
Felson, B. (1973) *Chest Roentgenology*.: W.B. Saunders.

5 Alcohol and Cigarettes – Pulmonary Complications

Alcohol

Airways

- Aspirated foreign body +/– associated atelectasis
- Bronchiectasis from recurrent aspiration or pneumonias
- Exacerbation of obstructive sleep apnea

Parenchyma

- Acute aspiration pneumonia from impaired sensorium
- Other pneumonias, e.g. klebsiella, anaerobes, actinomycosis, *Rhodococcus equii* (upper lobe cavitary disease simulating TB)
- Lung abscess
- Tuberculosis/atypical mycobacteria
- Sporotrichosis ('alcoholic gardener's syndrome' – simulating TB)
- Foreign body granuloma from aspiration
- Metastatic hepatoma
- Pulmonary edema from alcoholic cardiomyopathy

Pleura

- Transudate, e.g. cirrhosis, CHF from alcoholic cardiomyopathy
- Exudate, e.g.
  - Tuberculosis, parapneumonic/empyema,
  - Ruptured esophagus
  - Pancreatitis
  - Metastatic hepatoma
- Hemothorax secondary to trauma
- Chylothorax secondary to trauma

Neuromusculoskeletal

- Rib fractures post falls

- Elevated hemidiaphragm secondary to ascites/hepatomegaly
- Hyperventilation and respiratory alkalosis with cirrhosis
- Seizures with DTs

Mediastinum

- Acute mediastinitis from prolonged vomiting and ruptured esophagus
- Posterial mediastinal mass from varices

Vascular

- Hepatopulmonary syndrome with acute or chronic alcoholic liver disease
- Pulmonary artery hypertension with cirrhosis and portal hypertension
- Tumor emboli with hepatoma complicating cirrhosis

Cigarettes

1. Lung cancer
2. Upper airway cancers, e.g. mouth, larynx
3. Non-respiratory cancers with pulmonary metastases, e.g. bladder, pancreas, stomach, eosphagus
4. Asthma
5. COPD
6. Eosinophilic granuloma
7. Respiratory bronchiolitis – interstitial lung disease
8. Desquamative interstitial pneumonitis
9. Spontaneous pneumothorax

Fraser R.S., Muller N.L., Colman N., Paré P.D. (1999) Diagnosis of Diseases of the Chest 4th Edn., WB Saunders.
Baum, G.L., Crapo, J.D., Celli, B.R., Karlinsky, J.B. (eds) (1997) *Textbook of Pulmonary Diseases*, 6th edn.: Lippincott-Raven.
Fishman, A.P., Elias, J.A., Fishman, J.A., Grippi, M.A., Kaiser, L.R., Senior, R.N. (1998) *Fishman's Pulmonary Diseases and Disorders*, 3rd edn.: McGraw-Hill.

6 Alveolar Hemorrhage

Syndrome (AHS)

Definition: Alveolar hemorrhage can result from diseases affecting the bronchial circulation (e.g. bronchogenic cancer, bronchiectasis) or the pulmonary circulation, involving the large (e.g. pulmonary arteries) or small vessels (e.g. capillaritis, see p. 846)

Pathologic findings include

1 Capillaritis
2 Bland hemorrhage
3 Diffuse alveolar damage, the finding in ARDS

*Often misdiagnosed as pneumonia or pulmonary edema at initial presentation

DIFFERENTIAL AND DIAGNOSTIC WORK-UP

I

Define the presence of AHS by

1 History of hemoptysis varying from massive to spotty, accompanied by dyspnea
   - Hemoptysis is occasionally completely absent
   - Presentation can be chronic and insidious or acute and fulminating, with rapid progression to respiratory failure requiring mechanical ventilation
   - Often an early manifestation of a systemic disease and

seen in a wide range of immunologic or idiopathic disorders (see below)

2 Physical exam can reveal focal or diffuse rales on auscultation with occasional evidence of a systemic disease, e.g. vasculitis, arthritis, etc.
3 Chest X-ray finding is airspace disease with air bronchograms indistinguishable from edema or infection
   - The distribution can be bilateral and diffuse or asymmetric and focal
   - With blood resorption, the airspace consolidation is replaced by an interstitial reticular pattern which resolves completely if bleeding does not recur
   - Recurrent bleeding can result in interstitial fibrosis
4 Labs include hypoxemia, anemia and increased ESR
   - Renal function and urinalysis may suggest a pulmonary-renal syndrome
5 PFTs reveal an elevated D_{LCO} for carbon monoxide
6 Bronchoscopic findings are those of no gross bleeding sites but increasingly bloody returns on BAL, associated with high RBC counts and hemosiderin-laden macrophages (if hemorrhage is more chronic)

The above can be caused by multiple disorders and therefore the following work-up will narrow the differential diagnosis

II

Determine the presence of **isolated pulmonary disease**, e.g. IPH, *vs.* associated **renal disease**, e.g. Goodpasture's *vs.* **extra-renal disease**, e.g. Wegener's – by history, physical and labs

III

In the presence of renal disease (urinalysis, bloods), R/O AGBM antibody disease, vasculitis, collagen vascular disease or other causes of the **pulmonary-renal syndrome** of alveolar hemorrhage accompanied by glomerulonephritis on history, physical, labs

Immunologic

- Vasculitis of Wegener's microscopic polyarteritis, Churg-Strauss (see p. 843)
- Systemic lupus erythematosus (see p. 144)
- AGBM disease (Goodpasture's syndrome) (see p. 708)
- Idiopathic rapidly progressive glomerulonephritis (RPGN)

Non-immunologic

- IgA nephropathy
- Idiopathic RPGN

IV

R/O any cause of **massive bleeding** with aspiration of blood

1 Airways diseases, e.g. bronchiectasis, carcinoma
2 Parenchymal diseases, e.g. necrotizing pneumonia, primary or metastatic cancer, abscess, mycetoma, tuberculosis
3 Bronchial or other systemic arterial bleed, e.g. aortic rupture
4 Pulmonary arterial disorders, e.g. infarct (septic/bland), AV malformation, angiosarcoma
5 Pulmonary venous hypertension, e.g. left atrial myxoma, mitral stenosis or insufficiency, LAM, tuberous sclerosis, pulmonary veno-occlusive disease
6 Pulmonary capillary disorders, e.g. isolated capillaritis, pulmonary capillary hemangiomatosis

V

R/O exposure to **exogenous agents**

- Inhaled, e.g. cocaine, trimetillic anhydride
- Ingested, e.g. penicillamine
- Injected, e.g. post-lympangiography

VI

R/O **hematologic disorders**, e.g. coagulation abnormalities, post bone-marrow transplant, DIC, antiphospholipid syndrome

VII

R/O **Idiopathic pulmonary hemosiderosis**

Clinically, a disease of children under age 10 with equal sex distribution or seen in young adults (~20% of reported cases) with a 2 to 1 male predominance

- The thoracic manifestations are clinically and radiologically identical to Goodpasture's syndrome (see p. 708) with presentations including
  - Hemoptysis varying from blood-tinged to massive
  - Subclinical alveolar hemorrhage with iron-deficiency anemia
  - Repeated episodes of alveolar hemorrhage and hemoptysis leading to interstitial fibrosis, dyspnea, clubbing and cor pulmonale
  - May co-exist with celiac sprue (in children)
- Prognosis is quite variable with survival of 20 years or more described
- Labs may reveal an iron-deficiency anemia
- Biopsy demonstrates bland pulmonary hemorrhage without immune complexes and may be confused with capillaritis pathologically
- Radiologic features are those of Goodpasture's syndrome

Diagnostic criteria

1 Compatible clinical and radiologic features
2 Normal renal function and structure with negative immunofluorescence
3 Absent AGBM antibodies in the blood
4 Exclusion of other diseases causing alveolar hemorrhage such as infection, coagulopathy, hemodynamic abnormality or a systemic disease, e.g. Wegener's, SLE

VIII

Lab tests including

- BUN, Cr, urinalysis, LFTs, CBC, iron studies, cryoglobulins, serum complement, hepatitis B surface antigen
- ANA, AGBM antibodies, lupus anticoagulant, anticardiolipin antibody, antibodies against double-stranded DNA, c-ANCA, (e.g. Wegener's) or p-ANCA, (e.g. Churg-Strauss/microscopic polyarteritis)
- Drug screening for cocaine
- Blood cultures, e.g. bacterial endocarditis

IX

Radiologic studies

1 Chest X-rays for evaluation of a disease process other than alveolar hemorrhage, e.g. cardiomegaly, neoplasm, Kerley B lines, etc.
2 +/– chest CT
3 +/– sinus X-rays (may suggest Wegener's)
4 +/– pulmonary angiography, left and right heart catheterization, bronchial arteriography

X

Echocardiography for suspected mitral valve, left atrial or left ventricular disease resulting in pulmonary venous hypertension

XI

Bronchoscopy

- BAL to R/O underlying infection, neoplasm
- Transbronchial biopsy

XII

Open lung biopsy for patients with unexplained alveolar hemorrhage plus

1 No extrapulmonary disease and non-diagnostic blood tests, as in
    - Isolated pulmonary capillaritis
    - Idiopathic pulmonary hemosiderosis (diagnosis of exclusion)

- Goodpasture's syndrome confined to the lung where AGBM antibodies in serum are negative

2 Non-specific systemic vasculitis – R/O Wegener's
3 Non-immunologic RPGN – R/O pulmonary vasculitis

Biopsies should be sent for
- Light microscopy
- Electron microscopy for electron dense material characteristic of immune complexes
- AGBM antibodies
- Immunofluorescence patterns
  - *Linear*: diagnostic of Goodpasture's
  - *Negative*: Wegener's, microscopic polyarteritis, isolated pulmonary capillaritis
  - *Granular*: SLE, Henoch-Schonlein purpura (IgA)

XIII

Renal biopsy when kidney disease is present by urinalysis, BUN, Cr, antibody testing
- Document and describe glomerulonephritis
- Establish the presence or absence of vasculitis and its impact on differential diagnosis
- Immunofluorescence patterns
  - *Linear*: Goodpasture's
  - *Granular*: SLE
  - *Pauci-immune*: Wegener's, microscopic polyarteritis

XIV

Skin biopsy demonstrating nonspecific vasculitis or the characteristic findings of Henoch-Schönlein, i.e. leucocytoclastic vasculitis and IgA deposition

Fraser R.S., Muller N.L., Colman N., Paré P.D. (1999) Diagnosis of Diseases of the Chest 4th Edn., WB Saunders.

Baum, G.L., Crapo, J.D., Celli, B.R., Karlinsky, J.B. (eds) (1997) *Textbook of Pulmonary Diseases*, 6th edn.: Lippincott-Raven.

Fishman, A.P., Elias, J.A., Fishman, J.A., Grippi, M.A., Kaiser,

L.R., Senior, R.N. (1998) *Fishman's Pulmonary Diseases and Disorders*, 3rd edn.: McGraw-Hill.

Green, R., Ruoss, S., Kraft, S. *et al.* (1996) Pulmonary capillaritis and alveolar hemorrhage. Update on diagnosis and management. *Chest* **110**: 1305–1316.

Leatherman, J., Davies, S., Hoidal, J. (1986) Alveolar hemorrhage syndromes: diffuse microvascular lung hemorrhage in immune and idiopathic disorders. *Medicine* **63**: 343–361.

Green, R., Ruoss, S. *et al.* (1996) Pulmonary capillaritis and alveolar hemorrhage. *Chest* **110**: 1305–1316.

Jemmings, C., King, T., Tuder, R. *et al.* (1997) Diffuse alveolar hemorrhage with underlying isolated pauciimune pulmonary capillaritis. *Am. J. Resp. Crit. Care Med.* **155**: 1101–1109.

7 Alveolar Proteinosis

Definition: Rare lung disorder of unclear etiology – ? altered surfactant metabolism – characterized by alveolar filling with a periodic acid-schiff positive proteinaceous material, the alveolar walls being preserved.

Alveolar proteinosis may be primary or secondary to

1. Infection, e.g. nocardia, aspergillus, cryptococcus, pneumocystis, others
2. Impaired immunity with HIV, lymphoma, leukemia
3. Exposure to minerals or chemicals including silica, aluminum dust, titanium, insecticides

Clinically, reported in all age groups with most patients between 30–50 years, a male to female ratio of 3:1 and presentations including

- Asymptomatic radiologic findings in ~$^1/_3$ of patients
- Non-specific respiratory symptoms of dry cough and dyspnea, usually subacute in onset, rarely a fulminant course
- Cough productive of gelatinous material, casts, or mucous secondary to superinfection or smoking
- Systemic features of malaise and weight loss with fevers, the latter prompting a search for superinfection
- Absence of extrapulmonary involvement except for clubbing in <$^1/_3$ of patients
- Radiologic picture of pulmonary edema without clinical evidence of heart disease (should suggest that diagnosis)

Disease course is variable and includes

- Spontaneous resolution in ~25% of cases
- Stability

- Progressive disease with respiratory failure or superimposed infection with nocardia, tuberculosis, atypical mycobacteria, pneumocystis or other organisms
- 30% mortality from the above in untreated patients with a good response to whole lung lavage

Restrictive disease is present on **PFTs** with a disproportional reduction in DCO, while hypoxemia is common

Radiologic features

1 Bilateral symmetrical airspace disease on chest X-ray, often perihilar (bat's wing) in distribution, resembling cardiogenic pulmonary edema
   - Unilateral involvement seen in <20% of cases
2 Interstitial pattern (rarely)
3 HRCT features of
   - 'Ground glass' or airspace consolidation with sharp demarcation from normal lung creating a 'geographic' pattern
   - Intralobular and interlobular septal thickening (due to incorporation of the phospholipid-proteinaceous material into the interstitium), without architectural distortion, creating typical polygonal shapes ('crazy-paving')
   - Absence of pleural effusion and mediastinal lymphadenopathy

Differential diagnosis will include those diseases characterized radiologically by alveolar filling, where specific causes of airspace disease can be excluded, e.g. inhalational injury, aspiration, CHF, etc.

1 Alveolar cell carcinoma
2 Lipoid pneumonia
3 Chronic infection, e.g. TB, atypicals, fungi, nocardia, pneumocystis
4 Sarcoid
5 Drug reaction
6 Amyloid
7 Atypical pulmonary edema
8 Lymphoproliferative disorders, e.g. LIP, lymphoma
9 BOOP

10 Chronic eosinophilic pneumonia
11 Alveolar hemorrhage
12 Vasculitis, e.g. Wegener's, Churg-Strauss, microsopic polyarteritis

Diagnostic gold standard is transbronchial or open lung biopsy, where alveolar spaces and respiratory bronchioles are filled with an acidophilic surfactant-like material staining bright pink with PAS reagent.

Strongly supportive findings include

- Compatible chest X-ray/HRCT
- Blood tests revealing hypoxemia, increased LDH and elevated levels of surfactant proteins A and D
- Elevated levels of surfactant proteins A and D in BAL fluid
- 'Milky' or 'muddy' effluent on BAL with PAS positive staining of the proteinaceous material and alveolar macrophages containing granular eosinophilic material

Fraser R.S., Muller N.L., Colman N., Paré P.D. (1999) Diagnosis of Diseases of the Chest 4th Edn., WB Saunders.

Baum, G.L., Crapo, J.D., Celli, B.R., Karlinsky, J.B. (eds) (1997) *Textbook of Pulmonary Diseases*, 6th edn.: Lippincott-Raven.

Fishman, A.P., Elias, J.A., Fishman, J.A., Grippi, M.A., Kaiser, L.R., Senior, R.N. (1998) *Fishman's Pulmonary Diseases and Disorders*, 3rd edn.: McGraw-Hill.

Wang, B., Stern, E., Schmidt, R. *et al.* (1997) Diagnosing alveolar proteinosis. A review and update. *Chest* **111**: 460–466.

Goldstein, L.S. *et al.* (1998) Pulmonary alveolar proteinosis: clinical features and outcomes. *Chest* **114**: 1357–1362.

Goadwin, J.D., Kavuru, M., Curtis-McCarthy, P. *et al.* (1988) Pulmonary alveolar protenosis: CT findings. *Radiology* **169**: 609–613.

8 Arteriovenous Fistulas – Pulmonary (PAVF)

Definition: Refers to an abnormal vascular communication between a pulmonary artery and pulmonary vein, most often congenital in origin although acquired causes include hepatic cirrhosis, mitral stenosis, trauma, metastatic tumors, schistosomiasis, others

- 90% of cases involve a single feeding artery and vein (simple) versus 10% with two or more feeding arteries or draining veins (complex)
- PAVFs are usually 1 to 5 cm in size, occasionally greater than 10 cm but can be microscopic, often in association with radiologically visible lesions
- 50–70% of cases are associated with hereditary hemorragic telangiectasia (HHT)
- 10% of patients present in childhood with an increasing incidence through later decades

Clinical and laboratory presentations include

- Abnormal chest X-ray in >90% of patients, with or without pulmonary symptoms, which often develop between ages 40–60

  Dyspnea is seen in patients with large or multiple PAVFs or diffuse microvascular disease and congestive heart failure can develop
- Platypnea, i.e. dyspnea when upright but improving when lying flat
- Orthodeoxia, i.e. a fall in arterial oxygen when changing from supine to the upright position
- Hemoptysis (reflecting parenchymal or endobronchial lesions) which may vary from mild to massive
- Hemothorax with ~⅓ of cases described in the last half of pregnancy

- Unexplained hypoxemia (relates to the size and number of PAVFs)
- Polycythemia (secondary to hypoxemia) or anemia (secondary to bleeding)
- Paradoxical (systemic) emboli
- CNS disease develops in about 30% of patients and presentations include stroke, transient ischemic attacks, seizures, migraine, brain abscess, meningitis, encephalitis
  - Underlying etiologies include primary neurologic disease from associated HHT, hypoxemia, paradoxical bland emboli, septic emboli, polycythemia, cerebral thrombosis
- Feature of HHT, an autosomal dominant disease characterized by arteriovenous malformations in skin, mucous membranes and visceral organs
  - About 25% of patients have PAVFs which are uncommonly manifest before adulthood
  - Usual presentation is epistaxis or cutaneous telangiectases although visceral involvement with GI bleed, dyspnea or CNS disease may be the initial presentation
  - The two mutated genes that have been discovered are the Endoglin gene on chromosome 9 and the ALK-1 gene on chromosome 12

Physical findings can include
- Cyanosis (~⅓)
- Clubbing (~⅓)
- Murmur over the lesion (~½)
- Skin or mucosal telangectases with HHT

Radiologic features
1. Single or multiple nodules (⅓ of cases), one to several cm in size, with lower lobe predominance
2. Feeding artery relating to the hilum and a draining vein relating to the left atrium
3. Enlargement with time (~25% of cases), in pregnancy, in the supine position or with a Mueller maneuver and a decrease in size with a valsalva

4 Microvascular telangiectases can present with a normal chest X-ray or increased markings at the lung bases

Diagnostic features

1 Diagnosis of HHT with at least two of the following
   - Recurrent spontaneous epistaxis
   - Telangiectases over the skin or mucosa
   - Visceral AVMs
   - Positive family history
2 Respiratory findings as above
3 Hypoxemia with demonstration of an intrapulmonary right-to-left shunt by
   - Contrast echography
   - Passage of technetium-labelled macroaggregates of albumen through the lung with entrapment in other organs
   - Calculation of the shunt fraction breathing 100% oxygen
4 Chest X-ray abnormalities as above in addition to other radiologic studies including
   - Enhancement with contrast CT
   - Digital subtraction angiography
   - MRI
5 Pulmonary angiography remains the gold standard

Fraser R.S., Muller N.L., Colman N., Paré P.D. (1999) Diagnosis of Diseases of the Chest 4th Edn., WB Saunders.

Baum, G.L., Crapo, J.D., Celli, B.R., Karlinsky, J.B. (eds) (1997) *Textbook of Pulmonary Diseases*, 6th edn.: Lippincott-Raven.

Fishman, A.P., Elias, J.A., Fishman, J.A., Grippi, M.A., Kaiser, L.R., Senior, R.N. (1998) *Fishman's Pulmonary Diseases and Disorders*, 3rd edn.: McGraw-Hill.

Gossage, J., Kanj, G. (1998) Pulmonary arteriovenous malformations. *ARRD* **158**: 643–661.

Gutmacher, A., Marchuk, D., White, R. (1995) Hereditary hemorrhagic telangiectasia. *NEJM* **333**: 918–924.

9 Aspiration Injuries

GASTRIC ASPIRATION (ACUTE/CHRONIC) – COMPLICATIONS

Upper airways

1 Hoarseness
2 Pharyngitis
3 Choking episodes

Lower airways

4 Asthma
5 Bronchitis
6 Bronchiectasis
7 Acute bronchiolitis which can progress to bronchiolitis obliterans or BOOP
8 Foreign body aspiration and localized airways obstruction
9 Chronic cough

Parenchyma

10 Acute aspiration pneumonia (chemical pneumonitis)
11 Lipoid pneumonia
12 Organizing pneumonia (inflammatory pseudotumor)
13 *Mycobacterium fortuitum-choleonae*
14 Miliary granulomatosis – granulomas developing around meat or vegetable material and manifest as multiple lung nodules resembling hematogenous or endobronchial tuberculosis

15 Atelectasis from airway material
16 Foreign body granuloma
17 Pulmonary fibrosis seen with chronic aspiration, typically lower lobe, often bilateral and can simulate UIP
18 Bacterial infection from oropharyngeal flora, often anaerobes

*The above should be suspected in patients with:

- Altered sensorium: functional, e.g. alcohol, drugs, or structural, e.g. CVA
- Dysphagia: functional, e.g. myasthenia, or structural, e.g. stricture
- Gastro-esophageal reflux disease (GERD) including medications that can decrease lower esophageal sphincter pressure
- Tracheo-esophageal or broncho-esophageal fistula
- Chronic debilitating disease

LIPOID PNEUMONIA – EXOGENOUS

Definition: A pulmonary parenchymal disorder due to aspiration or inhalation of animal, vegetable or mineral oil

- Microscopic findings and fat stains can distinguish endogenous from exogenous fat with other causes of fat in the lungs including
  - Endogenous lipoid pneumonia
  - Fat emboli
  - Alveolar proteinosis
  - Lipid storage diseases

Clinical presentations

1 Asymptomatic radiologic finding in approximately 50% of cases (see below)
2 Non-specific respiratory symptoms of cough, dyspnea
3 Acute presentation suggestive of bacterial pneumonia

Complications

1 Recurrent bacterial pneumonia

2 Superinfection with atypical mycobacteria, particularly *M. chelonei-fortuitum*
3 Colonization with *Cryptococcus neoformans*
4 Progressive disease with cor pulmonale and respiratory failure
5 Hypercalcemia secondary to granulomatous inflammation
6 ? Bronchioloalveolar cell cancer developing in areas of fibrosis
7 Systemic dissemination of free oil and lipophages to the scalene and intra-abdominal lymph nodes as well as to the liver, spleen, kidneys, etc.

Radiologic features

1 *Air space consolidation, focal or diffuse, unilateral or bilateral, in an aspiration segment
2 *Mass-like lesion with irregular and spiculated margins resembling lung cancer (fat attenuation may be identified on CT)
3 Multiple mass-like opacities
4 Interstitial reticular pattern, unilateral or bilateral, developing in the later stages (may simulate UIP)
5 Atelectasis from endobronchial granulation tissue or oil (rare)
6 Pleural effusion (rare)
7 Fat attenuation in areas of airspace consolidation on chest CT

Diagnostic gold standard is lung biopsy (TTNA, transbronchial) which demonstrates lipid-laden macrophages in the alveoli or interstitium

Diagnosis should be suspected with

1 History of
   - Psychiatric disorder or illness predisposing to aspiration
   - Oil ingestion, e.g. laxatives
   - Aspiration, e.g. nose or throat application, lip balms
   - Inhalation, e.g. occupational or home exposure
2 Lipid-laden macrophages in sputum or BAL
3 Radiologic findings as above

CHEMICAL PNEUMONITIS

Definition: Lung reaction due to aspiration of substances which are toxic to the lower airways and parenchyma in the absence of bacterial infection

Clinically, patients present with the acute onset of dyspnea, fever, diffuse rales, frequent wheezing and cyanosis if severe

- Hypoxemia is accompanied by radiologic infiltrates in the 'aspiration segments', the latter seen within a few hours

Course of disease includes

1. Rapid clinical improvement and radiologic clearing
2. Progression to ARDS
3. Initial improvement followed by worsening infiltrates, secondary to superimposed bacterial pneumonia

ASPIRATION – SOLID FOREIGN BODY

Multiple **etiologies** described

- Endogenous, e.g. tooth
- Exogenous vegetable matter, e.g. peanuts, or mineral, e.g. bone

Usually solitary but multiple foreign bodies are seen in a small percentage of cases

Clinical presentations

1. Acute: 'cafe coronary' with aphonia, sudden dyspnea and cyanosis
   - Typically described during aspiration of meat in a restaurant and simulates an acute myocardial infarct
2. Subacute/chronic
   - Cough, wheezing, hemoptysis, bronchitis, bronchiectasis, recurrent pneumonia, empyema
   - There is usually a history of choking at the time of aspiration, the cough dating back to a specific time, although in a significant percentage of cases aspiration is not clinically recognized

- Localized wheezing may be found on auscultation and occasionally the foreign body can become incorporated into the bronchial wall simulating a neoplasm

Radiologic findings

Most frequent in the lower lobes (most often RLL) and include

1. Opaque foreign body in an airway, either in a main bronchus or peripheral airway
2. Obstructive pneumonitis
3. Volume loss which may be accompanied by oligemia
4. Expiratory air trapping and contralateral mediastinal shift
5. Bronchiectasis
6. Bronchostenosis
7. Abscess formation/empyema
8. Fistula formation

Diagnostic features

1. History of choking or of a severe coughing spasm after 'swallowing' food
2. Localized wheeze on auscultation
3. Chest X-ray findings as above
4. Hypoperfusion of a normal or minimally abnormal lung on X-ray
5. CT demonstration of an intralumenal foreign body (localized area of high attenuation)
6. Bronchoscopy

DROWNING/NEAR-DROWNING

Definition: Drowning is defined as death from asphyxiation due to submersion

- Usually, but not always, accompanied by aspiration with ~10% of cases classified as **dry drowning** – laryngospasm preventing the inhalation of water, with subsequent cerebral anoxia and paralysis of the respiratory center

Near-drowning is defined as survival following a submersion episode

Pulmonary complications

- Upper airways
  - Opacified sinuses
  - Laryngospasm
- Lower airways
  - Bronchospasm
  - Foreign body aspiration including a 'sand bronchogram' of calcium carbonate
- Parenchyma
  - Fluid aspiration
  - Pneumonia (bacterial or fungal infection) from the aspirated water
  - Pneumonia from host flora or hospital
  - ARDS from pollutants or organisms in the water
- Pleura
  - Pneumothorax
- Chest wall
  - Abdominal distension from swallowed water
- Abnormal central drive
  - Anoxic brain damage
  - Underlying predisposing cause of the near drowning including *alcohol, *drugs, cervical trauma, head injury, seizures, other

Arterial blood gas abnormalities

- Hypoxemia and metabolic acidosis

Systemic complications include

- Anoxic encephalopathy (main determinant of mortality)
- Multiple organ failure
- Septicemia
- Rhabdomyolysis and myoglobinuria
- Intravascular hemolysis and hemoglobinuria
- Hyponatremia (fresh water) or hypernatremia (salt water)

Chest X-ray findings

Similar with both fresh and sea water aspiration and include

1. Bilateral symmetric airspace edema
2. Resolution within 1–2 days

3 Occasionally normal films due to 'dry near-drowning'
4 Suspect pneumonia when films worsen 3–4 days following the acute episode

Fraser R.S., Muller N.L., Colman N., Paré P.D. (1999) Diagnosis of Diseases of the Chest 4th Edn., WB Saunders.

Baum, G.L., Crapo, J.D., Celli, B.R., Karlinsky, J.B. (eds) (1997) *Textbook of Pulmonary Diseases*, 6th edn.: Lippincott-Raven.

Fishman, A.P., Elias, J.A., Fishman, J.A., Grippi, M.A., Kaiser, L.R., Senior, R.N. (1998) *Fishman's Pulmonary Diseases and Disorders*, 3rd edn.: McGraw-Hill.

Spickard, A., Hirschman, J.V. (1994) Exogenous lipoid pneumonia. *Arch. Int. Med.* **154**: 686–691.

10 Asthma

Definition: An airway disorder with

1 Persistent or paroxysmal symptoms of cough, wheezing, dyspnea
2 Variable airways obstruction as defined by
  - 12% increase in FEV_1 post BD (>180 ml)
  - 20% change in FEV_1 over time (>250 ml)
  - 20% diurnal variation in PEFRs
3 Airway hyper-reactivity
  - Defined as exaggerated airway narrowing in response to inhalation of various materials and can be quantified by the use of pharmacologic agents
  - Thought to be an acquired (*vs.* congenital) abnormality although exact pathogenesis is unknown
  - Bronchial provocation with histamine or methacholine can confirm the diagnosis of asthma when symptoms are suggestive but routine lung function is normal
  - Airway hyper-responsiveness is present when FEV_1 falls >20% at a concentration of 8 mg/ml or less of methacholine
  - The above can vary depending upon exposures the patient has had, can change daily, and may only be demonstrable following a specific exposure, e.g. occupational or seasonal asthma
  - False negative tests can be seen in patients on

bronchodilators or antihistamines (when histamine is used) while positives can be seen in an asymptomatic subset of the population (~5%) as well as in patients with baseline airway narrowing, e.g. COPD, bronchiectasis

Reversible disease is present in most patients but progressive airways obstruction is seen in some, usually those with the most severe disease, but unpredictable for individual cases

- The latter presumably reflects airway remodeling and narrowing due to chronic uncontrolled inflammation

AMBULATORY ASTHMA – DIFFICULT TO CONTROL

1 **Aspiration**
   - Gastro-esophageal reflux disease (GERD) where history includes heartburn, regurgitation, hoarseness, as well as worsening symptoms when supine or following food or alcohol
   - Allergic rhinitis or sinusitis with improvement of asthma symptoms following antibiotics and nasal steroids

2 **Inhalational exposures**
   - Respiratory irritants
     - Indoor: cigarette smoke; personal products, e.g. hair spray, deodorant, cologne, etc.; household products, e.g. bleaches, cleaners, air deodorizers, etc.
     - Outdoor: respirable particulates, sulfur dioxide, ground-level ozone
   - Aero-allergens
     - Indoor: cats (or other animal allergics), dust mites, alternaria, cockroaches
     - Outdoor: as for indoor plus pollens and other molds
   - Occupational exposures: irritants, sensitizers

3 **Infections**
- Viral, mycoplasma or chlamydia – bronchitis, bronchiolitis, pneumonia
- Fungal, e.g. allergic bronchopulmonary aspergillosis
- Parasitic, e.g. tropical eosinophilia
- Allergic reaction to skin fungal infection trychophyton

4 **Ingestions**
- Food additives, e.g. metasulfite salts, tartrazine, monosodium glutamate

5 **Asthma complications**
- Mucus plugs/atelectasis
- Bronchopulmonary aspergillosis
- Pneumothorax – pneumomediastinum
- Chronic eosinophilic pneumonia
- Churg-Strauss vasculitis

6 **Medication related**
- Inadequate bronchodilators prescribed
- Non-compliance (one of the commonest causes)
- Technical factors re inhalers
- Laryngeal candidiasis from steroids
- Methotrexate induced pneumonitis or opportunistic infection
- Drug-induced bronchospasm e.g. salicylates, NSAIDs β-blockers (oral or ophthalmic)

7 **Steroid 'resistance'** defined as <15% increase in FEV_1 or mean PEF above baseline values of <75% predicted after 2 weeks of high dose prednisolone, e.g. 40 mg daily, although the mechanism is unclear.

8 **Weight gain** from oral steroids +/– obstructive sleep apnea, which can worsen asthma control

9 **Thyrotoxicosis** (mechanism unclear)

10 **Diseases simulating asthma** (see below)

DISEASES SIMULATING ASTHMA

Upper airways

- Vocal cord dysfunction/tumors/paralysis
- Tracheal narrowing – intralumenal, endotracheal or extramural
- Tracheomalacia
- Tracheobronchomegaly
- Tracheo-esophageal fistula
- Anaphylaxis

Lower airways

- COPD
- Bronchiectasis
- Bronchiolitis
- Localized bronchial narrowing – intralumenal, intramural, extramural
- Broncho-esophageal fistula
- Recurrent aspiration

Parenchyma

- Parasitic infections, e.g. tropical eosinophilia, schistosomiasis

Vasculature

- Pulmonary edema secondary to pulmonary venous hypertension
- Pulmonary emboli
- Lymphangitic carcinoma
- Carcinoid syndrome

CNS

- Anxiety attacks

CHEST X-RAY FINDINGS

1 Often normal
2 Reversible hyperinflation with flat diaphragms, increased retrosternal and retrocardiac airspaces, dorsal kyphosis

3 Enlargement of the main pulmonary artery and hilar branches
4 Reversible oligemia
5 Bronchial wall thickening manifest as 'ring signs' or 'tramlines'
6 Occasional long and narrow cardiac silhouette

Complicating Radiologic Infiltrates

1 Mucus plugs
2 Allergic bronchopulmonary aspergillosis
3 Bronchocentric granulomatosis
4 Atelectasis
5 Loeffler's syndrome
6 Chronic eosinophilic pneumonia
7 Mycoplasma, viral or chlamydial pneumonia with exacerbation of asthma
8 Opportunistic infection, e.g. invasive aspergillosis, when on immunosuppressive treatment
9 Drug toxicity, e.g. methotrexate
10 Allergic granulomatosis of Churg and Strauss – nodules/airspace consolidation
11 Bronchiectasis
12 Pneumothorax, pneumomediastinum, pneumopericardium

ASPIRIN-INDUCED ASTHMA (AIA)

ASA sensitivity is seen in 5–25% of asthmatics and clinical presentations include

- Cutaneous – hives, urticuria
- Respiratory – upper and lower airways disease
  - Samter's triad is the combination of ASA sensitivity, nasal polyps and asthma in patients not previously sensitive to ASA

Upper airways disease

- May precede lower respiratory symptoms and characterized by inflammation of the nasal mucosa and paranasal sinuses

- Sinus opacification is seen in >90% of cases accompanied by the frequent occurrence of nasal polyps

Lower airways disease

AIA differs from atopic asthma as follows

1. Usually presents in the fourth decade versus classic atopic asthma under age 20
2. Family history is rarely positive
3. Normal IgE levels
4. Negative aeroallergen skin tests

Seen in 5–10% of asthmatics where symptoms develop 30 minutes to 4 hours post ASA ingestion with profuse rhinorrhea, flushing of the head and neck, conjunctivitis and wheezing

- Severe reactions can result in hypercapneic respiratory failure and death
- Simultaneous skin and respiratory reactions are uncommon

Diagnosis of AIA is made by *in vivo* testing with a placebo controlled oral challenge in suspected patients while monitoring spirometry or an aspirin challenge with simultaneous assay of urinary leukotrienes

REACTIVE AIRWAY DYSFUNCTION SYNDROME (RADS)

Definition: The persistence of hyper-reactive airways following acute exposure to a respiratory irritant (irritant-induced asthma), usually the result of a spill or accident

- The exposure is usually single and intense, can occur at home or work, with numerous irritants described including smoke, household cleaners, ammonia, acids, chlorine, etc. resulting in
  - Symptoms of airways disease, i.e. cough, wheezing and dyspnea, in patients with no previous history of respiratory disease, beginning within 24 hours of exposure without a latent period of prior 'sensitization'

a. Re-exposure to low dose of the irritant will generally not trigger asthma
b. If work-related, patients can continue to work in the same building after measures have been applied to avoid exposure to the irritant as completely as possible

- PFTs ranging from normal to obstructive
- Bronchial hyper-reactivity as demonstrated by, e.g. methacholine challenge test
- The above potentially persisting from months to years

PREDICTORS OF LIFE-THREATENING ASTHMA

1 History of near-fatal asthma requiring intubation
2 History of severe asthma, e.g. recurrent ER visits or hospitalizations
3 Poor compliance with medication
4 Denial of disease
5 Delay in seeking treatment
6 'Labile' airways, i.e. >50% variability in PEFRs daily
7 Poor perception of severity

OCCUPATIONAL ASTHMA

Definition: Asthma caused by exposure to an agent specific to the workplace

- Asthma is usually of new onset (but can pre-exist) with bronchial hyperresponsiveness usually acquired versus existing previously
- The response is usually allergic-mediated through IgE antibodies (or other unknown immunologic reactions) while in ~5% of cases a high level respiratory irritant exposure is responsible with no latency period

- 'Sensitization' to a high (e.g. animal/plant protein) or low molecular weight agent (e.g. isocyanates) occurs over weeks to years with further exposure at even low levels triggering asthma
- atopy and smoking are host factors, especially for high molecular weight agents

- Irritant aggravation of coincidental asthma is the most common differential
  - Typically there is no worsening of bronchial hyper-reactivity as measured on challenge tests, e.g. HCT, before and after exposure

Diagnostic features

1 History of asthma beginning during a working lifetime with worsening of symptoms on working days, manifest as an immediate (minutes) or delayed (hours) response or both
  - Rhinitis and conjunctivitis may precede lower respiratory symptoms

2 Confirmation of the diagnosis of asthma by history, physical and airways obstruction on spirometry pre- and post-bronchodilator when symptoms are present

3 Measurement of PEFRs or spirometry several times daily at and off work for more than two weeks, looking for diurnal variability >20% in PEFRs on working days *vs.* days off

4 With normal spirometry, challenge tests should demonstrate bronchial hyperreactivity changes before and after work exposure
  - Significant improvement in airway hyper-reactivity on challenge testing after being away from work for a few weeks, or deterioration on returning to work, is supportive of occupational asthma
  - A normal challenge test in a symptomatic patient who is working rules out occupational asthma
  - Worsening of PEFRs at work without an accompanying change in airway hyper-reactivity is more suggestive of work-related aggravation of prior asthma

5 Identification of specific IgE antibodies to a workplace allergen by skin tests, a negative test excluding that particular antigen (while a positive test may reflect only sensitization without asthma)
6 Specific challenge testing done in specialized centers

In conclusion, all individual investigations for occupational asthma can have false positives or negatives and therefore a combination of tests is required (see Cartier, A (1998) Seminars in Asthma Management)

- The diagnosis is difficult to establish if patients have left work, cannot, or will not return, making early referral and evaluation of occupational asthma essential
- The major factor determining recovery, persistence or death relates to the duration of symptoms after clinical disease has occurred, making early diagnosis important
- The 'index case' should prompt consideration of the existence of occupational asthma in other exposed workers, with medical screening of co-workers coordinated by the plant physician or a public health agency

Is the patient in a high risk employment for OA?

Crab or prawn / processing plant worker
Isocyanates / industrial spray painter, foundry worker
Epoxy curing agents / manufacture of plastics and adhesives
Psyllium / health care worker
Western red cedar / carpenter or woodworker
Laboratory animals / technician or research assistant
Flour / baker
Latex / health care worker
Colophony / electronic soldering

Fraser R.S., Muller N.L., Colman N., Paré P.D. (1999) Diagnosis of Diseases of the Chest 4th Edn., WB Saunders.
Baum, G.L., Crapo, J.D., Celli, B.R., Karlinsky, J.B. (eds) (1997) *Textbook of Pulmonary Diseases*, 6th edn.: Lippincott-Raven.
Fishman, A.P., Elias, J.A., Fishman, J.A., Grippi, M.A., Kaiser, L.R.,

Senior, R.N. (1998) *Fishman's Pulmonary Diseases and Disorders*, 3rd edn.: McGraw-Hill.

Tarlo, S., Boulet, L.P., Cartier, A. *et al.* (1998) CTS guidelines for occupational asthma. *Can. Resp. J.* **5**: 280–300.

Chan-Yeung, M., Malo, J.L. (1995) Occupational asthma. *NEJM* **333**: 107–112.

Brooks, S.M., Weiss, M., Bernstein, I.L. (1985) RADS: persistent asthma syndrome after high level irritant exposure. *Chest* **88**: 376–384.

Alberts, W.M., DoPico, G.A. (1996) Reactive airways dysfunction syndrome. *Chest* **109**: 1618–1626.

Chan-Teung, M. (1995) Assessment of asthma in the workplace. ACCP consensus statement. American College of Chest Physicians. *Chest* **108**: 1084–1117.

Lynch, D. (1998) Imaging of asthma and allergic bronchopulmonary mycosis. *Radiol. Clin. North Am.* **36**: 129–142.

Cartier, A. (1998) Occupational asthma. *Seminars in Asthma Management* October, **2**(3): 1–15.

11 Atelectasis

Definition: Loss of alveolar volume

DIFFERENTIAL DIAGNOSIS

Includes:

1. Pulmonary consolidation, but fissures are not displaced, associated X-ray findings are absent (see below) and an air bronchogram may be seen
2. Loculated pleural fluid
   - Lower chest posteriorly simulates lower lobe collapse
   - Left upper anterior hemithorax simulates LUL collapse
   - Minor or lower major fissures simulates RML or lingular collapse but demonstration of nearby fissures, thickened pleura elsewhere and rounded contours are clues to fluid
3. Mediastinal lesion

ETIOLOGIES

Non-obstructive Atelectasis

- Compressive, e.g. pneumothorax, pleural effusion, bullae
- Adhesive, e.g. radiation pneumonitis, pulmonary emboli

- Cicatrization, e.g. old tuberculosis, RML syndrome, silicosis
- Plate atelectasis, e.g. splinting
- Rounded atelectasis, e.g. asbestos exposure

Obstructive Atelectasis – Bronchial Stenosis or Occlusion

Intralumenal

- Foreign body aspiration, broncholithiasis, mucoid impaction, misplaced E-tube

Intramural

- Congenital, e.g. bronchial atresia
- Traumatic, e.g. bronchial laceration
- Inflammatory, e.g. sarcoid, plasma cell granuloma, relapsing polychondritis
- Infectious, e.g. tuberculosis, actinomycosis, fungal
- Infiltrative, e.g. amyloid, tracheobronchopathia osteochondroplastica
- Vasculitis, e.g. Wegener's
- Neoplastic, e.g. primary (benign/malignant) or metastatic

Extramural

- Torsion of a bronchus
- Congenital, e.g. bronchogenic cyst
- Neoplastic, e.g. mesothelioma, parenchymal tumor
- Vascular, e.g. aortic aneurysm, anomalous origin of the left pulmonary artery from the right pulmonary artery, enlarged left atrium
- Lymphadenopathy, e.g. neoplastic, inflammatory
- Mediastinal, e.g. neoplastic, inflammatory

CHEST X-RAY FINDINGS

1. Displacement of interlobar fissures bounding the affected lobe
2. Hemidiaphragmatic elevation
3. Tracheal and mediastinal shift to the affected side
4. Narrowing of rib spaces

5 Compensatory hyperinflation of the remaining lobe/lung
6 Hilar displacement
7 Crowding of the bronchovascular markings
8 Local increased density of the involved lung
9 Herniation across the midline of the opposite lung if atelectasis is unilateral

CT SIGNS OF 'MALIGNANT ATELECTASIS'

1 Obstructed or narrowed airway
2 Central mass with bulging of the proximal portion of the collapsed lobe or segment on chest X-ray, e.g. 'S' sign of Golden with RUL collapse
3 Tumor is often difficult to distinguish from contiguous atelectasis or obstructive pneumonitis
   - Intravenous contrast results in vascular enhancement of the collapsed lung *vs.* little enhancement by the central tumor
   - Bronchogenic cancer is the most common cause of the above findings, with uncommon etiologies being lymphoma, sarcoid, tuberculosis, fungal infection and granulomatous mediastinitis

'FAILURE TO EXPAND'

1 Persistent airways obstruction
   - Intralumenal, endobronchial, peribronchial
2 Pleural peel
   - Pleural thickening
   - Primary or metastatic neoplasm
3 Persistent air leak
   - Bronchial, e.g. suture breakdown, infection, neoplastic erosion
   - Alveolar, e.g. ruptured bulla, abscess, neoplasm

RIGHT MIDDLE LOBE SYNDROME

Confusing term and used to describe **non-obstructive** atelectasis of the RML

- Bronchoscopy shows a patent bronchus as does bronchography, which often shows bronchiectasis
- **Diagnosis** should be made **only** after a patent bronchus is demonstrated
- Serial X-rays may show variable degrees of volume loss fluctuating over time

OBSTRUCTIVE PNEUMONITIS

Most common radiologic manifestation of an obstructed airway and comprised of:

1. Atelectasis
2. Bronchiectasis with dilated mucous-filled bronchi distal to the obstruction
3. Inflammatory infiltrate including mononuclear cells and lipid-laden macrophages

- The atelectasis can be segmental, lobar or involve the entire lung, without air bronchograms
- An obstructing tumor may be difficult to distinguish from atelectasis or obstructive pneumonitis and require an i.v. bolus of contrast (where enhancement is seen in the atelectatic or consolidated lung *vs.* the primary tumor)
- With high-grade central obstruction the accumulation of fluid and cells distal to an obstructing lesion compensates for absorbed alveolar air, limiting volume loss, and resulting in a drowned lung
- Distal infection (acute bronchitis, bronchiolitis, pneumonia, abscess formation) can result in the affected area of lung enlarging rather than decreasing in volume, an example of where bronchial obstruction does not always lead to volume loss

Fraser R.S., Muller N.L., Colman N., Paré P.D. (1999) Diagnosis of Diseases of the Chest 4th Edn., WB Saunders.
Naidich, D.P., Zerhouni, E.A., Siegelman, S.S. (1998) *Computed Tomography and Magnetic Resonance of the Thorax*, 3rd edn. New York: Raven Press.
Felson, B. (1973) Chest Roentgenology.: W.B. Saunders.

12 Axillosubclavian Vein Thrombosis (ASVT)

1 **Axillary lymphadenopathy** – malignant

2 **Pancoast's syndrome** +/– radiotherapy

3 **Fibrosing/granulomatous mediastinitis**

4 **Paget-Schroetter syndrome**
- Syndrome of spontaneous ASVT is seen in young healthy individuals, frequently following strenuous activity or trauma involving the arm/shoulder
- There is often a compressive anomaly at the thoracic outlet, unilateral or bilateral, with secondary perivenous fibrosis exacerbating the venous obstruction
- Symptoms and signs include:
  a. Shoulder/axillary pains
  b. Swelling of the hand/arm which is increased with exertion and improved with rest
  c. Subcutanous collateral veins over the upper arm and chest
  d. Features of pulmonary emboli
- Diagnostic tests include:
  a. Ultrasonography (screening test)
  b. Contrast venography of arm
  c. CT/MRI/digital subtraction angiography
  d. R/O hypercoagulable state

5 **Catheter-induced**
- Seen when central venous catheters have been placed into the subclavian vein for, e.g. chemotherapy, feedings, i.v. access
- Clinical features include:
  a. Asymptomatic finding
  b. Pain in the shoulder, neck or supraclavicular area

c. Hand/arm edema
d. Embolization to the lungs
e. Paradoxical emboli with, e.g. patent foramen ovale
f. Post-thrombotic syndrome of swelling, chronic pain and venous hypertension
g. Venous gangrene

- Investigations as above

6 **Hypercoagulable state**

7 **Direct vascular trauma**

8 **Septic thrombophlebitis**, e.g. drug addict

Haire, W. (1995) Arm vein thrombosis. *Clinics in Chest Medicine* **16**: 341–350.

Aburahama, A.F., Sadler, D.L., Robinson, P.A. (1991) Axillary-subclavian vein thrombosis: changing patterns of etiology, diagnostic and therapeutic modalities. *Ann. Surg.* **57**: 101–107.

Beeker, D.M., Phlibrick, J.T., Walker, F.B. (1991) Axillary and subclavian vein thrombosis. *Arch. Int. Med.* **151**: 1934–1943.

13 Azygous Shadows

Azygous Continuation of the IVC

- The normal azygous vein is the superior continuation of the ascending lumbar vein and ascends parallel and to the right of the esophagus
- It drains the lower intercostal veins, the hemi-azygous veins at about T8, via communicating vessels that cross the midline, is joined by the right superior intercostal vein superiorly, then arches anteriorly to join the posterior surface of the SVC
- Azygous continuation of the IVC is often asymptomatic unless there is associated congenital heart disease
- May be associated with asplenia or polysplenia

Chest X-ray features include:

1 Frequent intrathoracic IVC
2 Increased right tracheobronchial opacity
3 Displacement of the right mediastinal pleura laterally creating a right paraspinal interface, analogous to the left paraspinal interface from the aorta
4 'Second arch' seen on the lateral chest X-ray below the aortic arch

CT manifestations include dilatation of the ascending azygous vein in the retrocrural space equal to the aortic diameter

Azygous Opacity

1 **Increased azygous node** (any cause of mediastinal lymphadenopathy)
2 **Other mediastinal mass**
3 **Increased azygous vein** (normal <10 mm in diameter)
   - Volume effect, e.g. right heart failure, supine position (normal <14 mm), pregnancy
   - Congenital abnormalities, e.g. persistent left SVC,

azygous continuation of the IVC, anomalous pulmonary venous drainage
- Obstruction to SVC, IVC, portal vein, hepatic vein obstruction (intra- or extra-hepatic)
- Idiopathic dilatation of the azygous arch

4 **Pulmonary mass**

5 **Pleural mass**

Fraser R.S., Muller N.L., Colman N., Paré P.D. (1999) Diagnosis of Diseases of the Chest 4th Edn., WB Saunders.

Naidich, D.P., Zerhouni, E.A., Siegelman, S.S. (1998) *Computed Tomography and Magnetic Resonance of the Thorax*, 3rd edn. New York: Raven Press.

Felson, B. (1973) Chest Roentgenology.: W.B. Saunders.

14 Biopsy of Granulomas

GRANULOMAS ON LUNG BIOPSY

Definition: Granulomas are a non-specific inflammatory reaction developing in response to multiple infectious and non-infectious agents

- Pathologically they are a compact collection of mononuclear macrophages which may be accompanied by necrosis and inflammatory cells
- Sarcoid and infections are the two most common causes clinically

Differential Diagnosis

1 **Primary airways diseases**
   - Bronchocentric granulomatosis

2 **Primary parenchymal diseases**
   - Aspiration, e.g. oil aspiration, foreign body granulomatosis, miliary granulomatosis
   - Inhalational, e.g. allergic alveolitis, silicosis, berylliosis, hard metal disease
   - Infectious
     - *Bacterial*: tuberculosis, nocardia, actinomycosis
     - *Fungal*: blastomycosis, histoplasmosis, coccidioidomycosis, cryptococcosis, sporotrichosis, ABPA, pneumocystis
     - *Parasitic*: toxoplasmosis, schistosomiasis, visceral leishmaniasis, ascaris, toxocara, tropical eosinophilia

- Sarcoid/necrotizing sarcoid granulomatosis
- Drugs, e.g. methotrexate
- Plasma cell granuloma (inflammatory pseudotumor)
- Eosinophilic granuloma
- Hyalinizing granuloma
- Rheumatoid nodules

3 **Primary vascular diseases**
- Vasculitides, e.g. Wegener's, Churg-Strauss, lymphomatoid granulomatosis, Takayasu's
- i.v. talcosis

4 **GLUS syndrome**
- Granulomatous lesions of unknown significance seen in 15–20% of biopsies
- No etiology found in this group which is B-cell positive (versus sarcoid and mycobacterial infections which are B-cell negative)

Clues to Etiology

1 **History**
- Drug use/abuse, e.g. methotrexate, i.v. talcosis
- Dysphagia or altered level of consciousness, e.g. lipoid pneumonia, miliary granulomatosis
- Inhalational exposures at work or home, e.g. berylliosis, allergic alveolitis
- Country of origin and travel history, e.g. specific bacterial, fungal, parasitic infections
- Asthma, e.g. bronchocentric granulomatosis, Churg-Strauss
- New onset of wheezing, e.g. Wegener's granulomatosis, parasitic infection

2 **Presence of extrapulmonary disease**, e.g. sarcoid, vasculitis

3 **Bloods**
- Peripheral eosinophilia, e.g. Churg-Strauss, bronchocentric granulomatosis, rarely Wegener's granulomatosis
- Serology, e.g. fungal infections, brucella, tularemia

- Serum precipitins, e.g. allergic alveolitis, bronchocentric granulomatosis
- Parasitemia, e.g. leishmaniasis
- Elevated ACE level, e.g. sarcoid
- Lymphocyte transformation test, e.g. berylliosis

4 **Sputum** – for tuberculosis, mycology, parasites

5 **Radiologic abnormalities on chest X-ray/CT**

- Upper lobe distribution
  – e.g. tuberculosis, fungi, sarcoid, allergic alveolitis
- Patterns of disease
  – Cavitation, e.g. tuberculosis, fungi, Wegener's, Churg-Strauss, cystic disease
  – Cystic disease, e.g. eosinophilic granuloma
  – Large nodules, e.g. Wegener's, lymphoma, lymphomatoid granulomatosis, sarcoid
  – Miliary, e.g. tuberculosis, fungi
  – Localized disease, e.g. foreign body granuloma, plasma cell granuloma, hyalinizing granuloma, some infections
  – Diffuse disease, e.g. sarcoid, drugs, inhalational
- Associated extraparenchymal abnormalities
  – Mediastinal/hilar adenopathy, e.g. tuberculosis, fungi, sarcoid, beryllium, granulomatous response to a neoplasm
  – Pleural effusion, e.g. tuberculosis, fungi, Wegener's
  – Airways disease, e.g. endotracheal or endobronchial Wegener's

6 **Associated pathologic findings**

- Eosinophilia, e.g. Churg-Strauss
- Alveolitis, e.g. sarcoid
- Bronchiolitis, e.g. allergic alveolitis
- Vasculitis, e.g. Wegener's
- Inclusion bodies, e.g. sarcoid, beryllium
- Caseation necrosis, e.g. tuberculosis
- Coagulation necrosis, e.g. necrotizing sarcoid granulomatosis
- Non-caseating, e.g. sarcoid

GRANULOMAS ON MEDIASTINAL BIOPSY

1 **Granulomatous mediastinitis** secondary to *Histoplasma capsulatum* or *M. tuberculosis*
2 **Granulomatous lymphadenopathy**
- Infections – tuberculosis, fungal
- Inflammatory – sarcoid
- Inhalational – silica, beryllium
- Neoplasm-induced granulomatous response

Fraser R.S., Muller N.L., Colman N., Paré P.D. (1999) Diagnosis of Diseases of the Chest 4th Edn., WB Saunders.
Tarlo, S., Boulet, L.P., Cartier, A. *et al.* (1998) CTS guidelines for occupational asthma. *Can. Resp. J.* **5**: 280–300.
Chan-Yeung, M., Malo, J.L. (1995) Occupational asthma. *NEJM* **333**: 107–112.
Brooks, S.M., Weiss, M., Bernstein, I.L. (1985) RADS: persistent asthma syndrome after high level irritant exposure. *Chest* **88**: 376–384.
Alberts, W.M., DoPico, G.A. (1996) Reactive airways dysfunction syndrome. *Chest* **109**: 1618–1626.
Chan-Teung, M. (1995) Assessment of asthma in the workplace. ACCP consensus statement. American College of Chest Physicians. *Chest* **108**: 1084–1117.
Lynch, D. (1998) Imaging of asthma and allergic bronchopulmonary mycosis. *Radiol. Clin. North Am.* **36**: 129–142.
Haire, W. (1995) Arm vein thrombosis. *Clinics in Chest Medicine* **16**: 341–350.
Thompson, G., Utz, J., Rosenow, E. *et al.* (1993) Pulmonary lymphoproliferative disorders. *Mayo Clinic Proc.* **68**: 804–817.
Glickstein *et al.* (1986) Nonlymphomatous lymphoid disorders of the Lung. *AJR* **147**: 227–237.
Heitzman, Markarian, B., DeLise, C. (1975) Lymphoproliferative disorders of the thorax. *Semin. Roent.* **10**: 73–81.
Sharma, O.P., Flora, G. (1991) Diagnosis of pulmonary granulomas in the tropics. *Semin. Resp. Med.* **12**: 126–133.
Williams, G.T., Jones-Williams, W. (1983) Granulomatous inflammation: a review. *J. Clin. Pathol.* **36**: 723–730.

Boros, D.L. (1978) Granulomatous inflammations. *Drug Allergy* **26**: 184–243.

Sharma, O. (1991) Disease-a-month. *Hypersensitivity Pneumonitis* **XXXVII**: 415–471.

Brinker, H. (1994) Granulomatous lesions of unknown significance: the glus syndrome. In: *Sarcoid and Other Granulomatous Diseases*. New York: Marcel Dekker, pp. 69–86.

15 Biopsy of Lymphocytes – Typical/atypical

DIFFERENTIAL DIAGNOSIS

Differential diagnosis in non-HIV patients with no known underlying lung disease:

1. Lymphoid interstitial pneumonitis
2. Pseudolymphoma
3. Intrapulmonary lymph node
4. Primary pulmonary lymphoma
5. Secondary pulmonary lymphoma
6. Lymphomatoid granulomatosis
7. Post-transplant lymphoma
8. Inflammatory pseudotumor
9. Carcinoid syndrome
10. Small cell carcinoma
11. Hypersensitivity pneumonitis
12. Follicular bronchitis or bronchiolitis
13. Angioimmunoblastic lymphadenopathy
14. Intravascular lymphomatosis
15. Waldenstrom's macroglobulinemia

LYMPHOID INTERSTITIAL PNEUMONITIS (LIP)

Definition: A form of diffuse lymphoid hyperplasia occurring along the lymphatic pathways of the lung and characterized histologically by the interstitial proliferation of small lymphocytes, histiocytes and plasma cells distributed within alveolar septae and along bronchovascular bundles, fibrosis and honeycombing developing with disease progression

The polyclonal proliferation usually presents as diffuse lung disease but can be focal ? called pseudolymphoma, the polyclonality distinguishing LIP from lymphoma

HIV ⊖ Patients

Clinically LIP occurs most often between ages 40–60, female to male ratio of 2:1, and most patients symptomatic including:

- Non-specific respiratory symptoms of cough and dyspnea developing over months (rarely asymptomatic)
- Systemic features of fever, weight loss and night sweats in ~20% of cases, with adenopathy and splenomegaly being uncommon
- Associated Sjogren's syndrome as well as other autoimmune diseases including chronic active hepatitis, primary biliary cirrhosis, graft *vs* host disease, SLE, pernicious anemia
- May be an early manifestation of small cell lymphoma or progress to high grade lymphoma
- Diagnosis is made on thoracoscopic or open lung biopsy
- The course of disease is unpredictable and lung disease may resolve spontaneously or post-treatment, stabilize, evolve into progressive pulmonary disease with fibrosis, or develop as lymphoma

Labs are non-specific and include polyclonal hypergammaglobulinemia, hypogammaglobulinemia, ⊕ RF, ⊕ ANA

Radiologic features

1 *Bilateral lower lobe interstitial disease resembling lymphangitic carcinoma
2 Air space disease with air bronchograms as the interstitial process progresses
3 Nodules
4 End-stage interstitial fibrosis with a honeycomb lung
5 Lymphadenopathy and pleural effusion rarely seen
6 HRCT features of 'ground glass' opacities, airspace consolidation and thin-walled cysts

HIV ⊕ Patients

Clinically, seen more often in the pediatric age group where it is an AIDS-defining disease

- Presentation is of non-specific respiratory symptoms as well as systemic features of fevers, weight loss, hepatosplenomegaly and lymphadenopathy
- Important to R/O opportunistic infection in this group, particularly mycobacteria and pneumocystis

PSEUDOLYMPHOMA

Definition: Rare disorder consisting of a localized non-neoplastic mass of inflammatory tissue with a prominent lymphocytic component which is polyclonal

- Some investigators question its existence and feel it represents a malignant process
  - There is considerable overlap histologically with the low-grade lymphoma of MALT
  - Some patients diagnosed as pseudolymphoma develop true lymphoma years later
- A monoclonal B neoplasm must therefore be ruled out before the diagnosis is considered and patients should be investigated for evidence of extrathoracic or intrathoracic lymphoma initially, as well as in the following years, for evidence of disseminated lymphoma

Clinically, patients are usually over 40, show no sex preponderance, and can present with
- *Asymptomatic lung lesion
- Non-specific respiratory symptoms
- Systemic symptoms including fever or an associated autoimmune disorder, e.g. Sjogren's syndrome or systemic lupus (rarely reported)
- Surgical excision generally results in cure, with true pseudolymphoma having a benign course

Radiologically, it usually presents as a solitary nodule or localized airspace disease with air bronchograms, resembling alveolar cell carcinoma, and may be central or peripheral
- Intrathoracic lymphadenopathy is rare and suggestive of malignant lymphoma

INTRAPULMONARY LYMPH NODES

Definition: These are hyperplastic nodes which are biopsied or resected to rule out a neoplastic disorder

Clinically, they are usually asymptomatic, occur typically in smokers, males > females, and often seen with a history of dust exposure to asbestos or non-fibrous silicates

Radiologically, they are usually solitary nodules but multiple in ~30%, subpleural in location, and most often lower lobe in location
- Size varies from <1 cm to ~2 cm and often visualized only on CT scan
- there are no radiologic features distinguishing them from other causes of non-calcified intraparenchymal nodules

PRIMARY PULMONARY LYMPHOMA

Definition: Primary pulmonary lymphoma is an uncommon neoplasm, with controversy defining and distinguishing this from secondary pulmonary lymphoma with regard to the presence of hilar or mediastinal adenopathy or the time before extrathoracic involvement can be diagnosed, e.g. 3 months

Low-grade B-cell Lymphoma

80% of primary pulmonary lymphomas are low grade and the majority of these are small lymphocytic lymphomas of MALT (mucosa associated lymphoid tissue), B-cell neoplasms

Clinically, most patients are 60–70 years of age and present with

- Asymptomatic lung lesion in up to 50% of patients
- Non-specific respiratory symptoms
- Rarely as an endobronchial tumor
- Occasional systemic symptoms
- Sjogren's syndrome in ~10% of cases
- Associated lymphoid proliferation in extrapulmonary mucosal sites e.g. stomach, upper respiratory tract

Prognosis is excellent with

- Most patients having a complete remission post-resection or chemotherapy
- Stability of disease post-treatment
- Progressive disease in ~5% of patients, including transformation to intermediate or high grade lymphoma

Radiologic features

1 *Single/multiple nodules in ~70% of cases
2 Single/multiple areas of airspace consolidation in ~25%
3 Slow growth of the above over months to years
4 Tracheobronchial infiltration with airway narrowing or atelectasis
5 Pleural effusions (10%) or lymphadenopathy (<5%)

Diagnosis has been established from

1 Bronchial biopsy, TTNA, BAL
2 Pleural fluid and pleural biopsy

Intermediate/high Grade Lymphoma

Clinically, these are usually symptomatic with non-specific respiratory complaints, systemic symptoms reflecting extra-pulmonary disease and a poorer prognosis than low grade lymphocytic lymphoma

Most cases are of B-cell type and may be seen post-transplant, in AIDS or developing from low-grade B-cell lymphoma

Radiologic findings

1 *Single/multiple nodules
2 Interstitial pattern resembling lymphangitic cancer
3 Airspace opacities
4 Pleural effusions and lymphadenopathy

Primary Pulmonary Hodgkins' Disease

Diagnosis made by

1 Histologic features of Hodgkins' disease with Reed-Sternberg cells
2 Disease localized to the lung parenchyma without nodal involvement
3 Absence of extrathoracic disease clinically or pathologically

Clinically, most patients present with non-specific respiratory symptoms and B-symptoms of fevers, night sweats and weight loss

- Rare disorder compared to the pulmonary involvement seen in ~40% of patients with generalized Hodgkins' disease
- Open lung biopsy is required for definitive diagnosis with most cases being nodular sclerosis or mixed cellularity

Radiologic features

1 Nodular or mass lesion which can cavitate
2 Multiple nodules
3 Air space consolidation
4 Reticulonodular infiltrate

LYMPHOMATOID GRANULOMATOSIS

Definition: Rare disorder, histologically composed of

1 A polymorphic infiltrate of small lymphocytes, plasma cells, large cells with immunoblastic features
2 Predilection for vessel infiltration, the latter occasionally resulting in obliteration of the vascular lumen
3 Focal necrosis within the lymphoid nodules

EBV infection is suspected in many of the cases

Recently incorporated into the term angiocentric immunoproliferative lesion (AIL)

- Grade 1 lesion – benign lymphocytic angiitis and granulomatosis
- Grade 2 lesion – lymphomatoid granulomatosis
- Grade 3 lesion – lymphoma

Clinically, it occurs most often between ages 40–60 with a 2:1 male to female predominance and

- Non-specific respiratory symptoms
- Systemic involvement including fevers and weight loss
- Extrathoracic disease of the skin (rash, nodules), brain, cranial and peripheral nerves
- Rare involvement of the upper respiratory tract or clinical kidney disease (unlike Wegener's granulomatosis)
- Uncommon involvement of the reticulo-endothelial system including the liver, spleen, bone marrow or lymph nodes, early in the disease
- Poor prognosis with high mortality rates within 1–2 years if untreated

Lab studies are non-specific and include polyclonal hypergammaglobulinemia, hypogammaglobulinemia, ⊕ ANA, ⊕ RF

Radiologic features

1 Bilateral nodules which can increase, decrease, cavitate, rupture into the pleura or disappear
2 Patchy airspace consolidation

3 Pleural based opacities resembling pulmonary infarcts
4 Rarely, lymphadenopathy

POST-TRANSPLANT LYMPHOPROLIFERATIVE DISEASE (PTLD)

Definition: Seen in organ recipients after exogenous immunosuppression and reflects an EBV-related B-lymphocyte proliferation, rarely arising from T-cell lymphocytes

- Clinical spectrum varies from a mild polyclonal lymphoid hyperplasia to frank lymphoma, with patients who are seronegative pre-transplant more likely to develop PTLD than those who are EBV positive
- Incidence varies from <1% in bone marrow transplants to greater frequency with heart, liver or kidney transplant and highest incidence post-lung transplants (5–20%)
- Clinical presentation varies from asymptomatic to non-specific respiratory symptoms
- Pulmonary disease may be localized or disseminated, involving nodal or extranodal sites, including the GI tract, tonsils and cervical nodes
- Prognosis varies from a reversible disease with cessation or reduction in immunosuppressants plus antiviral agents, to death if untreated
- Most tumors are diagnosed within 1 year of transplant, but they can present from a few months to many years later

Radiologic findings

1 *Single or multiple pulmonary nodules
2 *Mediastinal/hilar lymphadenopathy presenting as discrete nodes or a mass lesion
3 Patchy airspace consolidation
4 Thymic enlargement
5 Pleuropericardial disease manifest as thickening or effusion

INFLAMMATORY PSEUDOTUMOR

Definition: An uncommon, reactive, non-neoplastic pulmonary lesion composed of variable proportions of plasma cells, lymphocytes, fibroblasts and histiocytes, synonyms including plasma cell granuloma, fibrous histiocytoma and organizing pneumonia, depending on the predominant cell type

- Anatomically, they are usually parenchymal in location but are also described within the trancheobronchial tree, mediastinum and pulmonary vasculature

Clinically, described in all age groups without sex predilection, and presentations include

- Asymptomatic parenchymal mass or nodule
- Non-specific respiratory symptoms following a chest infection
- Symptoms of tracheal or bronchial obstruction which may be accompanied by unilateral wheezing

Definitive diagnosis is established at pathology when a lesion is removed due to suspicion of neoplasia

Radiologic findings

1 *Solitary pulmonary nodule, mass or air space consolidation which can calcify – rarely multiple nodules
2 Endotracheal or endobronchial narrowing, the latter leading to obstructive atelectasis
3 Rarely, extraparenchymal extension or primary involvement of mediastinal and hilar structures including the central airways
4 Regression, stability, slow growth or rarely local aggressive behavior is seen on serial films

ANGIOIMMUNOBLASTIC LYMPHADENOPATHY

Defined histologically by

1 Proliferation of small vessels

2 Diffuse infiltrate of lymphocytes, plasma cells and immunoblasts, most often involving lymph nodes but also seen in other tissues

Clinically, patients are over age 40 and have prominent constitutional symptoms of fevers, night sweats and weight loss

- Physical exam reveals generalized lymphadenopathy as well as hepatosplenomegaly
- Recent drug ingestion or, less often, vaccination may predate symptoms
- Labs reveal polyclonal hypergammaglobulinemia as well as Coombs' positive anemia
- Prognostically, remissions are described spontaneously or with steroids but high mortality rates are described from infection or transformation to immunoblastic lymphoma

Radiologic features

1 *Mediastinal (usually paratracheal or hilar) lymphadenopathy
2 Interstitial infiltrates
3 Air space infiltrates or nodules
4 Pleural effusions

INTRAVASCULAR LYMPHOMATOSIS

Definition: Rare disorder characterized by the intravascular proliferation of neoplastic lymphoid cells

- Usually presents with CNS or skin involvement, although case reports describe pulmonary disease presenting with dyspnea and bilateral interstitial infiltrates

WALDENSTROM'S MACROGLOBULINEMIA

Definition: Rare disease characterized by malignant proliferation of plasmacytoid B-cell lymphocytes secreting IgM protein

Clinically, occurs in the elderly, lung involvement is uncommon and patients present with lymphadenopathy, hepatosplenomegaly, bleeding, neurologic symptoms, e.g. peripheral neuropathy visual disturbances and/or a full blown hyperviscosity syndrome

Pleuropulmonary manifestations include:

1 Non-specific respiratory symptoms
2 Asymptomatic radiologic findings (see below)
3 Infection from the immunosuppressive effect of the disease and/or therapy
4 Wheezing from diffuse endobronchial involvement
5 Exudative or chylous effusions

Radiologic features include

1 Diffuse > focal infiltrates, nodules or masses
2 Pleural effusion
3 Mediastinal lymphadenopathy
4 R/O superimposed infection

Diagnostic findings

1 Pleural fluid, BAL or lung biopsy demonstrating plasmacytoid lymphocytes expressing monoclonal IgM
2 IgM monoclonal spike in pleural fluid (and serum)
3 R/O infection

Fraser R.S., Muller N.L., Colman N., Paré P.D. (1999) Diagnosis of Diseases of the Chest 4th Edn., WB Saunders.

Thurlbeck, W., Churg, A. (eds) (1995) *Pathology of the Lung*, 2nd edn. (Place of publication): Thieme Medical Publishers.

Thompson, G., Utz, J., Rosenow, E. *et al.* (1993) Pulmonary lymphoproliferative disorders. *Mayo Clinic Proc.* **68**: 804–817.

Glickstein *et al.* (1986) Nonlymphomatous lymphoid disorders of the lung. *AJR* **147**: 227–237.

Heitzman, Markarian, B., DeLise, C. (1975) Lymphoproliferative disorders of the thorax. *Semin. Roent.* **10**: 73–81.

Agrons, G., Rosado-de-Christenson, M., Kiregczyk, W. *et al.* (1998) Pulmonary inflammatory pseudotumor: radiologic features. *Radiology* **206**: 511–518.

Filuk, R.B., Warren, P.N. (1996) BAL in Waldenstrom's macroglobulinemia with pulmonary infiltrates. *Thorax* **41**: 409–410.

Rausch, P.G., Herion, J.C. (1980) Pulmonary manifestations of Waldenstrom's macroglobulinemia. *Am. J. Hematol.* **9**: 201–209.

16 Breast and Genital Tract Diseases – Pulmonary Manifestations

BREAST CANCER

Pulmonary disease is the sole site of metastases in 10–15% of cases and can result from direct invasion, lymphatic and hematogenous dissemination

Airways

- Endobronchial metastases with secondary atelectasis, obstructive pneumonitis
- BOOP following radiotherapy

Parenchyma

- *Single or multiple nodules
- *Lymphangitic carcinomatosis
- 'Hyperlucent lung' post-mastectomy
- Miliary pattern
- Radiation pneumonitis

Pleura

- *Malignant pleural effusion
- Pleural thickening, nodules or masses

Vasculature

- Tumor emboli and pulmonary hypertension with enlarged pulmonary arteries

Chest wall
- Absent breast shadow
- Bone destruction of ribs, sternum
- Soft tissue axillary mass
- Subcutaneous metastatic nodules
- Chest wall sarcoma developing years post radiotherapy for breast cancer

Mediastinum
- Lymphadenopathy of the internal mammary or other nodal groups

CERVICAL CANCER

Pulmonary involvement usually occurs in association with intra-abdominal spread of disease but isolated metastases can occur
- Lung metastases are more common with adenocarcinoma than with squamous cell, and are seen clinically in 5–10% of patients

Airways
- Endobronchial metastases with secondary atelectasis, obstructive pneumonitis

Parenchyma
- *Solitary or multiple nodules
- Lymphangitic carcinomatosis

Pleura
- Malignant effusion

Mediastinum
- Hilar/mediastinal lymphadenopathy

THORACIC ENDOMETRIOSIS

Definition: Rare disorder whose exact incidence and pathophysiology are unknown

- Mean age at presentation is 35 years with approximately 85% of patients having associated pelvic endometriosis
- Symptoms develop 1–2 days after the start of menstruation and approximately 90% of cases (for unknown reasons) involve the right lung
- Diagnosis is usually made clinically but has been made from TTNA, BAL, pleural fluid analysis or surgery

Clinical Presentations

1. **Catamenial pneumothorax**
   - Responsible for the majority of cases (approximately 70%)
   - Patients present with dyspnea and/or chest pains temporally related to menstrual periods with recurrent pneumothoraces documented during menstruation
   - First episodes of pneumothoraces are most often described in women >30 years
   - Vast majority of pneumothoraces are right-sided, the remainder being left-sided or bilateral
   - Surgical examination of the pleura reveals endometrial implants in a small percentage of cases, with subpleural cysts, diaphragmatic defects or no abnormalities described in the majority
2. **Catamenial hemothorax**
   - Majority of surgical cases reveal pleural endometrial deposits
   - Hemothorax varies in size and may be accompanied by a pneumothorax
3. **Catamenial hemoptysis**
4. **Lung nodule**

CHORIOCARCINOMA – GESTATIONAL

Clinically, gestational choriocarcinoma usually follows within 6 months of a hydatidiform mole and rarely occurs post-abortion or following a normal pregnancy and pulmonary manifestations are

1 Asymptomatic radiologic finding
2 Non-specific respiratory symptoms of cough, dyspnea, hemoptysis, pleuritic pain
3 Pulmonary hypertension secondary to tumor emboli
4 Respiratory failure

- Spread is hematogenous with the lungs the most common site of metastases (~80%), followed by the vagina, pelvis, liver and brain
- Hypoxemia is common and secondary to shunting through highly vascular lesions
- Pleural effusions are usually bloody and can result in a hemothorax
- Diagnosis is established by elevated plasma β human chorionic gonadotrophin levels often exceeding 100 000 IU/L

Radiologic features

1 **Parenchymal disease**
   - *Single or multipe nodules, including 'canonball' lesions
   - *Diffuse miliary pattern
   - Residual "fibrotic" nodules post treatment
   - Normal X-ray (with tumor emboli)

2 **Pleura**
   - Malignant pleural effusions

3 **Vasculature**
   - Tumor emboli and secondary pulmonary infarction, simulating thromboembolism

OVARIAN CANCER

Intrathoracic metastases commonly occur with concurrent pelvic, peritoneal or liver metastases but rarely alone

Pleura

- *Malignant pleural effusion (most common intrathoracic manifestation)
- Pleural mass(es)

Parenchyma

- Single or multiple nodules
- Lymphangitic spread (uncommon)

Airways

- Endobronchial metastases (rare)

Mediastinum

- Lymphadenopathy

Vasculature

- Pulmonary emboli secondary to a hypercoagulable state
- Tumor emboli

TESTICULAR TUMORS

- **Seminomatous** tumors grow more slowly with local invasion prior to distant metastases, spread being via the lymphatic system
  - Localized testicular disease or minimal retroperitoneal node involvement makes pulmonary metastases unlikely but chest CT and serum markers, HCG and α-fetoprotein, should be obtained as non-seminomatous elements may be present
- **Non-seminomatous** tumors metastasize early to lung, with choriocarcinoma spreading hematogenously while the other cell types spread via the hematogenous and lymphatic pathways

Mediastinum

- *Lymphadenopathy (most common intrathoracic manifestation of seminoma)

Parenchyma

- *Solitary or multiple nodules, including ‘cannonballs’
- ‘Sarcoid-like’ granulomas
- BOOP secondary to bleomycin
- Alveolar hemorrhage from necrotic tumor, e.g. choriocarcinoma
- Lymphangitic pattern

Pleura
- Malignant pleural effusion
- Pleural mass

Airways
- Endobronchial metastases

PROSTATE CANCER

Pulmonary involvement typically occurs in association with other organ involvement, e.g. bones, and uncommonly as the sole metastatic site
- Serum prostate specific antigen (PSA) as well as immunohistochemical stains on lung biopsy for PSA and prostatic alkaline phosphatase can make the diagnosis
- Presentation varies from asymptomatic to non-specific respiratory symptoms, with radiologic manifestations as follows

Parenchyma
- Single or multiple nodules
- Lymphangitic carcinomatosis

Pleura
- Malignant effusions

Chest wall
- Osteolytic or osteoblastic metastases to the thoracic skeleton
- Extrapleural mass from rib metastases

Mediastinum
- Hilar or mediastinal lymphadenopathy

Airways
- Rarely endobronchial metastases
- Tracheobronchial compression (from mediastinal adenopathy)

Fraser R.S., Muller N.L., Colman N., Paré P.D. (1999) Diagnosis of Diseases of the Chest 4th Edn., WB Saunders.

Baum, G.L., Crapo, J.D., Celli, B.R., Karlinsky, J.B. (eds) (1997) *Textbook of Pulmonary Diseases*, 6th edn.: Lippincott-Raven.

Fishman, A.P., Elias, J.A., Fishman, J.A., Grippi, M.A., Kaiser, L.R., Senior, R.N. (1998) *Fishman's Pulmonary Diseases and Disorders*, 3rd edn.: McGraw-Hill.

Joseph, J., Sahw, S.A. (1996) Thoracic endometriosis syndrome. New observations from analysis of 110 cases. *Am J. Med*. 100: 164.

Elliot, D.L., Baker, A.F., Dixow, L.M. (1985) Catamenial hemoptysis. New methods of diagnosis and therapy. *Chest* 86: 687.

17 Bronchiectasis – Etiologic Investigations

Definition: Irreversible abnormal dilatation of the bronchial tree which may be local or generalized

- The classical **clinical triad** is that of
  1. Chronic cough/sputum
  2. Recurrent respiratory infections
  3. Recurrent episodes of hemoptysis
- Upper lobe 'dry bronchiectasis' is characterized by intermittent hemoptysis only
- Pulmonary complications include recurrent bronchitis or pneumonia, lung abscess, infected cyst with a new air–fluid level, empyema, hemoptysis, pneumothorax, cor pulmonale
- Extrathoracic manifestations include clubbing and, rarely, amyloid or a brain abscess
- Bronchiectasis is the end result of multiple pathologic processes with the following etiologies described in <50% of cases, the most common category being idiopathic

ETIOLOGY

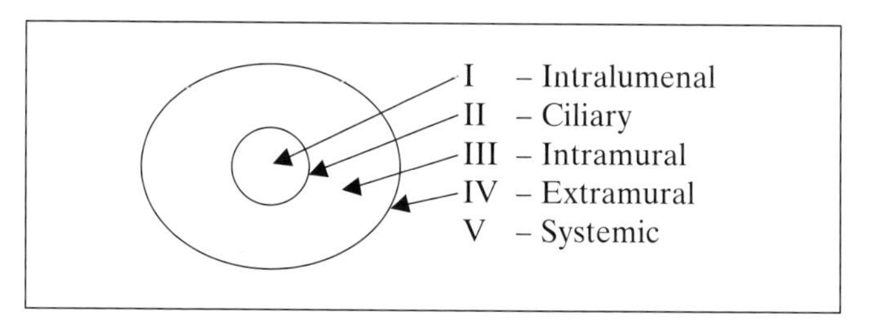

I – Intralumenal

1 **Allergic bronchopulmonary aspergillosis**
2 **Inhalation injury**, e.g. smoke, ammonia, sulfur dioxide
3 Recurrent **gastric aspiration**, most often in a dependent lung segment
4 **Post-obstructive** with localized airway narrowing – due to intralumenal (foreign body), intramural (endobronchial tumor) or extrabronchial disease (lymphadenopathy) and resultant focal disease
5 **Post-infectious** (important cause in countries with serious childhood infections)
   - Necrotizing bacterial infections, e.g. *Staph. aureus*, gram negatives, anaerobes, and whooping cough
   - Tuberculosis or atypical mycobacteria
   - Fungal, e.g. histoplasmosis
   - Viral, e.g. measles, adenovirus, HIV
   - Swyer-James syndrome
6 **Bronchiolitis**, e.g. diffuse panbronchiolitis, constrictive bronchiolitis
7 **Right middle lobe syndrome** – thought to result from remote infection of hilar nodes by tuberculosis or histoplasmosis with bronchial compression and recurrent pneumonia
   - As the lymphadenopathy resolves the right middle lobe bronchus becomes patent but non-obstructive atelectasis and bronchiectasis result

II – Ciliary Abnormalities

8 **Ciliary dyskinesia syndrome (CDS)** is a genetic disorder manifest by recurrent upper and lower respiratory infections usually beginning in childhood (although occasionally not apparent until the second or third decade) including rhinitis, otitis, sinusitis, bronchitis and bronchiectasis, as well as living but immobile spermatozoa
   - Ultrastructural defects are seen in cilia from a nasal or bronchial mucosal biopsy

- Male infertility and reduced female fertility occur as a consequence of dysmotility of the sperm tail and the oviduct cilia respectively

Kartagener's syndrome is a subset of the above and seen in ~50% of patients with CDS

- Autosomal recessive inheritance and characterized by the triad of sinusitis, bronchiectasis and situs inversus

Ciliary disorientation syndrome consists of recurrent otitis, chronic sinusitis, ± situs inversus

- There is normal structure and frequency of ciliary beating but the beating is incorrectly oriented

9 **Young's syndrome** is characterized by obstructive azoospermia due to involvement of the tail of the epididymis, bronchiectasis and sinusitis
   - There is a negative sweat chloride test and normal pancreatic function without dextrocardia, situs inversus or structural abnormality of cilia

III – Intramural

10 **Tracheobronchomalacia** (Williams-Campbell syndrome) is a form of familial congenital bronchiectasis characterized by cartilage deficiency in the 4th to 6th order bronchi, resulting in abnormal dilatation and ballooning of bronchi on inspiration and collapse with expiration as demonstrated on bronchography
   - Central areas of cystic bronchiectasis and peripheral lucencies (reflecting air trapping) are seen on CT
   - The cough mechanism becomes inefficient with retained secretions, recurrent pneumonia and bronchiectasis
   - Symptoms usually begin in infancy with the development of chronic cough, wheezing, clubbing, short stature and ~25% mortality by age 5 years

11 **Tracheobronchomegaly** (Mounier-Kuhn syndrome – see Tracheobronchial Disease, p. 766)

IV – Extramural

12 **Tracheo-esophageal** or **broncho-esophageal fistula**
13 **α_1-protease inhibitor deficiency** is characterized by emphysema but a minority of patients have co-existing bronchitis and bronchiectasis
14 **Bronchopulmonary sequestration**
15 **Interstitial fibrosis** and secondary traction bronchiectasis, e.g. UIP

V – Systemic Disorders

16 ***Cystic fibrosis** (most common cause in North America and Europe)
17 **Autoimmune disorders** including rheumatoid arthritis, Sjogren's syndrome, ankylosing spondylitis, relapsing polychondritis, systemic lupus, Marfan's syndrome
18 Associated with **ulcerative colitis**
19 **Yellow nail syndrome**
20 **Immunodeficiency states**
- Congenital/acquired immunoglobulin deficiencies including hypogammaglobulinemia, agammaglobulinemia, selective immunoglobulin deficiency
- Complement deficiencies
- WBC abnormalities including absolute leucopenia, qualitative dysfunction, T or B cell reductions

21 **Sarcoid** with bronchiectasis secondary to 'traction' from interstitial fibrosis or endobronchial involvement (which also results in bronchostenosis)
22 **Post-transplant**, e.g. bone marrow, lung

RADIOLOGY

1 **Chest X-rays** reveal the basal segments of lower lobes to be most commonly involved, with bilateral disease in 30–50%, the frequency of abnormalities correlating with the severity of disease
- Increased bronchovascular markings with loss of definition (peribronchial fibrosis/secretions)

- 'Tram lines' representing thickened dilated bronchi
- Volume loss of involved segment with compensatory hyperinflation of remaining lung
- Cystic spaces which may contain an air–fluid level or mycetoma
- 'Honeycomb' lung
- Tubular structures composed of mucus-filled bronchi

2 **Bronchographic** studies demonstrate remodeling of airways with
- Cylindrical bronchiectasis → uniform dilatations
- Varicose bronchiectasis → dilatations with an irregular contour
- Cystic bronchiectasis → dilated segments with pus-filled cavities

This previous radiologic gold standard is uncommonly used today, e.g. patients with recurrent hemoptysis and normal or equivocal findings on HRCT

3 **HRCT** has replaced bronchography as the diagnostic method of choice with one or more of the following radiologic signs, but is rarely able to distinguish the idiopathic variety from known secondary causes

Bronchial wall abnormalities
- Bronchial wall thickening, with visualization of bronchi within 1 cm of the lung periphery
- Bronchial dilatation, with the internal bronchial diameter greater than that of the accompanying pulmonary artery and manifest as:
  - 'Tramlines': cylindrically dilated bronchi visualized along their length
  - 'Signet ring': cylindrically dilated bronchi seen in cross section and accompanied by a branch of the pulmonary artery
  - 'String of cysts': sectioning bronchi that are irregularly dilated along their length

  - 'Cluster of cysts': multiple dilated bronchi lying adjacent to each other in atelectatic lung
- Lack of peripheral tapering

Bronchial content abnormalities
- Air: cystic/cavitary disease, honeycombing
- Fluid: air–fluid level
- Fungus: mycetoma
- Mucus-filled
  - Linear (gloved finger) or tubular opacities
  - Branching 'V' or 'Y' opacities
  - Multiple nodules (cluster of grapes)
  - Solitary nodule or mass-like lesion (mucocele)

Associated abnormalities
- Atelectasis, e.g. RML syndrome
- Findings of bronchiolitis (see p. 101)
- Mediastinal/hilar lymphadenopathy (uncommon)

4 **Associated radiologic abnormalities**
- *Airways disease*
  - Narrowing or obliteration of the bronchial lumen proximal to the area of bronchiectasis, secondary to an intralumenal (e.g. foreign body) endobronchial (e.g. neoplasm) or extramural lesion (e.g. mass, lymphadenopathy, mediastinitis)
  - Proximal airway calcifications which can be intralumenal (e.g. broncholith, foreign body) or extramural (e.g. calcified nodes compressing an airway)
  - Tracheobronchomegaly
  - Diffuse endotracheal and endobronchial lesions, e.g. laryngeal papillomatosis, tracheobronchopathia osteochondroplastica
- *Parenchymal disease*
  - Emphysema with α_1-antitrypsin deficiency
  - Centrilobular nodules and branching linear opacities in bronchiolitis
  - Parenchymal nodules in laryngeal papillomatosis

- *Pleural disease*
  - Effusion in yellow nail syndrome
- *Mediastinal disease*
  - Dextrocardia in Kartagener's Syndrome
  - Associated esophageal disease e.g. fistula, obstruction, documented aspiration
- *Vascular disease*
  - Anomalous feeding artery in bronchopulmonary sequestration
  - Diminutive main pulmonary artery and oligemia in Swyer-James

DIAGNOSTIC CLUES AND WORK-UP

1 History of
   - Remote lung infection, e.g. measles, whooping cough, bacterial pneumonia, TB, fungal
   - Associated extrapulmonary infections to suggest an underlying immunologic disorder, e.g. γ-globulin abnormality
   - Toxic inhalation
   - Acute foreign body aspiration, recurrent aspiration or mineral oil use
   - Congenital or familial disease, e.g. CF, BPS, Williams-Campbell, ciliary dyskinesia, α_1-antiprotease deficiency, hypogammaglobulinemia
   - Male infertility, e.g. Young's syndrome
   - Asthma, e.g. ABPA
2 Evidence of systemic disease, e.g. cystic fibrosis, yellow nail syndrome, collagen vascular disease, immunodeficiency state with multisystem infections
3 Associated chest X-ray or CT scan findings to diagnose
   - Endobronchial obstruction
   - Extrinsic narrowing

- BPS
- Mounier-Kuhn
- Emphysema
- Situs inversus

4 Blood tests
- Serum protein electrophoresis with immunoglobulin quantification
- WBC and differential
- Absolute eosinophil count
- Precipitins and IgE to aspergillus
- Serum complement, RF, ANA
- α_1-protease inhibitor quantification
- HIV serology

5 Sputum for tuberculosis, atypical mycobacteria, fungi, bacteriology
6 Sweat chloride
7 Bronchoscopy
- If localized disease is suspected and obstruction must be ruled out
- Bronchial biopsy with electron microscopic assessment of ciliary morphology

8 Nasal biopsy for ciliary morphology
9 PFTs
10 ABGs

Fraser R.S., Muller N.L., Colman N., Paré P.D. (1999) Diagnosis of Diseases of the Chest 4th Edn., WB Saunders.

Naidich, D.P., Zerhouni, E.A., Siegelman, S.S. *Computed Tomography and Magnetic Resonance of the Thorax*, 2nd edn. New York: Raven Press.

Moss, A., Gamsu, Genant (1992) Thorax and neck. In: *Computed Tomography of the Body with Magnetic Resonance Imaging*, 2nd edn, vol. 1.: W.B. Saunders.

Baum, G.L., Crapo, J.D., Celli, B.R., Karlinsky, J.B. (eds) (1997) *Textbook of Pulmonary Diseases*, 6th edn.: Lippincott-Raven.

Fishman, A.P., Elias, J.A., Fishman, J.A., Grippi, M.A., Kaiser, L.R.,

Senior, R.N. (1998) *Fishman's Pulmonary Diseases and Disorders*, 3rd edn.: McGraw-Hill.
Hansell, D. (1998) Bronchiectasis. *Radiol. Clin. North Am.* **36**: 107–128.

18 Bronchiolitis – Diagnosis and Differential

CLASSIFICATION AND DIAGNOSTIC FEATURES

A	Acute bronchiolitis
B	BOOP, primary or secondary
C	Chronic bronchiolitis
C	Cigarette-induced respiratory bronchiolitis
C	Constrictive bronchiolitis (= bronchiolitis obliterans), primary or secondary
D	Diffuse panbronchiolitis
E	Extrabronchiolar disease primarily, associated with bronchiolocentric infiltrates
F	Follicular bronchiolitis

Clinically, bronchiolitis presents with non-specific respiratory symptoms of cough and dyspnea which can progress to cyanosis and respiratory failure

- Some forms of bronchiolitis present acutely, e.g. smoke inhalation, whereas others present over years, e.g. diffuse panbronchiolitis
- Physical findings include hyperinflation as well as a combination of bilateral wheezes, rales and inspiratory 'squeaks'
- Multiple etiologies can result in similar pathology in addition to a given pathology, e.g. acute bronchiolitis, progressing to another, e.g. bronchiolitis obliterans

The **chest X-ray** findings depend upon the underlying etiology and pathology, but are non-pathognomonic and must be interpreted in the clinical context

- Normal to hyperinflated lungs
- Bronchial wall thickening
- Bilateral small nodules
- Diffuse interstitial disease
- Peripheral patchy airspace consolidation (BOOP)

HRCT findings – direct or indirect

- *Centrilobular nodular densities with characteristic V and Y-shaped configuration, reflecting inflammatory cells in the bronchiolar walls as well as mucus and exudate in the airways – typical of acute bronchiolitis (direct)
- *Mosaic perfusion with low attenuation areas (secondary to bronchiolar obstruction and air trapping) and redistribution of perfusion to normal areas of lung
- 'Tree-in-bud' pattern reflecting bronchiolar distension, mucus plugs and peribronchiolar inflammation
- Bronchiolectasis i.e. dilated airways in the secondary lobules (direct)
- *'Ground glass' opacities and consolidation – seen with BOOP (direct)
- Signs of bronchiectasis

Diagnosis

Bronchiolitis should be suspected in a patient presenting with dyspnea, cough and hypoxemia in the absence of known obstructive lung disease

plus

1 Combination of diffuse rales and wheezes on auscultation

plus

2 Normal chest X-ray or chest X-ray/HRCT abnormalities as above

plus

3 Restrictive or obstructive abnormalities on PFTs

plus

4 Predisposing conditions as listed below

ACUTE BRONCHIOLITIS

Pathologically, there is acute (but also chronic) cellular inflammation primarily involving the terminal and respiratory bronchioles with an intralumenal exudate

Etiologies include

- Acute infections, e.g. viral, mycoplasma, chlamydia, hemophilus, legionella
- Inhalation injuries, e.g. toxic fumes, smoke, cocaine, gases

Clinically, acute bronchiolitis may develop within hours, e.g. smoke inhalation, or days, e.g. mycoplasma and may be accompanied by

- Inflammation of the larger airways with signs of diffuse bronchospasm
- Pulmonary edema, e.g. smoke inhalation
- Clinical and radiologic features of pneumonia

Obstruction and hyperinflation on PFTs is typical with the sequelae of acute bronchiolitis including
1 Resolution
2 BOOP
3 Bonchiolitis obliterans
4 Swyer-James syndrome (post-viral)
5 ? Asthma following childhood viral bronchiolitis

Chest X-ray findings
1 Normal films
2 Hyperinflation
3 Bilateral small nodular shadows
4 Heavy bronchovascular markings with a reticulonodular pattern

HRCT findings
1 Centrilobular nodules and centrilobular branching linear structures
2 Pattern of mosaic alternation with air trapping on an expiratory CT
3 Associated findings may be present, e.g. focal areas of consolidation with pneumonia

BRONCHIOLITIS OBLITERANS ORGANIZING PNEUMONIA (BOOP) – IDIOPATHIC

(Cryptogenic Organizing Pneumonia)

A clinicopathologic syndrome occurring mainly in patients between 40 and 70 years of age, with equal frequency in males/females, and unrelated to smoking

Pathologically, there are polypoid masses of new granulation tissue within the lumina of bronchioles and alveolar ducts extending into the alveolar spaces, as well as a mixed interstitial cellular infiltrate

Clinically, it typically presents subacutely with a few weeks to months history of a flu-like illness including fever, weight loss and non-specific respiratory symptoms, especially cough and dyspnea

- Hemoptysis, bronchorrhea and chest pains are uncommon
- Physical exam is normal or may reveal rales
- Often misdiagnosed as pneumonia and referred for consultation due to lack of antibiotic response
- Symptoms may develop as patients are weaned off steroids which have been used to treat an unrelated disorder
- Rare manifestations include
  - Acute onset
  - Asymptomatic patient with an abnormal chest X-ray
  - Co-existence with chronic eosinophilic pneumonia
  - Fulminating and life threatening form presenting with an ARDS picture
    - Usually in current or former smokers, presenting over days to weeks
    - Physical exam (rales are frequent), laboratory tests and BAL are non-pathognomonic
    - Prognosis is poor with biopsies revealing a combination of BOOP, diffuse alveolar damage, honeycombing

Clinical course of the disease includes

- Good response to steroids within days to weeks in the typical or classic BOOP
- Relapses occur when prednisone dose is <10 mg daily and another diagnosis should be considered when disease worsens at doses >20 mg daily
- Spontaneous resolution
- Progressive disease and respiratory failure in approximately 10% of patients; seen mainly in the interstitial presentation with progression to honeycombing, similar to idiopathic pulmonary fibrosis

Chest X-ray findings include 4 distinct patterns (1–4)

1. Classic or typical pattern is bilateral patchy airspace disease
   - May be migratory with one opacity improving or disappearing while another appears

- Opacities vary in size from a few cm to an entire lobe and air bronchograms are common
- Peripheral distribution of airspace disease which resembles chronic eosinophilic pneumonia clinically and radiologically
- Differential diagnosis includes infections, alveolar cell cancer, lymphoma, chronic eosinophilic pneumonia, alveolar hemorrhage, alveolar proteinosis

2 Solitary focus of airspace disease
- Clinical suspicion is often that of malignancy resulting in a biopsy or resection
- Often upper lobe in location

3 Diffuse bilateral interstitial pattern
- Pattern varies from reticular to nodular
- Differential diagnosis is extensive, including UIP

4 Multiple large nodules or masses

5 Rarely pleural effusion, cavitation

HRCT findings

1 Unilateral or bilateral airspace consolidation or 'ground glass' opacities, often subpleural or peribronchovascular in distribution
- Air bronchograms are common

2 Small nodular opacities often peribronchiolar in location

3 Bronchial wall thickening in abnormal areas

4 Honeycombing is absent initially

5 Cavitary mass or nodule rarely occurs

6 Subpleural bands are common in the healing phase (similar to eosinophilic pneumonia)

PFTs reveal a restrictive picture with reduced lung volumes and diffusing capacity

- Airflow obstruction is absent except in smokers

The **diagnostic gold standard** is an open lung biopsy with the clinical and pathologic features distinguishing the primary from the secondary causes

- In a classic case the combination of clinical and radiologic findings ± transbronchial biopsy would be adequate to institute a steroid trial

- Atypical cases require thoracoscopic or open lung biopsy for confirmation

When the diagnosis of BOOP is made, **secondary BOOP** should be ruled out as it can be caused by a wide variety of disorders including

1. Aspiration
2. Inhalation
3. Infections – bacterial, mycoplasma, viral, fungal, parasitic
4. Drugs, e.g. bleomycin, amiodarone, cocaine, others
5. Post-transplant, especially bone marrow and lung
6. Collagen diseases, e.g. polymyositis, RA, dermatomyositis
7. Organizing ARDS
8. Hypersensitivity pneumonitis
9. Organizing eosinophilic pneumonia
10. Diffuse panbronchiolitis
11. Post-radiation for breast cancer
    - Seen a few weeks to about one year following radiotherapy
    - Clinically and radiologically it is similar to idiopathic BOOP
    - Parenchymal infiltrates involve areas of lung both within as well as outside the radiation ports
12. Others

CHRONIC BRONCHIOLITIS

Pathologically, there is chronic inflammation, fibrosis +/– increased smooth muscle with etiologies including

1. Inhalation, e.g. cigarettes, grain dust, silica, asbestos, allergic alveolitis
2. Bronchiectasis, COPD
3. Gastric aspiration
4. Connective tissue diseases, e.g. RA, Sjogren's
5. Post-lung transplant
6. Idiopathic

PFTs are obstructive with normal chest X-ray or reticulo-nodular opacities and normal CT or centrilobular nodules

CIGARETTE-RELATED RESPIRATORY BRONCHIOLITIS – INTERSTITIAL LUNG DISEASE – RBILD (see ILD p. 429)

Respiratory bronchiolitis is the earliest lesion seen in cigarette smokers, typically when patients are young and asymptomatic, with pigmented macrophages in membranous and respiratory bronchioles

An exaggerated form of this bronchiolitis, RBILD, is characterized by pigmented macrophages in bronchioles and adjacent alveolar spaces as well as mild bronchiolar and peribronchiolar inflammation or fibrosis (thought to be an early stage of DIP)

Clinical manifestations include

- Cough, sputum and dyspnea in young smokers
- Bibasilar rales (*vs.* wheezes) on auscultation in the absence of clubbing

Restrictive picture or mixed restrictive and obstructive disease on PFTs

Routine lab studies are non-specific

Radiologic features

1 Normal chest X-ray
2 'Dirty chest' with increased fine reticulonodular interstitial markings diffusely
3 Bronchial wall thickening, 'ground glass' opacities, centrilobular nodules on HRCT

Important to distinguish from other forms of interstitial lung disease as there is an excellent prognosis with resolution on stopping smoking

CONSTRICTIVE BRONCHIOLITIS (BRONCHIOLITIS OBLITERANS)

Pathologically, characterized by submucosal and peribronchiolar fibrosis of the membranous and respiratory bronchioles, little or no inflammation, with subsequent concentric bronchiolar lumenal narrowing

Clinically, this is a disease of the small airways producing a rapidly progressive form of obstructive lung disease

- Patients present with cough and dyspnea that progresses rapidly over a period of months to years
- May be seen under age 40, in non-smokers, or those with <20 pack/year smoking history
- Rales and wheezes are uncommon on physical exam with variable degrees of hypoxemia and hypercapnia on arterial blood gas
- The clinical severity of disease is reflected in the proportion of bronchioles involved and the degree of narrowing

PFTS typically show progressive airways obstruction, but may reveal restriction or combined obstruction and restriction

Definitive diagnosis requires open lung biopsy, with some cases primary or idiopathic, but known causes include

1 *Inhalation of toxic fumes, e.g. ammonia, sulfur dioxide, oxides of nitrogen, smoke inhalation
2 *Post-infectious – viral, mycoplasma, Swyer-James syndrome
3 *Post-transplant – heart, heart-lung, bone marrow
4 *Collagen diseases, especially rheumatoid arthritis but also SLE, scleroderma, Sjogren's syndrome
5 GI disorders including GE reflux, charcoal aspiration, primary biliary cirrhosis
6 Drugs, e.g. penicillamine, gold
7 A component of other pulmonary diseases including healed ARDS, chronic bronchitis, bronchiectasis, chronic asthma, cystic fibrosis, chronic hypersensitivity pneumonitis
8 Diffuse panbronchiolitis
9 Associated with neuroendocrine cell hyperplasia

Chest X-rays may be normal but usually reveal hyperinflation with or without interstitial infiltrates which are nodular or reticulonodular, reflecting perbronchiolar inflammation and fibrosis

HRCT reveals areas of decreased attenuation either geographic or with ill-defined margins which are large, polylobular, and accentuated on expiratory CT due to gas trapping (occasionally the inspiratory HRCT may be completely normal)

- The pattern of mosaic perfusion is due to areas of gas trapping with resultant reduced perfusion and low attenuation, *vs.* the normal residual lung which has the redistributed blood supply and therefore has relatively higher attenuation
- Thickening and dilatation of the larger (segmental and subsegmental) airways, i.e. bronchiectatic, as well as bronchioles are common
- Centrilobular nodules or branching linear structures may also be present ('tree-in-bud')

Diagnosis of constrictive bronchiolitis should be suspected with

1. Young patient presenting with progressive dyspnea
2. Absent or modest smoking history
3. Deteriorating PFTs with severe airflow obstruction not attributable to other causes (see intrathoracic airways obstruction on PFTs – p. 168)
4. Hyperinflation ± increased interstitial markings on chest X-ray

DIFFUSE PANBRONCHIOLITIS (DPB)

Pathologically characterized by intraluminal and peribronchiolar inflammation with lymphoid hyperplasia as well as foamy macrophages – may be accompanied by intraluminal neutrophils and plugs of organizing pneumonia

Clinically, this is a sinobronchial syndrome of unknown etiology, usually in Japanese patients, occasionally in Chinese and Koreans, but rare in Western countries

- The majority of patients are non-smokers and present with a several year history of sinusitis, beginning in the second or third decade, followed by chronic cough, mucopurulent sputum, dyspnea and recurrent respiratory tract infections while physical exam reveals rales, wheezes and rhonchi
- Colonization with *P. aeruginosa* accelerates the downhill course
- Diffuse panbronchiolitis is a chronic and progressive disease where hypoxemia is followed by hypercapnia and cor pulmonale
- The 5-year survival is <50% and 10-year survival approximately 25%, although some patients respond clinically to erythromycin

The process of bronchiolitis eventually results in narrowing and constriction of the respiratory bronchioles, with PFTs showing a marked obstructive picture, but may be accompanied by a restrictive component

Labs often show persistent elevation of polyclonal cold agglutinins in the absence of antibody to mycoplasma and may reveal HLA-B54 antigen, positive rheumatoid factor

Chest X-rays typically reveal hyperinflation with nodular shadows <2 mm in diameter, mainly in the lower lobes

- Signs of bronchiectasis are often present

Sinus X-rays reveal sinusitis

HRCT findings

1. Mosaic perfusion pattern
2. Centrilobular nodules and branching linear opacities ("tree in bud")
3. Dilated small bronchi and bronchioles
4. Bronchiectasis

EXTRABRONCHIOLAR DISEASE WITH BRONCHIOLOCENTRIC INFILTRATES

Definition: These are disorders where **bronchiolitis** is seen on pathology but is only part of a more extensive disease process, etiologies including

1 Allergic alveolitis
2 Asbestosis
3 Silicosis
4 Giant cell interstitial pneumonia
5 Eosinophilic granuloma
6 Sarcoid

- The clinical and exposure history as well as the radiologic findings, including expiratory HRCT, should strongly suggest the above diagnoses

FOLLICULAR BRONCHIOLITIS

Definition: Classified as a benign lymphoproliferative disorder of the lung and defined as lymphoid hyperplasia of the bronchus-associated lymphoid tissue

- Characterized histologically by polyclonal hyperplastic lymphoid follicles with reactive germinal centers often accompanied by compression of the bronchiolar lumen which may contain an inflammatory exudate
- The mononuclear cell infiltrate is mainly peribronchiolar and peribronchial but can be mistaken for and merges with LIP, where the inflammatory infiltrate is more diffuse

Etiologies include

1 Chronic inflammatory diseases of the large airways, e.g. bronchiectasis, cystic fibrosis
2 Collagen diseases, e.g. rheumatoid arthritis, Sjogren's syndrome
3 Congenital or acquired immunodeficiency states, e.g. HIV
4 Hypersensitivity reactions

- Patients usually present with progressive dyspnea while X-ray findings characteristically are those of diffuse reticulonodular disease
- CT findings are those of nodular infiltrates (usually small but can be up to 1 cm or more) peribronchial, centrilobular or subpleural in location, occasionally associated with 'ground glass' opacities

Fraser R.S., Muller N.L., Colman N., Paré P.D. (1999) Diagnosis of Diseases of the Chest 4th Edn., WB Saunders.

Naidich, D.P., Zerhouni, E.A., Siegelman, S.S. (1998) *Computed Tomography and Magnetic Resonance of the Thorax*, 2nd edn. New York: Raven Press.

Moss, A., Gamsu, Genant (1992) Thorax and neck. In: *Computed Tomography of the Body with Magnetic Resonance Imaging*, 2nd edn, vol. 1. (Place of publication): W.B. Saunders.

Fishman, A.P., Elias, J.A., Fishman, J.A., Grippi, M.A., Kaiser, L.R., Senior, R.N. (1998) *Fishman's Pulmonary Diseases and Disorders*, 3rd edn.: McGraw-Hill.

Muller, N.L., Staples, C., Miller, R. (1990) Bronchiolitis obliterans organizing pneumonia: CT features in 14 patients. *Am. J. Roent.* **154**: 983–987.

Epler, G.R., Colby, T., McLoud, T. *et al.* (1985) Bronchiolitis obliterans organizing pneumonia. *NEJM* **312**: 152–158.

Wortly, S., Muller, N. (1998) Small airway diseases. *Radiol. Clin. North Am.* **36**: 163–173.

Lynch, D. (1993) Imaging of small airways diseases. *Clinics in Chest Medicine* **14**: 623–634.

Cordier, J.F. (1993) Cryptogenic organizing pneumonitis. Bronchiolitis obliterans organizing pneumonia. *Clinics in Chest Medicine* **14**: 677–692.

Nizami, I., Kissner, D., Visscherd, D. *et al.* (1998) Idiopathic BOOP: an acute and life-threatening syndrome. *Chest* **108**: 271–277.

Padley, S.P., Adler, B.D., Hansell, D.M. *et al.* (1993) Bronchiolitis obliterans: high resolution CT findings and correlation with pulmonary function tests. *Clinical Radiol.* **47**: 236–240.

Aguayo, S.M., Miller, Y.E., Waldron, J.A. *et al.* (1992) Brief report: idiopathic diffuse hyperplasia of pulmonary neuroendocrine cells and airways disease. *NEJM* **327**: 1285–1288.

Kraft, M., Mortenson, R.L., Colby, T.V. *et al.* (1993) Cryptogenic constrictive bronchiolitis – a clinicopathologic study. *Am. Rev. Resp. Dis.* **148**: 1093–1101.

Howling, S.J., Hansell, D.M., Wells, A.U. *et al.* (1999) Follicular bronchiolitis: thin-section CT and histologic findings. *Radiology* **212**: 637–642.

19 Broncholithiasis

Definition: Calcified or ossified material in the tracheobronchial lumen

Etiologies include

1. *Granulomatous lymphadenitis, most often due to histoplasmosis (supported by the presence of splenic calcifications) or TB with extension of calcified necrotic material through the tracheobronchial wall
   - Other fungi and silicosis are rarely described
2. Aspirated foreign body which has impacted into the airway mucosa +/– *in situ* calcifications
3. Mucosal erosion and extrusion of calcified cartilage from the tracheobronchial tree into the lumen
4. Calcification/ossification of an endobronchial carcinoid
5. Calcification of a bronchocele in ABPA
6. Nephrobronchial fistula
7. Extension from a pleural plaque

Clinical presentations

- Lithoptysis is pathognomonic (<20% of patients)
- Respiratory symptoms of cough, localized wheezing, dyspnea and hemoptysis
- Obstructive pneumonitis
- Bronchiectasis
- Tracheal obstruction
- Broncho-esophageal fistula
- Asymptomatic finding when bronchoscopy or X-rays are performed for an unrelated reason
- Broncho-arterial fistula to a pulmonary artery and life-threatening hemoptysis

Radiologic manifestations

1 *Change in position or disappearance of a calcific focus on sequential films
2 *Findings of airways obstruction (predilection for the right bronchial tree)
   - Obstructive pneumonitis
   - Bronchiectasis
   - Atelectasis
   - Mucoid impaction
   - Localized expiratory air trapping
3 Focal hilar/parenchymal calcifications suggesting old granulomatous disease
4 Normal chest X-ray
5 *HRCT demonstration of focal calcification at the origin of an area of atelectasis is pathognomonic

Diagnostic features

1 *Lithoptysis
2 *Radiologic findings as above
3 *Bronchoscopic identification of endobronchial broncholiths
4 Hilar/carinal calcifications presenting with the other clinical or radiologic features of broncholithiasis, in association with distortion of the bronchial tree on bronchoscopy is suggestive
5 May resemble the localized form of granulomatous/fibrosing mediastinitis, particularly when there is predominant or exclusive hilar involvement

Fraser R.S., Muller N.L., Colman N., Paré P.D. (1999) Diagnosis of Diseases of the Chest 4th Edn., WB Saunders.
Naidich, D.P., Zerhouni, E.A., Siegelman, S.S. (1998) *Computed Tomography and Magnetic Resonance of the Thorax*, 3rd edn. New York: Raven Press.
Fishman, A.P., Elias, J.A., Fishman, J.A., Grippi, M.A., Kaiser,

L.R., Senior, R.N. (1998) *Fishman's Pulmonary Diseases and Disorders*, 3rd edn.: McGraw-Hill.

Conces, D.J. (1991) Broncholithiasis. CT features in 15 patients. *Am. J. Radiol.* **157**: 249–253.

20 Bronchopulmonary Sequestration (BPS)

Definition: A congenital abnormality where a portion of lung is detached from the tracheobronchial tree and receives its blood supply from a systemic artery

	Intralobar	Extralobar
Occurrence	6×	1×
Male : female	1.5 : 1	4 : 1
Age at diagnosis	>20 years	<1 year
Location	$^2/_3$ in LLL, $^1/_3$ in RLL • Involved lobe is contiguous to normal lung parenchyma and within the same visceral pleural envelope • Disordered mass of lung tissue isolated from the normal bronchial tree (before infection)	90% relate to left hemidiaphragm • Involved lobe is within its own pleural envelope, above, below or within the diaphragm, or mediastinal in location
Arterial supply	Descending thoracic aorta or its branches	Abdominal aorta or its branches, with a single vessel or multiple small vessels responsible
Venous drainage	Pulmonary veins, rarely systemic	Systemic and usually the azygous system
Diaphragmatic abnormalities	Occasional	60% – paralysis, hernias
Associated congenital defects	Rare	>50% of cases, including heart disease, pericardial cysts, frequent malformations
Clinically	Often asymptomatic until acute or recurrent pneumonia develops in adulthood • Infections are usually pyogenic although TB and mycotic infections are reported	Presents with respiratory distress, infections being less common

	Intralobar	Extralobar
	• May rupture into the pleural space or esophagus • Massive hemoptysis, complicating carcinoma and aspergilloma are reported	
Chest X-ray	Reflects the volume of lung sequestered as well as the presence or absence of infection • Prior to infection and communication with the bronchial tree 1 Homogenous lobulated soft tissue mass 2 Bronchovascular bundles of normal lung are festooned around the sequestered lobe • Post-infection there are single/multiple cysts which may contain air–fluid levels • Anomalous artery (or arteries) from the aorta or its branches • May communicate with the upper GI tract on barium swallow (should be R/O) • Complicating aspergilloma (rare) • Carcinoma within the sequestration (rare) • Anomalous systemic feeding vessel may occasionally be seen without aortography	Homogenous soft tissue mass is most common • Infection and communication with the bronchial tree are uncommon
CT/MRI	• Soft tissue/cystic masses • Anomalous vessel	

Table 20.1

Differential diagnosis of the solid or cystic mass of BPS includes

1 **Bronchiectasis**
2 **Bronchogenic cyst**

3 **Lung abscess**
4 **Bochdalek hernia**
5 **Pulmonary, metastatic or mediastinal neoplasm**
6 **Pneumonia**
7 **Atelectasis**
8 **Pneumatocele**
9 **Congenital adenomatoid malformation**
- An intralobar mass of disorganized lung tissue,? hamartomatous, and characterized by overgrowth of bronchioles
- Lesions are often cystic although may be solid and often communicate with the bronchial tree
- Presentation is usually in infancy and rarely reported in adulthood
- Radiologically presents as a mass with several air-containing cysts
- An anomalous systemic blood supply is rarely reported

10 **Pseudosequestration**
- Acquired abnormality characterized by systemic arterialization of lung tissue due to neovascularization caused by inflammation – usually organizing pneumonia or bronchiectasis
- Bronchial arteries are most common but the intercostals, esophageal and subdiaphragmatic vessels may be responsible
- A similar radiologic picture can be seen with diaphragmatic defects where abdominal contents, e.g. herniated liver, are present in the hemithorax and supplied by a systemic vessel

Fraser R.S., Muller N.L., Colman N., Paré P.D. (1999) Diagnosis of Diseases of the Chest 4th Edn., WB Saunders.

Naidich, D.P., Zerhouni, E.A., Siegelman, S.S. (1998) *Computed Tomography and Magnetic Resonance of the Thorax*, 3rd edn. New York: Raven Press.

Webb, R., Muller, N.L., Naidich, D.P. (1996) *High Resolution CT of the Lung*. 2nd edn.: Lippincott-Raven.

Baum, G.L., Crapo, J.D., Celli, B.R., Karlinsky, J.B. (eds) (1997) *Textbook of Pulmonary Diseases*, 6th edn.: Lippincott-Raven.

Fishman, A.P., Elias, J.A., Fishman, J.A., Grippi, M.A., Kaiser, L.R., Senior, R.N. (1998) *Fishman's Pulmonary Diseases and Disorders*, 3rd edn.: McGraw-Hill.

21 Calcifications

Parenchymal Calcifications – Benign Lung Nodule

1 Homogeneous, e.g. granuloma
2 Central nidus, e.g. granuloma
3 Laminar or target ring, e.g. histoplasmoma
4 'Popcorn', e.g. hamartoma
5 Multiple punctate foci, e.g. granuloma, hamartoma

Parenchymal Calcifications – Focal

1 Remote infection e.g. preumonia, cavitary disease, granulomas (tuberculosis, histoplasmosis)
2 Hamartoma
3 Metastatic disease, e.g. osteogenic sarcoma, chondrosarcoma, carcinoid, thyroid papillary carcinoma, cystadenocarcinoma of ovary, mucinous adenocarcinoma of breast or colon
4 Primary peripheral adeno- or squamous carcinoma (rare)
5 Amyloid

Parenchymal Calcifications – Diffuse

1 **Alveolar microlithiasis**
   - Rare disorder of unknown etiology, mainly in patients between 30–50, characterized by the accumulation of tiny calculi (calcium phosphate) in the alveolar airspaces, with interstitial fibrosis and apical bullae developing later in the course of disease
   - 50% of reported cases are familial
   - Majority of patients are asymptomatic, even with diffusely abnormal X-rays, although disease progression can result in respiratory insufficiency and cor pulmonale

Radiologic findings

a. Diffuse sand-like micronodulation, with sharply defined individual opacities <1 mm in diameter; the opacities can become confluent with a uniformly white lung field, but magnification reveals the discrete calcific densities
b. 'Black' pleural line between the ribs on one side and calcified subpleural parenchyma on the other
c. 'Lucent' mediastinum when compared to the lung density
d. Spontaneous pneumothorax from the rupture of apical bullae

Diagnostic features

a. Disease in siblings
b. Marked dissociation between symptoms and radiologic findings
c. Pathognomonic radiology
d. Recovery of microliths from sputum, BAL or transbronchial Bx
e. Open lung biopsy rarely needed

2 **Calcinosis**
- Typically seen in hypercalcemic patients, e.g. renal failure with secondary or tertiary hyperparathyroidism, multiple myeloma
- The clinical manifestations vary from asymptomatic to acute respiratory failure
- Chest X-rays most often show poorly-defined nodular opacities but range from normal (see only at pathology) to dense alveolar infiltrates resembling pneumonia or pulmonary edema, with upper lobe predominance
- Diagnosis is confirmed on CT scan as well as on bone scan which reveals pulmonary and other soft tissue uptake of the tracer

3 **Remote infections**
- Histoplasmosis, miliary tuberculosis, varicella

4 **Silicosis**

5 **Lymphoma – post-radiotherapy**

6 **Ossifications**
   - Mitral stenosis
   - Metastatic bone tumor
   - Idiopathic pulmonary fibrosis
7 **Amyloid**

Calcified Lymphadenopathy

1 Granulomas, e.g. tuberculosis, histoplasmosis
2 Sarcoid
3 Silicosis
4 CWP
5 Hodgkin's Disease (post-radiotherapy or chemotherapy)
6 Metastatic cancer, e.g. colonic adenocarcinoma, osteogenic sarcoma
7 Pneumocystis, especially on pentamidine treatment
8 Amyloid

Calcified Pleura

1 Remote hemothorax, pyothorax, tuberculosis
2 Asbestos exposure
3 Calcified fibrous pseudotumor

Calcified Tracheobronchial Tree

1 Aging
2 Tracheobronchopathia osteochondroplastica
3 Relapsing polychondritis

Calcified Vasculature

1 Pulmonary arteries in pulmonary hypertension
2 Mitral stenosis
3 Aortic calcifications

Fraser R.S., Muller N.L., Colman N., Paré P.D. (1999) Diagnosis of Diseases of the Chest 4th Edn., WB Saunders.
Naidich, D.P., Zerhouni, E.A., Siegelman, S.S. (1998) *Computed Tomography and Magnetic Resonance of the Thorax*, 3rd edn. New York: Raven Press.

22 Cardiac Diseases – Pulmonary Manifestations

MITRAL STENOSIS

Clinical presentations

1 Recurrent pulmonary edema
2 Recurrent bronchitis and pneumonia
3 Episodic hemoptysis secondary to bronchial varicosities
   - Usually spotty, but hemoptysis can be massive and present as diffuse alveolar hemorrhage
4 Cor pulmonale, right heart failure and pulmonary emboli

Radiologic findings

1 Signs of pulmonary venous hypertension
   - Upper lobe pleonemia
   - Lower lobe oligemia
   - Interstitial pulmonary edema with Kerley A & B lines progressing to interstitial fibrosis
   - Diffuse nodularity, mainly lower lobes, from hemosiderin-laden macrophages in alveoli (hemosiderosis)
   - Parenchymal ossifications manifest as densely calcified 2–5 mm nodules
   - Pleural effusions
2 Enlarged left atrium
3 Signs of pulmonary artery hypertension

- Enlarged main and hilar pulmonary arteries with rapid tapering
- Cor pulmonale
- Pulmonary emboli complicating right heart failure

ATRIAL MASS – LEFT OR RIGHT-SIDED

Differential diagnosis of the mass includes

1. Benign neoplasms, e.g. myxoma
2. Malignant neoplasms, e.g. primary sarcoma, metastases
3. Thrombus
4. Vegetations
   - Infectious, e.g. bacterial, fungal, rickettsial
   - Non-infectious, e.g. marantic endocarditis

Pulmonary manifestations of a **left-sided mass** include

1. Pulmonary venous hypertension with dyspnea, hemoptysis and pulmonary infiltrates
2. Pulmonary artery hypertension simulating mitral valve disease
3. Pulmonary thromboembolic disease and infarction secondary to
   - Pulmonary vein occlusion at entry into the left atrium
   - Left-to-right intracardiac shunts

Pulmonary manifestations of a **right-sided mass** include

1. Pulmonary emboli
2. Septic emboli

PLEURAL EFFUSION – POST-CARDIAC SURGERY

Etiologies

1. **Transudate**, e.g. CHF, constrictive pericarditis
2. **Exudate**, e.g. pulmonary embolus, traumatic, parapneumonic, post-cardiac injury syndrome
3. **Bloody**, e.g. traumatic

4 **Pus**, e.g. empyema
5 **Chyle**, e.g. disruption of the thoracic duct

POST-CARDIAC INJURY SYNDROME (PCIS)

Definition: The PCIS is characterized by a combination of clinical and radiological features developing 2–4 weeks post-cardiac surgery, myocardial infarction, blunt chest trauma or pacemaker implantation

Clinical findings include fever, pleuritic chest pain, dyspnea and hemoptysis with findings of pericarditis and pleural fluid/ pleuritis on physical exam

Radiologic findings

1 Left-sided or bilateral effusions, uncommonly unilateral right-sided
2 Pulmonary infiltrates, usually LLL
3 Enlarged cardiac silhouette

There are no pathognomonic findings and therefore the PCIS is a diagnosis of exclusion

1 Compatible clinical features
2 Compatible chest X-rays
3 Bloody or blood-tinged pleural effusion, negative cultures and a neutrophil predominance eventually replaced by mononuclear cells
4 Concurrent pericardial effusion on echocardiography
5 Elimination of CHF, pneumonia or pulmonary emboli to explain the above abnormalities

HEART TRANSPLANT

1 **Pneumonia**
- Bacterial: common community-acquired organisms in addition to legionella, nocardia, mycobacteria
- Viral: CMV

- Fungal: aspergillus, pneumocystis
- Parasitic: toxoplasmosis

2 **Post-transplant lymphoproliferative disorders**
3 **Pulmonary edema** secondary to rejection or accelerated atherosclerosis
4 **Left lower lobe atelectasis** secondary to phrenic nerve dysfunction
5 **Mediastinal lipomatosis** from steroids

Fraser R.S., Muller N.L., Colman N., Paré P.D. (1999) Diagnosis of Diseases of the Chest 4th Edn., WB Saunders.
Baum, G.L., Crapo, J.D., Celli, B.R., Karlinsky, J.B. (eds) (1997) *Textbook of Pulmonary Diseases*, 6th edn.: Lippincott-Raven.
Fishman, A.P., Elias, J.A., Fishman, J.A., Grippi, M.A., Kaiser, L.R., Senior, R.N. (1998) *Fishman's Pulmonary Diseases and Disorders*, 3rd edn.: McGraw-Hill.

23 Chest Wall Disorders

CHEST WALL MASS

1 Primary chest wall infection
   - Skin or soft tissue abscess
   - Osteomyelitis
2 Primary pleuropulmonary infection with chest wall invasion
   - Actinomycosis, nocardia
   - Empyema necessitas from tuberculosis
3 Primary chest wall neoplasm
   - Soft tissue tumors, benign or malignant
   - Bony lesions
     - Benign, e.g. eosinophilic granuloma, osteomyelitis, tumors
     - Malignant, e.g. myeloma, lymphoma, chondrosarcoma, osteogenic sarcoma, Ewing's sarcoma
4 Local direct neoplastic invasion, e.g. lung, pleura, breast, mediastinum, lymphoma
5 Metastatic tumor, e.g. lung, breast, kidney, thyroid

PECTUS CARINATUM

Definition: Congenital or acquired abnormality where the sternum protrudes more anteriorly than normal

- Congenital variety may be associated with a family history of chest deformity and is usually asymptomatic
- Acquired form is seen with ASD, VSD as well as severe asthma dating from childhood, with symptoms and clinical findings reflecting the underlying disease

PECTUS EXCAVATUM

Definition: Sporadic or inherited disorder characterized by sternal depression, resulting in the ribs on each side protruding more anteriorly than the sternum

- May occur in isolation or be associated with connective tissue disorders, e.g. Marfan's syndrome, Poland's syndrome, scoliosis or other congenital defects

Clinical features

- Usually asymptomatic other than the physical deformity
- Heart murmur common, often simulating pulmonary stenosis (kinking of PA)
- ? ↑ incidence of mitral valve prolapse
- PFTs usually normal with variable degrees of restrictive disease reported

Radiologic features

1. Cardiac displacement to the left and resulting in a nitral configuration
2. Silhouetting of the right heart border posteriorly due to the displaced right parasternal tissues, creating a density over the inferomedial portion of the right hemithorax
3. Sternal depression on lateral films
4. Abnormal mediastinal contours simulating a mass lesion

ANKYLOSING SPONDYLITIS (AS)

Definition: A seronegative inflammatory disease of the axial spine and adjacent soft tissues with the sacroiliac, hip and shoulder joints most often involved

- Males predominate (10:1) with symptoms developing between the ages of 20–40 and associated with the histocompatibility antigen HLA-B27 in ~95% of whites

Pulmonary disease is often asymptomatic with the following described

1. Fibrobullous apical lesions are seen in a variable percentage of patients depending whether chest X-ray or CT scan is used
    - The male to female ratio is ~50:1 with most cases presenting in adulthood, several years after the onset of arthritis
    - Usually asymptomatic unless secondary infection has occurred, with prognosis mainly determined by the nature and extent of the infection
    - They begin as non-specific linear infiltrates on X-ray, cystic or cavitary changes develop in some patients, with CT findings including bullae, mycetomas, fibrosis, bronchiectasis and pleural thickening
    - Superinfection of the bullae is described including aspergillus, *M. avium* and *M. kansasii*, others
    - Bronchopleural fistula and empyema frequently complicate surgery
2. Cricoarytenoid arthritis can result in hoarseness, sore throat, upper airways obstruction, acute respiratory failure and cor pulmonale
3. Pleural effusions and pleuritis described
4. Ankylosis of the costovertebral joints can result in reductions (usually mild) of TLC and VC with increased RV & FRC
5. Dyspnea is uncommon but can occur with severe reductions in chest expansion
6. Musculoskeletal chest pains secondary to arthritic involvement of the costovertebral joints as well as anterior chest involvement, e.g. sternoclavicular joints
7. Rarely, bronchiectasis, BOOP

KYPHOSCOLIOSIS

Definition: Lateral displacement (scoliosis) or excessive anterior angulation (kyphosis) of the spine is quantified by the Cobb angle, a value >100° being considered severe disease

- 80% of cases are idiopathic, while most secondary cases are due to neuromuscular disease (e.g. polio, muscular dystrophy) although vertebral disease, (e.g. tuberculous spondylitis) connective tissue disease, (e.g. Marfan's) or thoracic cage abnormalities, (e.g. thoracoplasty) may be responsible

Pulmonary problems include

1. Dyspnea and repeated respiratory tract infections usually developing after age 35
2. Hypoxemia, pulmonary hypertension, cor pulmonale and right heart failure
3. Respiratory failure with hypercapnia which may be secondary to a spinal deformity >100°, sleep apnea, inspiratory muscle weakness, other factors
4. Inspiratory muscle weakness, reduced chest wall/lung compliance and restrictive PFTs
5. Nocturnal hypoventilation with further arterial desaturation exacerbating the pulmonary hypertension
6. Difficulty interpreting chest X-rays including the mediastinum, cardiac size and presence of pulmonary infiltrates

THORACOPLASTY

Definition: Surgical procedure where a variable number of ribs and accompanying intercostal muscles are resected to induce lung collapse or obliterate the pleural space, e.g. empyema

Pulmonary complications can develop secondary to

1. Chest wall deformity with scoliosis
2. Underlying lung disease or resection

3 Associated fibrothorax
4 Phrenic nerve damage and diaphragmatic paralysis
5 Associated diffuse airways obstruction from old TB or smoking

Clinical problems include

1 Dyspnea on exertion
2 Restrictive PFTs
3 Hypoxemia, hypercapnia and respiratory failure
4 Pulmonary hypertension, cor pulmonale and right heart failure

CT findings can include

1 Diffuse or focal pleural thickening which is often calcified
2 Bronchiectasis
3 Underlying lung disease or evidence of resection
4 Residual loculated fluid collections

OBESITY – PULMONARY COMPLICATIONS

1 Obstructive sleep apnea
2 Obesity hypoventilation syndrome, defined by the combination of severe obesity and alveolar hypoventilation when awake
   - May be secondary to hypothalamic dysfunction or a low normal ventilatory response to CO_2 where hypoventilation occurs when faced with the mechanical load of obesity
   - Patients complain of dyspnea on exertion and hypoventilate but do not meet the criteria of OSA
   - Hypoxemia results in polycythemia, cyanosis, cor pulmonale and right heart failure
   - Left ventricular failure, myxedema, COPD and OSA (commonly present) should be ruled out
   - a common clinical scenario is the combination of obesity and airways obstruction resulting in alveolar hypoventilation
3 Abnormal physiology with

- Normal to reduced arterial PO_2
- Elevated pCO_2 which can be normalized with voluntary hyperventilation
- Normal to restrictive PFTs
- Variable reductions in chest wall and lung compliance

4 Mediastinal widening secondary to lipomatosis
5 Chest X-ray finding of poor inspiratory films with elevated hemidiaphragms (R/O subpulmonic effusions secondary to LV failure), as well as cardiomegaly reflecting an enlarged RV
6 Increased incidence of CAD and hypertension with CHF
7 Poor physical conditioning and resultant dyspnea

POLAND'S SYNDROME

Definition: Congenital abnormality characterized by hypoplasia or aplasia of the pectoralis major muscle and ipsilateral syndactyly, intrathoracic manifestations including

1 Hyperlucent ipsilateral chest (simulating mastectomy)
2 Absence or atrophy of ipsilateral ribs two to five
3 Aplasia of the ipsilateral breast
4 Increased incidence of lung hernias
5 Increased incidence of neoplasms including leukemia, neuroblastoma, others

Fraser R.S., Muller N.L., Colman N., Paré P.D. (1999) Diagnosis of Diseases of the Chest 4th Edn., WB Saunders.

Baum, G.L., Crapo, J.D., Celli, B.R., Karlinsky, J.B. (eds) (1997) *Textbook of Pulmonary Diseases*, 6th edn.: Lippincott-Raven.

Fishman, A.P., Elias, J.A., Fishman, J.A., Grippi, M.A., Kaiser, L.R., Senior, R.N. (1998) *Fishman's Pulmonary Diseases and Disorders*, 3rd edn.: McGraw-Hill.

24 Chylothorax

Definition: The accumulation of chyle (lymphatic fluid from the GI track) in the pleural space, and identified by

1 Triglyceride levels >110 mg/dL, with low cholesterol levels
2 Chylomicrons on lipoprotein electrophoresis
3 Lymphocytic exudate

- Fat normally enters the blood via the thoracic duct in the form of triglycerides or chylomicrons
- Fluid accumulation in chylothorax is due to disruption of the thoracic duct, its collaterals, or less often as the result of chylous ascites tracking from the peritoneum
- Dyspnea is common with large effusions and may require repeated thoracenteses and chronic chest tube drainage, which can result in malnutrition and immunosuppression
- In those patients without a history of trauma, the mediastinum and retroperitoneum should be imaged to rule out lymphoma

Diagnostically, the pleural effusion grossly usually has a milky appearance but may be serous or serosanguinous, especially if the patient has a poor fat intake, with the differential including

1 Pseudochylothorax
   - Milky appearance
   - Low triglycerides
   - Cholesterol >200
   - Usually secondary to tuberculosis, rheumatoid or other longstanding effusions
2 Empyema, which has a clear supernatant on centrifugation, unlike a chylothorax and pseudochylothorax

Etiologies include

1 Neoplastic, e.g. *lymphoma, mediastinal metastases
2 *Trauma, e.g. cardiac, pulmonary, esophageal or spinal

surgery, neck hyperextension, penetrating trauma, central line placement

3 LAM
4 Pancreatitis
5 Mediastinal infection, fibrosis or radiation
6 Noonan's syndrome
7 Idiopathic

Radiologic findings are those of non-chylous effusions with CT occasionally able to diagnose a chylothorax as a result of its fat content

- Bipedal lymphangiography can detail the abnormal anatomy
- Chest and abdominal CT will often identify the etiology of a chylothorax, whether nontraumatic, e.g. lymphoma, or traumatic

Fraser R.S., Muller N.L., Colman N., Paré P.D. (1999) Diagnosis of Diseases of the Chest 4th Edn., WB Saunders.
Fishman, A.P., Elias, J.A., Fishman, J.A., Grippi, M.A., Kaiser, L.R., Senior, R.N. (1998) *Fishman's Pulmonary Diseases and Disorders*, 3rd edn.: McGraw-Hill.
Staats, B.A., Ellefson, R.D., Budahn, L.L. *et al.* (1980) The lipoprotein profile of chylous and nonchylous pleural effusions. *Mayo Clinic Proc.* **55**: 700–704.

25 Collagen Diseases – Pulmonary Manifestations

RHEUMATOID ARTHRITIS (RA) – CLINICOPATHOLOGIC SYNDROMES

Chest disease is an important cause of morbidity and mortality

- 80% of patients will have a ⊕ RF
- Pleuropulmonary manifestations are twice as common in men as in women and in both sexes may antedate clinical joint disease
- Radiologic and pulmonary function abnormalities are very common compared to the incidence of clinical disease

Airways Disease

1 **Follicular bronchiolitis** (see p. 111)
   - Clinical symptoms are cough and dyspnea with a diffuse reticulonodular pattern or more focal, ill-defined nodular opacities described on chest X-ray
   - Gold or penicillamine therapy have been implicated etiologically in some patients
   - Distinguish from the interstitial inflammation and

fibrosis of RA as there may be greater steroid responsiveness

2 **Bronchiolitis obliterans** presents with rapidly worsening dyspnea, hyperinflation on chest X-ray and airways obstruction on PFTs, definitive diagnosis being made on biopsy
- HRCT findings are those of mosaic perfusion (+/– accompanying bronchiectasis) with the areas of reduced attenuation and vascularity accentuated on an expiratory scan
- Gold and penicillamine have been implicated in some patients

3 **BOOP**, with pathologic and radiologic findings identical to the idiopathic variety
- Distinguish from the interstitial inflammation and fibrosis of RA as there may be greater steroid responsiveness

4 **Bronchocentric granulomatosis** (rarely described)

5 **Bronchiectasis**
- Unrelated to the severity of the RA, often subclinical and may precede the development of arthritis
- Typically lower lobe in distribution with diagnosis established on HRCT

6 **Upper airways obstruction** from:
- Cricoarytenoid arthritis manifest by chronic sore throat, hoarseness and abnormal vocal cord motion, with fixation in the adducted position, often manifest only following an upper respiratory infection, or post-intubation with laryngeal edema
- Rheumatoid nodules in the laryngeal region

Parenchymal Disease

1 **Interstitial lung disease (ILD) – rheumatoid lung**
Most serious pulmonary complication, the reported incidence varying according to the diagnostic criteria used to define the disease

- The frequency of abnormalities reported varies depending upon whether chest X-ray, HRCT scan, physiology (PFTs, hypoxemia) or BAL alveolitis is used to detect abnormalities, chest X-rays being the least sensitive
- Clinically silent disease is far more frequent than clinically significant ILD, e.g. restrictive PFTs can be seen in the absence of symptoms, although individual cases are unpredictable with regard to disease development
- Seropositive males between 50 and 60 are statistically more likely to develop ILD but no association has been found between the severity of the joint or other extra-articular manifestations of RA and the development of pulmonary disease
- Disease spectrum is quite variable and ranges from subclinical disease detected only by one of the above studies, to the full blown picture of ILD identical clinically, pathologically and radiologically (HRCT findings) to usual interstitial pneumonitis
- Other pathologies are occasionally found including DIP, BOOP
- Overall prognosis and disease progression are variable, difficult to predict and vary from subclinical to progressive interstitial fibrosis, leading to the typical 'honeycomb' lung, in association with disabling symptoms of dyspnea, cough, respiratory failure and cor pulmonale

2 **Rheumatoid nodules**

Pathologically identical to subcutaneous nodules, are the only specific pleuropulmonary manifestation of RA, and usually seen in patients with advanced seropositive RA and multiple nodules involving the elbows or other sites.

- May develop in the lungs prior to the development of symptomatic arthritis and also described in the absence of clinical RA
- Usually asymptomatic with a benign course although cavitation can result in hemoptysis as well as rupture

into the pleural space with resultant pneumothorax, empyema, pyopneumothorax, bronchopleural fistula
- Open lung biopsy is required for definitive diagnosis, although TTNA can rule out tumor or infection which can have a similar appearance radiologically

Radiologic features
- Single or multiple nodules, a few mm to several cm in diameter, resembling metastases
- Peripheral subpleural location
- Cavitation is common, often with a thick wall which becomes thinner prior to disappearance
- Aspergillomas may develop in the cavities
- The course of the nodules is unpredictable as they can appear, enlarge, cavitate or regress independent of the joint disease

3 **Caplan's syndrome**

Defined as rheumatoid nodules occurring in the lungs of patients with a pneumoconiosis
- Originally described in coal workers, but other dust exposures, e.g. silica, asbestos, etc. can give a similar picture
- Pathologically, they are similar to other rheumatoid nodules except for a pigmented ring of dust which distinguishes these from uncomplicated rheumatoid disease

Clinically, the nodules can appear at any time in the course of arthritis and are unrelated to severity or chronicity

Radiologically, they are similar to the nodules occurring without pneumoconiosis
- 0.5–5.0 cm in diameter
- May evolve rapidly and appear in 'crops'
- Nodules may resolve, cavitate, calcify or fibrose

4 **Upper lobe fibrobullous disease** is characterized radiologically by upper lobe scarring and bullae similar to ankylosing spondylitis
- May be complicated by mycetoma formation

5 **Pneumonia** is an important cause of morbidity and should be distinguished from BOOP, UIP, drug-induced disease

6 **Secondary amyloid** (rare)

Pleural Disease

1 **Pleural effusion/pleuritis**

Clinically, it is the most common intrathoracic manifestation of rheumatoid arthritis

- Unrelated to the severity or chronicity of the joint disease and may antedate any arthritis by months although typically seen in patients with subcutaneous nodules, active arthritis and high rheumatoid factor titers
- Presentation varies from asymptomatic (~⅓ of patients) to symptoms of acute pleuritis
- Thoracocentesis should be done to R/O infection, neoplasm or other causes of an effusion

Radiologic features

- Usually unilateral but variable in size
- No associated parenchymal disease in the majority of cases, although rheumatoid nodules may be present
- Effusions may persist unchanged for months to years, resolve or recur
- Residual pleural fibrosis may develop

Pleural fluid characteristics

- Exudate with low glucose, low complement, pH < 7.2, elevated adenosine deaminase
- ⊕ rheumatoid factor (low titers may be seen in non-rheumatoid effusions)
  - Patients with known RA can leak RF into the pleural fluid from serum in the presence of a non-rheumatoid effusion, e.g. parapneumonic
- Cells vary from lymphocytic to neutrophilic predominance with total WBC < 10000 mm^3
- As with other chronic effusions, rheumatoid effusions may be milky or chyliform in appearance and due to high cholesterol levels, unlike a true chylous effusion which is characterized by elevated triglycerides

Pleural biopsy usually reveals non-specific pleuritis but may contain diagnostic rheumatoid nodules

2 **Empyema** is frequently described and may be secondary to rheumatoid nodules discharging necrotic contents into the pleural space as well as to steroid therapy

3 **Pneumothorax, pyopneumothorax** and **BPF** secondary to cavitation of a necrobiotic nodule and its rupture into the pleural space

Vascular Disease

1 Pulmonary hypertension in association with diffuse interstitial fibrosis
2 Isolated pulmonary hypertension (very rare)
3 Vasculitis (very rare)
4 Hyperviscosity syndrome (very rare) where conglomerates of rheumatoid factor obstruct small vessels, dyspnea being a component of the syndrome

Drug-Induced

1 Methotrexate (see p. 213)
2 Gold (see p. 209)
3 Penicillamine (see p. 216)

SCLERODERMA (PROGRESSIVE SYSTEMIC SCLEROSIS – PSS)

Clinically, the majority of patients will develop non-specific respiratory symptoms

- Lung disease typically occurs late in the course of disease and varies from mild to severe, with complications including the following

Pleura

1 Spontaneous pneumothorax secondary to rupture of a 'honeycomb' cyst
2 Pleural thickening or effusion, the latter secondary to scleroderma involving the pleura, myocardial fibrosis or renovascular hypertension

Mediastinum

3 Air esophagogram
- Air in the esophagus (without an air–fluid level) as well as air in the gastric fundus, in combination with a 'UIP picture' is characteristic of scleroderma

Vasculature

4 Pulmonary edema secondary to scleroderma cardiomyopathy
5 Pulmonary hypertension is seen in about ⅓ of patients with diffuse scleroderma
- May be secondary to interstitial lung disease and subsequent hypoxemia or due to primary vascular involvement of the pulmonary arteries, the latter being the common mechanism in the CREST syndrome
- Direct proliferative involvement of small and medium-sized pulmonary arteries and arterioles is manifest by smooth muscle hyperplasia, medial hypertrophy, intimal proliferation and is seen in 10–15% of patients with CREST
- Natural history is that of progression and death

Parenchyma

6 Aspiration pneumonia secondary to esophageal dysfunction
- May be recurrent and responsible for some cases of interstitial fibrosis
- May be complicated by abscess formation and empyema

7 Alveolar cell or bronchogenic cancer
8 Interstitial lung disease
- Chronic progressive pulmonary fibrosis is the most common pulmonary complication of PSS and seen in up to ⅔ of patients
  - Early disease may be asymptomatic, but evidence of alveolitis is reflected in BAL, positive gallium scan and 'ground glass' abnormalities on CT scan
  - Most patients present with the symptoms of

fibrosing alveolitis but this is rarely the initial presentation of scleroderma
- Radiologic features are those of UIP with the earliest changes seen in the lower lobes and manifest as a fine reticular pattern evolving into coarse reticulation and finally into a honeycomb lung
  - Disease distribution is peripheral with progressive volume loss, cyst formation and an increased incidence of pneumothorax
  - The HRCT findings are those of UIP with 'ground glass' areas early, progressing to features of fibrosis
- The earliest change on PFTs is a reduction in DCO, which can reflect the presence of either interstitial or pulmonary vascular disease
  - Patients with fibrosis eventually develop progressive restrictive disease with reductions in the subdivisions of lung volume

9 Pulmonary renal syndrome and alveolar hemorrhage secondary to penicillamine treatment

Airways

10 Hemoptysis from bleeding telangiectasias of the bronchial tree

11 BOOP

CREST SYNDROME

Variant of PSS with

1. Anticentromere antibody found in >50% of patients *vs.* <10% with PSS
2. Lower incidence of joint disease
3. Less skin involvement (distal extremities)
4. Pulmonary hypertension occurs more frequently in the absence of ILD
5. Chest X-ray may be normal or reveal similar abnormalities to those found in PSS

SYSTEMIC LUPUS ERYTHEMATOSUS (SLE)

Over 80% of cases occur in women during their childbearing years, with most patients presenting with joint or skin lesions

- Pulmonary involvement is seen in ~50% of patients and ranges from asymptomatic to an acute or chronic presentation
- The above may reflect primary pulmonary involvement or a secondary manifestation from infection, drugs, cardiac or renal disease

Pleural Disease

Clinically, pleural disease is the most common abnormality of the respiratory system in SLE and may be the first clinical manifestation of lupus

- Patients may present with pleuritic pains or be asymptomatic
- Pleural effusions can be unilateral or bilateral with equal frequency in both hemithoraces, tend to be recurrent and rarely may be massive
- A dry pleuritis and pleuritic pain but normal chest X-rays may occur
- Other causes of effusion must be ruled out – infection, congestive heart failure, uremia, emboli – and therefore a diagnostic thoracocentesis is warranted
- Pleural biopsy usually shows non-specific inflammation
- The fluid is exudative, usually serous and occasionally serosanguinous, with hemothorax rarely described
- Transudative effusions are due to associated nephrotic syndrome, congestive heart failure, or cirrhosis
- Immunologic testing reveals ⊕ ANA ≥ 1:160, ratio of pleural fluid to serum ANA > 1, and low levels of total complement C_3 and C_4
- ⊕ LE cells are specific for lupus but of variable sensitivity in pleural fluid

- The predominant cell is the neutrophil acutely with a subsequent lymphocytic effusion after 1–2 weeks
- Glucose levels are of no diagnostic value

Parenchymal Disease

1 **Acute lupus pneumonitis** (**ALP**) is seen in less than 5% of patients with SLE but may be the presenting feature
   - Case reports describe an increased risk in the immediate post-partum period
   - Patients present with the acute onset of cough, dyspnea, fever and pleuritic pain which may be accompanied by hemoptysis
   - ALP is a diagnosis of exclusion with the differential diagnosis including pulmonary embolism, alveolar hemorrhage, and particularly infection, which often requires bronchoscopy and BAL to exclude
   - Alveolitis is suggested by a combination of 'ground glass' opacities on HRCT, positive gallium scan and BAL findings
     – Radiologic infiltrates are similarly non-specific, patchy or diffuse, unilateral or bilateral, often lower lobe in distribution, and may be accompanied by an elevated hemidiaphragm and pleural effusion
   - Lung biopsy reveals non-specific inflammation but will exclude infection
   - Prognosis is often poor with a clinical course which includes
     – Resolution on steroids
     – Relapses
     – Progression to acute respiratory failure
     – Development of chronic interstitial lung disease

2 **Pulmonary hemorrhage** or **alveolar hemorrhage syndrome** (**AHS**) is an uncommon manifestation of SLE and patients may initially be misdiagnosed as primary pulmonary hemosiderosis

- Rarely the presenting feature but more typically seen in patients with active extrapulmonary disease and high titers of circulating anti-DNA antibodies
- Both AHS and ALP are thought to represent acute injury to the alveolar-capillary unit with the two entities overlapping with regard to their clinical, radiologic and biopsy features
- Features supporting a diagnosis of AHS include
  - Falling hematocrit
  - Elevated DCO secondary to alveolar hemorrhage
  - Frequent occurrence of hemoptysis
  - No gross bleeding site visualized but bloody BAL with hemosiderin-laden macrophages
  - Lack of purulent sputum or infectious agents identified in bronchial secretions
- The clinical spectrum varies from mild and chronic to acute and massive, with potential progression to acute respiratory failure and high mortality
- Differential diagnosis includes infection, pulmonary edema and pulmonary infarction
- Radiologic features include unilateral or bilateral opacities, ranging from 'ground glass' to consolidation, and may resolve over a few days with cessation of bleeding

3 **Chronic interstitial lung disease** (**CILD**) is a rare manifestation of SLE
- Exact incidence of disease depends upon the diagnostic criteria used with asymptomatic involvement on HRCT being more common than clinically significant disease
- CILD may develop *de novo* with insidious onset or follow episodic acute lupus pneumonitis and is rarely the presenting feature of SLE
- The clinical, radiologic and physiologic features are similar to those of UIP with the spectrum varying from 'alveolitis' (as measured by gallium, BAL or CT scan) to end-stage honeycomb lung
- Natural history is unclear with the clinical presentation

and response to treatment quite variable;? heterogeneous group of disorders

4 **LIP/pseudolymphoma**
- Rare associations

5 **Lung nodules +/– cavitation**
- Rarely described and may occur secondary to vasculitis with ischemic necrosis
- Diagnosis of exclusion after ruling out cavitary pulmonary infarcts as well as infections, e.g. tuberculosis, nocardia, fungi

Airways Disease

1 **Bronchiolitis obliterans** and **BOOP** are rarely described in SLE
- Clinical and radiologic features are previously described with the definitive diagnosis made on lung biopsy

2 **Upper airways obstruction** and stridor can occur due to epiglottitis, sublglotic stenosis or laryngeal inflammation from SLE

Chest Wall

1 **Diaphragmatic dysfunction** is a common cause of dyspnea in SLE and should be suggested by complaints of orthopnea in the absence of congestive heart failure
- Signs and symptoms of generalized muscle weakness are absent with diagnostic features including
- Reduced lung volumes without pleuroparenchymal disease radiologically (small lung volumes and elevated hemidiaphragms)
- Reduced mouth pressures
- Low transdiaphragmatic pressures
- Absence of phrenic nerve dysfunction
- Steroid use, malnutrition and pleural adhesions may also contribute to limiting diaphragmatic movement and generating subnormal pressures

- Thought to explain the restrictive pattern of PFTs in patients without obvious lung disease
- Course of disease is variable with spontaneous stabilization in some patients or improvement on treatment

2 **Musculoskeletal pain** is common, pleuritic in nature and duplicated by palpation of the painful areas? costochondritis? muscular in origin

Vascular Disease

1 **Pulmonary emboli**, acute or chronic, are seen in patients with antiphospholipid antibody e.g. lupus anticoagulant, the full syndrome including
   - Venous and arterial thromboses
   - Thrombocytopenia
   - Neuropsychiatric disorders
   - Recurrent fetal loss
   - Pulmonary hypertension
   - Livedo reticularis

2 **Pulmonary artery hypertension** may develop secondary to other disease processes, e.g. emboli, or be primary with histopathologic features identical to those of idiopathic pulmonary hypertension
   - Typically occurs in young women who have associated features of Raynaud's phenomenon, renal disease and autoantibodies including rheumatoid factor, ribonucleoprotein and lupus anticoagulant
   - Clinical features are those of primary pulmonary hypertension with a poor prognosis and 50% 2-year mortality reported

3 **Vasculitis of the small pulmonary arteries** is rarely described

4 **Acute reversible hypoxemia** is thought to represent a leuko-occlusive vasculopathy where complement activation and leukoagglutination occur in the pulmonary circulation in the absence of chest X-ray abnormalities or pulmonary embolic disease

Mediastinum

1 Mediastinal and hilar adenopathy on CT (very rare)

Secondary Pulmonary Manifestations

1 **Infection** is the most common cause of pulmonary infiltrates and may be due to underlying disease or immunosuppressive medication, with responsible agents including
   - Common bacteria which may present with atypical clinical and radiologic features
   - Opportunistic organisms
     – mycobacteria, nocardia, legionella
     – aspergillus, cryptococcus
     – pneumocystis
     – herpes viruses

2 **Drug toxicity**
   - Direct effects of immunosuppressives or steroids
   - Drug-induced lymphoma or infection

3 **Cardiac failure**

4 **Renal disease** with nephrotic syndrome or end-stage renal failure

DRUG-INDUCED LUPUS

Patients present with features of arthralgias, pericarditis, pleuroparenchymal lung disease, fever, skin rashes, anemia and leucopenia

- ANA is positive but antibodies against double-stranded DNA are absent
- Antihistone antibody is present in >95% of cases (seen in about 20% of SLE) and therefore its absence makes drug-induced lupus unlikely
- Pulmonary, renal and central nervous system disease are uncommon resulting in milder disease
- Multiple drugs have been described to give disease, most commonly *procainamide, hydralazine, INH, methyldopa, diltiazem, chlorpromazine, minocycline, others

Pulmonary involvement is manifest as

1 Pleural effusion or pleurisy
2 Diffuse parenchymal lung disease
3 Others e.g. pulmonary emboli, pulmonary artery hypertension, etc.

Diagnostic features

1 History of drug ingestion
2 Above presentation
3 ⊕ ANA and antihistone antibodies
4 Resolution of signs and symptoms within 4–6 weeks on discontinuation of the drug, although ANA may remain positive for 6–12 months

SJOGREN'S SYNDROME

Originally described as the triad of keratoconjunctivitis sicca, xerostomia and recurrent swelling of the parotid gland, and characterized by lymphocytic infiltrates of mainly the salivary and lacrimal glands but extraglandular infiltrates are seen in 5–10% of patients, involving many organs including the lungs

- clinically the 'sicca syndrome' may be found alone, i.e. primary, in association with another collagen vascular disease, (e.g. RA, SLE, PSS) or following bone marrow transplantation

Pulmonary manifestations

1 **Airways disease**
   - Laryngeal involvement with hoarseness, cough
   - Atrophy of the tracheobronchial mucus glands with dry cough, recurrent infections, bronchiectasis
   - Follicular bronchiolitis with extraglandular lymphocytic infiltration of the small airways
   - Bronchial hyper-reactivity in ~50% of patients

2 **Interstitial lung disease** occurs in up to 25% of patients, with cough and dyspnea being the usual symptomatology
   - Chest X-rays may be normal or show bibasilar

reticular or nodular disease, abnormalities being found more commonly on HRCT
- Subclinical alveolitis may be found on BAL in the presence of normal chest X-rays and no pulmonary symptoms whereas abnormal BAL findings and a positive gallium scan are typical of clinical disease
- Histologically the above can represent
  – UIP in various stages
  – lymphoid interstitial pneumonitis (see p. 73)
  – BOOP
  – recurrent pneumonia
  – amyloid

3 **Pulmonary artery hypertension**
4 **Pleural effusion** – rare and seen more often with secondary Sjogren's syndrome
5 **Associated collagen vascular disease**
6 **Lymphoproliferative disorders**
   - Pseudolymphoma representing tumor-like aggregates of lymphoid cells and often presenting as a mass lesion
   - Increased incidence of non-Hodgkin's lymphoma, sometimes primary in the lung

7 **Asymptomatic BAL lymphocytosis**, reflecting ? alveolitis; ? lymphocytic bronchitis/bronchiolithis

POLYMYOSITIS – DERMATOMYOSITIS

Definition: Inflammatory disease of skeletal muscle characterized by symmetric weakness of proximal muscles and neck flexors, elevated serum muscle enzymes, EMG and biopsy evidence of myositis as well as skin involvement in dermatomyositis
- Autoimmune serologic findings include ⊕ ANA and anti-Jo-1 antibody, a myositis-specific autoantibody

Pulmonary involvement may precede, be concurrent with or follow the inflammatory myopathy and be manifest as

1 *Recurrent **aspiration pneumonia** secondary to dysphagia

2 **Airways disease** with obstructive sleep apnea secondary to upper airway muscle weakness
3 Primary **lung cancer** or **metastatic** disease
4 **Interstitial lung disease** is seen in ~30% of patients but the frequency is quite variable in different series depending upon the diagnostic criteria used, e.g. HRCT, BAL or chest X-ray
   - Can be asymptomatic or present with non-specific symptoms of cough and dyspnea in association with bilateral interstitial infiltrates
   - Lung disease may precede, be concurrent with or follow the dermatologic and myopathic manifestations and is unrelated to their extent or severity
   - presents insidiously with cough and dyspnea, the pathology being that of UIP, varying from a cellular phase of alveolitis to a fibrotic, honeycomb lung
   - Response to treatment reflects the underlying pathology with the more cellular and less fibrotic reactions having the best prognosis
5 **Acute lung disease** developing over a few weeks, presenting with cough, fever and dyspnea in the absence of CHF
   - Chest X-rays reveal bilateral airspace disease, superimposed on an interstitial pattern, underlying pathology including
     – BOOP
     – DAD
     – Pulmonary capillaritis and hemorrhage
6 **Pulmonary edema** secondary to cardiac disease
7 **Respiratory muscle weakness** from the underlying disease or steroids can result in hypoventilation and respiratory failure
   - Less severe involvement can result in impaired cough and small lung volumes on chest X-ray
   - May rarely be the presenting feature of disease without peripheral muscle involvement
   - Restrictive disease is seen on PTFs without evidence of pleuropulmonary disease on chest X-ray
8 **Pulmonary artery hypertension** can be primary (rare) or

secondary to LV failure, respiratory muscle weakness or hypoxemia from ILD

9 **Pulmonary vasculitis/capillaritis** (rare)
10 **Pleural effusions** (rare)
11 **Associated collagen vascular disease**
12 **Immunosuppressive drug-induced** infection or lymphoma

MIXED CONNECTIVE TISSUE DISEASE

Definition: Term coined in 1972 to describe patients with clinical features of systemic lupus (SLE), scleroderma (PSS), polymyositis-dermatomyositis and high titers of anti-ribonucleoprotein antibody and speckled ANA (>1:1000)

- There is a marked female predominance with the average age at presentation 35 to 40
- Pleuropulmonary complications are those seen in the individual underlying diseases and tend to reflect the severity or predominance of the SLE, PSS or PM-DM, including

Parenchyma

1 Interstitial fibrosis – findings are those of UIP with the degree of fibrosis being severe if the predominant clinical feature is PSS
2 Aspiration pneumonia secondary to dysphagia in patients with features of scleroderma or polymyositis
3 Opportunistic infection in patients on steroids or other immunosuppressives
4 Alveolar hemorrhage syndrome in patients with SLE

Vascular

5 Pulmonary hypertension is the most common cause of death, disease being primarily vascular, with little associated interstitial fibrosis present
6 Thromboemboli are seen in patients with lupus anticoagulant

Pleural effusion

7 Reported frequency is variable although pleuritic pains are often described

Neuromuscular

8 Respiratory muscle weakness may occur when PM-DM predominates, leading to respiratory failure

MARFAN'S SYNDROME

Definition: Autosomal dominant abnormality of connective tissue manifest as abnormalities of the ocular (subluxation of the lens), cardiovascular (aortic aneurysm/dissection, aortic and mitral regurgitation) and respiratory systems, the latter including

1 **Pleural disease**
   - *Pneumothorax (most common pulmonary abnormality)
2 **Parenchymal disease**
   - Apical bullae
   - Diffuse emphysema
   - Upper lobe or diffuse interstitial fibrosis
   - Recurrent pneumonia from bronchiectasis
3 **Airways disease**
   - Bronchiectasis
   - Congenital malformations of the bronchus
4 **Chest wall disease**
   - Pectus excavatum
   - Scoliosis
5 **Vascular disease**
   - *Aortic aneurysm/dissection
   - Cystic medial necrosis of a pulmonary artery
   - Aneurysm of the ductus anteriosus

Fraser R.S., Muller N.L., Colman N., Paré P.D. (1999) Diagnosis of Diseases of the Chest 4th Edn., WB Saunders.

Moss, A., Gamsu, Genant (1992) Thorax and neck. In: *Computed Tomography of the Body with Magnetic Resonance Imaging*, 2nd edn, vol. 1. (Place of publication): W.B. Saunders.

Thurlbeck, W., Churg, A. (eds) (1995) *Pathology of the Lung*, 2nd edn. (Place of publication): Thieme Medical Publishers.

Baum, G.L., Crapo, J.D., Celli, B.R., Karlinsky, J.B. (eds) *Textbook of Pulmonary Diseases*, 6th edn. (Place of publication): Lippincott-Raven.

Fishman, A.P., Elias, J.A., Fishman, J.A., Grippi, M.A., Kaiser, L.R., Senior, R.N. (1998) *Fishman's Pulmonary Diseases and Disorders*, 3rd edn.: McGraw-Hill.

Fenlon, H.M., Doran, M., Sant, S.M. *et al.* (1996) High-resolution chest CT in SLE. *AJR* **166**: 301–307.

Mills, J. (1994) Systemic lupus erythomatosus. *NEJM* **330**: 1871–1879.

Condemi, J. (1992) The autoimmune diseases. *JAMA* **268**: 2882–2892.

Wiedemann, H.P., Matthay, R.A. (1989) Pulmonary manifestations of the collagen vascular diseases. *Clinics in Chest Medicine* **10**: 677–699.

Remy-Jardin, M., Remy, J., Wallaery, B. *et al.* (1993) Pulmonary involvement in progressive systemic sclerosis: sequential evaluation with CT, pulmonary function test and BAL. *Radiology* **188**: 499–506.

Sullivan, W., Hurst, D., Harmon, C. *et al.* (1984) A prospective evaluation emphasizing pulmonary involvement in patients with MCTD. *Medicine* **63**: 92–107.

Wiedemann, H.P., Matthay, R.A. (1992) Pulmonary manifestations of systemic lupus erythematosus. *J. Thor. Imag.* **7**: 1–18.

Haupt, M.N. *et al.* (1981) The lung in systemic lupus erythematosus: analysis of the pathologic changes in 120 patients. *Am. J. Med.* **71**: 791–798.

Wilcox, Stein, H., Clarke, S. *et al.* (1988) Phrenic nerve function in patients with diphragmatic weakness and systemic lupus erythematosus. *Chest* **93**: 352–358.

Remy-Jardin, M., Remy, J., Cortet, B. *et al.* (1994) Lung changes in rheumatoid arthritis: CT findings. *Radiology* **193**: 375–382.

Murns, S., Wiedermann, H.P., Matthay, R.A. (1998) Pulmonary manifestations of systemic lupus erythematosus. *Clinics in Chest Medicine* **19**: 641–665.

Tanoue, L. (1998) Pulmonary manifestations of rheumatoid arthritis. *Clinics in Chest Medicine* **19**: 667–685.

Cain, H., Noble, P., Matthay, R. (1998) Pulmonary manifestations of Sjogren's syndrome. *Clinics in Chest Medicine* **19**: 687–699.

Schwarz, M. (1998) The lung in polymyositis. *Clinics in Chest Medicine* **19**: 701–712.

Miller, L., Greenberg, D., McLarity, J. (1995) Lupus lung. *Chest* **88**: 265–269.

Minai, O., Dweik, R., Arroliga, A. (1998) Manifestations of scleroderma pulmonary disease. *Clinics in Chest Medicine* **19**: 713–731.

Prakash, N. (1998) Respiratory complications in mixed connective tissue disease. (*Journal Name*) **19**: 733–746.

Tomioka, H., King, T. (1997) Gold-induced pulmonary features, outcome and differentiation from rheumatoid lung disease. *Am. J. Resp. Crit. Care Med.* **155**: 1011–1020.

26 COPD

COMPLICATIONS

Cardiovascular

1 Pulmonary artery hypertension, cor pulmonale and right heart failure
   - Mild to moderate pulmonary hypertension in most patients at rest but can become severe with exercise
2 Arrythmias – supraventricular and ventricular arrythmias occur with MAT being the most characteristic
   - Predisposing features include hypoxemia, hypercania, hypokalemia, hypomagnesemia, drugs (e.g. theophylline, digoxin, β agonists), coronary artery disease, CHF
3 Left ventricular dysfunction and failure occurring independently, secondary to hypoxemia or possibly related to right ventricular dysfunction
   - History, physical and radiologic studies are often equivocal with the most useful criteria being
     – Rapidly changing pattern of bronchovascular markings on serial chest X-rays
     – Bilateral pleural effusions
     – Echocardiogram to assess LV function
     – Measurement of wedge pressure
4 Acute myocardial infarction from hypoxemia

5 Acute arterial hypotension
   - Respiratory: tension pneumothorax from ruptured bullae; large pulmonary embolus from stasis in the legs or right heart
   - Cardiac: hypoxemia-induced arrythmias, failure, infarction
   - Hypovolemia: high incidence of upper GI bleed
   - Sepsis: pneumonia or extrapulmonary source
   - Anaphylaxis: drugs, food
   - Addisonian: patients unknowingly on steroids at home
   - Drug-induced: diuretics
   - Neurogenic: vasovagal
6 Bacteremias from infected intravascular devices, with or without infective endocarditis
7 Polycythemia secondary to hypoxemia and elevated carboxyhemoglobin levels in smokers

Respiratory

1 Progressive deterioration in lung function leading to respiratory failure, with repeated episodes of acute-on-chronic failure
   - The rate of decline in lung function in smokers is ~65 ml/yr *vs.* ~35 ml/yr in patients who stop smoking
   - Hypercapnia typically occurs with $FEV_1 < 1$ L (in some patients only)
   - Acute respiratory failure is characterized by a reduced PO_2 and/or elevated PCO_2 with decrease in pH, from baseline values
   - Each acute increase of 10 mmHg in PCO_2 results in 1 mEq ↑ HCO_3 and 0.08 ↓ pH
   - Each chronic increase of 10 mmHg in PCO_2 results in a 3.5 mEq ↑ HCO_3 and a 0.03 ↓ pH
2 Pulmonary emboli arising in the legs from stasis, in a dilated right heart, or from a pulmonary artery catheter
   - septic emboli may develop following infection of bland emboli or from a septic focus, e.g. IV site, right heart valves
3 Acute bronchitis or pneumonia – community-acquired or nosocomial

- opportunistic infection can be seen, e.g. cryptococcus, particularly with the use of high dose steroids for prolonged periods of time

4 Colonization with resistant organisms, e.g. MRSA
5 Aspergillus infection
- Aspergilloma in a pre-existing bulla
- Mucoid impaction – ABPA
- Subacute necrotizing pulmonary aspergillosis
- Invasive aspergillosis

6 Reactivation tuberculosis secondary to steroids
7 Atypical mycobacterial infection
8 Chronic pulmonary histoplasmosis infecting pre-existing bullae
9 Pneumothorax from a ruptured bulla
10 Bronchogenic cancer from smoking
11 Hemoptysis – R/O neoplasm
12 Mucous plugs/atelectasis

Gastrointestinal

1 Peptic ulceration/upper GI bleed
2 Antibiotic-induced pseudomembranous colitis
3 Colonization with resistant organisms, e.g. VRE

Metabolic

1 Metabolic alkalosis from diuretics or steroids, with a secondary respiratory acidosis
2 Hypokalemia secondary to diuretics, steroids, β-agonists
3 Hypophosphatemia secondary to poor oral intake, diuretics, antacids
4 Hyponatremia secondary to salt and water retention, pneumonia, lung cancer, diuretics
5 Muscle weakness secondary to hypokalemia, hypophosphatemia, steroids, hypoxemia
6 Malnutrition
7 Osteoporosis with vertebral fractures (secondary to steroids, inactivity)

Neurologic

1 Altered sensorium reflecting hypoxemia, acidemia
2 Seizures secondary to hypoxemia, theophylline

3 Depression
4 Impaired neuropsychologic function secondary to hypoxemia

WORSENING COPD

Triggers include:

Upper airway	• Stricture from prior tracheostomy or intubation • Cigarette-induced carcinoma • Obesity and obstructive sleep apnea
Lower airway	• Infections of bacterial, mycoplasma, viral or chlamydial origin and manifest as epiglottitis, laryngitis, tracheitis, bronchitis or bronchiolitis • Non-compliance with bronchodilator meds • Bronchogenic cancer • Increasing bronchospasm from – Environmental triggers – β Blockers – Smoking – Recurrent gastro-esophageal reflux • Mucus plugging – ABPA
Parenchyma	• Lung cancer • Pneumonia – community-acquired or nosocomial • Reactivation of tuberculosis or atypicals
Pleura	• Pneumothorax
Vasculature	• Pulmonary edema from hypoxemic cardiac dysfunction, arrythmias or concurrent heart disease • Pulmonary emboli from leg edema and stasis or right ventricular mural thrombi
Chest wall	• Rib fracture from coughing • Abdominal distension from aerophagia or obesity
Neuromuscular	• Central depression from sedative drugs or metabolic alkalosis • Muscle weakness from steroids, malnutrition, electrolyte disturbances, e.g.: ↓K, ↓Ca, ↓PO_2, ↓Mg
Systemic	• Systemic infection • New onset anemia with reduced O_2 carrying capacity to the respiratory muscles

Table 26.1

Manifestations

- Increasing **respiratory symptoms** of dyspnea, cough, etc.
- **CNS** changes in **sensorium** ranging from delirium to coma; morning headaches suggesting hypercapnia
- **Cardiac** disease including arrythmias, syncope, increasing angina/myocardial infarction, left heart failure, cor pulmonale with right heart failure

Physical Findings

1. Tracheal findings
   - Reduced length of trachea palpable above the sternal notch (normally 3–4 fingers)
   - Tracheal descent with inspiration
2. Use of accessory muscles – scalene, sternomastoids and parasternals
3. Excavation of suprasternal and supraclavicular fossae during inspiration with nasal flaring
4. Intercostal indrawing
5. Cardiovascular findings
   - Jugular vein filling during expiration
   - Pulsus paradoxus
   - Findings of pulmonary hypertension with a right ventricular heave, ↑P_2, right-sided S_3 gallop, jugular venous distension
6. Tachypnea, orthopnea, ↑ A-P chest diameter, hyperresonance, reduced breath sounds, expiratory > inspiratory wheezes and ronchi
7. Reduction in cardiac and liver dullness
8. Loss of bucket-handle movement of upper ribs
9. Paradoxical diaphragmatic motion
10. Paradoxical movement of costal margin (Hoover's sign), i.e. downwards and inwards
11. Prolonged forced expiratory time (normal duration <4 seconds)
12. Peripheral findings
    - Cyanosis
    - Asterixis secondary to hypercapnia
    - edema
    - altered sensorium

ACUTE EXACERBATION OF CHRONIC BRONCHITIS (AECB)

Definition: Patients who present with increasing dyspnea and/or sputum volume and/or purulence of sputum, in the absence of pneumonia

- Increased neutrophils and bacteria are seen in sputum although the exact role of bacteria has been debated
- The bacterial spectrum most often is that of *Haemophilus influenzae*, *S. pneumoniae*, *Moraxella catarrhalis* and *Haemophilus parainfluenzae*, but with increasing severity of underlying lung disease, gram negatives become increasingly important

Sequelae of AECB range from spontaneous remission to requirement for hospitalization and acute respiratory failure

Factors to identify high risk patients include:

1. Advanced age
2. Severity of airways obstruction
3. Associated bronchiectasis
4. Poor performance status
5. History of frequent exacerbations annually
6. Co-morbidity, e.g. CHF, diabetes, chronic renal or liver disease

INTUBATION – INDICATIONS

Respiratory

- Respiratory arrest
- Respiratory pauses with loss of consciousness
- Gasping for air
- Worsening hypoxemia – O_2 saturations <90% on 100% O_2
- Progressive acidemia
- Inability to clear secretions

Cardiac

- Bradycardia with decreased level of consciousness
- Hypotension

CNS

- Coma
- Psychomotor agitation requiring sedation
- Progressive encephalopathy with asterixis, confusion

RADIOLOGY

Chest X-Ray Findings

1 **Chronic bronchitis** cannot be diagnosed radiologically but suggestive features include
   - Bronchial wall thickening manifest as a 'ring' sign on cross-section or as 'tramlines' when seen longitudinally
   - Heavy bronchovascular markings ('dirty chest')

2 **Emphysema** – 'arterial deficiency' type
   - Hyperinflation with flattened diaphragm exhibiting superior concavity, increased AP diameter, increased retrosternal and retrocardiac airspaces, anterior bowing of the sternum and accentuation of the dorsal kyphosis
   - Oligemia with decreased caliber of vessels, rapidity of tapering distally and frequent asymmetric distribution
   - Bullae
   - Long narrow cardiac silhouette
   - May be accompanied by enlarged central pulmonary arteries

3 **Emphysema** – 'increased markings'
   - Hyperinflation
   - Enlarged hilar pulmonary arteries
   - 'Dirty chest'
   - Cardiomegaly
   - Bullae are uncommon

4 **Prominent hilar shadows** (pulmonary hypertension) and encroachment of the cardiac silhouette on the retrosternal space (RV enlargement)

HRCT Scan Findings

Centrilobular emphysema is characterized by focal areas of low attenuation, with or without visible walls which reflect areas of fibrosis or compressed adjacent lung parenchyma

- Upper lobe predominance and centrilobular in distribution
- Severe disease results in the areas of decreased opacity becoming confluent, the focal centrilobular distribution no longer apparent, and the lungs resembling panlobular emphysema

Panlobular emphysema results in uniform destruction of the pulmonary lobules with reduction in the number and size of vessels, i.e. 'simplification' of lung structure

- Lower lobe predominance
- The focal lucencies of centrilobular emphysema are absent as are visible walls
- Early disease may not be apparent

Paraseptal emphysema results in subpleural lucencies with thin but visible walls

- May occur in isolation or in association with centrilobular emphysema

Role of HRCT

1. **Pre-op evaluation** for patients undergoing bullectomy
    - Assessment of adjacent lung tissue should help distinguish otherwise normal but compressed lung from emphysematous lung
2. **Pre-op evaluation** for LVRS
    - Can evaluate the severity and distribution of emphysema with identification of 'target zones'
    - Can identify exclusion criteria for surgery, e.g. bronchogenic cancer, extensive pleural disease or other parenchymal process
3. **Diagnosis of emphysema** at an early stage where patients present with dyspnea and a low DCO but little or no airways obstruction on PFTs
    - The differential diagnosis will include interstitial or pulmonary vascular disease, particularly when chest X-rays are not helpful, as occurs in early emphysema,

early interstitial lung disease or primary pulmonary vascular disorders

4 **Confirmation of emphysema** and **exclusion** of other disorders e.g. ILD in smokers who are dyspneic, have low DCO and airways obstruction on PFTs, but may have abnormal lung markings on chest X-ray in addition to hyperinflation
5 **Detection of paraseptal emphysema** in young adults with spontaneous pneumothorax, manifest as subpleural bullae which are apical in distribution
6 **Diagnosis** of **complicating bronchiectasis**

Radiologic Complications

1 **Airways**
- Mucus plugs
- ABPA
- Endobronchial narrowing (from a smoking-related neoplasm)

2 **Parenchyma**
- Pneumonia
- Pulmonary edema (LV dysfunction)
- Chronic histoplasmosis in upper lobe bullae
- Reactivation tuberculosis (from steroids)
- Superinfection with atypical mycobacteria
- Aspergilloma in a pre-existing bulla
- Lung cancer secondary to smoking
- Enlargement of bullae over time

3 **Vasculature**
- Pulmonary emboli and infarction
- Pulmonary artery hypertension
- Cor pulmonale

4 **Pleura**
- Pneumothorax
- Pleural effusion secondary to associated CHF, pneumonia, metastatic lung cancer

5 **Mediastinum**
- Pneumomediastinum

COPD VS. BULLOUS DISEASE

(see bullae p. 178)

	Bullous Disease	COPD + Bullae
Occurrence	Sporadic or familial	Sporadic or familial
Clinically	Often asymptomatic	Usually symptomatic
Radiology	• Upper lobe predominance • May be localized and small or occupy an entire hemithorax • Intervening lung is ± normal except for compression as well as displacement and distension of vessels	• Bullae can be seen with any type of emphysema but most often centrilobular or paraseptal • Intervening parenchyma is abnormal with narrowed and attenuated vasculature
PFTs	N to ↓ VC usually ↑ FRC, RV N to ↓ DCO (if adjacent lung is compressed) Normal flow rates (unless chronic bronchitis is present)	↓ VC ↑ RV, FRC ↓ DCO ↓ Flow rates
Surgery	Large bullae occupying > ⅓ of a hemithorax with • Compression of underlying lung, dyspnea and poor response to medical therapy • Recurrent pneumothoraces • Recurrent infection	Controversial (see LVRS)

Table 26.2

LUNG VOLUME REDUCTION SURGERY (LVRS)

Rationale is to increase the elastic recoil pressure of the lung in patients with emphysema (usually in smokers +/– α_1 anti-trypsin deficiency), ideally resulting in

1 Increased driving pressure
2 Increased tethering of the airways

3 Reductions in lung volumes and chest wall inflation with subsequent improved muscle function and reduced work of breathing

Resection of non-giant bullae or generalized emphysema is more controversial with patient selection required to choose those COPD patients most likely to respond, i.e.

- Areas of emphysematous lung and preserved lung
- Marked hyperinflation
- Relatively little intrinsic airways disease
- Surgical benefits are highly dependent on patient selection with no clear consensus on the definition of a 'successful outcome,' i.e. which parameters should be measured and followed
- Several different surgical procedures have been used to remove 20–40% of the emphysematous lung

Potential Surgical Candidates

Clinical features of

1 Severe dyspnea affecting daily activities and not responding to maximal medical therapy
2 Ability to participate in a post-op pulmonary rehabilitation program
3 Age < 75 years
4 Discontinuation of smoking
5 $PCO_2 < 55$
6 Absence of
  - Predominant airways disease/purulent secretions, e.g. asthma, bronchiectasis
  - Pleural disease from prior surgery or pleurodesis
  - Chest wall disease, e.g. marked deformity from kyphoscoliosis
  - Left heart dysfunction and significant CAD
  - Significant systemic disease
  - Ventilator dependence

Radiologic imaging on chest X-ray, CT scan, V/Q scan

1 Severe emphysema with heterogenous disease, i.e. large 'target areas' (minimal perfusion/parenchymal

destruction) as well as large 'reserve areas' (well perfused/little parenchymal destruction)

2 Marked hyperinflation
3 Absence of associated disease involving the pleura, parenchyma or mediastinum

Physiologic studies revealing severe obstruction (FEV_1 < 35%), hyperinflation (TLC > 125%), air trapping (RV > 250%), $PCO_2 < 55$

INTRATHORACIC AIRWAYS OBSTRUCTION ON PFTS – DIFFERENTIAL

1 Localized or generalized tracheal obstruction (see Upper Airways Obstruction p. 829)
2 Tracheobronchomegaly
3 Tracheomalacia
4 Localized major bronchial narrowing
5 Generalized bronchial narrowing
   - Asthma
   - Allergic bronchopulmonary aspergillosis
   - Bronchocentric granulomatosis
   - Chronic bronchitis
   - Bronchiectasis
   - Bronchiolitis
6 Parenchymal diseases
   - LAM
   - Eosinophilic granuloma
   - Emphysema, including α_1 antitrypsin deficiency
   - Bullous disease
   - Silicosis
   - Sarcoid
   - Chronic eosinophilic pneumonia
7 Vascular diseases
   - Churg-Strauss
   - i.v. talcosis

α_1 ANTITRYPSIN DEFICIENCY (AAT)

AAT, also known as α_1 protease inhibitor, is a glycoprotein produced in the liver, secreted into the blood, that then diffuses into the lung protecting lung tissue from damage by enzymes, its main substrate being neutrophil elastase

- AAT deficiency is seen in about 2% of emphysema patients and is an inherited disorder where the Pi (protease inhibitor) phenotype consists of two autosomal co-dominantly inherited alleles, carriers having one normal gene and one deficient gene, contributing 50% and 10% respectively to the total α_1 protease inhibitor concentration
- PiMM is present in about 90% of patients of European descent with normal AAT serum levels
- More than 75 alleles of the gene have been identified, PiZZ being responsible for the vast majority of cases of emphysema (>95%)
- The PiZ phenotype is a point mutation in a single nucleotide with lysine replacing glutamic acid
- The change in tertiary structure of the molecule results in dimerization with another molecule and aggregation in the hepatic endoplasmic reticulum, impeding the secretion of protein from the cell (usually remains subclinical) and resulting in low plasma levels
- Liver disease is seen with the alleles Z and M (Malton) which cause intrahepatocyte accumulation of AAT
- The PiZ phenotype is also less effective as an inhibitor of neutrophil elastase
- The threshold protective level for AAT is greater than 35% of normal, the PiZZ phenotype averaging about 15%

Clinical features

Patients with PiZZ are caucasian, the Z allele being rare in blacks and orientals

- Dyspnea usually develops between ages 25 and 40 although not every deficient individual will develop emphysema
- Majority of symptomatic patients are current or ex-smokers, smoking resulting in more severe disease with an

earlier age of presentation, although there is significant variability in the severity of lung function in both smokers and non-smokers
- Emphysema is panacinar, more marked in the lower lobes and reflected on chest X-ray and CT scan
- Reports of an association with bronchiectasis (rarely the presenting features) and asthma

PFTs show airflow obstruction (reflecting loss of elasticity and airway narrowing), gas trapping and low DCO, with an accelerated rate of decline in lung function and decreased survival compared to the overall population, mortality rates rising dramatically when $FEV_1\% < 35$

Liver complications include neonatal hepatitis and jaundice in about 10% of patients, unexplained chronic liver disease in older children, as well as adult cirrhosis and hepatoma in ~10–15% of patients, the latter often occurring without childhood liver disease
- A rare skin manifestation is necrotizing panniculitis

AAT is **frequently undiagnosed** and therefore should be suspected with
1. COPD in a non-smoker or premature onset of moderate-severe disease in smokers < 50 years of age
2. Family history of emphysema
3. Family history of AAT
4. Unexplained bronchiectasis
5. Non-resolving 'asthma' in patients < 50 years of age
6. COPD with unexplained cirrhosis or liver disease
7. Bullous emphysema more prominent at the lung bases than the upper lobes

Diagnostic features
1. Serum protein electrophoresis will reveal a flat baseline (in homozygotes) in the α_1 globulin region instead of a small peak
2. The α_1 protease inhibitor level in serum will be less than 35% of normal
3. Phenotyping is subsequently performed to identify the specific alleles

Fraser R.S., Muller N.L., Colman N., Paré P.D. (1999) Diagnosis of Diseases of the Chest 4th Edn., WB Saunders.

Moss, A., Gamsu, Genant (1992) Thorax and neck. In: *Computed Tomography of the Body with Magnetic Resonance Imaging*, 2nd edn, vol. 1. (Place of publication): W.B. Saunders.

Campbell, E.J.M. (1969) Physical signs of diffuse airways obstruction and lung destruction. *Thorax* **24**: 1–3.

Pingleton, S. (1988) Complications of acute respiratory failure. (Journal Name) **137**: 1463–1493.

Roné, C., Mal, H., Sleiman, C. *et al.* (1996) Lung volume reduction in patients with severe diffuse emphysema. *Chest* **110**: 28–36.

Brenner, M., Yusen, R., McKenna, R. *et al.* (1996) Lung volume reduction surgery for emphysema. *Chest* **110**: 205–218.

Webb, R. (1994) HRCT of obstructive lung disease. *Radiol. Clin. North Am.* **32**: 745–752.

Takasugi, J., Goodwin, J. (1998) Radiology of chronic obstructive pulmonary disease. *Radiol. Clin. North Am.* **36**: 29–55.

Webb, R. (1994) HRCT of obstructive lung disease. *Radiol. Clin. North Am.* **32**: 745–755.

American Thoracic Society (1999) Guidelines for approach to the patient with severe hereditary alpha 1-antitrypsin deficiency. *Am. J. Resp. Crit. Care Med.* **140**: 1494–1497.

27 Cough

CHRONIC COUGH – NORMAL CHEST X-RAY

Definition: Variable, usually greater than 3–4 weeks in duration

Upper airways disease

1 *Post-nasal drip is usually secondary to a viral RTI, sinusitis or rhinitis
   - Frequent throat-clearing, rhinorrhea, sneezing and nasal itch are typical
   - Cobblestoning of the oropharyngeal mucosa, nasal polyps, rhinitis or sinus tenderness are found on physical
   - Response to antihistamines, decongestants, nasal steroids or antibiotics (for acute sinusitis)
   - Investigations would include sinus X-rays ± sinus CT demonstrating mucosal thickening +/– fluid levels

2 Ear disorders, e.g. otitis, wax, hairs, foreign body

3 Pharyngeal/laryngeal inflammation, infection, neoplasm

Lower airways disease

1 *Tracheitis/tracheobronchitis/bronchitis
   - Typically follows a 'viral' RTI and manifests as a dry, hacking cough, day or night, which can continue for several weeks
   - Bronchial provocation is negative

2 *Asthma

3 Bronchiectasis
4 Intralumenal, e.g. foreign body, broncholith
5 Peribronchial, e.g. nodes, thyroid
6 Endobronchial neoplasm
7 Smoking
8 Eosinophilic bronchitis
    - Sputum eosinophilia >3% of non-squamous cells
    - No history of asthma
    - No evidence of airways obstruction on spirometry or PEFRs
    - Negative methacholine challenge test
    - Good response to inhaled steroids

Parenchyma

- Interstitial lung disease, e.g. early UIP, sarcoid, pneumocystis

Pulmonary vascular disease

- Pulmonary venous hypertension with early interstitial edema, e.g. mitral stenosis, LV failure

Gastro-esophageal

1 *Gastro-esophageal reflux
2 Dysphagia, structural or functional, with recurrent aspiration
3 Tracheo-esophageal/broncho-esophageal fistula

Drugs, e.g. ACE inhibitors, β-blockers, others

Psychogenic

Work-Up

1 History, physical, chest X-ray, PFTs
2 Evidence of asthma
    - Serial peak expiratory flows with >20% diurnal variation
    - Airways obstruction on spirometry with bronchodilator response
    - Positive methacholine challenge test with >20% decrease in FEV_1 at 8 mg/ml or less
    - Positive allergen skin prick tests

3 GI assessment with barium swallow, endoscopy, esophageal pH and manometry
4 CT scan for
   - Early ILD
   - Bronchiectasis (HRCT)
   - Endobronchial, e.g. carcinoma or intralumenal disease, e.g. broncholiths
5 Bronchoscopy
   - Normal chest X-ray with absence of improvement in cough on treatment for post-nasal drip, asthma, GERD; discontinuation of smoking; patient not taking ACE inhibitors
6 Echocardiogram to assess LV function, mitral valve
7 Sputum for eosinophils (asthma, eosinophilic bronchitis), lipid-laden macrophages (chronic aspiration)

'COUGHED UP SOMETHING'

Intralumenal

1 Foreign body, e.g. tooth, bone, peanut
2 Worm, e.g. ascaris, hydatid
3 Mucus plug
   - Expectoration of casts of the bronchial tree is termed 'plastic bronchitis' and can be seen with
     - Asthma
     - ABPA
     - Bronchiectasis
     - Cystic fibrosis
     - Pneumonia
     - Alveolar proteinosis
     - Idiopathic
4 Blood clot
5 Purulent material

Intramural

6 Tissue from a polyp, benign or malignant neoplasm

Extramural

7 Broncholith
8 Food or secretions secondary to a tracheo-esophageal or broncho-esophageal fistula
9 Hair from a mediastinal cystic teratoma

Parenchymal

10 Bronchorrhea with alveolar cell carcinoma
11 Gelatinous material in alveolar proteinosis
12 Microliths in alveolar microlithiasis
13 Melanoptysis (jet-black sputum), e.g. progressive massive fibrosis of CWP, cocaine inhalation, melanoma, *Aspergillus niger* infection

Gibson, P.G., Hargreave, A., Girgis-Gabardo, M. et al. (1995) Chronic cough with eosinophilic bronchitis: examination for variable airflow obstruction and response to corticosteroid. *Clin. Exp. Allergy* **25**: 127–132.

Irwin, R.S., Curley, F.G., French, C.L. (1990) Chronic cough: the spectrum and frequency of causes, key components of the diagnostic evaluation, and outcome of specific therapy. *Am. J. Resp. Crit. Care Med.* **141**: 640–647.

Brightling, C., Ward, R., Kah Lay Goh et al. (1999) Eosinophilic bronchitis is an important cause of chronic cough. *Am. J. Resp. Crit. Care Med.* **160**: 406–410.

28 Cyanosis

Definition: Blue discoloration of the skin with a differential diagnosis which includes

1. **Central cyanosis** where arterial hypoxemia is present with 5 gm % of reduced hemoglobin and caused by
   - Pulmonary disease, i.e. shunt, V/Q mismatch, diffusion impairment, hypoventilation
   - Right-to-left shunts, cardiac or extracardiac
2. **Peripheral cyanosis** where arterial oxygen level is normal and seen with
   - Hypotension or shock
   - Peripheral arterial obstruction
   - Raynaud's
3. **Cold agglutinins** can cause acrocyanosis from blood agglutination in veins with purplish discoloration of nose, ears and extremities
4. **Methemoglobinemia** occurs when >1% of hemoglobin is oxidized to the ferric form (which cannot bind oxygen), resulting in normal P_aO_2, low O_2 sats, ↑ methb levels
   - Methb levels >1.5 gm % result in cyanosis (i.e. 10% of a normal Hb level) and causes include:
     - Congenital, e.g. cytochrome b5 reductase deficiency, M – hemoglobins
     - Acquired, e.g. drugs, toxins
5. **Sulfhemoglobinemia** from drugs, toxins
6. **Pseudocyanosis** from hemochromatosis, argyria, fluorescent lighting

Baum, G.L., Crapo, J.D., Celli, B.R., Karlinsky, J.B. (eds) (1997) Textbook of Pulmonary Diseases, 6th edn.: Lippincott-Raven.
Fishman, A.P., Elias, J.A., Fishman, J.A., Grippi, M.A., Kaiser, L.R., Senior, R.N. (1998) *Fishman's Pulmonary Diseases and Disorders*, 3rd edn.: McGraw-Hill.

29 Cystic-cavitary Disease

Definition: Areas of lucency with well-defined walls and can be caused by a diverse group of pathologies including

- Blebs
- Bullae
- Cysts
- Cavities
- Pneumatoceles
- Lung gangrene
- Cystic bronchiectasis
- Honeycombing

*Bullae, cysts and thin-walled cavities are difficult or impossible to distinguish at times

Radiologically they can be completely air-filled, air–fluid, or fluid-filled, the latter not being distinguished from a mass lesion on chest X-ray

Clues to identification of the above include size, shape, number, wall thickness, location, central versus peripheral distribution, as well as associated radiologic findings, e.g. nodules, fibrosis, cavity contents

1 **Blebs** are collections of air within or contiguous to the visceral pleura, synonymous with subpleural bullae, and associated with spontaneous pneumothorax formation

2 **Bullae** are defined as thin-walled air containing spaces greater than 10 mm in diameter with walls <1 mm thick. They are seen in parenchymal disorders including
   - Primary bullous disease (see p. 166)
     – Defined as multiple bullae in otherwise normal lung
     – Seen in the upper lobes > lower lobes but pathophysiology is unclear

- Bullous emphysema
- Post-infectious
- i.v. drug abuse
- ankylosing spondylitis
- Late stage fibrosis, e.g. sarcoid, pneumoconiosis (PMF)
- In otherwise normal lungs

Sequelae include

- Progressive but unpredictable enlargement
- Chronic respiratory failure and cor pulmonale
- Spontaneous pneumothorax
- Hemorrhage
- Fungal colonization with aspergillus
- Bacterial superinfection manifest by increasing cough, sputum, often pleuritic chest pain and a new air–fluid level on X-ray, the differential including
  - Lung abscess
  - Fungal infection
  - Tuberculosis
  - Pulmonary hemorrhage
  - Cavitary carcinoma
  - Hydropneumothorax
- Bronchogenic cancer arising within the bullous wall
- Air emboli and sudden death (airliner, scuba diving)
- Disappearance post infection

Chest X-rays are insensitive in diagnosing bullae *vs*. those found on CT scan or at autopsy and are characterized by areas of increasing lucency sharply delineated by fine radiopaque lines (composed of compressed lung +/– pleura)

3 **Pneumatoceles** are defined as thin-walled air containing spaces indistinguishable radiologically from a bulla, cyst or thin-walled cavity

- Most widely used to describe the lesions which develop during the course of staph pneumonia, most often in children

- Similar lesions are seen with other pneumonias, e.g. legionella, gram negatives, as well as post trauma and following hydrocarbon aspiration

4 **Lung gangrene** is defined as ischemic necrosis (usually 2° to pulmonary artery thrombosis) and can involve a portion or an entire lobe
- Typically develops during the course of pneumonia from klebsiella, less commonly pneumococcus, other gram negatives, anaerobes, tuberculosis, aspergillus but also described post trauma or torsion
- Usual presentation is that of an acute bacterial pneumonia which fails to improve on antibiotics, the patient often having severe hemoptysis and features of sepsis

Radiologic features
- Airspace consolidation with small foci of cavitation which coalesce to form a large cavity
- A crescent-shaped lucency which marks the beginning of the separated necrotic material from the cavity wall
- A mass, separated from the wall, sitting within the cavity and changing position as the patient shifts position

5 **Cystic bronchiectasis**

6 **Honeycombing** is defined as multiple ring shadows in close proximity representing airspaces of 5–10 mm in diameter with wall thickness of 2–3 mm

It is typically peripheral in distribution without intervening areas of normal lung and can be seen in the following
- Airways disease, e.g. bronchiectasis
- Parenchymal disorders including
  - UIP
  - Inherited disorders, e.g. neurofibromatosis, familial fibrocystic pulmonary dysplasia, Hermansky-Pudlak syndrome
  - Asbestosis
  - Collagen diseases, e.g. RA, scleroderma

- Drug reactions
- LAM, tuberous sclerosis
- Eosinophilic granuloma
- End-stage sarcoid
- End-stage allergic alveolitis

7 **Cysts** are **defined** as thin-walled air containing spaces whose diameter is >10 mm with a wall thickness between 1–3 mm and can be seen with

Parenchymal disease

- LAM (multiple)
- Eosinophilic granuloma (multiple)
- Traumatic lung cyst
- Echinococcus
- Post-infectious
- LIP
- Pneumocystis
- Honeycombing e.g. UIP (multiple)

*Advanced centrilobular emphysema can mimic multicystic lung disease, e.g. LAM, eosinophilic granuloma, but the areas of low attenuation do not have distinct walls and often contain a "centrilobular dot"

Airways disease

- **Bronchogenic cysts** are congenital anomalies due to a portion of tracheobronchial tree becoming separated during the branching process
  - They are usually asymptomatic until infection supervenes, this occurring in approximately 75% of cases, resulting in one or more of the following
    a. Communication with the tracheobronchial tree and change in radiologic appearance
    b. Hemoptysis
    c. Progressive cyst enlargement and compression of adjacent structures
    d. Rarely, pneumothorax and air embolism
    e. Loss of the respiratory epithelial lining of the cyst with difficulty in identifying its true nature and distinguishing it from an infected bulla or abscess

- Radiologically prior to rupture it is a solitary (rarely multiple), fluid-filled lesion of variable density ranging from water to soft tissue, depending on the cyst contents
- Usually located in the medial third of the lung and often in a lower lobe
- When infection develops, the fluid is replaced with a combination of air and/or pus with the appearance mimicking a bronchopulmonary sequestration or an infected lung bulla

- **Bronchopulmonary sequestration** (see p. 117)
- **Cystic adenomatoid malformation**
  - Congenital malformation, unilateral and usually involving only one lobe
  - Characterized by an abnormal proliferation of terminal respiratory elements resulting in hyperinflation and presentation in the neonate with acute respiratory distress
  - Less commonly presents in infancy or childhood with recurrent infections or an abnormal chest X-ray
  - Radiologically presents as a hyperinflated lobe with a well-defined mass containing air-filled cysts of varying sizes and wall thickness
  - Differential diagnosis includes
    a. Bronchopulmonary sequestration
    b. Multiple bronchogenic cysts
    c. Congenital diaphragmatic lesions

8 **Cavities** are **defined** as thin or thick-walled gas containing spaces, whose walls are >1 mm in thickness

Thin-Walled Cavities

Parenchymal diseases

1 Infectious

- Chronic bacteria – active tuberculosis (often thick-walled); post-treatment tuberculosis; atypical mycobacteria (often thick-walled)

- Fungal – coccidioidomycosis, sporotrichosis, pneumocystis
- Parasitic – echinococcus, paragonimiasis

2 Inflammatory
- Rheumatoid nodules
- Sarcoid

3 Neoplastic
- Cavitary bronchogenic cancer (usually thick-walled)
- Lymphoma (often thick-walled)
- Metastases – cavitate in approximately 4% of cases; usually head and neck primary in males and a genitalia primary in females; upper > lower lobes; multiple other cell types can cavitate including adenocarcinoma, sarcoma, others; may be thin or thick-walled and often associated with lung nodules radiologically

Airways disorders

4 Laryngeal papillomatosis

5 Rarely in BOOP, bronchoalveolar cell cancer

Vascular disorders

6 Septic emboli (thick or thin-walled)

7 Wegener's granulomatosis (initially thick-walled)

8 Rheumatoid nodules (initially thick-walled) but can become thin-walled with resolution

Thick-Walled Cavities – Single or Multiple

Parenchymal diseases

1 *Neoplastic, e.g. carcinoma, lymphoma, metastases, lymphomatoid granulomatosis

2 *Infectious
- Acute bacterial – *Staph. aureus*, gram negatives, anaerobes, rhodococcus, legionella
- Chronic bacterial – tuberculosis, atypicals, nocardia, actinomycosis, *Pseudomonas pseudomallei*
- Fungal – histoplasmosis, coccidioidomycosis, paracoccidioidomycosis, blastomycosis (uncommon), sporotrichosis, mucormycosis, aspergillus, cryptococcus (uncommon)
- Parasitic – amebiasis

3 Inhalational, e.g. silicosis, coal workers' pneumoconiosis
4 Sarcoid
5 Amyloid
6 Inflammatory, e.g. rheumatoid

Vascular disorders

7 Septic emboli (thin or thick-walled)
8 Wegener's granulomatosis
9 Churg-Strauss granulomatosis

Airways disorders

10 Bronchopulmonary sequestration (thin or thick-walled)
11 Bronchocentric granulomatosis (rarely)

Cavitary Contents

1 Air–fluid level, air containing or fluid-filled
2 Mycetoma
3 Blood clot (rapidly developing intracavitary foreign body radiologically resembling a mycetoma)
4 'Water-lily' sign of echinococcus
5 Lung gangrene (irregular mass in a lung cavity developing during the course of pneumonia)

Fraser R.S., Muller N.L., Colman N., Paré P.D. (1999) Diagnosis of Diseases of the Chest 4th Edn., WB Saunders.

Naidich, D.P., Zerhouni, E.A., Siegelman, S.S. (1998) *Computed Tomography and Magnetic Resonance of the Thorax*, 3rd edn. New York: Raven Press.

Moss, A., Gamsu, Genant (1992) Thorax and neck. In: *Computed Tomography of the Body with Magnetic Resonance Imaging.* 2nd edn. vol. 1.: W.B. Saunders.

Webb, R., Muller, N.L., Naidich, D.P. (1996) *High Resolution CT of the Lung*, 2nd edn.: Lippincott-Raven.

Takasugi, J., Goodwin, J. (1998) Radiology of chronic obstructive pulmonary disease. *Radiol. Clin. North Am.* **36**: 29–55.

Webb, R. (1994) HRCT of obstructive lung disease. *Radiol. Clin. North Am.* **32**: 745–755.

Goodwin, D., Webb, W.R., Savoca, C., Konstan, M. et al. (1980) Review of multiple thin-walled cystic lesions of the lung. *AJR* **135**: 593–604.

30 Cystic Fibrosis (CF) – Diagnostic Features

Most common lethal autosomal recessive disease affecting caucasians

- Monogenic disease with the carrier frequency ~1 in 25 in the white population but rare among Asians and African blacks
- Disease is caused by mutations in the cystic fibrosis gene on the long arm of chromosome 7 encoding for the cystic fibrosis transmembrane regulator (CFTR) protein
- The latter normally functions as a chloride channel at the apical membrane of secretory epithelial cells
- More than 700 mutations of the CF gene have been described, 70% being the Δ F508 mutation
- Individuals born today can expect a survival of ~40 years and therefore CF is no longer a pediatric disease
- Pulmonary disease is responsible for most of the morbidity and mortality

Clinical features of respiratory disease

Lung disease is the presenting feature of CF in ~40% of cases, with ~70% of patients diagnosed by age 1

- Cough is initially intermittent, then chronic and productive, with acute exacerbations
- Airways inflammation and infection, particularly with *Staph. aureus*, pseudomonas, aeruginosa, *Haemophilis influenzae* and *Burkholderia cepacia*, result in bronchitis, bronchiolitis and bronchiectasis
- The above, plus superimposed bronchial hyper-reactivity, result in clinical features of airways obstruction with dyspnea, wheezing, air trapping, and a 'barrel' chest
- Hemoptysis is common and varies from mild to life-threatening

- ABPA is seen in 5–10% of patients
- Findings of pulmonary hypertension and cor pulmonale result from chronic hypoxemia
- Upper airways disease includes pansinusitis and nasal polyps
- ~10% of patients are diagnosed only as adults, many of whom may not appear chronically ill, the classic features of disease being absent
- Respiratory disease continues to dominate the clinical picture as patients grow older however
  - Sinopulmonary disease may be milder with a slower rate of decline in pulmonary function
  - Gastrointestinal and pancreatic symptoms may be mild or absent
  - Rarely, sweat chlorides may be borderline (40–60 mmol/L) or normal (<40 mmol/L)

Extrapulmonary disease includes

- GI – pancreatic insufficiency, rectal prolapse, meconium ileus, pancreatitis, cholelithiasis, liver disease
- Endocrine – delayed puberty, diabetes mellitis
- Obstructive azospermia
- Sweat chloride >60 mEq/L
- Heat stroke

PFTs reveal obstructive disease with intrapatient variability reflecting fluctuating airways inflammation and mucous plugs

- Lung function deteriorates with age but the pattern and extent are quite variable
- FEV_1 has been correlated with survival and need for a lung transplant (when clinical deterioration documented)

Diagnosis of CF in adults should be considered when the following **respiratory manifestations** are present

1. Bronchiectasis – chronic cough and sputum, recurrent acute respiratory infections, episodes of hemoptysis, which vary from streaking to massive
2. Airways obstruction and wheezing with features of 'asthma' in the presence of diffuse reticular or reticulonodular densities on chest X-ray

3 Persistent colonization/infection with mucoid and non-mucoid *Pseudomonas aeruginosa*, *Burkholderia cepacia*, as well as *Staphylococcus aureus* and non-typable *Haemophilus influenzae*
4 Pneumothorax, often recurrent and due to rupture of sub-pleural blebs
5 Clubbing (universal) and hypertrophic pulmonary osteoarthropathy (5%)
6 Respiratory failure and cor pulmonale as a result of the underlying bronchitis, bronchiolitis, bronchiectasis and fibrosis
7 Sinusitis is seen in >90% of patients and nasal polyps in ~20%
   - Normal sinus films are very unusual in CF
8 Allergic bronchopulmonary aspergillosis is seen in ~10% of patients with CF
9 Radiologic (chest X-ray and HRCT) features as below

Radiologic Findings

1 Chest X-rays may be normal early in the disease
   ↓
2 Small airways inflammation and obstruction
   - Chest X-ray
     – Hyperinflation, initially intermittent and then persistent
     – Nodular or reticulonodular infiltrates, beginning in the upper lobes and extending diffusely
   - HRCT
     – Expiratory air trapping
     – Pattern of mosaic perfusion
     – Centrilobular nodules (secretions in branching terminal airways, i.e. 'tree-in-bud' pattern)
   ↓
3 Bronchial wall thickening, i.e. 'tramlines' and 'ring' signs
   ↓
4 Bronchiectasis (upper lobe predilection) and cyst formation with central bronchi alone involved in about ⅓ of

cases *vs.* central and peripheral bronchi in about ⅔ of cases

5 Associated abnormalities can include
- Mucus plugs with subsegmental, segmental or lobar atelectasis
- Cystic spaces due to bronchiectasis or emphysematous cysts
- Pneumothorax in ~10% secondary to rupture of the above
- Upper lobe predominance, particularly the RUL
- Hilar enlargement due to pulmonary hypertension or lymphadenopathy (~40%) secondary to chronic infection
- Mediastinal adenopathy
- Hyperinflation, mainly in lower lobes

Pathologic Findings

The above are seen in adults dying with CF
1. Organizing pneumonia
2. Areas of acute bronchopneumonia and lung abscesses
3. Mucus plugs
4. Bronchiectasis
5. Bronchiolitis
6. Areas of atelectasis
7. Cyst-like spaces
8. Right ventricular hypertrophy

Sweat Chloride

1. Diagnosis of CF should be made only if there is an elevated sweat chloride concentration (>60 mmol/L) on two separate occasions in a patient with one or more clinical features consistent with the CF phenotype or a history of CF in a sibling
2. 1–2% of patients with the clinical syndrome of CF have a normal sweat chloride
3. Sweat chloride >60 mmol/L are seen in about 4% of normal adults

4 In adults, a value >70 mmol/L discriminates between CF patients and those with other lung disease
5 Elevated levels seen with endocrine disorders, e.g. hypothyroidism, adrenal insufficiency, nephrogenic diabetes insipidus, etc., as well as skin disease, e.g. ectodermal dysplasia, atopic dermatitis

Criteria for Diagnosis

1 Compatible clinical features or history of CF in a sibling **plus**
2 Laboratory evidence of CFTR abnormality
   - Increased sweat chloride concentration by pilocarpine iontophoresis on two or more occasions, **or**
   - Identification of two mutations in each CFTR gene known to cause CF, **or**
   - Demonstration of abnormal nasal epithelial ion transport (*in vivo* increase in nasal potential difference)

Evaluation of Atypical Cases

1 Respiratory microbiology
2 Radiologic assessment for bronchiectasis
3 Evaluation of paranasal sinuses on plain X-rays and CT
4 Quantitative assessment of pancreatic function
5 Male genital tract evaluation with absence of the vas deferens
6 Exclusion of other diagnoses

Fraser R.S., Muller N.L., Colman N., Paré P.D. (1999) Diagnosis of Diseases of the Chest 4th Edn., WB Saunders.

Baum, G.L., Crapo, J.D., Celli, B.R., Karlinsky, J.B. (eds) (1997) *Textbook of Pulmonary Diseases*, 6th edn. Lippincott-Raven.

Davis, P., Drumm, M. (1996) Cystic fibrosis. *Am. J. Resp. Crit. Care Med.* **154**: 1229–1256.

Stern, R. (1997) The diagnosis of cystic fibrosis. *NEJM* **336**: 487–491.

Rosenstein, B. (1998) What is a cystic fibrosis diagnosis? *Clinics in Chest Medicine* **19**: 423–441.

31 Diaphragm

ELEVATED HEMIDIAPHRAGM – DIFFERENTIAL DIAGNOSIS

1 **Supradiaphragmatic**
 - Any cause of reduced lung volume, e.g. atelectasis, infarction, splinting, fibrothorax

2 **Diaphragmatic paralysis**
 - The etiologies of unilateral diaphragmatic paralysis include
   - *Idiopathic in about 60% of cases
   - *Lung cancer
   - Trauma
     a. Non-surgical
     b. Surgical, neck or thoracic
     c. Phrenic nerve cooling
   - Cervical disc disease
   - Primary neurologic diseases
   - Post-infectious, e.g. herpes zoster, polio
   - Vasculitis (mononeuritis multiplex)
   - Mediastinal diseases, e.g. goitre, aneurysm, calcified nodes
 - **Clinically**, about 50% are asymptomatic with the remainder complaining of resting (often underlying

lung disease) or exertional dyspnea, +/– cough, +/– chest pain, +/– orthopnea

- Course of the idiopathic variety is unpredictable with some patients improving significantly
- The presence of symptoms should prompt a search for underlying cardiorespiratory disease or bilateral diaphragmatic involvement

Diagnostic work-up

- Typical radiologic appearance of an elevated, paralysed hemidiaphragm as an accentuated dome configuration on PA and lateral X-rays
- Ultrasound evaluation demonstrating a lack of thickening on inspiration (related to diaphragmatic muscle shortening)
- Sniff test where upward paradoxical motion of the affected diaphragm is seen under fluoroscopy in ~90% of patients
- Absent EMG response to phrenic stimulation in the neck
- CT scan of chest +/– neck +/– abdomen
- Abnormal lung function with slightly reduced vital capacity (~70–80% of normal), reduced $P\mathrm{di}_{\mathrm{max}}$, $P_{\mathrm{I_{max}}}$ ~60% of predicted, as well as increasing hypoxemia and further reduction in vital capacity when supine
- R/O other causes of an elevated hemidiaphragm

3 **Diaphragmatic eventration**

- Congenital absence of all or part of the diaphragm muscle
- Usually asymptomatic with a thin, atrophic and smooth elevated hemidiaphragm on X-ray
- When complete, may be difficult to distinguish from a paralysed hemidiaphragm as it shares the same radiologic signs
- Eventrations are usually partial, right-sided and located anteromedially, with liver filling in the space

- Total eventrations consist of a thin membranous sheet, are less common than partial eventrations, and are almost exclusively left-sided

4 **Subdiaphragmatic**
- Organomegaly, e.g. liver, spleen, stomach, bowel
- Fluid, e.g. ascites, subphrenic abscess (acute or chronic and may be calcified)
- Inflammation, e.g. pancreatitis, cholecystitis

5 **'Pseudodiaphragmatic' mass**, i.e. non-diaphragmatic disease simulating an elevated hemidiaphragm and including
- *Subpulmonic effusion
- Ruptured diaphragm
- Pleural tumor
- Diaphragmatic tumor
- Parenchymal tumor
- Chest wall tumor
- Mediastinal tumor

6 **Scoliosis**
- The raised hemidiaphragm is on the side of the concavity

7 **Decubitus film**
- The raised hemidiaphragm is dependent

BILATERAL ELEVATED HEMIDIAPHRAGMS

1 **Supradiaphragmatic**
- Poor inspiratory effort, e.g. splinting
- Bilateral pulmonary volume loss, e.g. acute pulmonary infarcts, chronic pulmonary fibrosis, bilateral fibrothoraces

2 **Diaphragmatic paralysis or weakness**
- usually seen in association with generalized skeletal muscle weakness due to diffuse neuromuscular disease, e.g. amyotrophic lateral sclerosis, rarely the initial or only muscle involved and etiologies include

- Spinal cord damage, e.g. trauma above C5
- Motorneuron disease, e.g. polio, remote bulbar polio with post-polio syndrome, ALS
- Phrenic nerve involvement, e.g. Guillain-Barré
- Neuromuscular junction disorders, e.g. myasthenia gravis
- Diaphragmatic muscle disease, e.g. SLE, acid maltase deficiency, limb-girdle muscular dystrophy, hypothyroidism, hyperthyroidism

Diagnostic features and workup

- Clinical symptoms of dyspnea and orthopnea which can progress to cor pulmonale and right heart failure
  - Orthopnea may be severe with poor sleep pattern and daytime somnolence
  - Resting tachypnea is worsened when supine, along with signs of paradoxical abdominal motion and often generalized muscle weakness
- Radiologically, there is diaphragmatic elevation with low lung volumes and bibasilar atelectasis but the sniff test under fluoroscopy may not demonstrate paradoxical motion, as active expiration below FRC and relaxation of abdominal musculature during inspiration can result in passive diaphragmatic descent
- Physiological features
  - Reduced transdiaphragmatic pressure is the gold standard (several methods described)
  - Reduced VC with a 25–50% further reduction when supine (*vs.* <10% in normals)
  - Low P_{Imax}
  - Hypoxemia which worsens when supine (secondary to atelectasis)
  - +/– hypercapnia which worsens during sleep
  - Secondary polycythemia
- Diaphragmatic electromyography and phrenic nerve stimulation to distinguish phrenic nerve disease from muscle disease

- R/O systemic disorders which have diaphragm paralysis as a manifestation
- R/O other causes of bilateral elevated hemidiaphragms

3 **Subdiaphragmatic** – any cause of abdominal distension
- Fat
- Feces
- Fetus
- Flatus or pneumoperitoneum
- Fluid, e.g. ascites, bilateral subphrenic abscesses
- Fatal growth (i.e. tumor)
- Organomegaly of the GI tract, GU tract, retroperitoneal structures

4 **R/O bilateral subpulmonic effusions**

DIAPHRAGMATIC HERNIAS

Definition: Transdiaphragmatic evisceration of abdominal contents into the thorax and may be congenital or acquired

1 **Hiatal hernia**
- Most common diaphragmatic hernia and caused by gastric herniation through the esophageal hiatus
- Often asymptomatic but may present with retrosternal burning, hematemesis, melena, anemia or strangulation
- Mass with an 'air–fluid' level is seen in the posterior inferior mediastinum, often projected on PA film as a smooth well-defined shadow in the right lower hemithorax in the plane of the cardiophrenic angle
- Barium study is diagnostic

2 **Morgagni hernia**
- Uncommon in clinical practice, developmental in origin and most often seen in obese middle-aged women
- Majority are right-sided, usually asymptomatic and present as a mass in the right cardiophrenic angle on PA film and retrosternal area on the lateral

- The shadow is occasionally inhomogenous due to air-containing bowel or fat, CT demonstrating herniation of omental fat through the parasternal region
- Most contain only omentum and patients usually remain asymptomatic, although they may present with non-specific respiratory or GI symptoms as well as with strangulation

3 **Traumatic hernias** (see p. 789)
- Trauma may be external, e.g. auto accident, falls, sports injuries, stab/gunshot wounds, or internal, e.g. hyperemesis
- May be diagnosed at the time of injury or its recognition delayed for months or years as patients are often asymptomatic
- Size and position of the rupture determine the hernial contents, which in turn determines its density
- Colon and stomach are most often involved, sometimes accompanied by the spleen and left kidney
- Responsible for ~10% of diaphragmatic hernias but 90% of strangulated hernias
- An alteration in the diaphragmatic contour with visualization of stomach or bowel in the chest is the major clue to diagnosis but other findings include:
  - A curvilinear visceral shadow simulating an abnormally high hemidiaphragm or inability to visualize the diaphragm
  - Contralateral shift of the heart and mediastinum in the absence of a large effusion or pneumothorax
  - Volume loss in the overlying lung with a basilar opacity reflecting atelectasis or parenchymal disease
  - Rib fractures – recent or remote, which may be accompanied by a pleural effusion

Diagnosis confirmed by
- CT or MRI revealing
  - Discontinuity of the diaphragm
  - Herniation of bowel, stomach, liver, omental fat, kidney or spleen
  - Focal constriction of bowel or liver

- Barium studies of the upper or lower GI tract
- Liver scan showing an intrathoracic location
- Pneumothorax following a diagnostic pneumoperitoneum

4 **Bochdalek hernia**

Clinically, they are usually asymptomatic in adults, although complications include bowel obstruction, bowel strangulation and bowel perforation with a resultant pyopneumothorax

Chest X-ray is that of a smooth bulge, 5 cm anterior to the posterior diaphragmatic insertion, left > right, with its density often less than that of the adjacent soft tissues due to its fat contents

- Bochdalek hernia usually contains fat from the omentum or retroperitoneum, as well as abdominal structures herniating through this defect, e.g. kidney, and can simulate an intrathoracic mass
- CT appearance is that of a rounded mass of fat density on the thoracic diaphragmatic surface posteromedially; there is discontinuation of the soft tissue line of the diaphragmatic muscle adjacent to the mass with continuity of the sub- and supradiaphragmatic densities through the diaphragmatic defect

Differential diagnosis includes a diaphragmatic lipoma or eventration (in both the diaphragmatic muscle is intact), a pleural-based pulmonary mass, mediastinal or paravertebral mass

ABNORMAL DIAPHRAGMATIC CONTOUR

1 **Scalloping**

- Smooth arcuate elevations replace the normal diaphragmatic contour
- Results from visibility of the muscle fascicles near their insertion on the lower ribs and seen with hyperinflation and a flat hemidiaphragm
- Asymptomatic and benign

2 **Muscle slips**
   - Meniscus-shaped shadows extending laterally from each hemidiaphragm due to muscle slips originating from the lateral and posterior ribs
   - Caused by the abnormally low descent of the diaphragm on inspiration and disappearing on expiration

3 **Cysts**
   - Congenital intradiaphragmatic, i.e. extralobar sequestration
   - Cystic teratoma
   - Invasive liver cysts, e.g. hydatid, amebic
   - Simple cyst of the diaphragm or liver

4 **Neoplasms**
   - Benign – often asymptomatic with lipoma being the most common
   - Malignant – fibrosarcoma is the most common primary and presents with non-specific respiratory symptoms; metastatic spread occurs via the hematogenous route or by direct extension.

5 **Traumatic rupture**

6 **Bochdalek** or **Morgagni hernia**

7 **Contiguous disease** – pleural, parenchymal, chest wall, mediastinal or subdiaphragmatic

8 **Partial eventration** (hepatic herniation)

9 **Accessory diaphragm**
   - Partial duplication of the right hemidiaphragm with a part or all of the lower lobe between it and the true hemidiaphragm
   - Often seen with the scimitar syndrome

Radiologic Clues to Diagnosis

1 CT demonstration of diaphragmatic defects of traumatic or non-traumatic origin
2 Identification of the thinned diaphragm of eventration on CT

3 Signs of paralysis or eventration
   - Abnormal elevation of a hemidiaphragm
   - Reduced, absent or paradoxical motion
   - Paradoxical movement with the sniff test
   - Mediastinal swing
   - ? Ultrasound
4 Location of hernias
   - Bochdalek hernias are usually left-sided with a 'bump' on the superior aspect of the hemidiaphragm posteriorly
   - Right cardiophrenic angle mass seen with Morgagni hernias
   - Postero-inferior mediastinal mass with esophageal hiatus hernias
5 Density features
   - Air, e.g. bowel identified on barium swallow or barium enema
   - Fat, e.g. lipoma
   - Cystic, e.g. extralobar sequestration, teratoma, invasive liver cyst
   - Kidney (IVP diagnosis) or other soft tissue density
6 R/O diseases of the pleura, parenchyma, chest wall or mediastinum simulating an abnormal hemidiaphragm with the diaphragm itself being normal
7 Identify associated abnormalities involving the airways, parenchyma, pleura, vasculature or chest wall
8 Abdominal ultrasound to R/O subdiaphragmatic pathology
9 Liver scan to diagnose a partial eventration on the right side with hepatic herniation

INCREASED SPACE BETWEEN GASTRIC FUNDUS AND DIAPHRAGM

1 Normal variant with distance <1 cm in ~90% of the population
2 Subpulmonic effusion

3 Diaphragmatic tumor
4 Subdiaphragmatic fluid, e.g. ascites, subphrenic abscess
5 Organomegaly involving the spleen, left lobe of liver, kidney, adrenal, pancreas

Fraser R.S., Muller N.L., Colman N., Paré P.D. (1999) Diagnosis of Diseases of the Chest 4th Edn., WB Saunders.

Naidich, D.P., Zerhouni, E.A., Siegelman, S.S. (1998) *Computed Tomography and Magnetic Resonance of the Thorax*, 3rd edn. New York: Raven Press.

Moss, A., Gamsu, Genant (1992) Thorax and neck. In: *Computed Tomography of the Body with Magnetic Resonance Imaging*, 2nd edn., vol. 1.: W.B. Saunders.

Felson, B. (1973) *Chest Roentgenology*.: W.B. Saunders.

Gottesman, E., McCool, D. (1997) Ultrasound evaluation of the paralyzed diaphragm. *Am. J. Resp. Crit. Care Med.* **155**: 1570–1574.

32 Drug-induced Lung Disease

DIAGNOSTIC CRITERIA

Diagnosis of drug-induced lung disease is more often suspected than proven, as there are no pathognomonic clinical, laboratory, radiologic, lung function, BAL or biopsy findings

Criteria supporting the diagnosis include

1 Temporal relationship, i.e. an appropriate latency period with the diagnosis suspected after exposure to a wide variety of cytotoxic, non-cytotoxic and illegal drugs, particularly if accompanied by a peripheral eosinophilia
   - May be immediate, e.g. heroin-induced pulmonary edema, or delayed making the diagnosis more obscure
2 An appropriate clinical presentation which becomes clearer as more cases are reported for a specific agent
3 Improvement with discontinuation of the drug

Shortcomings of Diagnosis

1. Disease onset can be acute, subacute or chronic, without a relationship between the duration of prior drug exposure and an adverse reaction
2. Adverse reactions may progress after the drug has been stopped and in some cases may occur only years after drug exposure, e.g. BCNU in children
3. Co-factors may interact to produce lung disease, e.g. high FiO_2 and bleomycin leading to ARDS
4. Only a small percentage of pulmonary drug reactions come to biopsy, with numerous drugs producing a similar reaction pattern as well as an individual drug being able to produce more than one pathologic pattern
5. The diagnosis of drug-induced disease is one of exclusion, having ruled out the underlying disease as well as infection

Role of Lung Biopsy

1. Document the histologic pattern, e.g. BOOP, etc.
   - Can be altered by therapy, e.g. steroids reducing eosinophils and making the biopsy atypical
2. Attempt to identify features characteristic of a specific drug, e.g. kayexalate
3. Rule out other processes, e.g. infection, underlying disease
4. Estimate the likelihood of drug responsibility as causative (rare), probable or possible, when clinical and radiologic information are available, otherwise only a histologic pattern will be given

INTERSTITIAL LUNG DISEASE

Interstitial pneumonitis/fibrosis is the most common form of drug-induced lung disease

- Nitrofurantoin, amiodarone and methotrexate are most common but multiple other drugs are described including sulfasalazine, alkylating agents, e.g. busulfan, and cytotoxic agents, e.g. bleomycin

- Correlation with drug dosing or duration is poor and lung disease can develop following any route of administration, e.g. intravesical
- Underlying disease may affect the likelihood of drug-induced injury, e.g. methotrexate-induced disease is more common with underlying rheumatoid arthritis

The **diagnosis** is based upon

1 Clinical features of cough, dyspnea and bibasilar rales developing over days to months
2 Interstitial infiltrates on chest X-ray and HRCT
   - The above can be variable and reflect the underlying pathology, that of UIP, DIP, Hypersensitivity Pneumonitis, Non-specific Interstitial Pneumonitis, rarely BOOP
3 Restrictive pattern on PFTs
4 Exclusion of other causes, e.g. infection
5 Open lung biopsy occasionally

AMIODARONE PULMONARY TOXICITY (APT)

Amiodarone is an iodinated benzofuran derivative used to treat certain life-threatening cardiac arrythmias

- Toxicity is associated with phospholipid cytoplasmic inclusions in many organs, including the lungs, although the above inclusions may be present without toxicity
- Pulmonary toxicity seen in 5–10% of patients with 5–10% of these dying
- Blood levels are neither diagnostic nor predictive of toxicity with risk factors including
  - Pre-existing lung disease as defined by chest X-ray and/or pulmonary function tests
  - Dose of drug given (uncommon with less than 400 mg daily) and the duration of therapy (several months), although there is marked variability in case reports

- Surgery
- Pulmonary angiography

Clinically, it is often difficult to evaluate non-specific respiratory symptoms in patients on amiodarone, as underlying cardiac disease, pulmonary emboli or pneumonia can mimic drug toxicity, presentations including

1 Subacute illness with cough, dyspnea, weight loss and occasionally fever
   - Seen in ~⅔ of cases of toxicity and usually in patients on 400 mg daily for at least two months
   - Chest X-rays show bilateral diffuse interstitial disease

2 About ⅓ of patients present acutely with fever, cough, pleuritic chest pains and dyspnea, simulating infection
   - Differential usually involves pneumonia and thromboembolic disease
   - Chest X-rays reveal airspace disease, generalized or localized
   - The latter distribution can be predominantly peripheral resembling eosinophilic pneumonia, or upper lobe simulating tuberculosis
   - Focal area(s) of consolidation resulting in a mass-like lesion(s) resembling a neoplasm can also be seen
   - Necrotizing lesions and pleural effusions are rarely described

3 Post-operative ARDS within 18–72 hours of surgery (? synergistic effect of high FiO_2) or within 30 minutes of pulmonary angiography

Diagnostic criteria

1 Compatible clinical and radiologic picture

2 Pulmonary function tests reveal restrictive disease, with a 15–20% reduction in DCO from baseline values being the most sensitive indication
   - DCO greater than 85% of predicted excludes toxicity and therefore baseline PFTs are suggested

3 Hyperdensity seen in the lung and liver on CT scan due to the high iodine content of amiodarone, but this does not distinguish toxicity from normal drug accumulation

4 Gallium scan is usually positive (versus the negative scan of CHF)
5 Foamy alveolar macrophages with intracytoplasmic lamellar inclusions on BAL (also seen in the absence of toxicity)
   - Similar lipid-filled inclusions may be found on lung biopsy specimens which may also reveal chronic interstitial pneumonia with fibrosis, diffuse alveolar damage, or BOOP
6 Exclusion of congestive heart failure, pneumonia and pulmonary emboli (often difficult)
7 Beginning resolution of symptoms and findings within days of stopping the drug, with or without the addition of corticosteroids
   - Complete resolution may take a month or more due to the half life of 40–70 days
8 Associated extrapulmonary toxicity may be present including skin rash or discoloration, thyroid dysfunction, neurotoxicity, corneal deposits

BCNU (Carmustine)

BCNU is a nitrosurea, widely used for central nervous system tumors as well as other neoplasms

Risk factors for pulmonary toxicity
- Total dose given with increasing risk over 1400 mg/m^2 but seen after a single dose
- pre-existing lung disease
- abnormal lung function

Pathologically, there is interstitial fibrosis with little inflammation

Clinical presentations
1 Insidious onset of dry cough and dyspnea, developing from one month of initial therapy to after drug cessation
2 Rare reports of fulminant disease with an ARDS picture
3 Rare reports of veno-occlusive disease
Pulmonary function is restrictive with low DCO

BLEOMYCIN

Clinically, the incidence of pulmonary disease is variable depending upon

1. Diagnostic criteria used
2. Underlying risk factors in the patient population including
   - Age greater than 70
   - Cumulative dose greater than 450 units
   - Concomitant radiotherapy
   - High FiO_2 and the use of other chemotherapeutic agents
   - Decreased renal function

Overall incidence of lung disease is about 10% with 10% of this group dying of pulmonary toxicity and presentations including

1. *Insidious onset of cough, dyspnea and fever with bibasilar rales, potentially progressing to chronic progressive fibrosis
2. Acute 'hypersensitivity pneumonitis' picture with cough, dyspnea, fever and peripheral eosinophilia – rare
3. ARDS 18–48 hours post-surgery, ? FiO_2 dependent
4. Acute chest pain syndrome
5. Asymptomatic findings on chest X-ray or biopsy

The course of established disease includes

- Radiologic resolution in 6–12 months and functional resolution in 1–2 years on discontinuing bleomycin
- Steroid responsiveness, particularly those with the acute form of disease
- Slowly progressive interstitial fibrosis or rapidly progressive disease seen in ~2% of patients

Radiologic pattern classically is that of bilateral interstitial reticular disease with lower lobe predominance, which can progress to extensive airspace consolidation

- Often peripheral with frequent involvement of the costophrenic angles

- Less commonly, subpleural nodular densities simulating metastases are seen, with BOOP histologically

PFTs are used to (1) predict subclinical toxicity and (2) monitor fibrosis

- A falling DCO is the most sensitive indicator, followed by reductions in vital capacity and lung volumes
- A 15–20% reduction in the above from baseline values should warn of toxicity

Diagnostic features

1 Compatible history, X-rays, PFTs, histology
2 Atypical cells on BAL may be present
3 Exclusion of infection and tumor recurrence

BUSULFAN

Clinically, pulmonary toxicity is seen in <5% of patients and loosely correlates with total dose >500 mg although other chemotherapy and radiation may enhance toxicity

- Latent period between initiation of therapy and pulmonary disease is quite variable, from months to years, but is often greater than 4 years
- Onset is insidious with symptoms of cough, dyspnea, fever and weight loss
- Progressive disease is frequent with development of fibrosis and mortality rate ~50% reported

Radiologically, there is diffuse bilateral disease with lower lobe predominance

- An interstitial reticulo-nodular pattern is typical and may be associated with airspace consolidation

Diagnostic features

1 Total drug dose usually exceeding 500 mg
2 Compatible clinical and radiologic features
3 Atypical cytology on sputum or BAL
4 Absence of infection or neoplasm on open biopsy, with associated cytologic atypia

CHLORAMBUCIL

Pulmonary toxicity is rarely reported and unrelated to the cumulative dose

- The interval between drug administration and symptoms has varied from months to years, with chronic interstitial pneumonitis being the usual presentation, although there are reports of acute disease
- X-rays reveal bibasilar interstitial reticular disease

Diagnosis is one of exclusion with

1. Compatible clinical and radiologic presentation
2. No evidence of infection or neoplasm
3. Improvement following drug withdrawal and recurrence upon retreatment

COCAINE

Pulmonary complications are described after i.v., snorting or smoking 'crack' cocaine

Parenchymal disease

Several names have been given to an **acute pulmonary syndrome** occurring 1–48 hours following cocaine use, i.e. 'crack lung', eosinophilic pneumonitis, hypersensitivity pneumonitis, interstitial pneumonitis

- Patients present with a combination of dyspnea, chest pain, fever, hemoptysis, hypoxemia and diffuse pulmonary infiltrates, peripheral/pulmonary eosinophilia
- The course of 'pneumonitis' is variable and includes:
  - Spontaneous resolution
  - Improvement with steroids
  - Progression to ARDS

Differential diagnosis is that of other cocaine-induced disorders which can vary from acute to chronic in presentation including

1 Non-cardiac pulmonary edema
2 Cardiac pulmonary edema (ischemia, arrythmias)
3 Infection
4 Alveolar hemorrhage syndrome
5 BOOP
6 Loeffler's syndrome
7 Interstitial pneumonitis

Airways disease

- Upper – sinusitis, septal perforation, epiglotitis
- Lower – cough, black sputum, hemoptysis, dyspnea, chest pains, wheezing, asthma exacerbation, tracheal stenosis from thermal burns

Vascular disease

- Pulmonary edema – cardiac or non-cardiac
- Pulmonary infarction
- Pulmonary artery hypertension
- Talc granulomatosis from adulterants, e.g. talc, silica

Pleural disease

- Pneumothorax, hemopneumothorax

Neurogenic

- Respiratory depression or arrest

Mediastinal disease

- Pneumomediastinum
- Pneumopericardium

Associated Pulmonary Diseases

1 HIV risk
2 Increased incidence of tuberculosis
3 Aspiration due to impaired consciousness

Cocaine-induced Chest Pains – Differential Diagnosis

1 Myocardial ischemia
2 Septic emboli
3 Rhabdomyolysis of chest muscles
4 Acute bronchitis

5 Aortic dissection
6 Pneumothorax
7 Pneumomediastinum
8 Pneumopericardium
9 Hemopneumothorax

CYCLOPHOSPHAMIDE

Clinically, lung disease is seen in <1% of patients and is a diagnosis of exclusion as the clinical, radiologic, biopsy and lung function findings are non-diagnostic

Presentation may be early or late onset with little correlation between drug dosage, duration of therapy, associated chemotherapy or radiotherapy and the development of pulmonary toxicity

1. Early-onset pneumonitis develops 1–6 weeks after drug exposure and patients present with a short duration of symptoms, i.e. cough, dyspnea, +/– fever and fatigue
   - Radiologically non-specific bilateral reticular or reticulonodular densities are seen
   - Clinical improvement is seen on stopping the drug +/– steroid use
2. Late-onset pneumonitis is seen in patients on treatment for months to years
   - Non-specific respiratory symptoms of fever, cough and dyspnea develop insidiously and are accompanied by a restrictive pattern on PFTs
   - Diffuse reticular or reticulonodular infiltrates are often accompanied by pleural thickening
   - A poor prognosis is reported in this group

GOLD

Gold-induced lung disease is manifest as chronic interstitial pneumonitis, bronchiolitis obliterans or BOOP

Chronic interstitial pneumonitis is unrelated to the cumulative dose of gold administered or the gold concentration in lung tissue

- Disease can appear from weeks to years following treatment with a female to male ratio of 4:1
- Symptoms of dyspnea and dry cough may be accompanied by fever and skin rash
- Most patients improve on cessation of therapy but prognosis is variable with occasional disease progression requiring steroid therapy

PFTs are restrictive and labs are non-specific with eosinophilia seen in ~⅓ of patients, liver dysfunction in ~20% and proteinuria in ~20%

Chest X-rays reveal bilateral interstitial or airspace opacities with mid and upper zone predominance while **CT** scans demonstrate alveolar opacities in a bronchovascular distribution

Biopsy is non-specific and the diagnosis is one of exclusion, the major differential being the interstitial lung disease of rheumatoid arthritis

ILLICIT i.v. DRUGS – PULMONARY DISEASE

Differential diagnosis is extensive with potential diseases affecting any anatomic component of the respiratory system (see below)

- These may be complicated by concurrent problems in drug abusers including
  - Smoking, e.g. obstructive lung disease
  - Alcoholism, e.g. cardiomyopathy and CHF
  - Other drug abuse, e.g. cocaine
  - Tuberculosis
  - HIV, e.g. infectious, inflammatory and neoplastic disorders
  - Asthma with increased risk of fatal asthma

Parenchymal disease

1 Infections, including aspiration or other community acquired pneumonia, necrotizing pneumonia, lung abscess
2 Tuberculosis including multidrug resistant disease
3 Bullous disease and precocious emphysema is seen in the HIV ⊕ and ⊖ population, bullae occurring in the upper lobes and lung periphery

Airways disease

4 Recurrent acute bronchitis leading to bronchiectasis
5 Bronchopleural fistula
6 ? BOOP

Vascular disorders

7 Pulmonary edema – cardiac or non-cardiac in origin
8 Septic emboli manifest as nodular or wedge-shaped densities that frequently cavitate
   - Source can be a septic thrombophlebitis or endocarditis
9 Pulmonary artery mycotic aneurysms
   - Thought to develop from septic emboli to the pulmonary arteries or vasa vasorum, the embolic source originating from tricuspid vegetations or a septic thrombophlebitis
   - Respiratory symptoms of fever, dyspnea, chest pains and hemoptysis may accompany chest X-ray findings of a perihilar mass, peripheral nodule, area of consolidation or cavitation, the latter two findings representing contiguous pneumonia
   - Blood cultures are usually positive and associated pulmonary hypertension or tricuspid endocarditis may be present
   - Proximal aneurysms may be seen on echocardiography, with spiral CT, MRI or angiography demonstrating central or peripheral aneurysms
   - The natural history is unclear although about ⅓ are thought to rupture
10 Pulmonary hypertension: primary, e.g. HIV related, or secondary e.g. foreign body granulomas, emphysema, cocaine

11 Silicone pneumopathy is seen in patients who take illicit silicone injections for aesthetic reasons and characterized by silicone emboli in the alveolar capillaries
  - Clinically, patients may be relatively asymptomatic or present acutely within days of the silicone injection with dyspnea, fever and chest pain, accompanied by hypoxemia
  - Massive embolization of silicone can result in death, but the long term sequelae of milder cases is unclear
  - HIV and subsequent opportunistic infection should be ruled out in this patient population
  - Chest X-rays show bilateral patchy infiltrates with low probability V/Q lung scans
  - Transbronchial biopsy of the affected areas can show foreign material within small vessels (foreign body granulomatosis)

12 **i.v. talcosis** is seen in i.v. drug abusers where the talc content, along with cellulose or cornstarch of drugs intended for oral use, cause pathologic findings of vascular thrombosis, interstitial fibrosis, foreign body granulomas, mass lesions and emphysema

   Clinical presentation varies from asymptomatic (most addicts) to sudden death from massive occlusion of the vascular tree
  - Non-specific respiratory symptoms develop in heavy users, reflecting the above pathology, with disease and disability progressing even after cessation of exposure
  - Physical exam may reveal glistening talc deposits in the retina with talc found on biopsy of the liver, spleen, lymph nodes or bone marrow

   Management problems encountered clinically include
  - Airways obstruction
  - Interstitial lung disease reflecting granulomatous inflammation and/or fibrosis
  - Pulmonary hypertension and cor pulmonale secondary to vascular occlusions, interstitial fibrosis and emphysema

- Mass-like parenchymal lesions
- AIDS and related complications

Radiologic findings

- Diffuse micronodulation resembling alveolar microlithiasis is the earliest change, followed by enlargement and coalescence of the opacities in the upper lobes – resembling the progressive massive fibrosis of silicosis
- Pulmonary artery hypertension and cor pulmonale
- Bullae and areas of emphysema developing late in the course of disease

Pleural disease

13 Pneumothorax secondary to attempted injection into the subclavian/interal jugular veins, ruptured bullae or septic emboli
14 Empyema secondary to a lung abscess, bronchopleural fistula, or pneumonia

Chest wall disease

15 Sternoclavicular osteomyelitis or pyoarthrosis

Neurogenic disease

16 Central alveolar hypoventilation progressing to respiratory arrest

Mediastinal disease

17 Lymphadenopathy secondary to tuberculosis or talc
18 Pneumomediastinum secondary to direct injection
19 Acute mediastinitis from chest wall infection

METHOTREXATE (MTX)

MTX is an antimetabolite used to treat neoplasms, psoriasis, and rheumatoid arthritis, with pulmonary disease secondary to

1 **Underlying disease** for which MTX was prescribed, e.g. rheumatoid arthritis and rheumatoid lung, breast cancer
2 **Infections**, either the usual community pathogens or opportunistic agents including
   - Viral, e.g. CMV

- Fungal, e.g. aspergillus, cryptococcus, disseminated histoplasmosis, pneumocystis

3 '**Hypersensitivity pneumonitis**' or a **UIP-like picture** are described unrelated to the dosages used or duration of therapy

- Toxicity is seen with various modes of delivery of the drug including i.v., i.m., intrathecal, local and oral, most cases occurring within 2 years of therapy
- Lung disease rarely progresses to interstitial fibrosis
- There are no pathognomonic clinical, radiologic or laboratory features and diagnosis is based upon
  - Non-specific respiratory symptoms of fever, cough and dyspnea with a subacute more common than an acute onset
    - symptoms can develop days to years following initiation of therapy
  - Clinical and radiologic pleuritis in ~10% of patients
  - Radiologic features of bilateral diffuse/patchy interstitial disease or combined interstitial and airspace disease, lymphadenopathy being rare
  - Granulomatous reaction with bronchiolitis and pneumonitis on biopsy without organisms being seen or cultured
  - Absence of infection on BAL
  - Eosinophilia in about 50% of patients
  - Cinical and radiologic improvement following withdrawal of MTX +/– institution of steroid treatment, but fatalities are occasionally described
  - Restrictive PFTs

MITOMYCIN

Incidence of pulmonary toxicity is <10% and often described when mitomycin is used with other agents, typically in treatment of disseminated gastric or pancreatic adenocarcinoma

- unrelated to the dosage used with reports after an initial course of therapy

Clinical presentations

1 *Subacute dyspnea and dry cough with interstitial pneumonitis and fibrosis radiologically
2 'Hemolytic-uremic syndrome' with renal failure, microangiopathic hemolytic anemia and non-cardiogenic pulmonary edema in patients with adenocarcinoma
3 Sudden onset of dyspnea and acute respiratory failure in patients receiving vinca alkaloids after previous mitomycin therapy, with onset minutes to hours following treatment

NITROFURANTOIN

Acute Nitrofurantoin Toxicity

Responsible for ~90% of cases with symptoms developing within hours to days (or weeks) of treatment and thought to be a hypersensitivity reaction

- Onset is acute and symptoms can include fever, chills, cough, dyspnea, pleuritic chest pain, arthralgias, skin rash
- Chest X-rays reveal diffuse interstitial reticular disease with lower lobe predominance; pleural effusion may accompany the parenchymal disease or occur alone
- Leucocytosis with peripheral eosinophilia in ~80% of cases may be accompanied by pleural fluid eosinophilia
- PFTs reveal restrictive disease
- Lung biopsy shows an acute interstitial pneumonitis which may contain eosinophils in addition to neutrophils and mononuclear cells
- Prognosis is excellent with low mortality and resolution in 4–8 weeks on stopping the drug

Chronic Nitrofurantoin Toxicity

Uncommon and responsible for ~10% of cases, with symptoms developing months to years after treatment

- Severity of the lung disease is related to the dose and duration of treatment
- Onset is insidious with cough and dyspnea

- WBC counts are normal with eosinophilia seen in ~40% of cases and pleural fluid eosinophilia described
- Chest X-ray findings are similar to the acute syndrome but pleural effusions do not occur in isolation
- PFTs reveal restrictive disease
- Lung biopsy may be similar to that seen acutely but may instead show fibrosing alveolitis
- Spontaneous resolution of disease can occur but progressive fibrosing alveolitis is described even after discontinuation of nitrofurantoin and an overall mortality of ~10% is described

PENICILLAMINE

Pulmonary disease is rarely described but reports include

1. Bronchiolitis obliterans with most cases described in rheumatoid arthritis
2. Drug-induced lupus
3. Pulmonary-renal syndrome with alveolar hemorrhage and a presentation similar to Goodpasture's syndrome but absence of AGBM antibodies
4. UIP-like reaction with clinical symptoms, PFTs and X-rays similar to those of fibrosing alveolitis
5. Hypersensitivity pneumonitis-like picture with eosinophilia

RETINOIC ACID SYNDROME

All-transretinoic acid is used to treat promyelocytic leukemia and can result in the retinoic acid syndrome 2–21 days after initiation of treatment

- Presentation is acute with dyspnea, fever, recent weigh gain
- Intrathoracic findings include diffuse alveolar hemorrhage as well as pleural or pericardial effusions

- Chest X-ray findings are those of bilateral diffuse alveolar or interstitial infiltrates, manifest histologically by neutrophilic or leukemic infiltrates with alveolar hemorrhage
- DIC often accompanies the lung disease in addition to associated fever, fluid retention, thrombotic events and multiple hemorrhages

STEROIDS

Airways

- Oropharyngeal and laryngeal candidiasis

Parenchyma

- Infections including tuberculosis, pneumocystis, aspergillus, cryptococcus, generalized varicella, others

Vasculature

- Fat emboli
- Systemic hypertension with secondary CHF

Chest wall

- Steroid myopathy
- Obesity

Mediastinum

- Mediastinal lipomatosis

Fraser R.S., Muller N.L., Colman N., Paré P.D. (1999) Diagnosis of Diseases of the Chest 4th Edn., WB Saunders.

Baum, G.L., Crapo, J.D., Celli, B.R., Karlinsky, J.B. (eds) (1997) Textbook of Pulmonary Diseases, 6th edn.: Lippincott-Raven.

Fishman, A.P., Elias, J.A., Fishman, J.A., Grippi, M.A., Kaiser, L.R., Senior, R.N. (1998) *Fishman's Pulmonary Diseases and Disorders*, 3rd edn.: McGraw-Hill.

Cooper, A., White, D., Matthay, R. (1986) Drug-induced pulmonary disease. *ARRD* **133**: 321–340.

Martin, W.J., Roseman, E.C. (1988) Amiodarone pulmonary toxicity. *Chest* **93**: 1067–1076.

Albertson, T., Walby, W., Derlet, R. (1995) Stimulant-induced pulmonary toxicity. *Chest* **108**: 1140–1149.

Rosenow, E.C. (1972) The spectrum of drug-induced pulmonary disease. *Ann. Internal Med.* **77**: 977–991.

Rosenow, E.C., Myers, J.L., Swensen, S., Pisani, R. (1992) Drug-induced pulmonary disease. An update. *Chest* **102**: 239–250.

Aronchick, J., Grefter, W. (1995) Drug-induced pulmonary disorders. *Semin. Roent.*: 18–34.

Haim, D., Lippmann, M., Goldberg, S. *et al.* (1995) The pulmonary complications of crack cocaine. *Chest* **107**: 233–239.

Cregler, L., Mark, H. (1986) Medical complications of cocaine abuse. *NEJM* **315**: 1495–1500.

Tashkin, D., Khalsa, M., Gorelick, D. *et al.* (1992) Pulmonary status of habitual cocaine smokers. *ARRD* **145**: 92–100.

Malik, S., Myers, J., DeRemee, R. *et al.* (1996) Lung toxicity associated with cyclophosphomide use. *Am. J. Resp. Crit. Care Med.* **154**: 1851–1856.

33 Dyspnea – Normal Chest X-ray

1 **Airways**
- Upper airways obstruction (see p. 829)
- Tracheomalacia
- Lower airways obstruction: localized, e.g. endobronchial lesion
  generalized, e.g. bronchiolitis obliterans, COPD, asthma

2 **Parenchyma**
- Interstitial disease, e.g. sarcoid, UIP, allergic alveolitis, early PCP
- Early acute airspace disease, e.g. pulmonary edema, ARDS, pneumonia
- Emphysema, bullous disease

3 **Pleura**
- Pleural effusions may be seen only on CT
- Subtle asbestos-related pleural plaques

4 **Vascular**
- Pulmonary
  - Arterial, e.g. emboli: thrombus, fat, tumor; pulmonary hypertension, vasculitis
  - Capillary, e.g. early miliary disease
  - Arteriovenous shunts, e.g. cirrhosis
  - Venous, e.g. veno-occlusive disease
- Great vessels, e.g. SVC or IVC obstruction

5 **Hematologic**
- Anemia
- CO poisoning
- Methemoglobinemia

6 **Neuromuscular**

- Neurologic, e.g. Guillain-Barré, diaphragmatic weakness/paralysis as in SLE
- Neuromuscular, e.g. myasthenia gravis
- Muscular
  - Inherited, e.g. muscular dystrophies, metabolic myopathies, familial periodic paralysis, congenital nemaline red myopathy
  - Acquired, e.g. SLE, polymyositis, hypo/hyperthyroidism, steroid induced, hypokalemia, rhabdomyolysis

7 **Chest wall**

- Any cause of abdominal distension and interference with normal diaphragm function, e.g. obesity, ascites

8 **Mediastinum**

- Fibrosing/granulomatous mediastinitis may present with a normal chest X-ray in spite of extensive disease

9 **Hyperventilation with normal or elevated PO_2**

- Psychogenic
- Metabolic, e.g. acidosis, fever, hyperthyroidism
- Cirrhosis
- Pregnancy
- Sepsis
- Drugs e.g. progesterone, ASA

10 **Cardiac disease**

- LV dysfunction from ischemia, hypertension, etc.
- Right → Left Shunts
- Left atrial myxoma, ball-valve thrombus, mitral stenosis

11 **Deconditioning**

Fraser R.S., Muller N.L., Colman N., Paré P.D. (1999) Diagnosis of Diseases of the Chest 4th Edn., WB Saunders.

Baum, G.L., Crapo, J.D., Celli, B.R., Karlinsky, J.B. (eds) (1997) *Textbook of Pulmonary Diseases*, 6th edn.: Lippincott-Raven.

Fishman, A.P., Elias, J.A., Fishman, J.A., Grippi, M.A., Kaiser, L.R., Senior, R.N. (1998) *Fishman's Pulmonary Diseases and Disorders*, 3rd edn.: McGraw-Hill.

34 Embolic Diseases

THROMBOEMBOLI

Sources	Clinical clues
90% from the deep veins of legs	DVT
10% from:	
Prostatic, uterine, internal iliacs	Pelvic disease
Renal veins	Hematuria, flank pains
Inferior vena cava	Often none
Right heart chambers	RV infarct, RA or RV dilatation
Right heart valves	i.v. drug abusers
Upper extremities	Trauma
Superior vena cava	SVC syndrome
Internal jugular vein	Anaerobic URI

Table 34.1

DVT Differential

- Superficial phlebitis
- Post-phlebitic syndrome versus recurrent DVT
- Cellulitis
- CHF with edema or other causes of chronic venous insufficiency
- Ruptured Baker's cyst
- Hematoma
- Femoral artery aneurysm
- Lymphadenopathy (groin)

Natural History of Venous Thrombosis

1 Resolution
2 Organization with development of varicose veins or a post-phlebitic limb with edema, pain, skin discoloration and ulceration
3 Proximal extension
4 Embolization with symptomatic pulmonary emboli in about 30% of patients and subclinical emboli in about 20% when acute proximal DVT is untreated

Natural History of Pulmonary Emboli

1 Resolution
2 Organization and recanalization
3 Fragmentation and embolization to more peripheral vessels
4 Thromboembolic pulmonary hypertension, acute or chronic
5 30% mortality if untreated (vs 2% if treated)

Common Underlying Clinical Conditions

1 **Primary or idiopathic**
- Comprises approximately 40% of cases of pulmonary emboli where diagnostic workup fails to identify predisposing factors
- Approximately 10% of patients within the primary or idiopathic group will be diagnosed as having an underlying neoplasm, usually a GI, GU or pulmonary adenocarcinoma
- Trousseau described thromboembolism as a complication of a known cancer or as the first clinical manifestation of an occult neoplasm
- Investigation for malignancy is indicated when there is a clinical suspicion from the history, physical findings or routine labs

2 **Surgery/trauma** characterized by endothelial damage, e.g. hip fracture or replacement, knee replacement, abdominal or pelvic cancer surgery

3 Stasis from **heart failure** or other states including pregnancy, obesity, varicose veins, stroke, paraplegia, intra-abdominal tumors, post-op, sickle cell, hyperglobulinemia

4 Identification of a **hypercoagulable** state should be suspected with
- Thrombosis in patients under age 50 with no obvious risk factor
- Thrombosis in an unusual site
- Recurrent thromboembolism
- Family history of thromboembolism

Patients with thrombophilia, i.e. a tendency to develop **recurrent** venous thromboembolism, fall into two categories (Table 34.2)

Measurable	Non-measurable
• *Resistance to activated Protein C • Anti-thrombin III deficiency • Protein C deficiency • Protein S deficiency • Lupus anticoagulant and anti-cardiolipin antibody • Hyperhomocysteinemia • Dysfibrinogenemias (very rare) • Fibrinolytic disorders (very rare) • Prothrombin 20210A allele • Myeloproliferative diseases with thrombocytosis	• Drugs, e.g. 'pill', chemotherapy • Inflammatory bowel disease • Pregnancy • Malignancy (pulmonary, GI, GU)

Table 34.2

Resistance to Activated Protein C

- Most common cause of heritable thrombophilia
- Protein C is an endogenous anticoagulant protein which normally inactivates factors V and VIII
- A single point mutation in the factor V gene, factor V Leiden, makes it resistant to inactivation by activated protein C (APC)
- Factor V Leiden is seen in ~4% of whites (rare in blacks

and Asians) and in ~20% of unselected patients with DVT, the latter being the most common clinical manifestation

- A heterozygote has about a 5-fold lifetime risk of developing DVT but the risk of thrombosis is only ~20%, with associated genetic and risk factors increasing the incidence, e.g. pregnancy, 'pill', strong family history
- Homozygous patients are at higher risk for thrombosis but only small numbers of patients have been studied
- Testing includes phenotyping (APC resistance) and genotyping (factor V Leiden)

Clinical Presentations

1 **Respiratory system**

Asymptomatic hypoxemia

- ABG or oximeter reveals hypoxemia in the absence of respiratory symptoms
- Workup of the hypoxemia confirms the diagnosis

**Pulmonary infarction*

- Patients present with the acute onset of pleuritic pains which may be accompanied by dyspnea and/or hemoptysis
- Represents occlusion of segmental or subsegmental vessels
- Splinting and a pleural friction are often present on exam
- Chest X-rays show features of infarction

**Dyspnea*

- Physical findings in the lungs are usually negative, typically with normal chest X-rays

Thromboembolic pulmonary hypertension – acute or chronic

- Seen when >50% of the vascular tree is obstructed
- Patients present with progressive dyspnea, cor pulmonale, right heart failure and frequent supraventricular arrhythmias
- Chronic pulmonary hypertension seen as a

complication of <1% of emboli and secondary to recurrent or unresolved pulmonary emboli

Wheezing – rarely

2 **Cardiovascular system**

Angina-like

- Patients present with a clinical picture suggestive of acute cardiac ischemia

Acute hypotension

- Presents with circulatory collapse and severe dyspnea, often with related retrosternal chest pain, occasional cyanosis and syncope
- Represents obliteration of >50% of the pulmonary vascular tree

Atrial fibrillation, new onset, or other supraventricular tachyarrythmia

Sudden death/cardiac arrest

3 **GI tract**

Acute abdomen

- Episodes of acute RUQ, LUQ or epigastric pains can simulate cholecystitis, splenic infarction or hemorrhage, and may be accompanied by an ileus and elevated serum bilirubin

4 **Central nervous system**

- May present with syncope, seizures, altered sensorium, coma, hemiplegia

5 **Paradoxical embolism**

- Paradoxical emboli should be considered in patients with systemic emboli plus
  - A known embolic source in the venous system
  - The presence of a known intracardiac (patent foramen ovale, ASD, VSD) or intrapulmonary (AV malformation) shunt
  - New and severe hypoxemia from the right-to-left shunt

Influences on clinical presentation of pulmonary emboli

- Patient age
- Level of physical activity
- Underlying cardiorespiratory disease and subsequent reserve
- Extent of pulmonary vascular obstruction secondary to embolization and subsequent resolution or organization
- Size and number of emboli as well as the time interval between embolic events

Cardiorespiratory consequences

- Hypoxemia, hypocapnia
- Wheezing
- Atelectasis
- Pulmonary edema
- Pulmonary infarction
- Pulmonary hemorrhage
- Pulmonary hypertension, acute or chronic
- Right ventricular ischemia
- Opening of a foramen ovale with right to left shunting

Mortality with Pulmonary Emboli

1 Pulmonary emboli (~50%)
   - Unsuspected pulmonary emboli typically in patients unable to communicate with MD
   - Suspected but undiagnosed pulmonary emboli, e.g. indeterminate lung scan
   - Diagnosed but inadequately anticoagulated
   - Properly diagnosed and treated but
     - Hemodynamic compromise, i.e. cardiac arrest, hypotension, RV dysfunction with normal blood pressure
     - Right heart thrombi (free-floating)
     - ? free-floating ileofemoral thrombi

2 Underlying heart or lung disease

3 Cancer

4 Stroke

5 Heparin-induced hemorrhage – spontaneous hemothorax, extrathoracic hemorrhage, e.g. GI, GU, retroperitoneum

6 Heparin-associated thrombocytopenia develops in ~5% of patients, 5–12 days after starting therapy
   - characterized by the presence of heparin dependent IgG antibodies which activate platelets and are responsible for the complications
   - 10–20% of these patients will develop thromboses, arterial (75%) or venous (25%), whereas spontaneous hemorrhage is uncommon
7 Other

Differential Diagnosis of Pulmonary Embolism

Vascular disease

1 Dressler's syndrome
2 Aortic rupture or dissection
3 Pericarditis
4 Pericardial tamponade
5 Primary pulmonary hypertension
6 Myocardial infarction
7 Pulmonary artery sarcoma

Parenchymal disease

8 Pneumonia

Pleural disease

9 Pneumothorax
10 Empyema
11 Viral pleuritis
12 Asbestos pleuritis
13 Collagen diseases – SLE, RA

Chest wall disease

14 Costochondritis
15 Rib fracture
16 Musculoskeletal pain

Airways disease

17 Asthma

Mediastinal disease

18 Esophageal rupture
19 Pleuropericardial fat pad necrosis

20 Fibrosing/granulomatous mediastinitis with pulmonary artery or venous thrombosis

Subdiaphragmatic disease

21 Perforated viscus
22 Infarction – spleen, kidney, bowel
23 Inflammatory – pancreatitis, cholecystitis
24 Splenic, subphrenic or pancreatic abscess

Neurologic

25 Anxiety

Diagnostic Work-Up

1 **History and physical** findings including
- Personal history with assessment of risk factors
- Family history
- Compatible presentation
- Embolic source
- Pulmonary hypertension
- Right ventricular dysfunction
- Signs of pulmonary infarction

2 **Chest X-ray** findings

Without infarction are usually normal but abnormalities can include
- Absolute or relative enlargement of a central pulmonary artery
- Abrupt tapering of a central pulmonary artery
- Enlargement of the azygous vein or superior vena cava
- Cardiomegaly secondary to right ventricular dilatation
- Atelectasis secondary to diaphragmatic elevation
- Oligemia

With infarction (seen in approximately 10% of pulmonary emboli) the findings may include the above, plus
- Pleural effusion which is usually small
  - A progressively increasing effusion developing after initiation of therapy should suggest

— Heparin-induced hemothorax
— Recurrent emboli
— Another diagnosis e.g. pneumonia, dissection

- Line shadows which can be secondary to pleural/ parenchymal scars, plate atelectasis or thrombosed arteries and veins
- Pulmonary opacity (Hampton's Hump) defined as a segmental, homogenous, pleural-based density in the form of a truncated cone with its apex pointed toward the hilum, appearing 12 hours to a few days post-pulmonary arterial occlusion
  - Posterior basal segment of the right lower lobe is the most common site
  - Air bronchogram rarely present due to filling of the airways with blood and edema
  - Cavitation is rare and often due to a septic embolus, although aseptic liquifaction of pulmonary infarcts is reported; can mimic the appearance of necrotizing pneumonia radiologically (and clinically)
  - The classic segmental opacity can represent hemorrhage or true tissue infarction but both entities look identical radiologically
  - Hemorrhage typically resolves within 4 to 7 days whereas true infarction may only clear in 3 weeks or more
  - The shadow of a resolving infarct maintains its density and shape while getting smaller (similar to a melting ice cube), and differs from resolving pneumonia where scattered areas of radiolucency render a previously homogeneous density inhomogeneous

3 **ECG changes** are non-specific and include

- T-wave inversion in the anterior leads V_1–V_4 is the most common finding
- S1 – Q3 – T3 pattern, new onset RBBB or right axis deviation, p – pulmonale, seen in <⅓ of patients with massive or submassive pulmonary emboli and acute cor pulmonale
- New onset atrial fibrillation

4 **ABGs** which classically reveal hypoxemia with low or normal PCO_2 but blood gases can be normal (particularly in young patients without underlying cardiopulmonary disease)

5 **V/Q scan** – 98% sensitive, safe, readily available

Shortcomings

- Indirect visualization of pulmonary blood flow with abnormal scans expressed in terms of probabilities only
- The majority of scans are neither normal or high probability and therefore indeterminate (with even high probability scans not demonstrating emboli in up to 40% of cases when the clinical suspicion is unlikely)
- PIOPED study has shown that patients with indeterminate or low probability scans can have angiographically demonstrated pulmonary emboli, especially when associated with a high clinical suspicion of disease
- False positive scan in a patient with a prior pulmonary embolus that has not completely resolved, leaving a residual perfusion defect
- Low specificity with non-embolic perfusion defects potentially secondary to:
  - Airways diseases
    - Local endobronchial lesion, Swyer-James
    - Generalized obstruction, e.g. asthma, COPD
  - Parenchymal diseases
    - Space-occupying process from pneumonia
    - Lung destruction from emphysema
  - Pleural diseases
    - Effusion, fibrothorax
  - Vascular disorders
    - Hypoplasia or absence of pulmonary artery
    - Extrinsic arterial obstruction from bronchogenic cancer, mediastinitis
    - Veno-occlusive disease, primary or extrinsic
  - Chest wall disorders
    - Splinting from rib fractures

6 **Spiral CT**

- Diagnosis of acute PE by non-invasive direct visualization of the pulmonary arteries to the level of the segments, with demonstration of filling defects and 'railway track' signs
  - High specificity with sensitivity for the main, lobar and segmental arteries but improvements in scanner technology are leading to detection of subsegmental emboli
- May demonstrate other diseases not suspected from chest X-ray or V/Q scan
- Follow-up of acute emboli with demonstration of the evolution of chronic changes, e.g. stenosed pulmonary arteries, persistent filling defects with eccentric thrombi, partial recanalization
- ? Diagnosis and assessment of chronic thromboembolic disease

Shortcomings

- Complications of i.v. contrast, e.g. allergic reactions, renal dysfunction
- Quality and speed of the scanner influence interpretations
- Unclear frequency of false negative scans due to emboli distal to segmental vessels, as well as their clinical significance, e.g. impaired cardiopulmonary reserve and an identifiable DVT may make these significant
- False negative scans due to parenchymal opacifications that obscure central vessels as well as possible 'blind spots' in the RML and lingular arteries
- False positive scans secondary to lymph nodes

7 **Gadolinium – enhanced MRI**

- Direct visualization of the pulmonary arteries to the level of the segments with high sensitivity and specificity
- Avoids nephrotoxic contrast, non-invasive, no radiation exposure

- Can demonstrate disease which is unsuspected on chest X-ray

Shortcomings

- Not readily available, claustrophobic, metallic implants, e.g. pacemakers
- Incidence and significance of false negative scans distal to segmental vessels is unclear

8 **Pulmonary angiography**
- Gold standard for diagnosis with direct visualization of the pulmonary arterial tree demonstrating cut-offs or filling defects
- Today it is mainly used in patients with a high clinical suspicion of PE, indeterminate lung scan, but negative leg dopplers and negative spiral CT (where only the central vessels were adequately visualized)
- As CT scanner technology improves and visualization of subsegmental vessels is appreciated, the role of pulmonary angiography may be questioned
- Differential diagnosis of filling defects includes pulmonary emboli, *in situ* thrombosis, pulmonary artery tumor (e.g. sarcoma), secondary tumors (e.g. intracardiac sarcoma, lung, mediastinum, extrathoracic), granulomatous or fibrosing mediastinitis

Shortcomings

- Invasive, requiring pulmonary artery catheterization, not universally available, radiation exposure
- Contrast material required with potential side-effects of nephrotoxicity, cardiotoxicity, hypersensitivity
- Associated with morbidity of approximately 1.5% and mortality of approximately 0.3%
- Underlying coagulopathy can result in bleeding
- Frequency and significance of undiagnosed emboli in the distal arterial tree are unclear

9 **Venous imaging** for patients with non-diagnostic pulmonary imaging and/or suspected DVT

a. *Contrast venography*

- Gold standard for diagnosis of venous thrombosis of the upper and lower extremities demonstrating an intralumenal filling defect (most reliable sign) or abrupt cut-off of a deep vein
- Most sensitive test for calf DVT and accurate for the iliac veins (versus IPG or U/S)

Shortcomings

- Invasive and requires i.v. contrast with potential complications of hypersensitivity reactions, nephrotoxicity, cardiotoxicity, phlebitis
- In patients with a history or prior DVT, it may be difficult to diagnose a superimposed acute thrombosis, i.e. identification of a constant intralumenal filling defect

b. *Impedance plethysmography*

- Non-invasive, safe, portable test for diagnosis of lower (not upper) extremity DVT
- Evaluates the rate of venous return from the lower extremity and can detect the increased venous outflow resistance in DVT
- Can also diagnose recurrent DVT if IPG normalization has been documented following a prior DVT

Shortcomings

- Operator dependent
- False negatives are seen with most calf thrombi (~20% positive) and proximal thrombi not reducing venous outflow
- False positives are seen in non-thrombotic disorders reducing venous return from the legs, e.g. pelvic or abdominal pathology, increased central venous pressure, reduced arterial flow

c. *Duplex ultrasound*

- Safe, portable, non-invasive test for symptomatic proximal DVT of the lower and upper extremity
- A transducer applied over the length of the vein

normally can demonstrate complete compression of normal opposing venous walls, with non-compressibility of a vein being the most reliable sign of acute DVT
- Can diagnose other pathology simulating DVT

Shortcomings
- Operator dependent
- Venous compression may be limited by obesity, edema, casts, extrinsic compression of a vein, e.g. pelvic mass
- Less sensitive for iliac veins, calf DVTs as well as asymptomatic proximal DVTs
- Diagnosis of recurrent DVT as ultrasound may not return to normal after an acute DVT

d. *MRI*
- Safe, specific, sensitive test for diagnosis of DVT involving the upper extremity, IVC, non-iliac pelvic veins, iliacs, proximal leg veins
- ? Distinguish acute from chronic DVT
- Can also diagnose pulmonary emboli

Shortcomings
- Those of MRI, i.e. claustrophobia, metallic devices, massive obesity
- Less accurate for calf DVT

10 **Echocardiography**
- Trans-esophageal echo can demonstrate thrombus in the main pulmonary artery
- Demonstration of intracardiac thrombi including
  - Immobile mural thrombus, which has a good prognosis
  - Mobile and 'snake-like' thrombi which carry a high mortality with heparin and require thrombectomy or thrombolysis
- Demonstration of a patent foramen ovale with the risk of a right-to-left shunt and subsequent paradoxical emboli

- Demonstration of RV hypokinesis and dilatation
  - As a predictor of high mortality from pulmonary emboli, in the absence of RV infarction
  - May support the clinical suspicion of an acute massive pulmonary embolus

11 **D-dimer**, a breakdown product of the action of plasmin on cross-linked fibrin, and therefore a marker for acute thrombosis
- Present shortcomings include: variability of the assays, overlap of values in normals and patients with thrombosis, elevated levels in many non-thrombotic disorders including infections, neoplasms, rheumatologic disorders, etc.
- Its role as a screening test is still unclear

FAT EMBOLI

Definition: Globules of free fat in the vasculature

The most common sources of fat emboli are
- Bone marrow, e.g. *long bone/pelvic/hip fractures, *external cardiac massage, sickle cell disease, seizures, replacement arthroplasty, acute osteomyelitis

Other sources include
- Liver secondary to alcohol, poisons, steroids
- Limbs, e.g. crush injury, liposuction
- Intravenous, e.g. hyperalimentation
- Others, e.g. pancreatitis, diabetes, extracorporeal circulation

Clinically, fat embolism is most common in the elderly post-hip fracture or anthroplasty, and in younger adults post-leg fracture
- Symptoms typically begin 1–2 days post injury with involvement of the following organ systems

Cardiorespiratory — Asymptomatic

	— Non-specific respiratory symptoms
	— Cyanosis, ARDS, cor pulmonale, systemic hypotension
CNS	— Varies from an altered sensorium to coma
Skin	— Petechiae mainly involving the anterior axillary folds
Kidneys	— Lipiduria
Eyes	— Conjunctival petechiae, retinal scotomata

Chest X-rays vary from normal (majority of cases) to patchy, bilateral diffuse airspace disease progressing to ARDS
- The distribution is diffuse and symmetric with resolution in 7–10 days

V/Q scans show mottled subsegmental perfusion defects with preservation of ventilation

Diagnosis is clinical-radiologic, the sensitivity and specificity of fat droplets in alveolar macrophages on BAL being unclear

Differential diagnosis includes lung contusion which appears immediately post-trauma, is often asymmetric in distribution, and resolves within 24–36 hours

SEPTIC EMBOLI

Definition: Embolized thrombus contaminated by bacteria, rarely fungi or parasites (although secondary infection of bland emboli can give similar pathologic and radiologic features)

Septic emboli can arise from
- Septic thrombophlebitis, central or peripheral
  - Skin infections
  - Infection of the pelvis, pharynx (see Lemierre's syndrome p. 614), bones or other organ systems

  - Infected in-dwelling line such as a catheter or dialysis shunt
- Heart
  - Tricuspid endocarditis, often in i.v. drug users
  - Congenital heart disease, e.g. VSD

Clinically, a predisposing factor is usually present including i.v. drug abuse, congenital heart disease, skin infection, immunocompromised host, with *Staph. aureus* and then streptococcus being the most common organisms

- Clinical features are those of pulmonary thromboembolic disease with accompanying fever, hemoptysis and purulent sputum

Chest X-ray findings

1 Multiple bilateral parenchymal nodules
2 Patchy airspace disease resembling bronchopneumonia
3 Migratory nature to the above infiltrates
4 Cavitation is frequent and may be associated with a 'target sign', i.e. pieces of necrotic lung within a cavity, simulating a mycetoma or invasive aspergillosis
5 Pleural effusions

CT findings

1 Multiple nodules or subpleural wedge-shaped opacities
2 Frequent cavitation
3 Feeding vessel to the nodule
4 Pleural fluid in ~$\frac{2}{3}$ of cases
5 Occasional hilar/mediastinal lymphadenopathy

TUMOR EMBOLI

Definition: Tumor cells in the pulmonary arteries or capillaries which are not contiguous with metastatic foci

- Tumor emboli seed the systemic circulation and embolize to the lungs via
  - Liver metastases and hepatic vein invasion
  - Venous invasion at the site of the primary tumor
  - The thoracic duct

- Most tumor emboli are microscopic with large emboli typically described in hepatoma or choriocarcinoma, although vascular obstruction occurs due to the tumor itself as well as thrombosis from tumor induction of the coagulation cascade
- The above may be accompanied by intimal proliferation, fibrosis and medial hypertrophy further occluding the pulmonary arterial tree
- May be the initial manifestation of a neoplasm but more often occurs with established malignancy
- Venous thromboembolism may complicate underlying neoplastic disease, making the diagnosis of tumor emboli very difficult
- Blockage of the pulmonary arteries by tumor can be seen with
  - Carcinomas, e.g. lung, breast, GI, GU, etc.
  - Sarcomas, e.g. pulmonary artery sarcoma, right atrial sarcoma, chondrosarcoma
  - Myxoma, e.g. cardiac
  - Melanoma

Clinical presentations

- Progressive dyspnea, ranging in duration from days to months
- 'Pulmonary infarct' with chest pains and hemoptysis
- Hypoxemia and unexplained pulmonary hypertension progressing to cor pulmonale
- DIC
- Sudden death
- Incidental finding at autopsy in about 50% of cases

Radiologic findings

1. Normal chest X-rays
2. Enlargement of the pulmonary arteries/right ventricle
3. Features of pulmonary infarction with infiltrates, atelectasis and pleural effusions
4. Lymphangitic carcinomatosis is often present concurrently

V/Q scan findings

1 Microemboli are manifest as multiple, small, peripheral, subsegmental defects with normal ventilation (similar to primary pulmonary hypertension)
2 Macroemboli present with larger perfusion defects as seen with venous thromboembolism and an accompanying normal ventilation scan
3 Normal scan

Pulmonary angiography

- Large emboli present as filling defects, but the typical microscopic emboli do not reveal any abnormality

Diagnostic Work-Up

1 Suspect the diagnosis in a patient with a known primary neoplasm presenting with
    - Dyspnea
    - Pulmonary infarction
    - Pulmonary hypertension
    - DIC
    - Non-resolution of perfusion defects on a V/Q scan after heparin therapy
2 HRCT scan to R/O accompanying lymphangitic cancer
3 Echocardiogram looking for intracardiac tumor/clot
4 Right heart and pulmonary artery angiogram to visualize
    - Thrombus
    - Tumor, e.g. right atrial myxoma, pulmonary artery sarcoma
5 Right heart catheter and sampling of pulmonary capillary blood for cytology
6 Angioscopy for direct visualization and biopsy of tumor in the central pulmonary artery
7 Abdominal ultrasound/CT visualizing the tumor source extending into the renal veins, hepatic veins or IVC
8 Gold standard is lung biopsy

AIR EMBOLISM

Systemic air embolism results from air entering the pulmonary venous circulation, e.g. status asthmaticus, thoracocentesis, needle biopsy, ascent while breathholding during scuba diving in patients with bullous disease

- Clinically, patients present with CNS disease, e.g. coma, convulsions, death, and/or cardiac disease, e.g. acute ischemia, hypotension, arrhythmias
- Radiologically, air is seen in the left heart chambers, intracerebrally or in other systemic arteries

Pulmonary air embolism results from air entering the systemic circulation, e.g. surgery (ENT, neurosurgery), air insufflation procedures, intravenous therapy, CVP insertion, obstetrics, and its passing into the pulmonary circulation

- Clinical features include increased permeability pulmonary edema, systemic hypotension, acute pulmonary hypertension, sudden death and paradoxical systemic emboli
- Air in the right heart chambers and pulmonary arteries as well as enlargement of the central pulmonary arteries may be seen on chest X-ray or CT
- Echocardiography can document air in the RV as well as pulmonary hypertension and RV enlargement

Fraser R.S., Muller N.L., Colman N., Paré P.D. (1999) Diagnosis of Diseases of the Chest 4th Edn., WB Saunders.

Baum, G.L., Crapo, J.D., Celli, B.R., Karlinsky, J.B. (eds) (1997) *Textbook of Pulmonary Diseases*, 6th edn.: Lippincott-Raven.

Fishman, A.P., Elias, J.A., Fishman, J.A., Grippi, M.A., Kaiser, L.R., Senior, R.N. (1998) *Fishman's Pulmonary Diseases and Disorders*, 3rd edn.: McGraw-Hill.

PIOPED Investigators (1990) Value of the ventilation-perfusion scan in acute pulmonary embolism. *JAMA* **263**: 2753–2759.

Hull, R.D., Hirsh, J., Carter, C. *et al.* (1985) Diagnostic value of ventilation perfusion lung scanning in patients with suspected pulmonary embolism. *Chest* **88**: 819–828.

Stein, P.D., Hull, R., Saltzman, H. *et al.* (1993) Strategy for diagnosis of patients with suspected acute pulmonary embolism. *Chest* **103**: 1553–1559.

Stein, P.D., Athanasoulis, C., Alavi, A. *et al.* (1992) Complications and validity of pulmonary angiography in acute pulmonary embolism. *Circulation* **85**: 462–468.

Carson, J., Kelley, M., Duff, A. *et al.* (1992) The clinical course of pulmonary embolism. *NEJM* **326**: 1240–1245.

Bassiri, A., Haghighi, B., Doyle, R. *et al.* (1997) Pulmonary tumor embolism. *Am. J. Resp. Crit. Care Med.* **155**: 2089–2095.

King, M.B. (1994) Unusual forms of pulmonary embolism. *Clinics in Chest Medicine* **15**: 561–568.

Remy-Jardin, M., Remy, J. (1999) Spiral CT angiography of the pulmonary circulation. *Radiology* **212**: 615–636.

(Authors) (1999) The diagnostic approach to acute venous thromboembolism. *Am. J. Resp. Crit. Care Med.* **160**: 1043–1066.

35 Empyema

Parapneumonic Effusion

Bacterial pneumonia with spread of infection to the pleura is the most common cause of empyema

1. Frequency of effusion depends upon
   - Underlying organism
   - Extent of investigations, with increasing sensitivity as we proceed from a PA and LAT chest X-ray to a lateral decubitus, chest ultrasound, and finally CT scan
2. Etiologically the majority of effusions are anaerobic or mixed anaerobe/aerobe, with aspiration being the most common pathophysiology
3. Aerobic infections present acutely with symptoms reflecting an underlying pneumonia whereas anaerobic infections often present more insidiously
4. Character of the fluid varies from a sterile exudate to gross pus, with 3 potential stages

Stage I

Exudative stage where the fluid is grossly thin with low fibrin and low WBC count

- pH > 7.4, glucose > 60, LDH < 500
- When fluid is free-flowing there are usually no complications, with good response to antibiotics, i.e. an uncomplicated parapneumonic effusion

Stage II

Fibrinopurulent stage where the fluid is thicker with increasing fibrin levels and higher WBC counts as bacterial invasion of the pleura occurs

- pH < 7.1, glucose < 40, LDH > 1000
- The increasing fibrin levels result in pleural adhesions with fluid loculation as well as pleural thickening and lung entrapment
- Consequences of the above include
  - Single or multiple chest tube requirements
  - Delayed radiologic resolution often with residual pleural fibrosis
  - Prolonged hospitalization
- The above and Stage III effusions are termed 'complicated' parapneumonic effusions

Stage III

Organizing stage is characterized by thicker fluid with increasing fibrin levels as well as fibroblastic proliferation

Associated findings and complications include

1 Pleural thickening which can result in a fibrothorax
2 Pleural calcifications
3 Thickening of the extrapleural soft tissues with increased extrapleural fat and subperiostal bone
4 Empyema necessitans, i.e. a pleurocutaneous fistula
5 Bronchopleural fistula

Diagnostic Work-Up

I. Diagnostic thoracocentesis, using pleural ultrasound if the fluid is loculated

1 Define the presence of an empyema by
  - Gross pus (often foul smelling) +/or
  - Positive gram stain +/or
  - Positive pleural fluid culture (aerobic/anaerobic) +/or
  - pH < 7.1, glucose < 40, LDH > 1000 = complicated parapneumonic effusion (? = empyema) +/or
  - TB, nocardia, fungal or protozoan studies if clinically suspected

2 Document associated findings of malignancy, food particles, elevated amylase, foul odor (50% of anaerobes), differential white count

II. Determine the responsible organism

Specific etiologic agents reflect the primary site of infection (lung is most common) as well as the underlying pathophysiology (aspiration most often)

- *Anaerobes, including actinomycosis
- *Mixed anaerobes and aerobes which include
  - **Strep pneumoniae*, *hemophilus, **Staph. aureus*, *gram negatives
  - Other strep species (e.g. *Strep. pyogenes*), nocardia, *Rhodococcus equi*, legionella
- Tuberculosis
- Fungi
- Amebae (rarely)

III. Document the radiologic features of empyema

Chest X-ray

1 Pleural fluid collections are usually vertically oriented
2 Pleural fluid collections are homogenous, have a convex medial border with tapering margins, and form an obtuse angle with the chest wall
3 Air is uncommon and may be secondary to
  - Bronchopleural fistula
  - Gas-forming organisms
  - Esophageal rupture
  - Iatrogenic
4 Air–fluid level widths are usually very different on PA and lateral films

CT scan

1 Characterizes the pleural fluid
  - Free, dependent, lenticular in appearance and conforms to the shape of the chest wall
  - More often loculated with demonstration of multiple individual pockets, the fluid being circumferential and non-dependent in distribution

2 Compression and distension of adjacent lung are common as an empyema enlarges and occupies over 10% of a hemithorax, resulting in displacement of airways and vessels
3 With i.v. contrast, the enhancing wall of an empyema cavity is smooth with uniform thickening of the separated visceral and parietal pleura, i.e. split pleura sign
4 Progressive thickening of the pleura occurs with time forming a thick pleural peel which can resolve medically or require surgery
5 Adjacent extrapleural soft tissue swelling is common with increasing extrapleural fat, subperiosteal new bone formation and pleural calcifications seen in a chronic empyema
6 CT features that indicate a possible source of the empyema
   - Parenchymal abscess, infected bulla or pneumonia
   - Bronchiectasis, obstructing lesion, bronchopleural, broncho-esophageal or tracheo-esophageal fistula, bronchopulmonary sequestration
   - Esophageal disease, e.g. rupture, obstruction, dilatation
   - Contiguous disease in the liver, spleen, bones, subdiaphragmatic region
   - Mediastinal disease, e.g. air, tumor, suppuration or lymphadenopathy
7 Guide interventional procedures

IV. Distinguish from an abscess cavity (see Abscess of Lungs, p. 12) and from **necrotizing pneumonia**, the latter characterized by
- Chest X-ray
  – Airspace consolidation with areas of cavitation
  – Poorly marginated
- CT scan
  – No surrounding wall seen after i.v. contrast
- Caveats
  – An abscess and an empyema may co-exist
  – In a small percentage of cases differentiation is impossible in spite of the radiologic features
  – Occasionally, even at surgery, differentiation is difficult

V. Determine the likely source of the empyema by history, physical, radiologic studies

- Airways
  - Bronchiectasis
  - Post-obstructive, e.g. malignancy
  - Tracheo-esophageal fistula
  - Broncho-esophageal fistula
  - Bronchopleural fistula
  - Bronchopulmonary sequestration
- Parenchyma
  - Abscess
  - *Pneumonia (most common cause)
  - Infected bulla or cyst
- Vascular
  - Septic emboli
  - Septicemia
- External causes
  - Post-thoracocentesis, thoracoscopy or thoracotomy
  - Trauma
- Contiguous spread
  - Esophageal rupture (elevated amylase and food particles)
  - Liver
  - Spleen
  - Subdiaphragmatic
  - Vertebral or rib osteomyelitis
  - Pharynx
  - Mediastinal suppuration

VI. Failure to respond to antibiotic and chest tube drainage should suggest

- Non-functioning chest tube due to improper position, obstruction, thick pleural fluid
- Multiloculated fluid collections which are not being drained
- Pleural peel with inability of the lung to expand and obliterate the pleural space

- Bronchial obstruction
- Bronchopleural fistula
- Inappropriate antibiotic choice or dose

Fraser R.S., Muller N.L., Colman N., Paré P.D. (1999) Diagnosis of Diseases of the Chest 4th Edn., WB Saunders.

Naidich, D.P., Zerhouni, E.A., Siegelman, S.S. (1998) *Computed Tomography and Magnetic Resonance of the Thorax*, 3rd edn. New York: Raven Press.

Moss, A., Gamsu, Genant (1992) Thorax and neck. In: *Computed Tomography of the Body with Magnetic Resonance Imaging*. 2nd edn, vol. I. (Place of publication): W.B. Saunders.

Alfageme, I., Munoz, F., Pena, N. *et al.* (1993) Empyema of the thorax in adults. Etiology, microbiologic findings, and management. *Chest* **103**: 839–843.

Sahn, S.A. (1993) Management of complicated parapneumonic effusions. *Am. Rev. Resp. Dis.* **148**: 813–817.

Stark, D.D., Federle M.P., Goodman, P.C. et al. (1983) Differentiating lung abscess and empyema: radiography and computed tomography. *AJR* **141**: 163–167.

Light, R.W. (1995) A new classification of parapneumonic effusions and empyema. *Chest* **108**: 299.

36 Endocrine Diseases – Pulmonary Manifestations

HYPERTHYROIDISM

1 Hypermetabolic state with tachypnea and dyspnea at rest
2 Tracheal obstruction from a goitre
3 Respiratory myopathy
4 Pulmonary edema and pleural effusions from a cardiomyopathy and atrial fibrillation
5 Thiourea induced granulocytopenia with secondary pneumonia
6 Thymic hyperplasia with an anterior mediastinal mass
7 Bulbar palsy with secondary aspiration pneumonia and respiratory failure

HYPOTHYROIDISM

1 Upper airways obstruction secondary to
  - Obstructive sleep apnea
  - Tracheal compression from a goitre
2 Pleural effusion, transudative or exudative, which may coexist with a pericardial effusion
3 Mediastinal goitre presenting as an asymptomatic anterior mediastinal mass or rarely with SVC syndrome
4 Hoarseness
5 Central hypoventilation with hypercapnia

6 Obesity
7 Phrenic neuropathy with secondary dyspnea

THYROID CANCER

Pulmonary involvement is most often seen with anaplastic thyroid cancer but can be seen in ~10% of patients with well-differentiated papillary or follicular tumor

Airways
- Direct tracheal invasion
- Neck mass
- Vocal cord paralysis from laryngeal nerve invasion
- Post-op upper airways obstruction secondary to
  - Hematoma
  - Damage to the recurrent laryngeal nerves
  - Hypocalcemia and stridor from parathyroidectomy

Parenchyma
- Single or multiple nodules
- Micronodular pattern resembling miliary tuberculosis
- Reticulonodular pattern
- Normal chest X-ray (abnormalities detected by CT scan or I^{131} uptake)

Mediastinum
- Hilar and mediastinal lymphadenopathy (may take up I^{131})

DIABETES MELLITUS

1 Acute pulmonary infections
   - Bacterial, e.g. *Strep. pneumoniae*, *Staph. aureus*, gram negatives
   - Fungal, e.g. mucormycosis manifest as cavitary lung disease or lesions in major airways
2 Aspiration pneumonia from gastroparesis and vomiting
3 Tuberculosis, including lower lobe disease in about 10% of patients

4 Pulmonary edema from ischemic heart disease
5 Uremia and secondary pulmonary disease (see p. 717)
6 Nephrotic syndrome with secondary pleural effusions or complicating thromboembolic disease

PHEOCHROMOCYTOMA (PARAGANGLIONOMA)

Neuroendocrine tumor arising from chromaffin tissues of the sympathetic nervous system; adrenal tumors called pheochromocytomas while those of extra-adrenal origin are termed paraganglionomas

- May be confused histologically with carcinoids or small cell carcinoma
- Tumors may be
  - Sporadic or familial
  - Unifocal or multicentric
  - Benign or metastatic
- Occasionally associated with other diseases affecting the lungs, e.g. neurofibromatosis, tuberous sclerosis, Carney's triad
- 90% arise in the adrenals (rarely in other subdiaphragmatic tissues) and are mainly epinephrine secreting, while 10% arise in the chest and predominantly secrete norepinephrine

Pulmonary manifestations

1 Mediastinal paraganglionoma
2 Metastatic parenchymal nodules
3 Metastatic hilar/mediastinal lymphadenopathy
4 Cardiac pulmonary edema secondary to hypertension, catecholamine cardiomyopathy, aortic insufficiency from dissection
5 Non-cardiogenic pulmonary edema
6 Catecholamine-triggered anxiety and respiratory alkalosis

Diagnostic work-up

1 High clinical suspicion with hypertension, arrythmias, pulmonary edema

2 Elevated urinary metanephrine and vanillymandelic acid
3 Elevated serum levels of norepinephrine
4 Radiologic studies including CT, MRI and MIBG-I^{131}

Fraser R.S., Muller N.L., Colman N., Paré P.D. (1999) Diagnosis of Diseases of the Chest 4th Edn., WB Saunders.

Baum, G.L., Crapo, J.D., Celli, B.R., Karlinsky, J.B. (eds) (1997) *Textbook of Pulmonary Diseases*, 6th edn.: Lippincott-Raven.

Fishman, A.P., Elias, J.A., Fishman, J.A., Grippi, M.A., Kaiser, L.R., Senior, R.N. (1998) *Fishman's Pulmonary Diseases and Disorders*, 3rd edn.: McGraw-Hill.

Brussel, T., Matthay, M., Chernow, B. (1989) Pulmonary manifestations of endocrine and metabolic disorders. *Clinics in Chest Medicine* **10**: 645–653.

37 Eosinophilic Granuloma *vs.* Lymphangioleiomyomatosis

EOSINOPHILIC GRANULOMA (EG)

Definition: Idiopathic disorder, usually localized to the lungs, bones or both organs, occasionally widely disseminated, and characterized histologically by clusters of histiocytosis-X (Hx) cells

- The above cells can be identified on light microscopy (characteristic clefted nuclei), immunohistochemistry (stains for S-100 protein and OKT-6) or electron microscopy where the characteristic Birbeck granules (tennis racket shaped) can be seen

Pathologically, the lung lesions evolve through various stages reflected on chest X-ray and CT scan

1 The earliest lesion is nodular (confluent granulomas) and peribronchiolar, with accumulations of Hx cells, eosinophils, and other inflammatory cells
2 The nodular lesion undergoes central scarring with extension of the cellular infiltrate peripherally resulting in discrete stellate-shaped lesions
3 The resultant stellate foci can resolve completely, undergo further scarring, form cysts which can coalesce, or progress to a honeycomb lung

- Biopsy late in the course of disease may reveal mainly interstitial fibrosis with few Hx cells and eosinophils, making diagnosis difficult

The **pathophysiology** of the characteristic cysts seen on HRCT is not clear but is believed to result from

1 Development of cavitation in the early nodular lesions which then progress to thick-walled and finally thin-walled cysts
2 Bronchiolar dilatation from the development of peribronchiolar fibrosis
3 Extension of fibrosis into the interstitial tissues with formation of a honeycomb lung

Clinically, it is a disease of young and middle-aged whites, rarely seen in blacks, with ~90% of patients being smokers, and presentations include

- Subacute to chronic non-specific respiratory symptoms of dyspnea and cough
- Chest pains from a pneumothorax or osteolytic rib lesion
- Constitutional symptoms of fevers and weight loss in ~30%
- Physical findings are non-pathognomonic with signs of cor pulmonale in advanced disease
- Extrapulmonary disease is most often manifest as osteolytic bone lesions in the skull, ribs, pelvis, or diabetes insipidus (minority of patients)
- Asymptomatic radiologic findings in ~25% of cases

Prognostically, asymptomatic patients tend to remain so

- Symptomatic patients can have partial or complete remission spontaneously, on stopping smoking, or with steroid treatment, although the efficacy of the latter is unclear
- 20% of patients can develop progressive interstitial fibrosis with honeycombing, pneumothoraces, pulmonary artery hypertension and respiratory failure
  - Radiologic correlation of the above is progressive cystic disease, honeycombing and pneumothoraces
  - The functional correlation is increasing airways obstruction and further reductions in DCO +/– lung volumes
- There are reports of an association of EG and bronchogenic cancer as well as extrapulmonary neoplasia developing many years later, but it is unclear whether

cigarettes are independently responsible for both diseases

PFTs can be obstructive, restrictive or a combination with reduced DCO out of proportion to the spirometric abnormalities

Chest X-ray findings

1 Bilateral, diffuse symmetric disease with upper lobe predominance and sparing of the costophrenic angles
2 Early disease is nodular with progression to reticulonodular, reticular, cystic and finally a honeycomb lung
3 The honeycomb lung preferentially involves the upper lobes with overall lung volume being normal to increased, unlike UIP
4 Pneumothorax is seen in ~10% of patients
5 Pleural effusions as well as mediastinal and hilar adenopathy are rare

HRCT scans demonstrate an upper lobe distribution with sparing of the costophrenic angles and the characteristic combination of nodules and cysts

- The earliest changes are nodules which pathologically represent peribronchiolar collections of inflammatory cells, centrilobular in location
- The nodules can either resolve or undergo fibrosis
- There is? evolution from nodules → cavitary nodules → thick-walled cysts → thin-walled cysts → confluent cysts
- Cystic lesions can remain stable, progress or become confluent with bizarre shapes
- Other cystic lesions form as the inflammatory nodule is replaced by fibrosis, with extension into the surrounding interstitium, creating a honeycomb pattern

Diagnostic features

1 Compatible clinical presentation
2 Characteristic radiologic findings
3 Associated diabetes insipidus in a patient with diffuse interstitial disease

4 BAL for Hx cells containing Birbeck granules on electron microscopy and cell block staining for S-100 protein and OKT-6 cells
5 Transbronchial biopsy and staining of tissue for neuropeptide S-100
6 Open lung biopsy (definitive)

LYMPHANGIOLEIOMYOMATOSIS (LAM)

Definition: LAM is a rare disorder, confined to females of child-bearing years or older women who have been exposed to estrogen, and characterized histologically by

1 Proliferation of immature smooth muscle within the parenchymal interstitium, in the walls of lymphatics, airways and pulmonary veins
2 Cystic lesions
3 Hemosiderosis

Histologically, LAM is indistinguishable from tuberous sclerosis, an autosomal dominant multisystem disease with equal sex distribution characterized by hamartomas in several organs but pulmonary disease in only ~3% of patients

Clinically, LAM has no known familial tendency

- Patients are generally symptomatic and present with dyspnea, cough, chest pains secondary to pneumothorax, recurrent hemoptysis due to pulmonary venous hypertension with secondary alveolar hemorrhage, or chyloptysis – the above reflecting smooth muscle proliferation in bronchioles, veins and lymphatics respectively
- Spontaneous pneumothorax is seen in ~80% of cases and chylothorax in ~25%
- Extrapulmonary disease may occur in the form of ascites (chyloperitoneum), chyluria, pericardial effusion (chylopericardium), lower extremity lymphedema, extrathoracic lymphadenopathy or systemic features of tuberous sclerosis
- Unilateral or bilateral renal angiomyolipomas, rare

hamartomatous renal tumors, are well described in LAM and may present with features of hematuria, flank pain and a mass or may be asymptomatic

- The natural history is not well defined for individual cases and ranges from relative stability to pulmonary hypertension, cor pulmonale, respiratory failure and death, with median survival of 10 years or less from onset of symptoms
- There are no good indicators of disease 'activity' but follow-up should include monitoring of PFTs, chest X-rays (may be normal and correlates poorly with physiology) as well as HRCT
- Exacerbation may occur during pregnancy, with stability of disease postoophorectomy or with administration of estrogen antagonists reported
- There are no pathognomonic findings on physical exam and no specific lab abnormalities
- As in other patients with cystic or bullous disease, air travel can result in pneumothorax, particularly in patients with extensive subpleural changes

PFTS usually reveal an obstructive picture with gas trapping, hyperinflation, and a low DCO, but restrictive disease or a mixed pattern is also reported

- Low FEV_1 % and increased TLC have been associated with a poor prognosis but there is a large variation in the rate of decline in lung function between patients

Chest X-ray findings

1 An initial diffuse, bilateral reticulonodular pattern evolving into a honeycomb lung resembling UIP, except that lung volumes are normal or increased
2 Normal chest X-rays are well described in spite an abnormal HRCT
3 Thin-walled cystic spaces
4 Kerley-B lines
5 Pneumothoraces are common
6 Pleural effusions are unilateral or bilateral and often large and recurrent

7 Lymphadenopathy may be seen
8 Signs of pulmonary artery hypertension and cor pulmonale eventually develop

HRCT is always abnormal at the time of diagnosis (even if chest X-rays are normal) with findings of

1 Thin-walled cysts present diffusely throughout both lungs without lobar preference
   - Cysts vary from 2 mm to 60 mm in diameter with normal intervening parenchyma, the cysts becoming larger and more numerous as the disease progresses
2 The irregular shaped cysts and associated nodules of eosinophilic granuloma are rarely seen
3 'Ground glass' opacities or areas of airspace consolidation ? hemorrhage are present in ~50% of patients
4 Mediastinal, hilar and retrocrural adenopathy may be present

Abdominal and pelvic CT may reveal

1 Renal angiomyolipomas
2 Lymphadenopathy

Diagnosis is strongly suggested by

1 Young females presenting with interstitial lung disease, a pneumothorax or chylothorax in association with:
2 Radiologic findings described above plus:
3 Obstructive and/or restrictive physiology on PFTs
4 Renal angiomyolipomas
   - Distinguishing LAM from EG or other interstitial lung disease is often difficult with definitive diagnosis usually requiring an open lung biopsy
   - Diagnosis has occasionally been made from biopsy of lymph nodes or masses taken from the abdomen or pelvis
   - The role of transbronchial biopsy and staining of LAM cells with HMB-45, a monoclonal antibody that binds to LAM cells (and recognizes antigens in melanoma cell lines), has been proposed as a less invasive procedure

Eosinophilic Granuloma vs. LAM

Eosinophilic Granuloma	LAM
Clinically	
• Rare disorder	• Rare disorder
	• Seen in 3% of patients with tuberous sclerosis
• Young to middle-aged adults	• Young to middle-aged adults
• Male or female	• Female only
• 90% are smokers	• Unrelated to smoking
• Asymptomatic in approximately 25%; non-specific respiratory symptoms; constitutional symptoms; chest pains secondary to pneumothorax or osteolytic bone lesions	• Dyspnea and hemoptysis are common; chest pains secondary to pneumothorax; rarely chyloptysis or chyluria
• Usually presents as localized lung and/or bone disease but may have systemic symptoms	• May present with systemic disease including chylous ascites, retroperitoneal nodes, angiomyolipomas of the kidney, chylopericardium
Chest X-rays	
• Bilateral symmetric upper and middle lobe disease with relative sparing of the costophrenic angles and lung bases	• Diffuse and bilateral involvement
• Lung volumes normal or increased	• Lung volumes normal or increased
• Early pattern is nodular, progressing to reticulonodular, reticular and finally honeycombing (or a combination)	• Areas of airspace disease may develop secondary to pulmonary hemorrhage; coarse reticulonodular pattern progressing to honeycombing
• Pneumothorax in about 20% of patients	• Pneumothorax common; chylous pleural effusions are common, unilateral or bilateral, often large and recurrent
• Prognosis varies and can include improvement, stability, worsening, or steroid responsiveness	• Progressive disease with eventual cor pulmonale
HRCT	
• Cysts, often with bizarre shapes and relative sparing of the costophrenic angles; nodules often variable in size and number and may occur without cysts; cavitary nodules may develop	• Cysts distributed diffusely throughout; nodules are rare

Continued

Eosinophilic Granuloma	LAM
• Lymphadenopathy is rare	• Hilar, mediastinal, and retrocrural nodes may be seen
PFT	
• Restrictive and/or obstructive disease	• Obstructive disease
BAL	
• Characteristic inclusions	• Non-diagnostic
Definitive diagnosis	
• Biopsy	• Biopsy

Table 37.1

Fraser R.S., Muller N.L., Colman N., Paré P.D. (1999) Diagnosis of Diseases of the Chest 4th Edn., WB Saunders.

Naidich, D.P., Zerhouni, E.A., Siegelman, S.S. (1998) *Computed Tomography and Magnetic Resonance of the Thorax*, 3rd edn. New York: Raven Press.

Moss, A., Gamsu, Genant (1992) Thorax and neck. In: *Computed Tomography of the Body with Magnetic Resonance Imaging*, 2nd edn, vol. I.: W.B. Saunders.

Webb, R., Muller, N.L., Naidich, D.P. *High Resolution CT of the Lung*, 2nd edn.: Lippincott-Raven.

Sullivan, E. (1998) Lymphangioleiomyomatosis. *Chest* **114**: 1689–1703.

Friedman, P., Liebon, A., Sokoloff, J. (1981) Eosinophilic granuloma of lung. *Medicine* **60**: 385–396.

Kitaichi, M., Nishmura, K., Itho, H. *et al.* (1995) Pulmonary lymphangio-leiomyomatosis: a report of 46 patients including a clinicopathologic study of prognostic factors. *Am. J. Resp. Crit. Care Med.* **151**: 527–533.

Johnson, S., Tattersfield, E. (1999) Decline in lung function in lymphangioleiomyomatosis. *Am. J. Resp. Crit. Care Med.* **160**: 628–633.

38 Eosinophilic Lung Disease

DEFINITION AND DIFFERENTIAL DIAGNOSIS

Definition: The combination of a pulmonary infiltrate plus

1 Peripheral blood eosinophilia and/or
2 Tissue eosinophilia on biopsy and/or
3 BAL eosinophilia (normal < 1%)

In the absence of peripheral eosinophilia, **suspect eosinophilic lung disease** as part of the differential diagnosis with the following

1 Wheezing (asthma, ABPA, bronchocentric granulomatosis, chronic eosinophilic pneumonia, Churg-Strauss, tropical pulmonary eosinophilia)
2 Pattern of changing pulmonary infiltrates (Loffler's syndrome)
3 Acute fulminating community-acquired pneumonia (acute eosinophilic pneumonia)
4 'Chronic' pneumonia (chronic eosinophilic pneumonia)
5 Systemic vasculitis (Churg-Strauss)

6 Drug reaction
7 Central bronchiectasis (ABPA)

Differential Diagnosis

Airways

1 Asthma
2 Allergic bronchopulmonary aspergillosis
3 Bronchocentric granulomatosis (BCG)

Parenchyma

1 Loeffler's – primary or secondary to drugs, parasites (= simple pulmonary eosinophilia)
2 Acute eosinophilic pneumonia (absent peripheral eosinophilia)
3 Chronic eosinophilic pneumonia
4 Hypereosinophilic syndrome (extrathoracic manifestations are common)
5 Tropical eosinophilia
6 Fungi, e.g. primary coccidioidomycosis
7 Drug-induced pulmonary disease
8 Lymphoma – rare
9 Tuberculosis – rare
10 Idiopathic pulmonary fibrosis – rare
11 Eosinophilic granuloma – rare

Vasculature

1 Churg-Strauss syndrome (extrathoracic manifestations are common)

ASTHMA

Peripheral or airway eosinophilia may accompany asthma

- The disorders that asthmatics are predisposed to and that can present with abnormal chest X-rays include
  - Mucus plugs
  - ABPA
  - Bronchocentric granulomatosis
  - Atelectasis

- Loeffler's syndrome
- Chronic eosinophilic pneumonia
- Bacterial, mycoplasma, viral, chlamydial or opportunistic infection (when on immunosuppressive treatment)
- Allergic granulomatosis of Churg-Strauss
- Drug toxicity, e.g. methyltrexate

BRONCHOCENTRIC GRANULOMATOSIS

This is a pathologic diagnosis made by surgical resection and not a specific clinical syndrome

- Biopsy reveals a necrotizing granulomatous reaction centered in the peripheral airways
- The diagnosis is one of exclusion of a known disorder, e.g. fungus, tuberculosis

Clinically, there are two groups of patients

1. Approximately ⅓ are asthmatic with tissue and peripheral eosinophilia
   - Fungal hyphae are present on biopsy and sputum cultures are often positive for aspergillus
   - The above patients are thought to be a subset of ABPA with similar radiologic features
2. Approximately ⅔ are non-asthmatic and either asymptomatic or present with an acute febrile illness resembling pneumonia, but tissue and blood eosinophilia are usually absent
   - The course of disease is variable and unpredictable, including
     - Stable or enlarging lesion
     - Spontaneous regression
     - Resolution on steroids

Radiologic findings are variable and include

1. Solitary mass lesions in ~60%
2. Areas of consolidation in ~30%
3. Obstructive atelectasis
4. Interstitial infiltrates

5 Cavitary lesions
6 Other

Histologically similar lesions can be seen in a variety of disorders including Wegener's, rheumatoid arthritis as well as infections caused by bacteria, tuberculosis, viruses, chlamydia and fungi

- Cultural, serologic and histologic pulmonary studies as well as search for a systemic disease should be undertaken, as this group is heterogeneous and the diagnosis of BCG does not imply a uniform pathogenesis

LOEFFLER'S SYNDROME

Definition: The combination of peripheral eosinophilia and radiologic features including

1 Single or multiple areas of airspace consolidation which are transient and change in from one to several days
2 Migratory nature of the infiltrates, disappearing in one area but appearing in another
3 Typically peripheral in location
4 Rarely appearing as nodules and simulating primary or metastatic cancer

Clinically, patients are atopic but often asymptomatic with the syndrome resolving spontaneously

- Rarely, patients are acutely ill with fever and dyspnea or present with asthmatic symptoms

Etiologies include

1 Drugs, (often in the form of single case reports) e.g. antibiotics, crack cocaine
2 Ascaris, most often *A. lumbricoides* and characterized by asymptomatic infiltrates, non-specific respiratory symptoms or coughing up an adult worm
   - Diagnosis is made by finding larvae in sputum and gastric washings as well as ova and adult worms in stool
   - Most common cause of Loeffler's syndrome worldwide
3 *Stronglyoides stercoralis* is endemic in rural tropical areas

- It can transform in the gut from non-infectious rhabditiform into filariform larvae and cause autoinfection manifest years after initial infection
- Clinical manifestations vary and can include an asymptomatic state, non-specific respiratory complaints, an asthma-like picture, or severe pneumonia in immunocompromised patients
- Diagnosed by finding larvae in sputum, gastric washings or stools

4 *Toxocara canis* and *catis* are seen worldwide with symptoms of cough and wheezing occurring mainly in children caused by swallowing soil contaminated with dog or cat feces
  - Diagnosed by positive serology and liver biopsy showing granulomas containing larvae

5 Other parasites or other inciting causes rarely reported

6 No etiology found in ~⅓ of cases

ACUTE EOSINOPHILIC PNEUMONIA

Definition: A constellation of clinical, radiologic and lab findings in the absence of a known inciting agent, e.g. drugs, infection, and therefore a diagnosis of exclusion

Clinical manifestations

- Acute febrile illness of 1–5 days duration
- Described in all age groups (most common in third decade) and both sexes
- The flu-like symptoms are accompanied by pleuritic chest pains and hypoxemic respiratory failure, the differential diagnosis including acute community acquired pneumonia or other causes of rapidly progressive airspace disease (see p. 22)
- *Should be considered in the differential diagnosis of fulminating community-acquired airspace disease, as it is treatable and curable
- No associated extrathoracic disease

- A rapid response to steroids is not followed by relapse after treatment cessation

Labs include a normal peripheral eosinophil count but pleural fluid, BAL and lung biopsy reveal eosinophilia

- BAL eosinophilia should suggest the diagnosis although this can be seen in a wide range of disorders including PCP, aspergillus, coccidioidomycosis, drugs, parasites, Churg-Strauss, BOOP, etc.

Radiologically, there are bilateral (rarely unilateral) diffuse interstitial and/or airspace infiltrates accompanied by small to moderate pleural effusions on chest X-ray while CT findings are those of 'ground glass' opacities and consolidation

CHRONIC EOSINOPHILIC PNEUMONIA (CEP)

Definition: Idiopathic disorder characterized by eosinophilia, pulmonary infiltrates and symptoms of greater duration and severity than those seen in Loeffler's syndrome, but lacking the fulminant course of acute eosinophilic pneumonia

Clinically, the majority of cases are seen in middle-aged women but all ages and both sexes are affected

- An atopic history is common and ~50% of patients are asthmatic, with some cases presenting during desensitization therapy for hay fever
- Onset is usually insidious with symptoms of fever, cough, dyspnea and weight loss developing months before the diagnosis is suspected
- Presentation varies from an asymptomatic finding to mild symptomatology or respiratory failure, accompanied by a peripheral eosinophilia, without extrathoracic manifestations
- Should be considered in the differential diagnosis of a non-infectious community acquired 'pneumonia-like' picture
- Spontaneous resolution occurs in <10% of patients

- A dramatic response to steroids is the rule with symptoms improving in 1–2 days and chest X-rays within ~10 days
- Relapses are common and steroid therapy must often be prolonged with symptoms and chest X-rays being the best guide for assessing treatment
- Multiple agents have been described to give similar clinical and radiologic features and therefore drugs, parasites, tuberculosis, aspergillus and other fungi must be ruled out

Lung biopsy reveals massive filling of airspaces with a mixture of eosinophils and macrophages

- Rarely, areas of bronchiolitis obliterans with intralumenal polyps may be prominent with hybrid features of CEP and idiopathic BOOP
- In the later stages of disease or during resolution interstitial changes may predominate

Labs reveal eosinophilia in the peripheral blood smear, sputum and/or BAL, often accompanied by elevated IgE levels

Chest X-ray findings

1 Peripheral, non-segmental homogeneous infiltrates, resembling the photographic negative of pulmonary edema in ~25% of cases
   - Unlike the more migratory and transient nature of Loeffler's syndrome, the infiltrates can persist for weeks
2 Disease distribution is unilateral or bilateral with upper and middle lobe predominance
3 Pleural effusion is seen in <10% of cases
4 Multiple other non-diagnostic patterns are described including interstitial disease

CT scan findings may better demonstrate the peripheral nature of the infiltrates

- Airspace consolidation is the predominant abnormality early on but a reticulonodular pattern may develop in the later stages
- Mediastinal adenopathy is described

HYPEREOSINOPHILIC SYNDROME

Rare and often fatal syndrome with **diagnostic** criteria of

1 Blood eosinophilia >1500 per mm^3 for >6 months
2 End-organ damage secondary to the increased eosinophils
3 Absence of a specific identifiable cause for the eosinophilia

Clinically, the disease peaks between ages 20–40 with a male to female ratio of 7:1

- Systemic symptoms of fevers, night sweats and weight loss are accompanied by non-specific pulmonary symptoms
- Cardiac involvement includes endocardial fibrosis, restrictive cardiomyopathy and mural thrombosis in addition to arterial and venous thromboembolism, neurologic, GI, skin and joint disease

Radiologic findings are non-specific including airspace infiltrates, interstitial infiltrates or pulmonary edema from cardiac involvement

Labs include bone marrow, BAL and peripheral eosinophilia as well as eosinophilic precursors on the peripheral smear

TROPICAL PULMONARY EOSINOPHILIA (TPE)

Definition: A filarial disease affecting people living in the tropics, mainly Southeast Asia, India, Sri-Lanka, as well as parts of China, Africa and the West Indies

- TPE is thought to be a hypersensitivity reaction to microfilariae liberated by mating of the adult worms of *Wuchereria bancrofti* or *Brugia malayi*
- The microfilariae induce an eosinophilic alveolitis in the lungs which can progress to interstitial fibrosis if untreated

Clinically, <1% of patients infected with lymphatic filarial parasites develop TPE, with disease thought to be more common in non-endemic, non-immune persons

- Indians and Pakistanis are particularly susceptible while whites are infrequently affected
- Most patients are 20–30 years of age with a male to female ratio of ~4 to 1
- Presentations include cough often worse at night, with dyspnea and wheezing, diagnosed as new onset bronchial asthma refractory to treatment
- Systemic symptoms of fevers and weight loss may be accompanied by nausea, vomiting and diarrhea

Lab findings

1 Peripheral eosinophilia >3000 mm^3
2 Elevated total IgE
3 Filarial – specific antibodies
4 Negative blood cultures for microfilariae

Radiologic findings

1 Diffuse nodular or reticulondular pattern
2 Normal in ~20%

Diagnostic criteria

1 Several months to year history of exposure in an endemic area
2 Clinical history and radiologic findings as above
3 Peripheral eosinophilia, total serum IgE >1000 u/mL, antifilarial antibodies
4 Detection of microfilarie in lung, liver or lymph node biopsies
5 Response to diethylcarbamazine in the majority of cases

DRUG-INDUCED PULMONARY EOSINOPHILIA

Multiple agents are described including ranitidine, crack cocaine, acetaminophen, L-tryptophan, antibiotics, (e.g. nitrofurantoin, ampicillin, minocycline, aerosolized pentamidine)

The **clinical spectrum** is quite variable and includes

1 A Loeffler-type picture with little or no symptomatology, e.g. penicillin

2 An acute presentation simulating hypersensitivity pneumonitis or bacterial pneumonia, e.g. nitrofurantoin, methyltrexate, cocaine
3 An insidious onset with chronic symptoms of dyspnea and cough, e.g. nitrofurantoin
4 ? Drug induced eosinophilic vasculitis, e.g. accolate

CHURG-STRAUSS SYNDROME

A rare clinicopathologic syndrome with 3 clinical stages

- Stage I – prodrome of asthma, allergic rhinitis, nasal polyps and sinusitis
- Stage II – eosinophilia and organ infiltration, e.g. eosinophilic pneumonia or gastroenteritis lasting months to years
- Stage III – systemic vasculitis developing from 3 to 20 or more years following the onset of asthma

Pathologically, the triad of (1) necrotizing vasculitis of small vessesl, (2) extravascular granulomas, and (3) tissue infiltration with eosinophils, will be present in Stage III but not in the pre or post-vasculitic phases

Clinically, respiratory symptoms relate to asthma or the presence of the pulmonary infiltrates, with most patients being between 30 and 45 years of age

- Prognosis is mostly determined by cardiac disease (acute or constrictive pericarditis, eosinophilic myocarditis, coronary arteritis *vs.* the endocardial fibrosis of hypereosinophilic syndrome), but involvement of the nervous system (central or peripheral), GI tract and skin also occur
- Focal segmental glomerulonephritis can occur but renal involvement is less frequent and severe compared to other small vessel vasculitides, e.g. Wegener's or microscopic polyangiitis
- Nasal and sinus disease may also suggest Wegener's but are non-destructive processes
- Mortality is due to congestive heart failure and

myocardial infarction (most commonly) followed by renal failure, CNS disease, GI complications and lung disease

Lab findings include a ⊕ ANCA, usually P-ANCA, in up to 70% of cases, in addition to pleural fluid and blood eosinophilia

Differential diagnosis includes other causes of eosinophilic lung disease in addition to Wegener's and microscopic polyarteritis

Radiologic findings

1. Normal X-rays in ~25% of cases
2. Airspace consolidation, non-segmental, transient, often peripheral and resembling eosinophilic pneumonia
3. Multinodular disease usually without cavitation
4. Interstitial disease, hilar adenopathy and pleural effusions are less commonly described
5. Pulmonary edema secondary to cardiac disease

Baum, G.L., Crapo, J.D., Celli, B.R., Karlinsky, J.B. (eds) (1997) *Textbook of Pulmonary Diseases*, 6th edn.: Lippincott-Raven.

Fishman, A.P., Elias, J.A., Fishman, J.A., Grippi, M.A., Kaiser, L.R., Senior, R.N. (1998) *Fishman's Pulmonary Diseases and Disorders*, 3rd edn.: McGraw-Hill.

Yookyung Kim, Kynny Sou Lee, Dong-Chull Choi, et al. The spectrum of eosinophilic lung disease: radiologic findings. *JCAT* **21**: 920–929.

Ong, R., Doyle, R. (1998) Tropical pulmonary eosinophilia. *Chest* **113**: 1673–1679.

Allen, J., Davis, B. (1994) Eosinophilic lung disease. *Am. J. Resp. Crit. Care Med.* **150**: 1423–1428.

Liebow, A.A., Carrington, C.B. (1969) The eosinophilic pneumonias. *Medicine* **48**: 251–285.

Allen, J., Davis, B. (1994) Eosinophilic lung diseases (State of the art). *ARRD* **150**: 1423–1438.

Tazelaar, H., Linz, L., Colby, T., et al. (1997) Acute eosinophilic pneumonia: histopathologic findings in nine patients. *Am. J. Resp. Crit. Care Med.* **155**: 296–302.

39 Gastrointestinal Diseases – Pulmonary Manifestations

ZENKER'S DIVERTICULUM

Clinical features

- Dysphagia
- Chronic cough and regurgitation of esophageal contents
- Recurrent pneumonia/bronchiectasis

Radiologic features

1 Superior mediastinal mass which may contain an air–fluid level, best seen on barium swallow
2 Anterior displacement of the tracheal air column
3 Recurrent and migratory pulmonary infiltrates representing repeated aspiration

ESOPHAGEAL FISTULAS

Tracheo-esophageal or broncho-esophageal fistulas may be congenital or acquired, the latter including

1. Esophageal or tracheal neoplasms (most common)
2. Infections including histoplasmosis and tuberculosis
3. Trauma or corrosive agents
4. Radiation
5. Foreign body
6. Crohn's disease of the esophagus
7. Broncholithiasis
8. Silicotic nodules

Clinical features

- Chronic cough which may contain food particles
- Asthma-like picture
- Recurrent bronchitis or pneumonia
- Bronchiectasis
- Hemoptysis

Diagnosis established by barium swallow, esophagoscopy and bronchoscopy

ACHALASIA

Clinical features

1. Dysphagia, weight loss and regurgitation of esophageal contents
2. Nocturnal cough/wheezing
3. Chronic cough and recurrent pneumonia, abscess formation or bronchiectasis from aspiration
4. Rarely dyspnea and stridor from tracheal compression and obstruction (by the megaesophagus) against the bony thoracic inlet
    - The above can develop insidiously or acutely, typically after a meal where presentation is that of acute shortness of breath that may be accompanied by features of the SVC syndrome as well as a soft, bulky supraclavicular mass that compresses with palpation

Radiologic features

1. Widened mediastinum caused by the esophagus bulging into the right hemithorax

2 Air–fluid level in the dilated esophagus
3 Anterior bulging and compression of the trachea on lateral chest X-ray

ESOPHAGEAL CANCER

Majority are squamous cell with early submucosal and transmural spread, followed by local spread, airways invasion (eliminating curative surgery) and distant metastases

- Tracheobronchial involvement may be suspected radiologically, but with the exception of fistula formation, documentation of invasion requires bronchoscopy and positive biopsy for patients who are potentially operable
- Evidence of direct tumor involvement of the airways, i.e. intralumenal tumor, wall infiltration or fistula formation, should be distinguished from the indirect signs, i.e. compression, distortion, posterior wall protrusion or rigidity, as the latter may still permit surgery

Pulmonary Manifestations

Airways

- Tracheal deviation
- Compression of posterior tracheal wall
- Thickening of posterior tracheal stripe (2.5–3.0 mm) or tracheo-esophageal stripe (approximately 3 mm), i.e. airway wall infiltration
- Exophytic intralumenal growth
- Tracheo-esophageal fistula
- Bronchial invasion
- Broncho-esophageal fistula

Parenchyma

- Aspiration pneumonia
- Metastases

Pleura

- Parapneumonic effusion
- Hydrothorax or hydropneumothorax secondary to esophageal rupture

Mediastinum

- Esophageal dilatation ± air–fluid level proximal to the cancer
- Intralumenal mass with an irregular esophageal lumen
- Localized or circumferential wall thickening
- Loss of the peri-esophageal fat planes with mediastinal invasion
- Local invasion of lymph nodes, aorta, left atrium, pericardium, tracheobronchial tree
- Acute mediastinitis secondary to rupture

ESOPHAGEAL CYST

Definition: Developmental abnormality characterized pathologically by smooth muscle, lack of cartilage and a lining of squamous or ciliated columnar epithelium (may occasionally be difficult to distinguish from a bronchogenic cyst)

Clinically, they are usually asymptomatic but can present with dysphagia or airway compression

Radiologically, they are within or adjacent to the wall of the esophagus with water or soft tissue density on CT

- Diagnosis has been made on gastro-esophageal ultrasound

INFLAMMATORY BOWEL DISEASE (IBD)

Pulmonary disease is uncommon in IBD with >80% of reported patients having ulcerative colitis and the remainder Crohn's disease

- In most patients, medical or surgical therapy has resulted in the bowel disease being inactive when lung disease develops, although pulmonary involvement may antedate, follow or be concurrent with the IBD
- Female to male ratio is approximately 60:40

Airways disease

1 70% of idiopathic lung involvement relates to airways disease with reports of
    - Tracheal or subglottic stenosis
    - Ulcerative tracheobronchitis
    - Bronchiectasis
    - Bronchiolitis – obliterative or diffuse panbronchiolitis
    - BOOP
2 Drug induced BOOP, e.g. sulfasalazine
3 Crohn's involvement of the esophagus with aspiration from strictures, ulceration or fistula formation

Vascular disease

1 Angiitis resembling Wegener's granulomatosis
2 Pulmonary edema secondary to hypoproteinemia

Parenchymal disease

1 Opportunistic infection in patients on steroids
2 Metastatic colon cancer with ulcerative colitis
3 Drug induced (sulfasalazine, 5-aminosalycilate) interstitial lung disease ± eosinophilia
4 Drug-induced lupus syndrome (sulfasalazine, 5-aminosalycilate) with parenchymal involvement
5 Idiopathic interstitial lung disease
6 Necrobiotic nodules
    - Idiopathic disorder characterized by a sterile accumulation of neutrophils with areas of necrosis, manifest radiologically as cavitary nodules
    - The suppurative nodules resemble the skin lesions of pyoderma gangrenosum which may co-exist

Pleural disease

1 Drug-induced lupus and secondary effusions
2 Drug-related, (e.g. sulfasalazine) eosinophilic pleural effusion
3 Idiopathic serositis, characterized by a neutrophilic exudate which may be recurrent with co-existent pericarditis

LIVER DISEASE – PULMONARY COMPLICATIONS

Parenchyma

- Metastatic hepatoma
- Aspiration pneumonia secondary to encephalopathy
- Emphysema in cirrhotics with α_1 antitrypsin deficiency
- LIP and interstitial fibrosis in chronic active hepatitis
- Several forms of interstitial lung disease in patients with primary biliary cirrhosis including
  - Fibrosing alveolitis
  - Lymphoid interstitial pneumonitis
  - Granulomatous inflammation
  - Diseases due to accompanying Sjogren's syndrome, scleroderma or CREST syndrome

Pleura

- Transudative effusions secondary to ascites
- Parapneumonic effusion
- Metastatic hepatoma
- Tuberculous pleurisy in alcoholics
- Pancreatic-related effusions
- Acute pleuritis and effusions in chronic active hepatitis

Chest wall

- Elevated hemidiaphragm secondary to ascites or hepatomegaly
- Rib or vertebral compression fractures from osteopenia due to vitamin D malabsorption

CNS

- Central hyperventilation

Mediastinum

- Posterior mediastinal mass secondary to varices

Vasculature

1 **Hepato-pulmonary syndrome (HPS)** is defined by the triad of
   - Liver disease
   - ↑ A-a O_2 gradient

- Intrapulmonary vascular dilatations representing arteriolar dilatations as well as direct arteriovenous communications

Clinically, HPS is seen in acute or chronic liver disease
- Patients complain of dyspnea on exertion and platypnea (dyspnea when upright and relieved when supine)
- Physical findings may include clubbing, cyanosis and cutaneous spider telangiectasias
- Arterial blood gases reveal hypoxemia and orthodeoxia (reduction in PaO_2 when changing from the supine to standing position)
- The above manifestations may resolve with improving liver function or post-liver transplant

Chest X-rays are usually normal but occasionally reveal increased bibasilar interstitial markings

Diagnostic tests
- Lung scan reveals radioactivity over the kidneys and brain due to shunting of the radioisotope through dilated intrapulmonary vessels
- Contrast echo showing microbubbles in the left heart 3–6 cycles after contrast in the right ventricle
- Pulmonary angiography which can directly demonstrate the vascular dilatations

2 **Pulmonary artery hypertension (PAH)** is seen in approximately 2% of patients with portal hypertension
- Cirrhosis is usually present but parenchymal hepatic disease is not necessary for PAH to develop
- Etiology is unclear ? unmetabolized substances in portal blood reaching the pulmonary vasculature through portosystemic shunts
- The histologic features are those of plexogenic pulmonary arteriopathy as seen in primary pulmonary hypertension

Clinically, the diagnosis is usually made after the onset of clinical hepatic disease
- Approximately 60% of patients are initially

asymptomatic but eventually develop symptoms of dyspnea, fatigue, chest pains and syncope
- Physical findings are those of pulmonary hypertension
- The diagnosis is one of exclusion as there are no pathognomonic findings

Radiologic features include right venticular enlargement, prominence of the main and central pulmonary arteries as well as peripheral vascular pruning
- The response of pulmonary artery hypertension to liver transplant is variable and unpredictable

HEMOCHROMATOSIS

Mortality is caused by congestive heart failure, liver failure, hepatoma and portal hypertension, but pulmonary manifestations include

1 Pulmonary edema and pleural effusions secondary to cardiomyopathy
2 Liver cirrhosis with complications of
    - Hepato-pulmonary syndrome
    - Portal and pulmonary hypertension
    - Hepatoma with pleuropulmonary metastases as well as tumor emboli

HEPATOMA

The lungs are the most common site of distant metastases and include

Parenchyma
- Single or multiple nodules
- Lymphangitic spread
- Miliary disease

Pleura
- Malignant effusions

Vasculature

- Pulmonary hypertension from tumor emboli

Chest wall

- Elevated right hemidiaphragm

LIVER TRANSPLANT – PULMONARY COMPLICATIONS

1 Lung disease seen in pre-transplant patients with **hepatic failure**

2 **Malignancy**
  - Post-transplant lymphoma
  - Metastatic lung disease from hepatoma or cholangiocarcinoma present in the pre-transplant liver
  - Lung cancer in smokers

3 **Pneumonia**
  - Bacterial – acute or chronic, e.g. tuberculosis
  - Viral – CMV, typically 4–6 weeks post-op with fever, myalgias, anthralgias, cough, dyspnea, hepatitis, neutropenia, thrombocytopenia and atypical lymphocytes
  - Fungal – endemic or opportunistic, e.g. aspergillus, cryptococcus, mucormycosis, pneumocystis

4 **Calcinosis** from calcium infusion in blood products and often superimposed, renal failure is uncommonly seen
  - Symptoms of cough and dyspnea in association with parenchymal opacities may be attributed to infection or edema, the diagnosis confirmed on technetium-99m phosphate scan or CT

5 **Pulmonary thrombosis** from massive platelet aggregation is a common cause of early death, within days of transplant

PANCREATITIS

1 **Hypoxemia** and a normal chest X-ray are common findings in acute pancreatitis, even in patients without

underlying cardio-respiratory disease, and thought to represent V/Q mismatch

- Narcotic control of pain and abdominal distension can exacerbate the impaired gas exchange

2 **ARDS** and multiorgan failure can occur in acute pancreatitis, although the exact pathophysiology is unclear

3 **Pleural effusions** secondary to

- **Acute pancreatitis** presents clinically with GI symptoms of abdominal pain, nausea and vomiting
  - The pleural effusions are small, of unclear pathophysiology, and can be left-sided (60%), right-sided (30%) or bilateral
  - Pleural fluid amylase is moderately elevated with levels <4000 IU/L
  - Typically the fluid is serosanguinous or grossly bloody with a neutrophil predominance microscopically
  - Effusions are self-limited and resolve as the GI symptoms regress
- **Pancreatic abscess** is a complication of acute pancreatitis and biliary tract surgery
  - High amylase pleural effusion may be accompanied by pneumonia
- **Pancreatic ascites** flows from the peritoneal to pleural cavities via diaphragmatic defects
- **Pancreatic pseudocyst** can result in a pleural effusion secondary to
  - Rupture into the peritoneal cavity with formation of pancreatic ascites and transdiaphragmatic spread
  - Direct extension into the pleural space with subsequent rupture
  - Posterior rupture into the retroperitoneum with extension into the mediastinum via the esophageal, aortic and IVC hiati; the mediastinal fluid may form a mediastinal pseudocyst and rupture into the pleura
- **Chronic pancreatitis**
  - Pleural effusions are due to direct extension of a pseudocyst across the diaphragm or from the

formation of a fistulous tract between the pancreas and pleural space
- Symptoms of chest pain and dyspnea can dominate the clinical presentation unlike acute pancreatitis, where GI symptoms predominate and pulmonary symptoms are minimal to absent
- There may be no preceding history of acute pancreatitis, although alcoholism is common
- CT or ERCP can demonstrate extension of a pseudocyst to the pleura but demonstration of a fistulous tract between the pancreas and pleura usually requires ERCP
- The effusions are left-sided > right-sided > bilateral and can be large
- Often recur rapidly post-thoracocentesis requiring more aggressive therapy
- Effusions are bloody or serosanguinous with neutrophil predominance
- Amylase levels may exceed 10 000 IU/L
- Complications include empyema and fibrothorax

PANCREATIC CANCER

Pulmonary involvement is common after liver metastases, with spread usually lymphangitic, through pleural lymphatics and into the pulmonary connective tissue septae

- Less common routes of spread are from tracheobronchial or mediastinal nodes as well as hematogenous spread though the splenic, portal and mesenteric veins

Radiologic features

1 Lymphangitic spread
2 Solitary nodule or mass
3 Multiple nodules
4 Cavitary lesions
5 Pleural effusions
6 Adenopathy

COLON/RECTAL CANCER

The primary route of spread is hematogenous although lymphatic involvement also occurs

- The lungs are second only to liver as the most common metastatic site, with rectal and left sided colonic lesions having a greater tendency for initial spread to the lungs
- Colon/rectal cancers are the most common source of a solitary metastatic nodule

Pulmonary Manifestations

Airways

- Endobronchial metastases with secondary atelectasis, obstructive pneumonitis
- Tracheal narrowing from endotracheal metastases

Parenchyma

- *Single or multiple nodules
- Lymphangitic carcinomatosis

Mediastinum

- Hilar/mediastinal lymphadenopathy

Pleura

- Malignant pleural effusion

Vasculature

- Tumor emboli
- Thrombo-emboli
- Pulmonary hypertension secondary to tumor emboli or thrombo-emboli

Fraser R.S., Muller N.L., Colman N., Paré P.D. (1999) Diagnosis of Diseases of the Chest 4th Edn., WB Saunders.

Baum, G.L., Crapo, J.D., Celli, B.R., Karlinsky, J.B. (eds) (1997) *Textbook of Pulmonary Diseases*, 6th edn.: Lippincott-Raven.

Rockey, D., Cello, J. (1990) Pancreaticopleural fistula. *Medicine* **69**: 332–344.

Shapiro, M., Dobbins, J., Matthay, P. (1989) Pulmonary manifestations of gastrointestinal disease. *Clinics in Chest Medicine* **10**: 617–643.

Camus, P., Piard, F., Ashcroft, T. *et al.* (1993) The lung in inflammatory bowel disease. *Medicine* **72**: 151–180.

Lange, P., Stoller, J. (1995) The hepatopulmonary syndrome. *Ann. Internal Med.* **122**: 521–529.

O'Brien, J., Ettinger, N. (1996) Pulmonary complications of liver transplantation. *Clinics in Chest Medicine* **17**: 99–114.

Castro, M., Krowka, M. (1996) Hepatopulmonary syndrome. *Clinics in Chest Medicine* **17**: 35–48.

Mandell, S., Groves, B. (1996) Pulmonary hypertension in chronic liver disease. *Clinics in Chest Medicine* **17**: 17–33.

40 Head and Neck Cancer – Pulmonary Manifestations

Most of the above are **squamous cell cancers** arising from the *larynx, *tongue, floor of mouth, tonsil, gums, pharynx, noses/sinuses, salivary glands

- Pattern of spread is typically to neck nodes with distant metastases often confined to the lungs
- A second primary malignancy develops in 15–30% of these patients, most often arising from
  - Head and neck
  - Lungs
  - Esophagus

Lung lesions which are more common than liver or bone metastases have been found

- During pre-treatment evaluation of the head and neck primary
- During routine follow-up
- At the time of local recurrence of the primary lesion

Metastatic head and neck carcinoma is suggested by

1 Multiple and bilateral lung nodules
2 Malignant cervical adenopathy

An independent lung primary is seen with

1 Different histology
2 The pulmonary lesion presenting more than 5 years following the head and neck lesion is suggestive

Radiologically, the usual pattern of spread is a single nodule or multiple nodules which may cavitate, CT being more sensitive than chest X-ray

- A solitary nodule is often difficult to diagnose as a primary or metastasis, even at pathology

Fraser R.S., Muller N.L., Colman N., Paré P.D. (1999) Diagnosis of Diseases of the Chest 4th Edn., WB Saunders.

Baum, G.L., Crapo, J.D., Celli, B.R., Karlinsky, J.B. (eds) *Textbook of Pulmonary Diseases*, 6th edn. (Place of publication): Lippincott-Raven.

Fishman, A.P., Elias, J.A., Fishman, J.A., Grippi, M.A., Kaiser, L.R., Senior, R.N. *Fishman's Pulmonary Diseases and Disorders*, 3rd edn. (Place of publication): McGraw-Hill.

41 Hematologic Diseases – Pulmonary Manifestations

AMYLOID

Definition: Rare multisystem disease of unknown etiology characterized by the abnormal deposition of extracellular fibrillar proteins derived from the light chains of monoclonal immunoglobulins

- Multiple classifications of disease are described reflecting the protein type, distribution, systemic *vs.* isolated pulmonary disease, predisposing conditions, etc.

Airways

Amyloid confined to the tracheobronchial tree is rare and may be localized, multifocal or diffuse, with the bronchoscopic appearance varying from submucosal plaques to tumor-like masses

Clinical spectrum includes

- Obstructive sleep apnea secondary to macroglossia
- Hoarseness, stridor and dyspnea secondary to laryngeal or subglottic infiltration

- Stridor, an asthma-like picture, hemoptysis, cough or dyspnea secondary to diffuse endotracheal/endobronchial disease
- Localized tracheobronchial mass-like lesion with recurrent pneumonia, bronchiectasis, atelectasis or hemoptysis
- Asymptomatic finding
- Associated with tracheobronchopathia osteoplastica
- Non-association with systemic amyloid

Radiologic findings

1 Heavy bronchovascular markings with hyperinflation
2 Localized airway narrowing
3 Atelectasis/obstructive pneumonitis

Parenchyma

Clinical spectrum includes

- Asymptomatic radiologic finding, common with nodular lesions which are not associated with systemic amyloid and usually have a benign course
- Dyspnea progressing to respiratory failure, reflecting parenchymal infiltration and/or pulmonary edema from cardiac amyloid
- Diffuse interstitial disease is usually associated with systemic involvement and may have unrecognized amyloid deposits in other organs

Radiologic findings

1 Nodule(s) or mass(es) with possible cavitation or calcification
2 Miliary pattern
3 Diffuse interstitial reticulo-nodular disease
4 Diffuse airspace disease
5 Pulmonary edema (from cardiac disease)

Pleura

Effusions may be secondary to amyloid infiltration (exudative and may be hemorrhagic) or associated CHF

Lymphadenopathy

Mediastinal or hilar node enlargement, unilateral or bilateral, may calcify, and may be localized or associated with systemic disease

Respiratory Muscles

Ventilatory failure due to an associated myopathy

Vascular

Pulmonary artery infiltration and dissection

Diagnostic features

1 Clinical-radiologic features as described
2 Associated extrapulmonary disease including hepatosplenomegaly, macroglossia, peripheral neuropathy, carpal tunnel syndrome, cardiomyopathy
3 Monoclonal light chains on serum or urine protein electrophoresis
4 Lung biopsy, e.g. TTNA, transbronchial, or other biopsy, e.g. rectal

ANTIPHOSPHOLIPID ANTIBODY SYNDROME (AAS)

Definition: A hypercoagulable state characterized by the presence of autoantibodies to membrane phospholipids, the immunoglobulins being anticardiolipin antibody and a lupus anticoagulant

- 60% of cases have both autoantibodies elevated while 40% have only one elevated
- AAS can be primary (50% of cases) or secondary to systemic lupus, other connective tissue disorders or rarely idiopathic thrombocytopenic purpura

Clinical features

- Arterial thrombosis involving the brain, heart, viscera and limbs
- Deep vein thrombosis

- Fetal loss
- Hematologic abnormalities including thrombocytopenia, Coomb's positive hemolytic anemia, livedo reticularis

Pulmonary manifestations

1 Pulmonary emboli and secondary pulmonary hypertension
2 Pulmonary arterial thrombosis
3 Pulmonary hemorrhage
4 ARDS

BLOOD TRANSFUSIONS – PULMONARY COMPLICATIONS

1 Pulmonary edema secondary to volume overload developing within hours and associated with other signs of CHF – R/O an acute MI
2 Non-cardiac pulmonary edema or transfusion-related acute lung injury is caused by the passive transfer of granulocyte or lymphocyte antibodies in the sera of donors who are usually multiparous
   - Seen with the transfusion of plasma-containing blood components, i.e. whole blood, RBCs, WBCs or platelet transfusions, but not simple plasma
   - Dyspnea develops within 2–4 hours with fever, chills, cough, tachycardia, blood eosinophilia, hypoxemia and hypotension
   - Bilateral patchy airspace disease with normal wedge pressure resolves with supportive therapy and carries a much better prognosis than ARDS, with low mortality
   - There are no pathognomonic findings but the diagnosis is suggested by
     – Lymphocytotoxic, HLA or granulocyte-specific antibodies in the serum of the donor or recipient
     – Positive cytotoxic lymphocyte cross-match
3 Anaphylaxis characterized by laryngeal edema and bronchospasm as well as urticaria beginning within minutes of the transfusion

4 Bacterial contamination by gram positive or negative organisms
   - Hypotension, often accompanied by a DIC picture, occurs within a few hours of transfusion and is confirmed with positive blood cultures
5 Hemolytic transfusion reaction
6 Delayed diseases, e.g. HIV infection, CMV pneumonia

BONE MARROW TRANSPLANT (BMT)

Pulmonary complications are seen in ~50% of transplant recipients and vary with

1 Underlying disease
2 Prior chemotherapy
3 Chest radiation
4 Development of chronic graft *vs.* host disease (GVHD)
5 Degree of immunosuppression used to treat the underlying disease or in conditioning regimens
   - Neutrophils usually return within a few weeks, but B cell and T cell function can take 6–12 months with normal immune function by ~1 year in the absence of chronic GVHD
6 Infectious history e.g. TB, fungal, CMV serology, exposures, prophylaxis taken
7 Autologous transplant (*vs.* allogeneic) characterized by
   - Absence of graft *vs.* host disease
   - Rarity of bronchiolitis obliterans
   - Rarity of CMV pneumonia and toxoplasma infection
   - Higher incidence of diffuse alveolar hemorrhage
   - Uncommon occurrence of idiopathic pneumonia syndrome

Specific complications can occur early (<100 days) or late (>100 days) and the timing is often a clue to etiology

- Pulmonary complications can arise in the airways, parenchyma or vasculature and are discussed below, followed by diagnostic clues and work-up

Airways

1 **Bronchiolitis obliterans** (BO) seen in <10% of allogeneic transplants but rare with autologous transplants
   - Etiology is unclear but thought to be a manifestation of chronic graft *vs.* host disease, although clinically active disease may not be seen in other organs at the time of diagnosis of BO
   - Usually seen 6–12 months post BMT but may be seen at any time after the 2nd month
   - Patients present with progressive cough, dyspnea, wheezing, inspiratory rales and have a mortality of ~40%
   - Associated features of chronic GVHD are often present, e.g. dryness of the mouth and eyes, dysphagia, scleroderma, serositis, hepatitis
   - Chest X-rays often reveal hyperinflation which may be complicated by recurrent pneumothorax and pneumomediastinum
   - HRCT findings reveal areas of reduced attenuation and perfusion, occasionally with centrilobular nodules, although inspiratory films may be normal with gas trapping seen on an expiratory CT
   - Diagnosis is based upon the above findings ± open lung or transbronchial biopsy

2 **BOOP** may be seen either early or late post BMT with unknown etiology in most cases, although it can follow infection, (e.g. CMV), aspiration, drugs, radiation, chronic GVHD
   - Patients present with fever, cough and dyspnea along with a restrictive pattern on PFTs

3 **Mucositis** is seen early post BMT and characterized by edema and inflammation of the upper airway, resulting in dysphagia, odynophagia, dyspnea and aspiration

4 **Lymphocytic bronchitis** characterized clinically by dry cough (usually in association with other features of GVHD) and pathologically by lymphocytic infiltration of the bronchi

Parenchyma

1 **Diffuse alveolar hemorrhage** (DAH) occurs within the first 4–5 weeks of BMT, is seen in ~20% of autologous recipients (less common in allogeneic transplants) and its onset frequently coincides with the onset of marrow recovery
   - Etiology is unclear but unrelated to coagulation parameters
   - Clinically the presentation mimics infection with cough, dyspnea, fever, hypoxemia and occasional hemoptysis
   - Chest X-rays and CT are non-specific and reflect parenchymal blood with bilateral interstitial and alveolar opacities
   - BAL reveals no gross bleeding from large airways, but progressively bloodier returns with abundant hemosiderin-laden macrophages, in the absence of an infectious agent identified
   - High mortality rate from respiratory failure is reduced with steroids

2 **Idiopathic pneumonia syndrome** (**IPS**) is defined by acute and diffuse lung injury post-BMT with no organisms identified on BAL or transbronchial biopsy and therefore a diagnosis of exclusion ? heterogenous group of disorders
   - Histologically characterized by an interstitial mononuclear infiltrate with diffuse alveolar damage
   - Etiology is unknown, but it is described in ~10% of patients, usually within 6 months of BMT, with an early peak in the first 2 weeks
   - Seen with both autologous and allogeneic transplant, but the latter are more frequent and severe
   - Presentation varies from asymptomatic to acute respiratory failure, usually with fever, dry cough, dyspnea, hypoxemia and diffuse infiltrates resembling CMV or pneumocystis
   - Mortality rates of ~70% are reported and are secondary to respiratory failure as well as secondary infection

3 **Pulmonary edema** is seen within the first few weeks post-BMT and is multifactorial, e.g. fluid overload, capillary leak from sepsis, chemotherapy-induced cardiac or renal dysfunction, prior radiotherapy
   - Also seen in association with hepatic veno-occlusive disease where a right pleural effusion may accompany the pulmonary edema
   - Chest X-rays reveal typical findings of edema with the presence of Kerley B lines supporting a cardiac etiology
   - Diagnosis is based upon the history, physical, X-rays and echocardiogram

4 **Drug reactions** can be seen any time post-BMT and present clinically with non-specific symptoms of fever, cough and dyspnea
   - Chest X-rays are also non-specific with bilateral diffuse or patchy infiltrates
   - Peripheral or BAL eosinophilia may be present
   - Diagnosis is based on clinical features, exclusion of other causes and compatible histology

5 **Recurrent malignancy**, leukemia or lymphoma, can result in non-specific respiratory symptoms and multiple patterns of pulmonary infiltrates
   - The presence of mediastinal or extrathoracic lymphadenopathy should suggest recurrence of the underlying malignancy

6 **Post-transplant lymphoproliferative disorder** (PTLPD) can occur at any time post-BMT and is a direct sequela of chronic immunosuppression resulting in the unchecked proliferation of EBV-infected B cells
   - The histologic changes range from polyclonal lymphoid hyperplasia to monoclonal B cell lymphoma
   - The chest can be the primary or metastatic site of involvement
   - Clinical presentation varies from asymptomatic to non-specific respiratory symptoms and extrathoracic disease

- Radiologically, single or multiple nodules or masses are the most common manifestation in addition to lymphadenopathy, thymic enlargement and pleuro-pericardial disease

7 **Secondary malignancy** (non-hematologic), primary pulmonary or metastatic to lung

8 **Pneumonia** can occur any time post-BMT and is a common (? most common) complication

a. **Bacterial** pneumonia is common during the neutropenic first weeks, with both gram positive and negative organisms responsible, although it is also seen later, particularly with chronic graft *vs.* host disease
   - Clinical presentation and chest X-ray abnormalities may be accompanied by positive blood cultures which confirm the diagnosis

   Mycobacterial infection, typical or atypicals, are described rarely

b. **Fungal** infection is most often due to **aspergillus** and seen during the early neutropenic stage as well as late with chronic graft *vs.* host disease
   - Radiologic findings are most often nodular or pneumonia-like opacities which can cavitate
   - CT findings include the ‘halo sign’, i.e. a nodular density surrounded by a rim of ‘ground glass’ attenuation (seen with neutropenia) as well as the ‘meniscus sign’, i.e. a crescentic cavity seen later in the course of disease and correlating with return of the WBC count to normal
   - Other fungi responsible include mucor, cryptococcus and endemic fungi

   Candida pneumonia can occur in association with *Candida* fungemia with areas of non-specific airspace consolidation on chest X-ray
   - CT features include nodules which may also demonstrate the ‘halo sign’ as well as ‘ground glass’ opacities or consolidation

Pneumocystis is seen less often due to antibiotic prophylaxis

c. **Viral** pneumonia can be seen early or late post-BMT with the greatest risk in seronegative recipients receiving marrow from a seropositive donor

CMV pneumonia is usually seen 2–6 months post-transplant in 15–40% of marrow recipients (see p. 636)

- Patients at highest risk have severe graft *vs.* host disease and therefore not a problem with autologous transplants
- The incidence has decreased with
  - Use of CMV-negative blood products in CMV-antibody-negative patients
  - Prophylactic use of acyclovir/gancyclovir
  - The administration of intravenous immune globulin containing CMV antibodies
- Endogenous reactivation or infusion from seropositive donors is responsible
- Clinical symptoms of fever, cough and dyspnea are accompanied by chest X-ray findings of reticular disease, nodular disease, airspace consolidation or a combination, although X-rays can be normal
- CT features include 'ground glass' as well as nodular opacities which can progress to airspace consolidation, localized or diffuse

Herpes simplex (HSV) is seen within the first few weeks post-BMT and should be suspected with skin, oral or esophageal lesions

- Acyclovir prophylaxis has reduced the incidence of disease
- X-rays reveal mixed interstitial and airspace disease
- HHV-6 and HHV-7 may account for some cases of idiopathic interstitial pneumonitis

Respiratory syncytial virus is seen in the first few weeks as well as late in patients with chronic graft *vs.* host disease

- Patients usually present with sinus, ear or other upper respiratory symptoms and X-rays are similar to HSV

Adenovirus and **parainfluenza virus** are described to cause fatal pneumonia

d. **Toxoplasmosis** usually occurs within the first six months post-transplant and is typically associated with GVHD
   - Reactivation of prior infection is thought responsible and should be suspected with a history of cat exposure
   - The brain is most often involved followed by cardiac and pulmonary disease

9 **Pulmonary alveolar proteinosis** is rarely described on BAL

Airways and Parenchymal Disease

Graft *vs.* host disease (GVHD), caused by donor T lymphocytes recognizing recipient tissue as foreign, can present as an acute or chronic disorder

1 **Acute GVHD** is seen in about half of allogeneic recipients (not seen with autologous transplants) and presents within the first 3 months
   - Characterized by the triad of skin, liver and GI disease, but pulmonary manifestations do not occur

2 **Chronic GVHD** is seen at least 3 months post BMT with ⅔ of cases occurring in patients who have had acute GVHD
   - There is multiorgan disease with pulmonary involvement, as well as opportunistic infection, sicca syndrome, malabsorption, liver disease, polyserositis and skin disease

   Airway manifestations
   - Bronchiolitis obliterans
   - Sino-pulmonary sicca syndrome with chronic bronchitis

Parenchymal disease

- Recurrent pneumonia from bacteria, TB, CMV, aspergillus, pneumocystis, toxoplasma
- Lymphoid interstitial pneumonitis

Vasculature

1. **Pulmonary infarcts**, septic or bland
2. **Bone marrow and fat emboli** seen during the infusion of donor marrow
3. **Pulmonary veno-occlusive disease** should be suspected in patients presenting with dyspnea, pulmonary edema and pulmonary hypertension

Diagnostic Clues and Work-Up

1. **Historical features** (Table 41.1)
   - Time of onset of pulmonary disease post-BMT
     - *BOOP, drug reactions, recurrent malignancy, PTLPD and pulmonary infarcts can be seen at any time
   - Rate of disease progression
   - Radiotherapy to the chest region with resultant radiation pneumonitis
   - Cytotoxic drug exposure
   - History of remote opportunistic fungal infection
   - CMV serologic status of donor and recipient
   - Prophylactic antibiotics and corresponding reductions in specific infections, e.g. PCP
   - Presence of CGVH disease (not seen with autologous transplants)
2. **Physical exam**
   - Skin or oral ulcers with HSV
   - Cardiac findings of CHF
   - Airways obstruction with bronchiolitis obliterans
   - Isolated pulmonary disease, e.g. DAH, IIP vs. extrathoracic disease, e.g. PTLPD, recurrent malignancy
3. **Blood tests**
   - Prolonged neutropenia predisposing to infection
   - Eosinophilia suggests a drug reaction

- Positive blood cultures for bacteria or fungi will definitively diagnose pneumonia

4 **Radiologic features**
- Nodular densities suggest BOOP, septic infarcts, bacteria, fungi, or neoplastic disease
- Diffuse disease can be secondary to pulmonary edema, DAH, IPS, drugs, infection e.g. PCP, CMV
- Lymphadenopathy suggests malignancy, less often infection
- Kerley-B lines suggest failure
- CT scan may reveal abnormalities not present on chest X-ray
  – e.g. 'halo' or 'meniscus' signs in fungal infection
  – e.g. 'ground glass' opacities with early pneumonia
  – e.g. peripheral distribution of disease suggestive of BOOP or eosinophilic drug reaction
- Hyperinflation seen with BO
- Extrathoracic nodules in the liver, spleen or kidneys suggest disseminated fungus or tumor

5 **Echocardiogram** to R/O LV dysfunction
6 **PFTs** to document airways obstruction in BO
7 **V/Q** or **spiral CT** to R/O thromboembolic disease
8 **BAL** of diagnostic value with infection, malignancy, DAH or drug-induced eosinophilia
9 **Transbronchial biopsy** or **TTNA** but yields are less than with open lung biopsy, the gold standard

LEUKEMIA – PULMONARY COMPLICATIONS

Parenchyma

1 **Opportunistic infection** is the **most common** cause of parenchymal infiltrates in leukemia
2 **Granulocytic sarcoma** is seen in acute myeloid leukemia where masses of myeloid precursor cells can present as a 'mass-like' lesion
3 **Leukemic cell lysis pneumopathy** is characterized by diffuse airspace disease triggered by chemotherapy, result-

ing in the lysis of large numbers of blast cells in the pulmonary circulation

4 **Drug-induced** lung disease
5 **Alveolar hemorrhage** which can be idiopathic or occur secondary to thrombocytopenia, aspergillus or other infections
6 **Pulmonary edema** triggered by anemia, i.v. fluids, cardiac leukemic infiltration or underlying heart disease
7 **Alveolar proteinosis** secondary to opportunistic infection
8 **Unrelated** disease
9 **Leukemic cell infiltrates** typically present as bilateral diffuse infiltrates, uncommonly localized
   - Seen with uncontrolled leukemia and a peripheral blast count > $6000/mm^3$
   - Pathologically the infiltrates are lymphangitic and vasocentric in distribution giving the radiologic picture of lymphangitic carcinoma or pulmonary edema
   - The diagnosis is one of exclusion of the preceding causes of parenchymal infiltrates
   - Definitive diagnosis can be established by open lung biopsy, transbronchial biopsy, or ? BAL, revealing leukemic cells in the absence of infection, hemorrhage or contamination by circulating blasts

Pleura

Pleural effusions secondary to direct leukemic infiltrates – R/O congestive heart failure, chylothorax, empyema, splenic infarction

Mediastinum

Hilar/mediastinal **lymphadenopathy** is the most common intrathoracic manifestation of leukemia, especially lymphatic leukemia

Airways

1 **Endobronchial** or **peribronchial** infiltrates
2 **Bronchiolocentric** infiltrates in chronic lymphocytic leukemia

3 **Endobronchial granulocytic sarcoma** in acute myeloid leukemia

Vascular

1 **Leukostasis** is defined as small vessel infiltration and occlusion by leukemic cell aggregates leading to microhemorrhages, alveolar edema and respiratory failure
- typically seen with WBC > 100 000/mm^3 and may develop shortly after the institution of chemotherapy
- Chest X-rays can be normal or demonstrate airspace edema

2 **Pseudohypoxemia** occurs as a laboratory artefact when patients with normal oxygen saturation on pulse oximetry demonstrate hypoxemia and low oxygen saturation on ABGs
- The above is due to consumption of oxygen by the marked leucocytosis (similar effects can be seen with extensive thrombocytosis and reticulocytosis), typically occurring with
  - WBC > 1 000 000/mm^3
  - Monocytes > lymphocytes > granulocytes
  - Elevated blood temperature
  - Delay between drawing an ABG and measuring O_2 levels

LYMPHOMA

Non-Hodgkin's disease

- Primary pulmonary lymphoma (see p. 75), i.e. lymphoma confined to the lungs +/– nodal involvement without extrathoracic disease for 3 months, e.g. low-grade B cell, intermediate/high-grade
- Secondary pulmonary lymphoma (much more common than above), i.e. pleuropulmonary disease in patients with concomitant or previous extrathoracic lymphoma
  - Develops by contiguous spread from mediastinal/hilar nodes or metastases

  - All histologic groups may be responsible, e.g. lymphoblastic, diffuse lymphocytic or histiocytic as well as specific secondary lymphomas including 'BMMW', i.e. Burkitt's, mycosis fungoides, malignant histiocytosis, Waldenstrom's
- Mediastinum
  - Prevascular and paratracheal adenopathy are the most common intrathoracic manifestations

Hodgkin's disease
- Primary pulmonary (vary rare)
- Secondary pulmonary (develops by direct extension from contiguous nodal disease)
- Mediastinum
  - Mediastinal and hilar node enlargement are the most common intrathoracic manifestations

The following can be seen with **Hodgkin's or non-Hodgkin's lymphoma**

Airways
- Tracheal narrowing from peritracheal or endotracheal disease
- Peribronchial or endobronchial disease with bronchial narrowing, leading to atelectasis or obstructive pneumonitis

Parenchyma
- Segmental/lobar consolidation or patchy airspace disease
- Reticulo-nodular or miliary pattern from interstitial infiltration
- Single or multiple nodules
- Mass-like lesions
- Cavitation
- Interstitial edema from lymphatic or venous obstruction

Pleura
- Focal or diffuse pleural thickening
- Pleural effusion which can be a transudate, exudate or chylous
- Pleural mass or nodule

Mediastinum/hilum

- Lymphadenopathy involving any mediastinal compartment
- Discrete mass due to confluence of nodes
- Thymic lymphoma manifest as thymic enlargement
- Mediastinal invasion with involvement of the superior vena cava, pericardium, esophagus or phrenic nerve

Chest wall

- Osteolytic/osteoblastic lesions of the sternum, ribs, vertebral column
- 'Extrapleural' lesions

MULTIPLE MYELOMA

Lung disease is rare, while liver, spleen, lymph nodes and pharynx are more commonly involved

Pulmonary disease may be seen as a manifestation of:

- **Multiple myeloma**, i.e. diffuse bone disease
- **Plasmacytoma of bone**, i.e. a plasma cell proliferation in the absence of a generalized plasma cell disorder
- **Extramedullary (extraosseous) plasmacytoma (EMP)** which may occur in isolation or accompany multiple myeloma, particularly in the aggressive terminal stage

Intrathoracic manifestations of **multiple myeloma** are quite variable and reflect

1 Direct plasma cell infiltration
2 Pulmonary edema from cardiac amyloid
3 Infection
4 Hypercalcemia
5 Thromboembolism

Chest wall (ribs, sternum, vertebrae)

- *Osteolytic bone lesions
- *Osteolytic bone lesions with an adjacent soft tissue mass extending into the thorax

- *Osteoporosis/fractures
- *Sternal mass
- Plasmacytoma of the thoracic skeleton
- Dense bones secondary to osteoblastic metastases

Airways

- Tracheal narrowing from endotracheal disease
- Endobronchial infiltrate or mass with resultant atelectasis (EMP)

Parenchyma

- *Superimposed pneumonia
- Localized mass or diffuse infiltrates (EMP)
- Pulmonary calcinosis from hypercalcemia
- Pulmonary amyloid
- Pulmonary edema from cardiac amyloid
- Pulmonary fibrosis from chemotherapy

Pleura

- Malignant pleural effusion or pleural mass (EMP)
- Transudative effusion from cardiac amyloid
- Parapneumonic effusion/empyema

Vasculature

- Pulmonary emboli secondary to a hypercoagulable state

Mediastinum

- Mediastinal mass (EMP)
- Lymphadenopathy (EMP)

MYELODYSPLASIA – PULMONARY COMPLICATIONS

1 Pneumonia, bacteremia or other infections
2 Secondary HIV infection from, e.g. transfusions
3 Rheumatic manifestations of vasculitis or a lupus-like syndrome and subsequent pulmonary involvement – few case reports
4 Sweet's syndrome (acute febrile neutrophilic dermatosis) – few case reports

5 Non-Hodgkin's lymphoma
6 Multiple myeloma and associated amyloidosis

SICKLE CELL LUNG DISEASE

Patients with sickle cell disease, usually hemoglobin SS and less commonly S/C or S/β-thalassemia, can develop acute or chronic lung disease

- Seen in ~⅓ of patients at risk with marked interindividual variation
- Rare when HbS is below 20%

Acute Chest Syndrome (ACS)

Definition: Acute onset of chest pains and pulmonary infiltrates often accompanied by fever, dyspnea, hypoxemia and bone pains, in patients with sickle cell disease

Etiology is unclear, although several potential causes include

1 **Infection** – bacterial, viral and mycoplasma are infrequently documented in spite of cultures and serologic studies, although antibiotics are often prescribed in these asplenic patients, especially with high fevers
2 **Lung infarction** – can be due to *in situ* thrombosis or sickling as well as to emboli from peripheral thrombi or infarcted bone marrow
    - HRCT scans occasionally demonstrate a paucity of arterioles and vessels in the lung periphery, suggesting occlusion of the microvascular circulation
3 **Thoracic bone infarction** involving the ribs, sternum or thoracic vertebrae can result in chest pains, secondary splinting and subsequent atelectasis, mainfest as unilateral or bilateral infiltrates
    - Clinically there may be bone tenderness
    - Bone scans done at least 72 hours post-acute event show increased uptake consistent with osteoblastic activity accompanying the repair process that follows marrow infarction

4 **Fat emboli** resulting from bone marrow necrosis is rarely diagnosed antemortem
   - Diagnosis can be made by finding alveolar macrophages with fat droplets in sputum or BAL as well as evidence of embolization to the skin, kidneys or retina

Sequelae of the ACS include
1 Resolution
2 Development of pulmonary edema
   - Cardiac, secondary to fluid overload from hydration or transfusions, LV dysfunction
   - Non-cardiac and secondary to narcotics, fat emboli
3 Progression to ARDS, the latter usually developing in hospital and uncommonly at the time of admission (pathophysiology is unclear)
4 Progression to chronic lung disease (see below)
5 HIV infection secondary to transfusions
6 Death, ACS responsible for 20–25% of all deaths in sickle cell disease with mortality rates up to 10% reported for individual acute episodes

Radiologic findings
1 Plate atelectasis
2 Pneumonia picture
3 Pulmonary infarction
4 Pulmonary edema
5 ARDS secondary to 2, 3, or 4
6 Pleural effusions seen in ~15% of patients
7 Manifestations of superimposed HIV infection

Diagnostic work-up can include
1 Chest X-ray, O_2 sats
2 Cultures, serology
3 Bone scan
4 Echocardiogram
5 V/Q scan ? HRCT scan
6 Sputum or BAL for lipid-laden macrophages

Chronic Lung Disease (CLD)

Definition: The combination of pulmonary hypertension and restrictive lung disease in sickle cell patients

- Clinically seen in patients who have had recurrent episodes of the ACS and present with progressive dyspnea, hypoxemia and chest pains
- Chest X-rays reveal increased interstitial markings bilaterally with signs of pulmonary hypertension
- PFTs reveal a restrictive picture with reduced lung volumes and DCO ± an obstructive component
- Histologically there may be little interstitial fibrosis but interstitial edema is seen with lymphatic dilatation
- Cardiac manifestations include
  - Cor pulmonale with RA + RV hypertrophy
  - LV fibrosis and myocardial infarcts without CAD

THALASSEMIA MAJOR

1. Extramedullary hematopoiesis with posterior mediastinal masses and rib lesions
2. Diaphragm elevation from massive hepatosplenomegaly
3. Congestive heart failure with episodes of pulmonary edema and transudative pleural effusions from repeated blood transfusions or myocardial involvement from hemochromatosis
4. Restrictive lung disease on PFTs which appear to correlate with increasing age and the burden of transfused iron

Fraser R.S., Muller N.L., Colman N., Paré P.D. (1999) Diagnosis of Diseases of the Chest 4th Edn., WB Saunders.

Baum, G.L., Crapo, J.D., Celli, B.R., Karlinsky, J.B. (eds) (1997) *Textbook of Pulmonary Diseases*, 6th edn.: Lippincott-Raven.

Fishman, A.P., Elias, J.A., Fishman, J.A., Grippi, M.A., Kaiser, L.R., Senior, R.N. (1998) *Fishman's Pulmonary Diseases and Disorders*, 3rd edn.: McGraw-Hill.

Utz, J., Swenson, S., Gertz, M. (1996) Pulmonary amyloidosis (1996). The Mayo Clinic experience from 1980–1993. *Am Internal Med.* **124**: 407–413.

Hilgebrand, F., Rosenow, E., Habermann, T. et al. (1990) Pulmonary complications of leukemia. *Chest* **98**: 1233–1239.

Edwards, J., Matthay, K. (1989) Hematologic disorders affecting the lungs. *Clinics in Chest Medicine* **10**: 723–746.

Campbell, J.H. *et al.* (1993) Investigation and management of pulmonary infiltrates following bone marrow transplantation. An 8-year review. *Thorax* **48**: 1248–1251.

Breuer, R. *et al.* (1993) Pulmonary complications of bone marrow transplant. *Resp. Med.* 1993; **87**: 571–579.

Ettinger, N., Trulock, E. (1991) Pulmonary considerations of organ transplant. Part 2. *ARRD* **144**: 213–223.

Winer-Muran, H., Gurney, J., Bozeman, P. *et al.* (1996) Pulmonary complications after bone marrow transplant. *Radiol. Clin. North Am.* **34**: 97–117.

Soubani, A., Miller, K., Hassoun, P. (1996) Pulmonary complications of bone marrow transplant. *Chest* **109**: 1066–1077.

Filuk, R.B., Warren, P.N. (1996) BAL in Waldenstrom's macroglobulinemia with pulmonary infiltrates. *Thorax* **41**: 409–410.

Rausch, P.G., Herion, J.C. (1980) Pulmonary manifestations of Waldenstrom's macroglobulinemia. *Am. J. Hematol.* **9**: 201–209.

42 Hemoptysis – NYD

NORMAL VASCULAR ANATOMY OF THE LUNG

- **Pulmonary circulation**
  - Systolic pressure < 20 mmHg
  - Diastolic pressure < 10 mmHg
  - The pulmonary arterioles interact with the airways at the level of the terminal bronchioles and distally giving rise to the pulmonary capillaries
- Bronchial circulation
  - Under systemic pressure
  - 1–2 bronchial arteries per lung and follow branches of the bronchial tree forming a sub-mucosal plexus
  - Beyond the terminal bronchioles, they anastomose with pulmonary arterioles and venules, accounting for the normal right to left shunt of 5% of cardiac output

Presentations of hemoptysis

1. Spotty hemoptysis/blood tinged sputum
2. Massive hemoptysis
3. Diffuse alveolar hemorrhage syndrome

DIAGNOSTIC WORK-UP OF HEMOPTYSIS

Hemoptysis can arise from multiple disorders which may primarily involve the airways, lung parenchyma or the lung vasculature – pulmonary or systemic

I. Eliminate an extrapulmonary cause of bleeding

1 R/O GI source, e.g. esophagus, stomach
2 R/O ENT origin, e.g. nose, pharynx, largynx
3 R/O factitious hemoptysis (Munchausen syndrome)

II. Determine the presence of an associated systemic disorder

1 Systemic vasculitis/collagen vascular disease testing for ANCA, ANA, RF, anti DNA AB, complement, hepatitis B surface Ag, circulating immune complexes
2 Pulmonary-renal syndromes, e.g. BUN, CR, urinalysis, anti GBM Ab, ANCA, ANA, anti DNA AB
3 Metastatic neoplasm, e.g. choriocarcinoma, angiosarcoma
4 AV malformations
5 R/O coagulopathy – platelets, PT, PTT, INR

III. Define the likely anatomic pulmonary origin of the bleeding as well as the **probable pathology**

1 **Airways** disease is the most common source in clinical practice and chest X-rays may or may not be normal
   - e.g. – Tracheitis/bronchitis
     – Bronchiectasis
     – Tuberculosis, atypicals, fungi
     – Broncholiths
     – Endometriosis
     – Endobronchial tumors
       — Benign/malignant
       — Metastatic from breast, colon, kidney, melanoma, esophagus
2 **Parenchymal** diseases where chest X-rays are typically abnormal
   - e.g. – Pneumonia (angioinvasive – aspergillus, mucor)
     – Mycetoma
     – Abscess
     – Neoplasms
     – Pulmonary-renal syndromes
     – Drug-induced (cocaine)

3 **Pulmonary vascular diseases** where chest X-rays are usually abnormal
- arterial, e.g.
  - Pulmonary artery hypertension
  - Emboli and infarction
  - Vasculitides/collagen/autoimmune disease
  - Vascular neoplasms
    - Hemangioma
    - Kaposi's,
    - Angiosarcoma
- Capillary, e.g.
  - Goodpastures, primary or secondary
  - Idiopathic pulmonary hemosiderosis
  - Isolated pulmonary capillaritis
  - Post-lymphangiogram
- Venous, e.g.
  - Cardiac or non-cardiac causes of pulmonary venous hypertension

4 **Systemic vessel as the cause of bleeding** where chest X-rays may be normal
- Origin of bleeding is usually from the bronchial arteries, but occasionally from the axillary, subclavian, intercostal, phrenics or aorta (see Systemic Blood Supply to Lung, p. 760)

IV. Radiologic

1 **Chest X-ray** looking for **associated** disease involving the airways, parenchyma, pleura, vasculature or mediastinum, in addition to the airspace disease secondary to hemorrhage

2 **CT scan** to document disease in the central airways as well as in airways distal to those seen with bronchoscopy, e.g. bronchiectasis, broncholithiasis
- CT scan can also demonstrate parenchymal disease not apparent on chest X-ray, e.g. lung nodule, mycetoma, endometriosis or diffuse interstitial disease, which may also be responsible for hemoptysis

3 **Arteriography** – bronchial/pulmonary

V. Bronchoscopy ± bronchial or transbronchial biopsy

HEMOPTYSIS – MASSIVE

Definition: Varies amongst different authors with regard to

1 Volume of blood coughed up and the time interval, e.g. >500 cc within 24 hours
2 Magnitude of blood loss as reflected in
  - Need for hospitalization
  - Hypotension
  - Requirement for transfusion
  - Aspiration
  - Upper airway obstruction from blood
  - Death

- Fatalities are secondary to asphyxiation or exsanguination and relate to the amount of blood expectorated, rate of bleeding, amount of blood retained in the lungs and the underlying pulmonary reserve

Sources of massive hemoptysis

1 *Bronchial arteries
2 Non-bronchial systemic collateral vessels, e.g. axillary, subclavian, intercostal, phrenic arteries
3 Pulmonary arteries – rare source with the exception of AV malformations and Rasmussen aneurysms
4 Alveolar hemorrhage syndromes
5 R/O the upper airway or a GI source of bleeding

Most common etiologies

1 Erosive tracheobronchitis
2 Bronchiectasis
3 Pulmonary carcinoma
4 Tuberculosis, active or inactive
5 Lung abscess/necrotizing pneumonia
6 Mycetoma
7 AV malformations
8 Bleeding diathesis
9 Vasculitis, e.g. Wegener's, Takayasu's
10 Capillaritis
11 Collagen disease, e.g. SLE

12 Septic emboli
13 Post-bone marrow transplant
14 Mitral stenosis
15 Aorticobronchopulmonary fistula, e.g. aneurysms secondary to TB, syphilis, mycotic, post-surgical, atherosclerotic, trauma, neoplastic

Fraser R.S., Muller N.L., Colman N., Paré P.D. (1999) Diagnosis of Diseases of the Chest 4th Edn., WB Saunders.
Baum, G.L., Crapo, J.D., Celli, B.R., Karlinsky, J.B. (eds) (1997) *Textbook of Pulmonary Diseases*, 6th edn.: Lippincott-Raven.
Fishman, A.P., Elias, J.A., Fishman, J.A., Grippi, M.A., Kaiser, L.R., Senior, R.N. (1998) *Fishman's Pulmonary Diseases and Disorders*, 3rd edn.: McGraw-Hill.

43 Hilar Shadows

BILATERAL SMALL HILA

1 **Congenital heart disease** including tetralogy of Fallot, tricuspid atresia, truncus arteriosus, transposition of the great vessels
2 **Acquired heart disease** with reduced pulmonary artery flow, e.g. cardiac tamponade, IVC syndrome
3 **Central pulmonary emboli**

UNILATERAL SMALL HILUM

1 **Proximal interruption of a pulmonary artery**
   - Rare congenital anomaly where the left or right pulmonary is absent but the intrapulmonary vessels are intact and present
   - Vascular supply to the lungs can arise from hypertrophied bronchial arteries, the aorta or a branch of the aorta
   - Congenital cardiovascular anomalies are present, particularly with left-sided lesions
   - Chest X-rays reveal a small hyperlucent lung with an absent hilar shadow resembling Swyer-James syndrome but differs as follows

- Absent air trapping on expiration
- Absent perfusion but normal ventilation *vs.* absent ventilation and perfusion in Swyer-James
- Absent pulmonary artery on angiography *vs.* a diminutive but present one in Swyer-James

2 **Scimitar syndrome**
3 **Swyer-James syndrome**
4 **Pulmonary embolus**
5 **Neoplastic invasion** of a pulmonary artery
6 **Lobar collapse** and hilar displacement behind the heart

UNILATERAL HILAR ENLARGEMENT

*Manifest as an alteration in the **size**, **contour**, or **density** of a hilum

Diagnostic Work-Up

1 Obtain previous films
2 Consider the potential anatomic origin (see below)
3 Determine the density characteristics on CT scan, i.e. soft tissue *vs.* fat, cystic, vascular or calcified
4 Document any associated abnormalities involving the airways, parenchyma, pleura, vasculature, mediastinum
5 CT with contrast is the initial imaging test of choice, although MRI may be of greater diagnostic value with pulmonary vascular disorders or for some bronchogenic cysts
6 Other investigations may include angiography, echocardiography

Anatomic Origins

1 **Airway** diseases including hamartoma, bronchogenic cyst, mucus plug, bronchogenic neoplasm
2 **Parenchyma**, i.e. any cause of localized airspace disease contiguous to the hilum
3 **Pleural** lesions including neoplasms or loculated fluid contiguous to the hilum

4 **Lymphadenopathy**, including lymphoma, bronchogenic or other secondary neoplasms, tuberculosis, fungal, sarcoid, other
5 **Mediastinal** lesions superimposed on a hilum
6 **Vasculature**
   - *Enlarged pulmonary artery*
     - Thromboembolic
     - Pulmonary artery hypertension
     - Pulmonary artery stenosis with post-stenotic dilatation on left
     - Pulmonary artery neoplasms – primary or metastatic (see below)
     - Idiopathic dilatation of the pulmonary artery
     - Pulmonary artery aneurysm (see below)
   - *Enlarged pulmonary vein*
     - Varix formation secondary to: mitral valve disease, congenital, idiopathic
       — Locations are RLL (60%) > LUL > RUL
       — Usually asymptomatic and discovered on routine X-ray
       — Diagnostic features
         a. Oval, round or tubular opacities in the hilum or perihilar region which changes in shape on valsalva or Mueller maneuvers
         b. CT with contrast demonstrating an enlarged vein draining into the left atrium
         c. Angiography
         d. Transesophageal echo
     - Left or right inferior pulmonary vein confluence
     - Left or right superior pulmonary vein pseudotumor
   - *AV malformation*

Pulmonary Artery Aneurysm

Definition: Rare vascular disorder that can involve the main, lobar or intrapulmonary branches of the pulmonary artery, with the following etiologies

1 Congenital heart disease, e.g. ASD, VSD, patent ductus arteriosus

2 Congenital abnormalities of the pulmonary valve, e.g. pulmonary stenosis
3 Congenital or acquired pulmonary vascular disorders
 - Pulmonary artery coarctation
 - Cystic medial necrosis
 - Hereditary hemorragic telangiectasia
 - Atherosclerosis
 - Infections, e.g. tuberculosis, fungal, pyogenic
 - Vasculitis, e.g. Takasayu's, Behcet's
 - Trauma
 - Pulmonary hypertension

Clinical presentations
- Asymptomatic radiologic finding
- Non-specific respiratory symptoms of dyspnea and chest pain
- Systemic symptoms of fevers, sweats and weight loss occurring when infection is responsible

Radiologically, the usual presentation is that of a hilar mass (if central) or a peripheral nodule
- Pulmonary artery may be better defined on echocardiography and infusion CT, with definitive diagnosis on angiography

Pulmonary Artery Sarcoma (PAS)

Definition: Rare tumors often confused with thromboembolic disease
- Arise from the pulmonary valve, central pulmonary artery or its main branches, with multiple histologic types described, but leiomyosarcoma is the most frequent

Clinical presentations are variable and should be suspected with
- Features of acute or chronic thromboembolic disease in a patient without risk factors as well as non-specific symptoms of dyspnea, chest pains, cough and hemoptysis, unresponsive to anticoagulants

- Perihilar mass in association with pulmonary artery hypertension
- Pulmonary, mediastinal or distant metastases

Physical findings are usually those of pulmonary hypertension and right heart failure

Sequelae include
- Right heart failure secondary to pulmonary outflow obstruction
- Lung infarct manifest as peripheral infiltrates due to tumor emboli or tumor associated thrombi
- Metastatic disease
- Sudden death

Resection rate is low with death often occurring within weeks to months of hospitalization

V/Q scans are non-specific and reveal the changes of thromboembolic disease

Echo may visualize the intravascular mass

Chest X-ray findings include
- Normal films
- Hilar mass with enlargement of the main pulmonary artery and proximal branches
- Findings of arterial occlusion with oligemia, infarction, pleural effusion

CT or **angiography** reveals an intralumenal filling mass in the central pulmonary artery or its main branches with differentiation from chronic thromboembolic disease often difficult, the differential features of sarcoma including

1 Vascular expansion and extravascular spread (*vs.* vascular narrowing and cut-offs in embolic disease)
   - Transmural growth can extend into the hilum, mediastinum, pericardium and lung parenchyma, simulating spread from primary tumors of the lung, mediastinum, heart or extrathoracic sites
2 Unilateral disease *vs.* the usual bilateral distribution of emboli

3 Heterogeneous density
4 Occasional enhancement post contrast

BILATERAL HILAR ENLARGEMENT (BHA)

1 **Vascular dilatation**
- Pulmonary artery hypertension
- Congenital heart disease with left-to-right shunt
- Mitral valve disease
- Left heart failure

2 **Lymphadenopathy**
- Idiopathic
  - *Sarcoid
- Neoplastic
  - *Lymphoma
  - *Metastatic cancer
- Infectious
  - Primary tuberculosis
  - Fungal, e.g. histoplasmosis, coccidioidomycosis
  - Viral
- Inhalational
  - *Silicosis
  - Berylliosis

SARCOID *vs.* MALIGNANCY – BHA

Sarcoid	Malignancy
• Responsible for the vast majority of cases • No history of prior malignancy • Symptomatic or asymptomatic • Normal or abnormal physical exam with uveitis or erythema nodosum being classical • Anemia is rare	• Lymphoma – always symptomatic • Lung cancer – extranodal lesions • Extrathoracic metastases – history of remote cancer – anemia is common

Table 43.1

Naidich, D.P., Zerhouni, E.A., Siegelman, S.S. (1998) *Computed Tomography and Magnetic Resonance of the Thorax*, 3rd edn. New York: Raven Press.

Moss, A., Gamsu, Genant (1992) Thorax and neck. In: *Computed Tomography of the Body with Magnetic Resonance Imaging*, 2nd edn, vol. 1.: W.B. Saunders.

Webb, R., Muller, N.L., Naidich, D.P. (1996) *High Resolution CT of the Lung*, 2nd edn.: Lippincott-Raven.

Felson, B. (1973) *Chest Roentgenology*.: W.B. Saunders.

44 HIV Pulmonary Disease

DIFFERENTIAL AND DIAGNOSTIC WORK-UP

The respiratory symptoms of HIV are generally non-specific and the radiologic abnormalities are rarely pathognomonic, with individual disorders having variable radiologic findings while multiple and diverse disorders can have a similar X-ray appearance

The differential diagnosis usually involves the following

Infections

1 Bacterial (bronchitis, bronchiolitis, pneumonia)
   - *Strep. pneumoniae*, *Staph. aureus*, hemophilus, legionella, pseudomonas, nocardia, rhodococcus, mycobacteria, others
2 Viral
   - CMV, herpes simplex, primary HIV infection
3 Fungal
   - Histo, blasto, coccidio, cryptococcus, aspergillus, pneumocystis
4 Parasitic
   - Toxoplasmosis, strongyloides

Inflammation

5 Non-specific interstitial pneumonitis
6 LIP
7 Lymphocytic alveolitis

Neoplasms

8 Kaposi's sarcoma
9 Non-Hodgkin's lymphoma
10 ? Increased incidence of lung cancer

Drug toxicity

11 Allergic alveolitis, e.g. septra
12 i.v. talcosis secondary to drug abuse
13 Neutropenia-induced infection
14 Drug-induced bleeding diathesis

Pulmonary edema

15 Cardiac disease, e.g. toxoplasma, CMV or HIV cardiomyopathy

Diffuse alveolar damage – fibrosis (biopsy diagnosis where no etiologic agent is identified)

Unrelated disease

Diagnostic Clues and Work-Up

1 **History**
- Country of origin and travel history reflecting the geographic distribution of infectious agents e.g. tuberculosis, endemic fungi such as histoplasmosis or coccidioidomycosis, pneumocystis
- HIV risk groups, e.g. Kaposi's in homosexual males, tuberculosis in i.v. drug abusers
- Prior infections as control of infection is more common than eradication, e.g. toxoplasmosis, CMV and cryptococcus are lifelong infections
- Animal contacts, e.g. toxoplasmosis from cats, rhodococcus from horses
- Tuberculosis risk factors, e.g. recent contact with tuberculosis, i.v. drug abusers, health care workers, urban minorities, incarceration, tuberculin status, contact with active tuberculosis cases
- Blood transfusions as a source of CMV
- Drug history, e.g.

- Chemoprophylaxis making specific infections unlikely
- Septra-induced allergic alveolitis
- i.v. talcosis with illicit drug use
- Drug-induced bleeding diathesis

2 **Presence of extrapulmonary disease**

- Lymphadenopathy, e.g. lymphoma, fungi, tuberculosis, atypicals
- CNS disease, e.g. toxoplasmosis, cryptococcosis
- Fundoscopic lesions, e.g. tuberculosis, viral, fungi
- Generalized systemic disease, e.g. tuberculosis, atypicals, fungi, CMV, Kaposi's, non-Hodgkin's lymphoma, rarely pneumocystis
- Skin lesions of Kaposi's, fungi, bacillary angiomatosis

3 **CD4 counts** reflecting the severity of immunosuppression

500
- URIs
- Bronchitis

400
- Tuberculosis
- Pneumonia

300
- Atypicals
- Recurrent pneumonia

200
- PCP
- Kaposi's sarcoma
- Sepsis
- Atypical manifestations of *M. tuberculosis* including dissemination

100
- Extrapulmonary cryptococcosis
- Breakthrough of PCP prophylaxis
- CMV
- Disseminated MAI, histoplasmosis, coccidioidomycosis
- Toxoplasmosis
- Pseudomonas

4 **Normal LDH** level makes PCP unlikely

5 **Chest X-ray findings**
- Normal
  - PCP, MAI
  - LIP, NSIP
- Nodules
  - Tuberculosis, fungi, nocardia
  - Kaposi's, lymphoma
  - Septic emboli
- Cavitation
  - Tuberculosis, *Staph. aureus*, nocardia, *Rhodococcus equii*, fungi, pneumocystis
- Cysts
  - Pneumocystis
  - i.v. drug users
- Diffuse infiltrates
  - Pneumocystis, tuberculosis, MAI, CMV, fungi
  - LIP, NSIP
  - Kaposi's sarcoma
  - Drug reaction
  - Pulmonary edema
  - Pyogenic pneumonia, e.g. hemophilus
  - Bronchiolitis
- Segmental/lobal infiltrates with air bronchograms
  - Often bacterial
- Other focal infiltrates
  - Pyogenic bacteria, tuberculosis, fungi, occasionally pneumocystis
- Lymphadenopathy
  - Tuberculosis, MAI, fungi, bacillary angiomatosis
  - Kaposi's, lymphoma
- Enlarged pulmonary arteries
  - i.v. talcosis
  - Idiopathic pulmonary hypertension
- Pleural effusions
  - Tuberculosis, parapneumonic, pneumocystis

  - Kaposi's, NHL
  - Transudates
- Pneumothorax
  - Pneumocystis

6 **CT scan** can detect abnormalities **not** appreciated on chest films including
- 'Ground glass' opacities or cystic changes in PCP
- Miliary pattern with tuberculosis or fungal dissemination
- Unsuspected lymphadenopathy
- Calcified nodes post-pentamidine treatment for PCP
- Rim enhancing and centrally necrotic nodes of tuberculosis
- Occult cavitation
- Pleural nodules in KS, NHL
- Evidence of bronchiolitis (centrilobular thickening, 'tree-in-bud', mosaic perfusion)

7 **Gallium scan**
- Diffuse parenchymal uptake is very sensitive but not specific for PCP except in patients with a normal chest X-ray and diffuse intense uptake
- Focal parenchymal uptake is seen with tuberculosis, bacteria, fungi
- Nodal uptake is seen with tuberculosis, fungi, NHL
- Diffuse low grade pulmonary uptake with extrapulmonary uptake is seen with
  - LIP: bilateral parotid gland uptake
  - CMV: esophagus, colon, adrenal uptake
- Negative galium but positive thallium scan with Kaposi's

8 **Sputum induction** for PCP or tuberculosis

9 **Smears and cultures** of pulmonary (sputum, lung, pleura) or extrapulmonary sites (blood, urine, stools, liver, bone marrow) for bacteriology, TB, atypicals, mycology, viruses

10 **Bronchoscopic visualization** and biopsy of Kaposi's, lung cancer and uncommonly tuberculosis, MAI, actinomycosis, nocardia, aspergillus, pneumocystis, bacillary angiomatosis, non-Hodgkins' lymphoma
   - *Transbronchial biopsy*
   - *BAL* for PCP, mycobacterial disease, fungi, viruses, ? bacteria

11 **Antigen detection** in
   - Serum or urine for acute infections e.g. histoplasma polysaccharide antigen, cryptococcal antigen
   - CSF for cryptococcal antigen

12 **TTNA** for focal peripheral lesions

13 **Thoracoscopy/thoracotomy**

INFECTIOUS DISEASES

Aspergillosis (see p. 618)

Infections caused by aspergillus can take the form of parenchymal invasion or tracheobronchial disease, are uncommon and often associated with other risk factors including neutropenia, broad spectrum antibiotics, steroid use and CD4 < 50

Pulmonary involvement is seen either in isolation or as part of disseminated infection

- Respiratory symptoms are non-specific but the diagnosis should be suspected with
  - Hemoptysis reflecting cavitary parenchymal disease or endobronchial disease
  - Expectoration of plugs representing bronchial casts and suggesting airway infection, the latter characterized by mucosal ulceration, tracheobronchial nodular thickening and pseudomembrane formation

Radiologic features

1 Focal infiltrates or nodules
2 Thick-walled cavitary lesions which may be large with little surrounding infiltrate

3 Diffuse bilateral interstitial or alveolar infiltrates resembling PCP
4 Patchy bilateral alveolar infiltrates
5 Tracheobronchial involvement with atelectasis, tracheobronchial irregularities impinging on the air column or dilated impacted airways
6 Pleural effusions

Diagnosis is often difficult as absolute proof requires histopathologic confirmation of tissue invasion or positive cultures from normally sterile fluids and tissues
1 Positive sputum or BAL cultures, a compatible pulmonary illness and no other infection detected is suggestive
2 Endobronchial biopsy showing mucosal invasion
3 Lung or other tissue biopsy, e.g. skin
4 ⊕ Urine cultures imply metastatic renal abscess

Bacterial Pulmonary Infections

Community-acquired bacterial pulmonary infection occurs commonly in HIV infected patients and is manifest as bronchitis, bronchiolitis, bronchiectasis or pneumonia

- Recurrent bacterial pneumonia is an AIDS-defining condition and frequently occurs before other AIDS-defining illnesses
- Seen at all CD4 counts, but is particularly common with CD4 < 200, as well as in i.v. drug users and smokers
- Pneumococcus is the most common cause of non-bacteremic bacterial pneumonia but others include hemophilus, *Staph. aureus*, legionella, nocardia, rhodococcus, pseudomonas, bartonella, others
- Recurrent tracheitis and bronchitis are seen in HIV with bacterial pneumonia frequently complicated by bacteremia and multilobar involvement

Clues to a bacterial etiology include
1 Acute onset of respiratory symptoms clinically
2 Purulent sputum with positive gram stain and absence of pneumocystis or acid-fast organisms

3 Segmental or lobar consolidation with air bronchograms is the most common radiologic manifestion of pneumonia in addition to the following
   - Hemophilus has been described to give diffuse interstitial disease simulating PCP
   - Rhodococcus can mimic TB with upper lobe nodules and cavitation
   - Cavitary disease is seen with gram negatives, e.g. pseudomonas
   - A diffuse interstitial pattern simulating PCP can be seen in acute bronchiolitis with CT scan features of
     – Bronchial wall thickening
     – Centrilobular densities with characteristic V and Y-shaped configuration (impacted bronchioles)
     – 'Tree-in-bud' pattern reflecting distended, mucus-impacted bronchioles
     – Pattern of mosaic perfusion with areas of decreased attenuation secondary to air trapping

4 CD4 < 200

5 Leucocytosis with a left shift

6 Normal or minimal elevation of serum LDH

7 Positive blood cultures (high incidence of bacteremia with *Strep. pneumoniae* being the commonest cause of bacteremia in bacterial RTIs)

Bacillary angiomatosis is seen predominantly in AIDS when CD4 is <200 (rarely in other immunocompromised patients)
Infectious disease caused by the genus Bartonella, *B. henselae* (the agent of cat-scratch fever) or *B. quintana* (trench fever), with the mode of transmission being a cat bite or scratch

- Gram negative rods with a characteristic trilaminar wall on electron microscopy
- Usually presents with skin lesions resembling Kaposi's, lymphadenopathy, anemia and fever
- Other organ systems can be involved with lytic bone lesions, low attenuation lesions in liver/spleen, soft tissue

masses, brain (aseptic meningitis, dementia) as well as systemic features of fever, chills, night sweats, weight loss accompanied by non-specific respiratory symptoms

Radiologic features

1 Lung nodules
2 Mediastinal/hilar adenopathy (nodule and soft tissue lesions enhance very strongly)
3 Pleural effusions
4 Polypoid endobronchial lesions

Diagnostic features

1 Histology showing foci of vascular proliferation
2 Warthin-Starry stains showing curved rods with trilaminar cell walls
3 Positive serology
4 PCR in tissue or body fluid
5 Blood or other cultures
6 Good response to antibiotics

Rhodococcus equi is a gram positive and variably acid-fast organism seen mainly in immunocompromised patients, especially AIDS

- Thought to be acquired by inhalation from soil, risk factors for infection including farm dust or horses

Clinically, lung disease is insidious in onset with non-specific respiratory and systemic symptoms, while extrapulmonary disease can involve lymph nodes, CNS, pericardium, eye and subcutaneous tissues

- High mortality is reported with illness frequently lasting several months prior to death

Radiologic findings can mimic tuberculosis and include

1 Upper lobe consolidation
2 Cavitation
3 Pleural effusions

Diagnostic findings

1 Positive blood cultures
2 Isolation from BAL, brushings, TTNA, endobronchial biopsy

Blastomycosis (see p. 625)

Rare in AIDS but should be suspected in the appropriate geographic areas, particularly with CD4 counts <200

- Disease can result from progression of primary disease or endogenous reactivation
- Usually presents as an acute illness with non-specific respiratory symptoms and purulent sputum
- Dissemination is seen in ~½ of cases with meningitis common as well as involvement of skin, bone and the male genitourinary tract
- Fulminating disease leading to an ARDS picture is described
- Prognosis is poor with death from progressive pneumonia or dissemination

Radiologic features are varied including a miliary pattern, nodules or non-specific infiltrates

Diagnostic features

1. Sputum and BAL smears showing the characteristic yeasts with single budding
2. Cultures of sputum, BAL
3. Skin biopsy
4. Serology is unreliable

Candidiasis (see p. 627)

Oral, esophageal and vaginal infections are common, representing impaired T cell immunity and resultant overgrowth of candida on mucosal surfaces

- Esophageal candidiasis is an AIDS-defining illness in ~15% of HIV-infected patients, ranges from an asymptomatic finding to dysphagia and odynophagia, and is generally accompanied by oral candidiasis
- Candidemia, disseminated candidiasis and pneumonia are rare, with candidemia typically occurring in the presence of the usual risk factors, e.g. neutropenia, multiple antibiotics, indwelling catheters
- Pulmonary candidiasis is a terminal manifestation of HIV

infection, often co-exists with other infections and is uncommonly diagnosed during life

Diagnostic features

1 Oropharyngeal candidiasis by examination and culture of scrapings
2 Esophageal candidiasis by barium swallow ('cobblestone' appearance) or endoscopy with biopsy (R/O CMV, herpes)
3 Disseminated disease by cultures of blood, usually sterile body fluids or tissue
4 Histopathologic evidence on tissue biopsy

Coccidioidomycosis (see p. 630)

Fungal infection caused by *C. immitis* endemic in parts of the South Western United States with disease in AIDS patients representing either recent infection or reactivation of latent infection

- In the earlier stages of AIDS the clinical and radiologic manifestations resemble those seen in normal hosts
- As immunosuppression worsens and CD4 counts are <250, the risk of acquiring disease increases and coccidioidomycosis presents as a progressive respiratory illness over days to weeks with non-specific respiratory symptoms
- Meningitis may occur with the above or less often alone, skin lesions are seen in ~5% of cases and dissemination to virtually any organ is described

Radiologic findings in patients with mild degrees of immunosuppression resemble those seen with primary infection in a normal host but advanced AIDS is characterized by

1 Diffuse macronodular infiltrates
2 Diffuse interstitial disease resembling PCP
3 Lymphadenopathy and pleural effusion can occur
4 Rarely, normal chest X-rays in association with extrathoracic disease

Diagnostic features

1 Bronchoscopic visualization and biopsy of endobronchial ulcers
2 Identification of spherules in lung biopsy, BAL or sputum
3 Culture of sputum, BAL, lung, blood
4 Serodiagnosis is unreliable

CMV Pneumonia

CMV infection is very common in advanced HIV disease with the respiratory system frequently involved (rarely alone) along with the adrenals, colon, liver, retina and CNS

- CMV pneumonia must be distinguished from CMV infection as the salivary glands are a frequent site of subclinical infection, with resultant positive cultures from respiratory secretions
- Pulmonary involvement can range from subclinical infection to respiratory failure but is rarely the sole cause of pneumonia and then only with late stage disease

Often undiagnosed during life due to co-existing infection and the absence of well-defined diagnostic criteria which might include

1 Radiologic disease
    - Airspace disease manifest as 'ground glass' opacities or consolidation
    - Interstitial opacities
    - Nodules/masses
    - Airways disease including bronchiolitis, bronchitis
2 Culture of CMV from sputum, bronchial washings or BAL
3 Detection of CMV inclusions in sputum or BAL by
    - Direct visualization
    - DNA probes to detect CMV DNA
    - Monoclonal antibody to detect CMV infected cells
4 Transbronchial or open lung biopsy demonstrating pneumonitis and histologic changes compatible with CMV
5 Worsening pneumonia despite no other pathogen found or adequate treatment of a co-pathogen
6 Response to antiviral therapy

Cryptococcosis (see p. 634)

Clinically, it is the most common systemic and life-threatening fungal infection in AIDS and can present at any time but usually when CD4 < 200 cells/mm^3

- Pathophysiology is that of inhalation of the organisms followed by hematogenous dissemination in immunocompromised patients
- Can be the initial opportunistic infection or occur with other infections
- Usually presents as a meningo-encephalitis with the skin being the second most common organ system involved
- Pulmonary disease may occur in isolation or in association with disseminated disease and presentations include
  - *Non-specific constitutional symptoms presenting over weeks, usually with fever, followed by neurologic symptoms of headache, neck stiffness, altered mental state, photophobia and focal neurologic defects
  - Acute meningitis
  - Non-specific respiratory symptoms suggesting PCP, often with subclinical meningitis
  - Isolated pleural effusion
  - Disseminated disease involving liver, spleen, GI tract, skin, eye, bone
  - Disease relapse if therapy is discontinued in patients with known disease

Radiologic features

1 *Diffuse interstitial reticular or reticulonodular infiltrates (resembling PCP)
2 Other infiltrates including cavitation, single or multiple nodules, mass-like lesion resembling carcinoma
3 Pleural effusion
4 Hilar/mediastinal adenopathy (which can occur without pulmonary infiltrates)
5 Normal chest X-ray

Diagnostic features

1 ⊕ Cryptococcal Ag in serum (98) > CSF > urine (negative serum test excludes cryptococcal meningitis)

2 ⊕ India ink stains on CSF
3 ⊕ CSF culture which may be present in the absence of WBCs, low glucose or elevated protein
4 ⊕ Blood cultures
5 Lung infection diagnosed by
   - Isolation of crytococcus from sputum, BAL, lung tissue or pleural fluid
   - Lung biopsy for histopathology
   - Detection of cryptococcal antigen >1:8 in BAL or pleural fluid
6 Biopsy of suspected skin or bone lesions

Herpes Simplex Virus Pneumonitis

Diagnosis is difficult as recovery from respiratory secretions may reflect contamination from oral lesions or asymptomatic shedding in saliva

Proposed criteria might include

1 Progressive pulmonary disease manifest as diffuse interstitial pneumonia or necrotizing tracheobronchitis with focal pneumonia
2 Positive cultures of lower respiratory tract secretions
3 Histopathologic evidence of disease (may be non-diagnostic)
4 No other pathogen identifiable
5 Response to antiviral therapy

Histoplasmosis (see p. 645)

Disease is acquired by inhalation and usually results from progression of a primary infection but can also represent reactivation of remote infection

- Dissemination is rare in normal hosts but common with HIV and the diagnosis should be suspected from the patient's country of origin or travel history

Clinically it is typically seen with advanced disease and presentations include

1 *Disseminated disease of subacute onset with non-specific complaints of fevers and weight loss

- Non-specific respiratory symptoms develop later in the course of disease and therefore localizing features are often absent early on

2 Acute onset with rapidly progressive disease and DIC
3 Chronic febrile diarrheal illness resembling a parasitic gastroenteritis
4 Upper GI bleed from gastric ulceration
5 Hepatosplenomegaly
6 Meningitis or intracerebral histoplasmosis
7 Disease relapse if therapy is discontinued in patients with known disease

Radiologic features

1 Normal chest X-rays in 25–50% of patients at disease onset
2 Non-specific nodular infiltrates or diffuse interstitial infiltrates resembling PCP
3 Hilar adenopathy and pleural effusions can develop

Diagnostic features

1 Epidemiologic features
2 Histoplasma polysaccharide antigen (HPA) in serum or urine, a negative test excluding disseminated disease
3 Smears of peripheral blood (positive in up to ½ of cases), bone marrow or BAL
4 Cultures of bone marrow, blood, BAL or lung biopsy
5 Wright-Giemsa stain of pleural fluid

Mycobacteria Tuberculosis

TB is the only complicating infection of AIDS transmitted from person to person

- Often occurs early in the course of disease due to the virulence of *M. tuberculosis* and is frequently the AIDS-defining illness

HIV is the most important risk factor for TB, seen in ~⅓ of cases and should therefore be screened for in all new cases, particularly with

1 Profound weight loss and diarrhea
2 Physical findings of oral thrush or Kaposi's sarcoma

3 Extrapulmonary TB
4 Atypical radiologic features (see below)

The rate of TB in HIV patients is affected by
1 PPD status of the population, representing latent infection
2 Exposure to active TB cases with rapid progression from recently acquired disease
3 Degree of immunosuppression

Differential features of TB in HIV positive individuals reflect the degree of immunosuppression (CD4 counts) and include
1 Increasing frequency of a negative PPD and cutaneous anergy as CD4 falls below 200
2 Positive blood cultures
3 Frequent occurrence of dissemination with involvement of bone marrow, GU tract, CNS and lymph nodes (cervical > axillary > retroperitoneal)
4 Poorly formed granulomas on biopsy with numerous AFB seen
5 Increasing multidrug resistance
6 The classic apical–posterior distribution of upper lobe infiltrates with cavitation becomes less frequent and is replaced by atypical changes including
   - Hilar/mediastinal adenopathy with low density centrally and rim enhancement following contrast
   - Lower lobe distribution or diffuse infiltrates including miliary disease
   - Pleural effusions
   - Reduced frequency of cavitary lesions
   - Normal chest X-rays in up to 15% of patients

Diagnostic studies
1 Chest X-ray
2 Positive PPD but a negative test (<5 mm) does not exclude active or latent TB when CD4 < 300
3 Smears of sputum, expectorated or induced
4 Cultures of blood, sputum, urine (first am sample on three consecutive days), BAL, lung biopsy, CSF, bone marrow,

liver, lymph nodes, pleura or other suspicious sites, with cultures positive in up to 90% of patients
5 ? Future role of PCR

Non-tuberculous Mycobacteria (NTM)

Clinically *Mycobacterium avium* complex (MAC) is responsible for the overwhelming majority of NTM disease and typically occurs when the CD4 count is less than 50

- With effective chemoprophylaxis for several other organisms, MAC may rarely present as the initial opportunistic infection
- Localized MAC has been described in several organs including the lungs but is rare
- Disseminated MAC is the most common systemic bacterial infection in HIV with the incidence of bacteremia increasing as CD4 counts drop, infection of a mucosal surface, e.g. lung, GI tract, being followed by bloodstream invasion

Clinically, patients present with several weeks to months of non-specific symptoms, signs and labs including

1. Increasing fatigue, fevers, night sweats, weight loss
2. GI symptoms of abdominal pains and diarrhea
3. Physical findings of hepatosplenomegaly and lymphadenopathy
4. Anemia and leukopenia reflecting bone marrow involvement
5. Respiratory symptoms are usually not prominent and if present non-specific

Chest X-rays are often normal, even with positive sputum cultures

- infiltrates when present are non-specific, e.g. nodules, patchy airspace disease, and may be associated with lymphadenopathy, pleural effusions and endobronchial lesions

Diagnostic features

1. Blood cultures are positive in over 90% of patients with MAC at autopsy

2 Positive cultures, +/– acid-fast organisms, +/– granulomas can be found from bone marrow, liver, lymph nodes
3 MAC pulmonary disease is diagnosed by positive cultures of respiratory secretions and a compatible radiographic picture for which no other cause is found
   - Positive cultures from sputum or BAL may reflect only colonization without evidence of localized or disseminated disease

Pneumocystis Carinii Pneumonia (PCP)

In the early to mid 1980s, PCP was the most common AIDS index diagnosis, but the incidence has been falling due to chemoprophylaxis and retroviral therapy

- Most cases are thought to represent reactivation of latent infection with ~75% of the population infected by age 4
- Incidence of PCP in HIV increases as the CD4 counts decrease, with clinical disease seen when CD4 < 200 cells/mm^3

Pathologically, there is usually an intra-alveolar exudate with mild interstitial pneumonitis which can resolve or progress to

1 Extensive alveolar exudation with diffuse alveolar damage and hyaline membrane disease
2 Chronic interstitial and intralumenal fibrosis

Less common pathologic features include

3 Absence of an alveolar exudate
4 DIP picture
5 Granulomatous inflammation
6 Cystic-cavitary disease
7 Vasculitis
8 Lymphocytic-plasma cell interstitial pneumonitis
9 Alveolar proteinosis

Clinical features

1 *Insidious onset of non-specific pulmonary and systemic symptoms developing over weeks
2 Uncommonly an acute fulminating course progressing to respiratory failure within 1 week, the usual presentation in non-HIV immunocompromised patients

3 Asymptomatic infection in ~5% of patients
4 Concurrent infectious diseases, most often CMV but including tuberculosis, atypicals, nocardia, cryptococcus and toxoplasmosis
   - Concurrent non-infectious diseases include Kaposi's and malignant lymphoma
5 Pleural effusion is uncommon ? more frequent with aerosolized pentamidine
   - Effusions are unilateral or bilateral and serous to bloody
   - Definitive diagnosis is made by demonstration of the trophozoite or cyst forms with appropriate stains, but presumptive when the effusion resolves under PCP treatment
6 Extrapulmonary disease is seen in ~1% of patients clinically, almost one half of these having concurrent PCP
   - Almost every organ system has been reported to be involved, most often lymph nodes, spleen, and liver, in part due to the role of aerosolized pentamidine
   - Manifestations vary from asymptomatic involvement, e.g. lymphadenopathy, to end-organ failure and death
   - CT scans typically show multiple low attenuation lesions as well as rim-like or punctate calcifications which are suggestive of the diagnosis

Radiologic features

Typical presentation

1 Diffuse, bilateral, symmetrical interstitial or airspace disease, perihilar in distribution, usually beginning in the lower lobes with spread to the upper lobes
   - Seen in ~80% of cases, but this picture is much less common in patients on pentamidine chemoprophylaxis
   - Can simulate diffuse pulmonary edema with air bronchograms

CT appearance is classically a mosaic distribution of bilateral, symmetric, 'ground glass' attenuation, which can be diffuse, perihilar or patchy

- Interlobular septal thickening may be seen acutely or can become more prominent with time, eventually resulting in interstitial fibrosis

Atypical presentation

2. Normal chest X-ray seen in ~15% of patients, unrelated to pentamidine prophylaxis, with HRCT demonstrating 'ground glass' opacities, a normal HRCT making PCP very unlikely
3. Upper lobe infiltrates, seen more commonly with pentamidine prophylaxis
4. Focal nodules or opacities, not involving the upper lobes
5. Dense consolidation
6. Cavitation within an area of consolidation, a mass or nodule is uncommon and thought to be secondary to vascular invasion, but superinfection should be ruled out
7. Pneumothorax may be the presenting feature of pneumocystis, reflecting subpleural necrosis and ruptured blebs
   - Risk factors include the presence of air-filled cysts, aerosolized pentamidine and cigarette smoking
   - Often bilateral, recurrent and associated with a poor prognosis
8. Cystic PCP (air-filled cysts or pneumatoceles) can be seen on chest X-ray but more commonly on HRCT in 5–35% of patients, developing with greater frequency in patients on pentamidine prophylaxis
   - Presentation is acute or chronic with complicating pneumothorax in ~⅓ of cases
   - Cysts are thin or thick-walled, regular or irregular in shape, usually multiple with an upper lobe predominance, 1–8 cm in diameter and with treatment can decrease in size or disappear over days to months

- Pathologically the cysts can be intraparenchymal containing pneumocystitis organisms or subpleural without evidence of active infection

9 Chronic PCP is typically seen in patients on prophylactic treatment and characterized by volume loss and scarring (often an upper lobe) radiologically as well as granulomas on biopsy, resembling tuberculosis
10 Pleural effusions are typically small, bilateral and resolve on therapy, although large, unilateral bloody effusions are described
11 Miliary disease (rare)
12 Endobronchial disease (rare)
13 Hilar/mediastinal adenopathy (rare)
14 Interstitial fibrosis

Gallium scan

Very sensitive in PCP with bilateral diffuse uptake seen, even in the presence of a normal chest X-ray

- The low specificity, cost and 2-day delay in results are drawbacks

Labs

PCP is unlikely with

1 DCO > 70% of predicted
2 Increasing oxygen saturation or a reduced A-aO_2 gradient with exercise
3 Normal LDH (elevated in 90% of cases)
4 CD4 count > 200

Diagnosis of PCP

1 Demonstration of pneumocystis on sputum induction (may be positive for weeks following appropriate Rx), BAL or transbronchial biopsy by
    - Silver stain (gold standard) to stain the cyst wall
    - Wright-Giemsa stain for the trophozyte (positive in ~80% of BAL specimens)
    - in patients on pentamidine prophylaxis, diagnostic yields from sputum induction and BAL are less

2 Monoclonal antibodies to the cyst wall (using immunofluorescent stains) on sputum or BAL
3 PCR (100% sensitive)

Toxoplasmosis

Toxoplasma gondii causes subclinical infection in most normal hosts with disease in AIDS patients thought to represent activation of latent infection

Clinically, pneumonia is uncommon and may occur in isolation or associated with CNS or disseminated disease

- Most common cause of focal brain lesions in HIV patients (encephalitis is the most common manifestation) but infection can disseminate with involvement of the lungs, liver, skeletal and cardiac muscle
- Pulmonary manifestations are non-specific with disease seen when CD4 counts <100

Radiologic features are variable with diffuse bilateral interstitial and alveolar infiltrates most common but nodules, cavities, lobar pneumonia and effusions are described

Diagnostic features

1 Compatible clinical picture, particularly with CNS disease
2 Positive serology with IgG antibodies to *T. gondii*, its absence making the diagnosis unlikely
3 Diffusely positive gallium scan
4 Smears or cultures of BAL/lung biopsy

NEOPLASTIC DISEASES

Kaposi's Sarcoma (KS)

Most common malignancy associated with HIV and probably caused by human herpesvirus 8

Clinically, it usually presents with cutaneous disease, but the initial presentation can be oral, visceral (GI tract, lungs, other) or nodal

- 95% of cases are seen in homosexual or bisexual males and typically present as immunity wanes (most cases seen with CD4 < 100), although it can appear at any time
- Lung disease is seen clinically in ~$\frac{1}{3}$ and at autopsy in ~$\frac{1}{2}$ of patients with known Kaposi's sarcoma
- Pulmonary disease typically follows cutaneous disease with initial presentation in the lungs in <15% of patients
- Intrathoracic involvement includes the airways, visceral pleura (percutaneous pleural biopsy is therefore negative) and lymph nodes in addition to the parenchyma
- Lung disease varies from asymptomatic to non-specific respiratory symptoms, with hemoptysis, hoarseness and stridor reflecting airways disease while dyspnea, hypoxemia and dry cough are manifestations of diffuse parenchymal involvement
- Prognosis is poor with survival in months in those patients with advanced lung disease

Radiologic findings

1. Bilateral, symmetric, focal or diffuse infiltrates on chest X-ray, often with perihilar predominance
2. Nodular infiltrates which can coalesce to airspace consolidation
3. Pleural effusions unilateral or bilateral, often large and associated with parenchymal disease in 90% of cases
4. Atelectasis from endobronchial obstruction
5. Hilar or mediastinal adenopathy in ~10%
6. Negative gallium but positive thallium scans
7. CT findings of
   - Peribronchovascular soft tissue thickening spreading from the hila and manifest as bronchial wall thickening as well as thickening of the interface between the vessels and lung
   - Airway findings ranging from wall irregularities to obstructed bronchi
   - Spiculated nodules

Diagnostic features include the patient with known Kaposi's sarcoma and a compatible chest X-ray, in addition to

1 Bronchoscopic findings of violaceous or red, irregularly-shaped lesions, flat or slightly raised, in the tracheobronchial mucosa in ~50% of patients with lung involvement
2 Negative gallium but positive thallium scans
3 Exclusion of infection with bronchoscopy
4 Transbronchial biopsy (yield ~10%) or open lung biopsy
5 ? Detection of human herpes virus-8 in BAL by PCR
6 Serosanguinous or bloody effusions which are exudative with negative cytology and occasionally chylous, the latter reflecting impaired lymphatic drainage

Non-Hodgkin's Lymphoma (NHL)

HIV-associated lymphoma is seen in 2–5% of HIV patients, in all risk groups, and is frequently extranodal in distribution including the CNS, bone marrow, liver, GI tract and mucocutaneous tissues

- Disease is usually seen with CD4 < 100 and EBV reported in up to 85% of cases
- Systemic symptoms of fevers, sweats and weight loss are present in ~75% of patients
- Intrathoracic manifestations variably reported in from 5–30% of HIV patients with NHL, in association with non-specific respiratory symptoms
- Thoracic involvement is rarely the initial or only disease site and is more commonly discovered during staging of the disease, involvement including the airways, parenchyma, pleura and lymph nodes
- Prognosis is poor with survival usually <6 months

Pathology is intermediate or high grade in 90% of cases, usually of B cell origin, with most patients presenting with stage III or IV disease

- Classification includes Burkitt's lymphoma, diffuse large cell lymphoma, anaplastic large cell lymphoma and primary effusion lymphoma or body cavity-based lymphoma

- The latter is a rare form of AIDS-related B cell lymphoma (human herpes virus-8 always present) where patients present with a pleural, pericardial or peritoneal effusions in the absence of a soft tissue tumor

Radiologic findings

1 *Single or multiple nodules (most common manifestation)
2 *Diffuse interstitial infiltrates
3 *Pleural effusions, unilateral or bilateral, often without associated parenchymal disease
4 Mass lesion(s) with cavitation
5 Endobronchial disease (uncommon)
6 Lymphadenopathy (uncommon)

Diagnostic features

1 Positive uptake of gallium and thallium
2 Thoracocentesis and pleural biopsy
3 Transbronchial or open lung biopsy

Primary Pulmonary Lymphoma (PPL) (see p. 75)

Definition: (1) Lymphomatous pulmonary involvement, (2) absence of mediastinal/hilar adenopathy, (3) absence of extrathoracic lymphoma before, during or three months after the diagnosis

- Related to severe immune deficiency and thought to result from reactivation of latent EBV infection within the lung, as in AIDS-related primary CNS lymphoma
- Histologically these are non-Hodgkin's lymphomas which are rare and described in the later stages of HIV disease when CD4 counts < 50
- Non-specific respiratory and systemic symptoms are common with the working diagnosis often that of infection
- The most common radiologic manifestions include a mass lesion or solitary/multiple nodules, with cavitation being common

Pulmonary Cancer

Increased risk is seen with cancer diagnosed at a younger age and displaying more aggressive behavior

- The clinical and radiologic features are those seen in non-HIV patients

INFLAMMATORY DISEASES

Lymphocytic Interstitial Pneumonitis (LIP)

Definition: Pathologically, a lymphoproliferative pulmonary disorder with diffuse infiltration of small lymphocytes, plasma cells and immunoblasts in alveolar septae and along lymphatics without an obvious cause

Clinically, it is uncommon in adults, occurs earlier rather than later in the course of HIV and presents with the insidious onset of dyspnea, cough and fever

- Prognosis varies from a benign course with spontaneous resolution or stability to respiratory failure

Radiologically, chest X-rays may be normal but typically reveal reticular or nodular infiltrates, predominantly basilar in location, with lymphadenopathy rarely described

- CT appearance is that of peribronchovascular nodules of 2–4 mm or 'ground glass' opacities

Diagnosis is confirmed on open lung biopsy with the above pathology and elimination of opportunistic infection

Non-specific Interstitial Pneumonitis (NIP)

Pathologic diagnosis characterized by a mononuclear cell infiltrate in the lungs, mainly lymphocytes and plasma cells, in the absence of a recognizable cause, e.g. infection, LIP, malignancy, drug effects, etc.

Clinically, seen in patients with advanced disease, CD4 < 200, and previous opportunistic infection or neoplasm

- Presentation varies from an asymptomatic finding on transbronchial biopsy to non-specific symptoms of cough, dyspnea, ± fever

- Chest X-rays vary from normal to reticular or nodular opacities, frequently with a positive gallium scan
- The symptoms, physical findings, blood gas abnormalities and X-rays can simulate pneumocystis infection
- The natural history is unpredictable with some cases showing spontaneous resolution of the radiologic abnormalities
- Diagnosis is one of exclusion as many patients have concurrent pulmonary disease or have had chemotherapy or remote PCP

Fraser R.S., Muller N.L., Colman N., Paré P.D. (1999) Diagnosis of Diseases of the Chest 4th Edn., WB Saunders.

Naidich, D.P., Zerhouni, E.A., Siegelman, S.S. (1998) *Computed Tomography and Magnetic Resonance of the Thorax*, 3rd edn. New York: Raven Press.

Moss, A., Gamsu, Genant (1992) Thorax and neck. In: *Computed Tomography of the Body with Magnetic Resonance Imaging*, 2nd edn, vol. 1.: W.B. Saunders.

Webb, R., Muller, N.L., Naidich, D.P. (1996) *High Resolution CT of the Lung*, 2nd edn.: Lippincott-Raven.

Baum, G.L., Crapo, J.D., Celli, B.R., Karlinsky, J.B. (eds) (1997) *Textbook of Pulmonary Diseases*, 6th edn.: Lippincott-Raven.

Fishman, A.P., Elias, J.A., Fishman, J.A., Grippi, M.A., Kaiser, L.R., Senior, R.N. (1998) *Fishman's Pulmonary Diseases and Disorders*, 3rd edn.: McGraw-Hill.

White, D., Matthay, R. (1989) Non-infectious complications of infections with the human immunovirus. *ARRD* **40**: 1763–1787.

Beck, J.M. (1998) Pleural disease in patients with acquired immune deficiency syndrome. *Clinics in Chest Medicine* **19**: 341–349.

Mylonakis, E., Barlam, T., Flanigan, T. *et al.* (1998) Pulmonary aspergillosis and immune disease in AIDS. *Chest* **114**: 251–262.

Heitzman, E.R. (1990) Pulmonary neoplastic and lymphoproliferative disease in AIDS. *Radiology* **177**: 347–351.

Beck, J. (1998) Pleural disease in patients with AIDS. *Clinics in Chest Medicine* **10**: 341–348.

McGuinness, G. (1997) Changing trends in the pulmonary manifestations of AIDS. *Radiol. Clin. North Am.* **35**: 1029–1080.

Levine, S. (1996) Pneumocystis carinii. *Clinics in Chest Medicine* **17**: 665–695.

Chin, D., Hopewell, P. (1996) Mycobacterial complications of HIV infection. *Clinics in Chest Medicine* **17**: 697–711.

Davies, S., Sarosi, G. (1996) Fungal pulmonary complications. *Clinics in Chest Medicine* **17**: 725–744.

White, D. (1996) Pulmonary complications of HIV-associated malignancies. *Clinics in Chest Medicine* **17**: 755–761.

Kuhlman, J. (1994) Pulmonary manifestations of AIDS. *Semin. Roent.* **xxix**: 242–274.

45 Hyperlucent Lung

UNILATERAL – PARTIAL OR COMPLETE

Airways disease (air trapping may be demonstrated)

1 Congenital bronchial atresia
   - Characterized by atresia or stenosis of a lobar, segmental or subsegmental bronchus, most often involving the apicoposterior segment of the left upper lobe but potentially affecting any area of lung
   - A mucocele or mucus plug develops distal to the site of obstruction in association with a normal bronchial tree beyond the point of obliteration

   Clinically, most patients are diagnosed prior to the age 25 and are usually asymptomatic although recurrent pneumonia may develop

   Radiologic features
   - A focal area of hyperlucency due to a combination of hyperinflation from collateral ventilation as well as oligemia
   - A mucocele, i.e. a distended mucus-filled obstructed bronchus, in the form of a tubular or branching structure, centrally located and forming the apex of a triangular zone of hyperlucency
   - Air-trapping on an expiratory CT or expiratory PA film

2 Partial bronchial obstruction, e.g. endobronchial neoplasm with air-trapping on expiration

3 Bronchogenic cyst

4 Bronchopulmonary sequestration
5 Swyer-James syndrome
  - Unilateral or bilateral disease characterized by a reduced density in one or several lobes reflecting underlying bronchitis, bronchiectasis, bronchiolitis, bronchiolitis obliterans and emphysema

  Etiologically thought to be due to a viral bronchiolitis, often adenovirus in early life

  Clinically, the presentation varies from an asymptomatic radiologic finding to symptoms of cough, dyspnea and recurrent chest infections, depending upon the extent of disease

  Radiologic features
  - Increased radiolucency of the involved lobes
  - Involved lung volume is normal or reduced at TLC
  - Air-trapping on expiration with mediastinal shift to the normal lung
  - Ipsilateral hilum is present but small, with attenuation of vessels throughout the radiolucent lung
  - Reduced ventilation and perfusion on scanning
  - Bronchiectasis of the involved lobe

Parenchymal disease (air trapping may be demonstrated)

6 Asymmetric emphysema
7 Compensatory hyperinflation post-lobectomy on lobar collapse
8 Congenital lobar emphysema
  - Neonatal lobar hyperinflation diagnosed within the first week of life

9 Bullae, cysts, cavities, pneumatoceles

Pleural disease

10 Pneumothorax

Chest wall disease (absence of air-trapping)

11 Asymmetric musculature, e.g. post-mastectomy, carpenters, butchers
12 Poland's syndrome
13 Poliomyelitis (pectoral muscle atrophy)

14 Patient rotation
15 Scoliosis

Vascular disease (absence of air-trapping)
16 Hypogenetic lung syndrome (Scimitar syndrome)
17 Proximal interruption of pulmonary artery
18 Anomalous origin of left PA from right
- The anomalous artery is located between the trachea and esophagus with compression of the right main stem bronchus and a hyperinflated right lung

19 Acquired obstruction of the PA, e.g. pulmonary emboli, pulmonary artery tumors (primary or secondary), extrinsic inflammatory disease

Technical factors
20 Patient rotation

BILATERAL HYPERLUCENT LUNG

Airways disease (lungs hyperinflated)
1 Asthma
2 Bronchiolitis
3 COPD
4 Tracheal or larnygeal obstruction
5 Bilateral bronchial stenoses

Parenchymal disease (lungs hyperinflated)
6 Bullous disease
7 Emphysema

Chest wall (normal lung volumes)
8 Bilateral mastectomy

Pleura
9 Bilateral pneumothoraces

Vascular disease (lung volumes normal or small)
10 Congenital cardiac disease
- e.g. Pulmonary valve stenosis, tetralogy, Ebstein's anomaly, persistent truncus type IV

11 Congenital pulmonary disease
   - e.g. pulmonary artery stenosis or coarctation

12 Pericardial tamponade

13 IVC obstruction

14 Primary pulmonary hypertension

15 Embolic occlusion of pulmonary arteries
   - e.g. thrombus, tumor, parasites

Fraser R.S., Muller N.L., Colman N., Paré P.D. (1999) Diagnosis of Diseases of the Chest 4th Edn., WB Saunders.

Naidich, D.P., Zerhouni, E.A., Siegelman, S.S. (1998) *Computed Tomography and Magnetic Resonance of the Thorax*, 3rd edn. New York: Raven Press.

Moss, A., Gamsu, Genant (1992) Thorax and neck. In: *Computed Tomography of the Body with Magnetic Resonance Imaging*, 2nd edn., vol. 1.: W.B. Saunders.

Felson, B. (1973) *Chest Roentgenology*.: W.B. Saunders.

46 Hypoxemia

Normal Chest X-ray

1 **Airways**
- Upper airways obstruction, acute or chronic
- Lower airways obstruction, localized or generalized

2 **Parenchyma**
- Interstitial disease, e.g. sarcoid, UIP, allergic alveolitis, early PCP
- Early acute airspace disease, e.g. pulmonary edema, ARDS, pneumonia
- Emphysema, bullous disease

3 **Vascular**
- Pulmonary
  - Arterial, e.g. emboli-thrombus, fat, tumor; pulmonary hypertension
  - Capillary, e.g. early miliary disease
  - Arteriovenous shunts
  - Venous e.g. early interstitial edema
- Cardiac, e.g. right-to-left shunts; mitral stenosis

4 **Neuromuscular**
- Neurologic, e.g. central alveolar hypoventilation – primary or secondary, Guillain-Barré
- Neuromuscular, e.g. myasthenia gravis
- Muscular, inherited or acquired

5 **Chest wall**
- Any cause of abdominal distension and interference with normal diaphragm function, e.g. obesity, ascites

6 **Pleural**
- (pleural effusion may be seen only on CT scan)

Mechanisms

1. V/Q mismatch
2. Anatomic shunt – pulmonary or cardiac
3. Diffusion impairment
4. Alveolar hypoventilation from neuromuscular disease
5. Reduced F_iO_2, e.g. altitude
6. Reduced mixed venous oxygen where underlying lung disease prevents compensation

Clinical Consequences

1 **Right heart**
- Pulmonary vasoconstriction and remodeling with subsequent pulmonary artery hypertension
- Cor pulmonale with right ventricular hypertrophy/ dilatation
- Right heart failure
- Effort syncope
- Exertional dyspnea

2 **Left heart**
- Angina/MI
- Arrythmias
- Failure
- Exertional dyspnea

3 **Respiratory system**
- Tachypnea and exertional dyspnea

4 **Skeletal muscle**
- Exercise intolerance
- Early shift to anaerobic metabolism
- Chronic malnutrition

5 **Secondary polycythemia**

6 **CNS**
- Impaired cognitive functions
- Altered mental status ranging from confusion to coma

Indications for O_2 – Acute

1 **Acute pulmonary disease** with $P_aO_2 < 60$ or O_2 sat < 90%

2 **Acute myocardial infarction** with reduced P_aO_2 which may be worsened by the use of vasodilator drugs

3 **Abnormal hemoglobins**
- CO poisoning with COHb
- Methemoglobin, e.g. nitrites, nitrates, sulfas
- Sickle cell with tissue hypoxia

4 **Inadequate tissue oxygenation**
- Severe anemia
- Shock with reduced cardiac output

5 **Pneumothorax** therapy where rapid lung expansion is required

Indications for O_2 – Chronic

Diseases most often requiring chronic oxygen include COPD, CF/bronchiectasis, interstitial lung disease, pulmonary vascular disease, neuromuscular disease

1 **Continuous** oxygen therapy with
- Resting $P_aO_2 \leq 55$ (O_2 sat ≤ 88%)
- Resting P_aO_2 55–59 and evidence of cor pulmonale,

right heart failure, secondary polycythemia or CNS dysfunction attributed to hypoxemia

2 **Non-continuous** oxygen with $P_aO_2 \leq 55$ (O_2 sat $\leq 88\%$) only on exertion and oxygen improving the measured exercise capacity (walk test with pulse oximetry)

3 **Nocturnal** oxygen in patients with suspected hypoxemia, e.g. pulmonary artery hypertension, polycythemia, left ventricular disease or CNS effects, who have daytime normoxemia but in whom $P_aO_2 \leq 55$ (O_2 sat $\leq 88\%$) is documented at night

Fraser R.S., Muller N.L., Colman N., Paré P.D. (1999) Diagnosis of Diseases of the Chest 4th Edn., WB Saunders.

Baum, G.L., Crapo, J.D., Celli, B.R., Karlinsky, J.B. (eds) (1997) *Textbook of Pulmonary Diseases*, 6th edn.: Lippincott-Raven.

Fishman, A.P., Elias, J.A., Fishman, J.A., Grippi, M.A., Kaiser, L.R., Senior, R.N. (1998) *Fishman's Pulmonary Diseases and Disorders*, 3rd edn.: McGraw-Hill.

47 Infiltrates

RECURRENT INFILTRATES – DIFFERENT AREAS OF LUNG

Airways

1 Tracheobronchomegaly (Mounier-Kuhn) with recurrent pneumonias
2 Tracheoesophageal fistula, e.g. neoplastic with recurrent aspiration
3 Mucus plugs, e.g. asthma
4 Allergic bronchopulmonary aspergillosis with central > peripheral infiltrates
5 COPD with recurrent pneumonia
6 BOOP
7 Bronchiectasis with recurrent pneumonia

Parenchyma

8 Aspiration, e.g. swallowing disorders
9 Inhalational, e.g. allergic alveolitis
10 Drug ingestion
11 Recurrent pulmonary edema, particularly with an atypical distribution

12 Recurrent pneumonias, e.g. Immunoglobulin deficiency, HIV, immunosuppressive drugs, leucopenias

Vascular

13 Eosinophilic infiltrates, e.g. Loefflers, chronic eosinophilic pneumonia
14 Alveolar hemorrhage syndromes
15 Pulmonary infarcts
16 Vasculitis/collagen vascular diseases

RECURRENT INFILTRATES – SAME AREA OF LUNG

1 Local bronchial narrowing, congenital or acquired
   - Intralumenal, e.g. foreign body, broncholith
   - Endobronchial, e.g. neoplastic
   - Peribronchial, e.g. nodes, mediastinal mass
2 Bronchiectasis, congenital or acquired
3 Broncho-esophageal fistula, e.g. neoplastic
4 Bronchopulmonary sequestration – recurrent infections
5 Bronchogenic cyst – recurrent infections

NON-RESOLVING PULMONARY INFILTRATE

Definition: A localized infiltrate present for **weeks to months** eliminating various acute lung injuries, e.g. acute infection

- May remain **stable**, **improve** or **worsen** over time, the differential diagnosis including

Airways

1 Post-obstructive – benign or malignant
2 Bronchiectasis
3 Bronchopulmonary aspergillosis
4 Bronchocentric granulomatosis
5 Bronchiolo-alveolar cell cancer

6 BOOP
7 Bronchopulmonary sequestration

Vascular

8 Pulmonary infarct
9 Vasculitides
10 Eosinophilic infiltrate
11 Vascular neoplasms

Parenchyma

12 Aspiration – lipoid pneumonia, miliary granulomatosis
13 Inhalation – progressive massive fibrosis
14 Infection – tuberculosis, atypical mycobacteria, anaerobes, actinomycosis, nocardia, fungal infections, melioidosis, paragonimiasis
15 Neoplasms – primary or secondary, including lymphoproliferative disorders
16 Pseudolymphoma
17 Inflammatory pseudotumor (organizing pneumonia)
18 Amyloid
19 Radiation pneumonitis
20 Calcinosis

ALVEOLAR INFILTRATES – PERIPHERAL

Definition: Infiltrates that are mainly subpleural in location with relative sparing of the perihilar areas

- Infiltrates may be chronic or recurrent and etiologies include:
  - Chronic eosinophilic pneumonia (CEP)
  - BOOP
  - Combination BOOP and CEP
  - Sarcoid
  - Drug reactions
  - Churg-Strauss vasculitis
  - Occasionally DIP
  - R/O TB
  - Pulmonary infarcts
  - Lung contusion

PULMONARY INFILTRATES – PERIPHERAL LYMPHADENOPATHY

1 Infectious
- Bacterial – tuberculosis, atypical mycobacteria, anthrax, brucellosis, tularemia, plague
- Mycoplasma
- Viral – CMV, Ebstein-Barr, HIV, adenovirus
- Rickettsial – Q-fever, Rocky Mountain spotted fever
- Fungal – blastomycosis, histoplasmosis, coccidioidomycosis, sporotrichosis
- Parasitic – toxoplasmosis

2 Neoplastic
- e.g. metastatic carcinoma, lymphoma, melanoma, leukemia, germ cell tumors

3 Immunologic
- e.g. collagen vascular disease (SLE, RA) graft *vs.* host disease

4 Drug reactions, e.g. dilantin
5 Eosinophilic granuloma
6 Sarcoid
7 Berylliosis
8 Castleman's disease
9 Kikuchi's syndrome

PULMONARY INFILTRATE/MASS – CONCURRENT CNS DISEASE

Airways

1 Malignant neoplasm with
- Metastases
- Paraneoplastic syndromes, e.g. non-bacterial thrombotic endocarditis

Parenchyma

2 Infections
- Bacterial, e.g. acute abscess, anaerobes, tuberculosis, actinomycosis, nocardia

- Fungal, e.g. cryptococcus, aspergillus, mucor
- Parasitic, rickettsial, mycoplasma, viral

3 Malignancy, e.g. carcinoma, lymphoma or vascular tumors with CNS metastases
4 Lymphomatoid granulomatosis
5 Aspiration pneumonia from an altered sensorium
6 Hypertensive encephalopathy and pulmonary edema
7 Sarcoidosis

Vascular

8 Vasculitis, e.g. Wegener's, Churg-Strauss
9 Collagen-vascular disease, e.g. SLE
10 AV malformations and CNS abscess or emboli
11 Pulmonary infarcts and paradoxical CNS emboli
12 Lung cancer with non-bacterial thrombotic endocarditis and CNS emboli

INFILTRATES AND WHEEZING

1 Asthma (see p. 52)
2 Allergic bronchopulmonary aspergillosis
3 Bronchocentric granulomatosis
4 Acute bronchiolitis
5 Bronchiectasis
6 Pneumonia secondary to mycoplasma, chlamydia, parasites, viruses
7 Acute gastric aspiration
8 Pulmonary emboli with infarction
9 Pulmonary edema secondary to pulmonary venous hypertension, cardiac or non-cardiac in origin
10 Lymphangitic carcinomatosis
11 Carcinoid tumor and carcinoid syndrome
12 Bronchogenic carcinoma or other tumor with localized airway obstruction
13 Any cause of pulmonary infiltrate in a patient with underlying airways obstruction
14 Tropical pulmonary eosinophilia

UPPER LOBE INFILTRATES/FIBROSIS

1 Tuberculosis
2 Histoplasmosis
3 Sporotrichosis
4 *Rhodococcus equi*
5 Radiation pneumonitis
6 Sarcoid
7 Allergic alveolitis
8 Progressive massive fibrosis of silicosis, CWP, talcosis
9 Ankylosing spondylitis
10 Rheumatoid arthritis
11 Eosinophilic granuloma
12 Calcinosis (metastatic calcifications)

INFILTRATES AND FEVER

Pneumonia is the most common cause, but the following should be considered

Parenchymal
1 Aspiration
2 Allergic alveolitis
3 Drug reaction
4 Lymphoma
5 Sarcoid
6 Alveolar proteinosis
7 Acute interstitial pneumonia (Hamman – Rich)
8 Radiation pneumonitis
9 Eosinophilic lung disease

Airways
10 BOOP

Vascular
11 Septic emboli
12 Sepsis and ARDS
13 Alveolar hemorrhage syndrome

14 Vasculitis
15 Collagen vascular disease

IMMUNOCOMPROMISED PATIENTS – DIFFERENTIAL DIAGNOSIS

Generalizations

- *X-rays are never specific for etiology of the infiltrates
- *Radiologic findings may result from two or more processes simultaneously or sequentially
- *Both infectious and non-infectious disorders can give similar patterns
- *Chest X-rays should be interpreted with as much clinical information as possible

1 **Underlying disease**
   - Neoplastic disease with evidence of tumor elsewhere, e.g. active extrathoracic lymphoma
   - Collagen disease/vasculitis of the lungs with known active disease
   - Rejection in transplant patients

2 **Infection** is most common cause of infiltrates and suggested by
   - **Concurrent infection** at other sites
     – e.g. Oropharyngeal lesions with herpes simplex, skin lesions in varicella-zoster, multiorgan disease is typical of CMV, candida, legionella, toxoplasmosis
   - **Granulocytopenia** below 500/mm^3 predisposes to gram negatives, staphylococcus, streptococcal species, fungal infections e.g. aspergillus, candida
     – The more severe and prolonged the neutropenia, the greater the chance of infection
   - **B cell defects**, e.g. CLL or myeloma with resultant hypogammaglobulinemia result in infection with encapsulated bacteria including *Strep. pneumoniae*, *Haemophilus influenzae*, *Neisseria meningitidis*

- **T cell defects**, e.g. steroids, chemotherapy, transplant, lymphomas, leukemias, result in
  - Bacteria – legionella, tuberculosis, atypicals, nocardia, salmonella, listeria
  - Viruses – CMV, HSV, HZV, RSV
  - Fungi – aspergillus, candida, cryptococcus, histoplasmosis, coccidioidomycosis, pneumocystis
  - Parasites – toxoplasmosis, strongyloides

3 **Sequelae of treatment** can result in
- Direct pulmonary toxicity secondary to drugs, radiation, oxygen therapy
- Lymphoma developing as a complication of immunosuppressive therapy
- Specific infections occurring less often due to the use of prophylactic drugs

4 **Alveolar hemorrhage** should be suspected with
- Falling Hb
- Elevated DCO
- Hemoptysis
- Bloody returns on BAL with hemosiderin-laden macrophages
- Absence of associated infection

5 **Pulmonary edema** – may be cardiac or non-cardiac in origin

6 **'Fibrosis/diffuse alveolar damage'** – pathologic diagnosis with no identified etiology

7 **Unusual causes** including alveolar proteinosis, veno-occlusive disease with bleomycin, sarcoid-like granulomas with testicular neoplasms

8 **Unrelated disease**

9 **BOOP** – can occur secondary to infections, drugs

10 **Bland thrombotic infarcts**

11 **Septic infarcts** may develop from a peripheral septic focus, e.g. in-dwelling line, septic thrombophlebitis, extrapulmonary abscess, or from the right heart valves
- Organisms responsible include staphylococcus, aspergillus and mucormycosis

Clues to Differential Diagnosis

1 Suspect the following **infections**
- Invasive fungal disease in hematologic malignancies or bone marrow recipients
- Candida pneumonia is rare but seen with leukemia and lymphomas
- CMV in solid organ and marrow recipients
- Pneumocystis as a cause of ground glass opacities and cystic spaces in HIV

2 Suspect **lymphoma** complicating HIV or transplants

3 **Extrathoracic disease**
- Skin
  - Vesicular lesions of *Herpes simplex*, *Varicella zoster*
  - Nodular lesions with dissemination of aspergillus, cryptococcus, nocardia, TB, candida
  - Ecthyma gangrenosum from pseudomonas
- CNS
  - Brain abscess from toxoplasmosis, aspergillus, cryptococcus
  - Meningitis from toxoplasmosis, cryptococcus, coccidioidomycosis
  - Encephalitis from *Herpes simplex*, toxoplasmosis
- Sinusitis
  - Aspergillus, mucormycosis
- Retina
  - Aspergillus, CMV, candida

4 **Disease onset, distribution and progression**

5 **PFTs** are usually non-specific and restrictive with low DCO and reduced subdivisions of lung volume but

- Elevated DCO is seen with alveolar hemorrhage
- Airways obstruction is seen with bronchiolitis

6 **Pattern recognition**

Nodules/masses
- Infections – staphylococcus or other lung abscess, tuberculosis, atypical mycobacteria, nocardia, aspergillus, cryptococcus
- Neoplasms – underlying disease or drug-induced lymphoma
- BOOP
- Infarcts – septic or bland
- Sarcoid-like granulomas

'Ground glass'/airspace consolidation
- Infections
- Lymphoma
- BOOP
- Infarcts
- Drug-induced
- Edema
- Hemorrhage
- Fibrosis – diffuse alveolar hemorrhage
- Alveolar proteinosis

Diffuse interstitial disease
- Infections, e.g. PCP, CMV, disseminated TB and fungi
- Drug-induced
- Lymphangitic carcinomatosis
- Pulmonary edema
- Non-specific interstitial pneumonitis

Miliary pattern
- Tuberculosis
- Disseminated histoplasmosis

Focal consolidation
- Bacterial or fungal infection
- Pulmonary infarct

- Lymphoma
- BOOP

Cavitation

- Bacterial abscess, TB, nocardia
- Fungi e.g. aspergillus, cryptococcus
- Septic emboli
- Neoplasms

7 **Associated radiologic abnormalities**
- Mediastinal adenopathy with neoplasms, mycobacterial infections
- Esophageal ulceration with HSV
- Nodular shadows in the liver, spleen or kidneys with disseminated fungus, neoplasms

8 **CT scan**
- Detection of unsuspected abnormalities
- 'Halo sign' with invasive fungal disease (non-specific)
- Low attenuation ring-enhancing lymph nodes with tuberculosis

Naidich, D.P., Zerhouni, E.A., Siegelman, S.S. (1998) *Computed Tomography and Magnetic Resonance of the Thorax*, 3rd edn. New York: Raven Press.

Baum, G.L., Crapo, J.D., Celli, B.R., Karlinsky, J.B. (eds) *Textbook of Pulmonary Diseases*, 6th edn.: Lippincott-Raven.

Fishman, A.P., Elias, J.A., Fishman, J.A., Grippi, M.A., Kaiser, L.R., Senior, R.N. (1998) *Fishman's Pulmonary Diseases and Disorders*, 3rd edn.: McGraw-Hill.

Primack, S., Muller, N. (1996) HRCT in acute diffuse lung disease in the immunocompromised patient. *Radiol. Clin. North. Am.* **32**: 731–742.

Brown, M., Miller, R., Muller, N. (1994) Acute lung disease in the immunocompromised host: CT and pathologic examination findings. *Radiology* **190**: 247–254.

48 Inhalational Diseases

ALLERGIC ALVEOLITIS

Definition: Syndrome characterized by the response of the lungs to repeated inhalation of and sensitization to a variety of organic dusts

- Exposures are most often occupational or hobby-related, being found at work, in the home, car, or associated with exposures to heating systems, air conditioners, other water sources, contaminated buildings, birds, trees, etc.
- The spores of thermophilic actinomycetes have been most often implicated, but antigens of fungi, bacteria, insects, animals, amebae, chemicals and proteins can also be responsible
- Attack rates are relatively low and reflect particle size, numbers, immunogenicity and host factors
- In spite of multiple and diverse inducing agents, the pulmonary symptoms, with or without systemic features,

are similar and can manifest as **acute**, **subacute** or **chronic** disease

Diagnostic criteria

1 ***History** of an exposure coincident with development of acute respiratory symptoms (nonsmokers ≫ smokers)
2 **Episodes**, often repeated, of cough, dyspnea, fever and malaise occurring hours after exposure, and resolving after removal from the environment
3 **Radiologic abnormalities** as described below – X-rays are occasionally normal (but disease can be confirmed on biopsy)
4 Bilateral lower lobe **rales**
5 **Restrictive pattern** occasionally with evidence of obstruction on PFTs, as well as resting or exercise-induced hypoxemia
6 Evidence of **exposure** from antigen specific antibodies (e.g. serum precipitins) or microbiologic investigation of the environment
7 **Lung biopsy** showing interstitial pneumonitis, bronchiolitis and granuloma formation
8 **Broncho-alveolar cell lavage** analysis demonstrating a suppressor T cell alveolitis
9 **Inhalation challenge**
10 **Exclusion** of other diseases with similar signs and symptoms

Acute Allergic Alveolitis

Patients present 2–8 hours post-antigen exposure, with symptoms peaking within 24 hours and resolving within 3 days

- May be misdiagnosed as 'atypical' pneumonia
- The presentation may be relapsing with re-exposure to the antigen
- Extrapulmonary disease is absent and the disease is mainly seen in non-smokers
- Prognosis is excellent following removal from the antigenic source

Clinical syndromes

1 'Flu-like' illness with fever, chills, myalgias, weakness (+/– recurrent)
2 'Pneumonia-like' with fever, cough and dyspnea (+/– recurrent)
3 Respiratory failure from inhalation of large quantities of antigen
4 'Asthma-like' picture with an immediate reaction followed 4–6 hours after by a 'late' response, typically seen in atopic patients (+/– recurrent)

Differential diagnosis

1 Atypical pneumonia
2 Idiopathic interstitial pneumonias including acute interstitial pneumonia, UIP, DIP
3 BOOP
4 Miliary disease
5 Drug reaction
6 Sarcoid
7 Pulmonary edema
8 Vasculitis
9 Collagen vascular disease

Chest X-ray features

1 Normal chest X-ray early in the course
2 *Airspace pattern – 'ground glass' or airspace consolidation
3 Interstitial disease – reticular, reticulonodular or nodular
4 Combination of interstitial and airspace disease, with the airspace disease eventually resolving and leaving residual interstitial disease
5 Disease is diffuse or has a lower lobe predominance
6 Uncommon lymphadenopathy and absence of pleural disease
7 Return of X-rays to normal in 1–4 weeks if patient is removed from the environmental antigen

HRCT features

1 Patchy 'ground glass' or airspace consolidation (reflecting the alveolitis) and centrilobular nodules (reflecting bronchiolitis)
2 Mosaic attenuation with the patchy areas of low attenuation between the 'ground glass' areas demonstrating air-trapping on expiratory scans (reflecting bronchiolar obstruction)

Sub-acute Allergic Alveolitis

Clinically uncommon with persistence of cough and dyspnea

- Biopsy reveals increasing granuloma formation with decreasing alveolitis and bronchiolitis
- Classic X-ray finding is a fine nodular pattern, less commonly 'ground glass' opacities, correlating with the above pathologies, although it can occasionally be normal
- HRCT findings are those of patchy areas of 'ground glass' opacities as well as nodular opacities, with middle and lower lobe predominance
  - Associated areas of decreased attenuation reflect hypoperfusion from bronchiolitis

Chronic Allergic Alveolitis

Clinically, the diagnosis of chronic allergic alveolitis is more difficult to make because

1 The dramatic presentation of acute disease (intermittent exposure to high antigen concentrations) is replaced with the insidious onset of cough and dyspnea due to chronic exposure to low antigen concentrations
2 Serum antibody levels become negative over 3 years if exposure is discontinued
3 Constitutional symptoms of fever, weight loss and fatigue may dominate the clinical picture
4 Late stage lung disease is similar to non-specific fibrosing alveolitis

Radiologic features

1 Coarse reticular pattern with honeycombing
2 Volume loss

3 Variable lobar predominance
4 Changes of superimposed acute disease in addition to the more chronic changes can be seen with recurrent antigen exposure
5 HRCT findings are those of fibrosis (honeycombing, architectural distortion, interlobular septal thickening, traction bronchiectasis) with superimposed areas of 'ground glass' opacity and scattered nodules

ALTITUDE-RELATED DISORDERS

High Altitude Illness

Definition: The symptoms and signs occurring in the setting of a recent gain in altitude

- ~25% of individuals ascending above 2500 meters develop manifestations of high altitude illness
- The spectrum of diseases relate to the maladaptation occurring in relation to hypoxia and include
  - Acute mountain sickness
  - High-altitude pulmonary edema (HAPE)
  - High-altitude cerebral edema (HACE)

Acute mountain sickness (AMS)

- Predominantly a neurologic syndrome secondary to cerebral edema with symptoms of headache, fatigue, dizziness, anorexia, nausea, vomiting and difficulty sleeping
- Occurrence depends upon the rate of ascent, the altitude attained, as well as individual susceptibility
- Typically seen with ascents >2500 meters, e.g. ski resorts
- Although pulmonary symptoms are generally absent, an ↑A-a O_2 gradient can be seen
- Gradual ascent can prevent the syndrome which generally resolves with descent if symptoms persist

High altitude pulmonary edema (HAPE)

- Seen in up to 15% of young, healthy individuals who are either arriving at high altitude (>2500 meters) for the first time or former residents returning after days to weeks at sea level

- Most common cause of death from high altitude
- Symptoms usually develop within a few days and include cough, dyspnea at rest, chest tightness and decreasing exercise tolerance, with the initial dry cough eventually productive of pink, frothy sputum
- Physical findings include tachypnea, tachycardia, rales, cyanosis and occasionally fever
- Physiologic studies demonstrate elevated pulmonary artery pressures, normal wedge pressure and a high protein pulmonary edema reflecting increased microvascular permeability
- Chest X-rays reveal a patchy distribution of infiltrates which may be unilateral or bilateral at the onset

High altitude cerebral edema (HACE)

- Reflects progression of AMS where the mild neurologic symptoms progress to ataxia and/or an altered level of consciousness leading finally to coma and death

AIR TRAVEL

Cabin pressures in commercial jet airliners are maintained between 560 and 690 mmHg, reflecting an altitude of about 8000 feet and FiO_2 of about 15% (*vs.* 21% at sea level)

- In normal individuals, an arterial PO_2 of about 95 mmHg at sea level will fall to about 60 mmHg at 8000 feet

Work-up should include

1. Identification of high risk patients
    - Chronic lung disease, obstructive or restrictive
    - Recent exacerbation of airways obstruction
    - History of hypoxemia-related symptoms
    - Chronically hypoxemic patients
2. PFTs and ABGs
3. Optimization of lung function
4. Stratification of patients
    - $PO_2 > 70$ will unlikely have problems
    - $PO_2 < 60$ will require supplemental O_2

- For borderline patients an estimate of arterial PO_2 during air travel can be made by
  - Measuring PO_2 with an FiO_2 of 15%, the hypoxia-altitude stimulation test (HAST)
  - Hypobaric chamber set to an altitude of 8000 feet

ASBESTOS-RELATED DISEASES

Pleural Diseases
Pleural plaques
Diffuse pleural thickening
Benign pleural effusion
Malignant mesothelioma

Parenchymal Diseases
Asbestosis
Bronchogenic carcinoma
Rounded atelectasis
Crow's feet
Benign pleural-based masses

Extrapleuropulmonary
Pericarditis
Pericardial mesothelioma
Peritoneal mesothelioma
Head and neck cancers
Gastrointestinal cancers

Pleural Plaques

Definition: Focal areas of pleural thickening involving mainly the parietal pleura

- No history of asbestos exposure, occupational or non-occupational, in approximately 20% of patients
- May be seen in up to 50% of asbestos-exposed workers

Clinically, pleural plaques are the most common radiologic manifestation of asbestos exposure as well as an important marker

- Mean latency period is approximately 30 years
- Patients are usually asymptomatic with the course of disease benign, although an increased incidence of dyspnea is seen ? secondary to sub-radiographic lung disease

- PFTs are usually normal although a mild restrictive pattern is occasionally reported

Chest X-ray features

1. Linear, elevated or pedunculated pleural thickening best seen along the lateral chest wall with relative sparing of the apices and costophrenic angles
2. Disease can involve the mediastinal pleura and pericardium as well as the interlobar fissures, where the appearance is that of a lung nodule
3. Bilateral > unilateral distribution
4. Plaques may calcify and appear as a thin white line of increased density in profile
5. Plaques may enlarge and/or coalesce simulating a neoplasm
6. Differential diagnosis includes subpleural fat, muscle slips, fractured ribs with pleural thickening, pleural tumor

HRCT is more sensitive for demonstrating pleural plaques not seen on chest X-ray

- A localized intrapulmonary pleural plaque simulating a neoplasm may be diagnosed by its location within a fissure

Diffuse Pleural Thickening (Pachypleuritis)

Definition: Variable, although general consensus is that of diffuse pleural thickening extending over >25% of the pleural surface and often involving the costophrenic angles

- The visceral pleura alone or visceral and parietal pleura are involved with adhesions between them that can obliterate the pleural space
- Associated pulmonary fibrosis may be present or absent

Clinically, patients are often dyspneic and may cough

- Onset of symptoms may be subacute or chronic, with stability or progression of symptoms
- May develop secondary to an asbestos effusion
- Clinical differentiation from mesothelioma may be difficult
- PFTs reveal mild to severe restrictive disease

Chest X-rays reveal diffuse pleural thickening which may be unilateral or bilateral

- Serial films may reveal stability, slowly progressive disease or rapidly progressive pleural thickening, often with a nodular configuration
- Differentiation from mesothelioma may be difficult radiologically

Benign Pleural Effusion

Clinically, benign asbestos-related effusions have the shortest latency period of all asbestos-related diseases and are often seen within 10 years of exposure

- They are frequently asymptomatic, although the presentation can be acute with pleuritic pain and fever
- Rarely associated with pericarditis but should be considered in the differential diagnosis of pleuropericarditis
- The effusions are typically small and self-limited but may be recurrent
- On thoracocentesis, the effusion is an exudate, often bloody, neutrophilic or mononuclear, and may have an eosinophilia

Radiologic features

1. Effusions are usually small and unilateral but may be large and bilateral
2. Can resolve completely
3. Can result in residual pleural plaques, pachypleuritis, rounded atelectasis
4. May be recurrent
5. Associated asbestosis or pleural plaques are uncommon at the time of the initial presentation

Diagnostic criteria

1. History of asbestos exposure
2. Absence of other causes of the effusion
3. Absence of malignancy developing during a 2–3 year follow-up
    - The above are supported by a recurrent nature of the effusion as well as other radiologic evidence of asbestos exposure

Malignant Mesothelioma

Clinically, an occupational history of asbestos exposure is frequent but epidemiologically not dose-related, unlike asbestosis or bronchogenic cancers

- The most common symptoms are dyspnea and pleuritic chest pain with <10% of patients being asymptomatic
- Chest wall invasion may be seen, especially at the site of thoracocentesis
- Systemic metastases are not usually diagnosed clinically but can be seen at autopsy
- Progressive invasion of the lung, mediastinum and nerves (spinal cord, brachial plexus, sympathetic chain) results in a poor prognosis with survival usually about 6 months, patients having severe hypoxemia and dyspnea
- Paraneoplastic syndromes have been described, e.g. DIC

Pleural effusions are large, exudative and grossly straw-colored to bloody with high hyaluronidase levels described

- Cytologic diagnosis is often difficult
- Diagnostically closed pleural biopsy is often unreliable in differentiating mesothelioma, mesothelial hyperplasia, and metastatic cancer, thoracoscopy being required with 1–2% false negatives
- Endobronchial disease on bronchoscopy suggests a lung primary as mesothelioma is rarely seen

Radiologic features are non-pathognomonic and similar to those of metastatic cancer

1 Moderate to large pleural effusion usually seen in association with pleural nodularity
2 Pleural mass or diffuse pleural thickening in the absence of free fluid
3 Encirclement and entrapment of the lung result in a small hemithorax with either lack of mediastinal shift to the opposite hemithorax or ipsilateral shift
4 Local invasion can involve the chest wall, ribs, heart, mediastinum, hilar nodes and diaphragm
5 Transdiaphragmatic spread with abdominal invasion

involving the peritoneum and liver as well as involvement of the contralateral pleura
6 Chest X-ray or CT scan can demonstrate associated pleural plaques or interstitial fibrosis in approximately 20% of patients

Pericardial Mesothelioma

Often diagnosed post-mortem and typically presents with advanced disease including
1 Pericardial involvement with constrictive pericarditis or a hemorrhagic effusion
2 Myocardial invasion with CHF or infarction
3 SVC syndrome

Asbestosis

Definition: Pulmonary interstitial fibrosis secondary to inhalation of asbestos fibers

Clinically, the factors affecting disease development include the degree of exposure, length of exposure and cigarette smoking, although the dose–response relationship is weaker in asbestosis than in many other pneumoconioses

- Symptoms usually develop 20 years or more after initial contact and are those of fibrosing alveolitis, namely cough and dyspnea
- Physical findings of bibasilar rales and finger clubbing are common with cor pulmonale and respiratory failure as complications
- Findings may also reflect the development of mesothelioma or bronchogenic cancer
- Hypoxemia occurs initially on exertion but later at rest

Chest X-rays are insensitive to early disease and may be normal with biopsy-proven asbestosis

- When abnormal, there are no pathognomonic features, but the findings of UIP with superimposed pleural disease are very suggestive and include
  - Bilateral, predominantly lower lobe disease, peripheral > central

- Reticulonodular pattern progressing to a honeycomb lung
- Associated pleural thickening or plaques
- Focal fibrotic masses, usually subpleural
- 'Shaggy heart' sign reflecting combined interstitial and pleural disease

Gallium scan is often positive and may be seen with a normal chest X-ray

- Correlates poorly with lung function or BAL cell profile

HRCT features

1 Findings of fibrosis
  - Traction bronchiectasis
  - Loss of lobular architecture
  - Honeycombing in advanced disease
  - Parenchymal bands
  - Subpleural lines
  - Interlobular septal thickening and irregular interfaces
  - Subpleural dot-like opacities (peribronchiolar fibrosis)
2 Pleural thickening or plaques
3 Focal fibrotic masses, usually subpleural, representing areas of conglomerate parenchymal fibrosis, round atelectasis or pleural plaques – associated neoplasia must be ruled out
4 Basal 'ground glass' opacities – uncommon but can be seen early in the course of disease

PFTs reveal a restrictive pattern with reduced lung volumes and DCO

- Associated obstruction may be present due to bronchiolar and peribronchiolar fibrosis

Diagnostic gold standard is the pathologic demonstration of fibrosis with mineralogic assessment of the number of asbestos bodies per gram of digested lung tissue while non-invasive diagnostic criteria include

1 Exposure history with an appropriate latent period between exposure and disease

2 Bilateral lower lobe inspiratory rales (may be present with normal chest X-ray)
3 Clubbing
4 Compatible radiologic changes
5 Restrictive disease on PFTs

Bronchogenic Carcinoma

Seen in 20–25% of heavily exposed asbestos workers

- Smoking and asbestos exposure increase the risk of cancer in a multiplicative fashion with 50 times the rate compared to non-smoking/non-asbestos exposed individuals
- The cell type and location of tumors are similar to those in smoking, non-asbestos exposed patients
- Asbestosis is often present radiologically and usually present histologically

Rounded Atelectasis

Definition: A benign mass associated with contiguous pleural thickening and seen in patients with a history of asbestos exposure

Clinically, rounded atelectasis is often asymptomatic

- TTNA is advocated by some to rule out a neoplastic lesion, particularly with an enlarging lesion or equivocal radiologic findings ? role of FDG-PET scanning showing metabolically inactive disease *vs*. lung cancer

Radiologic features

1 Sharply-defined pleural-based mass, 2–7 cm in diameter, usually in a lower lobe adjacent to an area of pleural thickening, unilateral or bilateral
2 Comet tail, i.e. a curvilinear structure extending from the mass to the hilum and containing bronchovascular structures
3 Slow progression radiologically
4 Enhancement following contrast CT

Crow's Feet (Transpulmonary Bands)

A possible early form of rounded atelectasis characterized by multiple fibrous strands within the lung, radiating to a focal area of pleural thickening, in the absence of a definable parenchymal mass

Benign Pleural-based Masses

Diagnosis of exclusion when a peripheral lung cancer or mesothelioma can be ruled out in a patient with features of asbestosis

BERYLLIOSIS

Definition: A chronic granulomatous disorder that affects the lungs as a result of a beryllium specific cell-mediated immune response

- Beryllium exposure is described in refineries, beryllium ceramics, the aerospace industry, manufacture of nuclear reactors and gyroscopes, fluorescent lamp manufacturing, exposure to the contaminated clothing of a spouse

Clinically, there are 2 forms of disease

1 Acute berylliosis (uncommon *vs.* the chronic form) is seen with high levels of dust exposure, often accidental
   - Characterized histologically by acute inflammation in the airways and lung parenchyma without granulomatous inflammation
   - Presentation may be fulminant, resembling pulmonary edema or more insidious developing over months

2 Chronic berylliosis is a systemic disease involving multiple organ systems and seen with at least 2 years of dust exposure and a latency period following exposure up to 15 years
   - Granulomatous inflammation is seen pathologically and thought to be immunologic in origin, with poor correlation between extent of exposure and disease, the lung content of beryllium lessening over time

Radiologic features are non-pathognomonic, similar to those of sarcoid, and can include

1. Normal chest X-ray
2. 'Ground glass' pattern
3. Reticular, reticulo-nodular or nodular interstitial infiltrates
4. Conglomerate masses
5. Honeycombing
6. Hilar/mediastinal lymphadenopathy

Diagnostic criteria

1. History of beryllium exposure
2. Hypersensitivity to beryllium on a patch test
3. Histologic evidence of non-caseating granulomas as well as beryllium content of the biopsy specimen
4. ⊕ Belt (beryllium lymphocyte transformation) test from blood or BAL

BUILDING-RELATED ILLNESSES (BRI)

Definition: BRI are reserved for illnesses attributed to non-industrial work environments, now representing the environment for more than 50% of the entire work force in North America and Western Europe

- They are characterized by recurrent symptoms with or without objective signs on physical exam and abnormalities on laboratory testing
- The health effects occur at work and are relieved when absent, meeting the traditional definition of work-related health problems
- Over time the most severely affected individuals may not experience relief when they leave work or the health effects may abate more slowly
- BRI are occupational illnesses caused by physical, chemical or biologic exposures within these building environments and can be divided into
    1. Specific illness with an identifiable cause and a fairly homogenous clinical picture, i.e. a number of individ-

uals are affected at the same time with similar signs and symptoms

Examples include

a. Legionnaire's disease/Pontiac fever
   – *L. pneumophilia*
b. Hypersensitivity pneumonitis/humidifier lung
   – Polymicrobial mixture
c. Asthma
   – Bio-aerosols
d. Rhinitis
   – Volatile organic compounds
   – Aero-allergens
e. Dermatitis
   – Carbonless paper
   – Fiberglass insulation
f. Mucosal irritation
   – Volatile organic compounds
   – Nitrogen oxide from auto exhaust fumes
g. Headaches
   – CO from auto exhaust fumes

2 Non-specific illness where no causative agent can be identified and workers have heterogenous clinical manifestations, i.e. widely different symptoms and usually no objective signs (formerly known as 'sick building syndrome')
   - The above are multifactorial and complex as it is likely that the indoor environment of large non-industrial buildings contains a wide range of exposures, the challenge being to identify the causative agents

Manifestations of Non-specific BRI

1 **Mucosal**
   - Includes irritation of the throat, nose and eyes
   - May be related to toxin exposure, e.g. formaldehyde, volatile organic compounds or nitrogen oxides
   - May also represent allergic manifestations from expo-

sure to bio-aerosols or inorganic complex compounds such as those released from carbonless paper

2 **Respiratory**
- Includes cough, chest tightness and shortness of breath
- May be related to allergen exposure or may be a form fruste of hypersensitivity pneumonitis

3 **Systemic**
- Includes symptoms of headache, fatigue, musculoskeletal pains and malaise
- This constellation of symptoms is reminiscent of organic toxic dust syndrome, humidifier fever or Pontiac fever
- May represent a reaction of a few highly sensitive workers to the same agents that cause specific building-related illnesses when present in higher concentrations

4 **Other**
- Some individuals may develop skin irritation or rash, nausea, poor appetite, etc.

Factors Associated with Non-specific BRI

Personal factors

1 **Atopic illness**
- May occur because individuals with a history of atopy are more sensitive to allergens and other exposures in the environment

2 **Younger age**
- May be due to a greater sensitivity

3 **Female gender**
- May be explained by work females are more likely to do and their consequent exposures

Work factors

1 **Secretarial and clerical work**
- Frequently associated with increased symptom reporting
- May reflect greater exposure to certain substances e.g. photocopier fumes, carbonless paper, etc.

– May also reflect that workers in these positions tend to remain at the same work location and within the building more hours than individuals in more senior jobs

2 **Ergonomic factors**
- Some problems, particularly musculoskeletal, may be the result of ergonomic factors, i.e. work injuries related to repetitive tasks, poorly designed furniture, etc.

3 **Job stress**
- A consistent finding is that job stress, however measured, is associated with increased symptom reporting, contributing to feelings of discomfort

Building factors

1 Typically seen in **mechanically ventilated** office towers with sealed windows
- The single most important factor appears to be air conditioning ? related to biologic contamination with bacteria and fungi

2 **Open concept offices**
- Particularly seen when there are no windows nearby
- The typical modern office has cramped, crowded, small work spaces which may contribute to a lack of workers' well-being

3 **Lack of personal control over ventilation**

4 **Outdoor air supply**
- A controversial topic
- If industry norms for minimum outdoor air supply are respected, symptoms will not be affected by further increase
- However if outdoor air supply is below the recommended minimum, symptoms may occur because of increased air pollutant levels

5 **Temperature and humidity**
- These have been considered 'comfort measures' but symptoms will increase dramatically if temperatures are above normal
- Mucosal irritation is more common when relative humidity drops below 20%

- Symptoms of malaise, fatigue and respiratory complaints increase when the humidity increases above 60% ? due to greater microbial contamination

Approach to Patient with Possible BRI

1 **History**
- Symptoms should be consistently work-related with relief when absent
- Whether the workers have identified any odors or can themselves identify any exposures – particularly new or changing exposures related to the time of onset of symptoms
- Ascertain if other workers in nearby work stations or in the same building are also affected, as well as whether symptoms are similar in these other affected workers
- A history of atopic illness or asthma is important
- Cigarette smoking may be protective for some forms of illness but increase the risk of others

2 **Other medical problems**
- BRI are a diagnosis of exclusion and therefore important to rule out other medical causes for the symptoms
- Other environments such as the home can give rise to similar symptoms, particularly if a delayed immunologic response is responsible

3 **Physical exam**
- In non-specific BRI physical exam is completely normal
- The above is also common with specific BRI but abnormalities may be detected for diseases such as hypersensitivity pneumonitis and asthma

4 **Laboratory exam**
- Hypersensitivity pneumonitis will manifest abnormalities in pulmonary function, chest X-ray and CBC
- Occupational asthma will demonstrate a consistent drop in peak flow at work or every evening after work, but not on weekends

Diagnosis of BRI

Identification of the causative agent in a suspected BRI is difficult, time consuming and requires the collaborative efforts of professionals with expertise in medicine, engineering and industrial hygiene

- Few practicing clinicians will have expertise in all these areas and therefore a stepwise approach should be followed

Step 1 – *Case definition*

- An accurate case definition is essential and should include the principal manifestations of the affected worker(s)
- Important to see other affected workers to define the extent of the problem and refine the case definition

Step 2 – *Walk-through inspection of the building*

- Inspect the ventilation system including cooling coils, strop pans and filter for evidence of biologic contamination and standing/stagnant water
- Examine the outdoor air intake for possible entrainment of automobile exhaust fumes
- Inspect the work station of the affected worker(s) for evidence of biologic contamination, e.g. water damage, mold spots in the carpet, ceiling or wall
- Look for sources of chemical contaminants such as photography development, photocopiers, special printers for graphics or technical drawings
- Look for local malfunctioning of the ventilation system
- Assess the physical layout for ergonomic factors or crowding

Step 3 – *Industrial hygiene measurements of indoor air quality*

- Based on the first two steps, decisions can be made in consultation with industrial hygiene experts as to what should be measured, where and when the measurement should be taken
  - Public Health/Occupational Health Departments are responsible for investigation of the work environ-

ment in most North American jurisdictions, although it can be very difficult to find the right person or organization
    — Publicly funded institutions responsible for a worker's health can provide invaluable assistance in the investigation of the work environment and may be instrumental in identifying additional affected workers
    — They may also ensure that corrective action is taken on the part of the building owners and/or employers
  – Private firms have sprung up devoted to indoor air quality measurement, the latter requiring expensive equipment and well-trained personnel

CARBON MONOXIDE POISONING

Normal carboxyhemoglobin (COHB) levels are <1% and related to the metabolism of hemoglobin and heme-containing compounds

- Elevated **endogenous** levels are seen with hemolysis or conversion from methylene chloride (which is present in paint strippers)
- **Exogenous** sources include vehicle exhausts, fires, indoor charcoal broilers, inadequate venting of heaters, air pollution (up to 2% COHB) and smokers (up to 9% COHB)

Toxicity results from

- Combination with hemoglobin at 230 times the oxygen affinity
- Shift of the oxyhemoglobin dissociation curve to the left and oxygen deprivation of the tissues
- Binding to heme-containing proteins at the cellular level
- Binding to cardiac myoglobin with levels 3 times greater than circulating COHB levels

- Binding to skeletal muscle myoglobin whose slower dissociation after exposure has ceased can result in a rebound elevation of blood COHB levels
- COHB levels of 20% result in headache, nausea, vomiting and poor manual dexterity
- Levels of 60% result in coma and seizures with death at 80% from cerebral anoxia and/or pulmonary edema

Clinical presentations are variable and can include

1 Flu-like illness with headaches, weakness
2 Prominent GI symptoms with nausea, vomiting and diarrhea
3 Acute CNS complaints including dizziness, headache, visual disturbances and altered mentation which can progress to seizures and coma
4 Cardiac disease including arrhythmias, acute infarction, syncope and cardiac arrest
5 Pulmonary edema of non-cardiac or cardiac origin
6 Chronic presentation with CNS features of mental deterioration, incontinence and gait disturbances, seen up to 240 days after large CO exposure

Physical exam may reveal cherry-red skin discoloration as well as fundoscopic hemorrhages

Radiologic findings may be normal or show signs of pulmonary edema, reflecting direct toxicity on the alveolocapillary membrane or cardiac edema

Lab abnormalities

1 Elevated COHB levels
2 Overestimation of oxygen saturation on pulse oximetry
   - At 660 nm, the absorption coefficient of COHB is similar to that of oxyhemoglobin; interpreting COHB as oxyhemoglobin and overestimating the true oxyhemoglobin level
3 Metabolic acidosis
4 Myoglobinuria

Prognostic features

- Level of COHB
- Rapidity and nature of the therapeutic intervention, i.e. hyperbaric chamber *vs.* 100% oxygen
- Spectrum of end-organ damage

COAL MINING – LUNG DISEASES

Coal Worker's Pneumoconiosis (CWP)

Definition: Lung disease due to inhalation and retention of carbon dust in the lungs as well as the lung tissue's reaction to its presence

- This contrasts with the 'benign anthracosis' of smokers or city dwellers where the carbon deposits have no pathologic or functional significance

Simple CWP is characterized by coal dust macules (non-palpable), coal dust nodules (palpable) and focal emphysema without associated fibrosis

- It is classified by the International Labour Office according to the number, size and shape of small opacities on chest X-ray
- The category is generally proportional to the intensity and duration of exposure to coal mine dust

Complicated CWP or **progressive massive fibrosis (PMF)** is defined by the development of foci of fibrosis >1 cm in diameter

Clinically, patients with simple CWP and mild disease are often asymptomatic without progression of their disease after removal from their environment

- Some patients have symptoms of cough and black sputum from 'industrial bronchitis' or smoking
- Progression of disease to PMF is unpredictable with postulated factors being the cumulative dust exposure, quartz contact of the coal dust, infection or immunologic factors
- Symptoms of PMF include increasing cough, sputum,

dyspnea, hemoptysis and expectoration of jet-black fluid, the latter reflecting cavitation of the 'mass-like' lesions with their rupture into the bronchial tree due to ischemia or infection
- Hypoxemia, pulmonary artery hypertension and cor pulmonale eventually result
- The conglomerate lesions must be distinguished from malignancy as well as infection

Lab abnormalities include hyperglobulinemia, positive rheumatoid factor and anti-nuclear antibodies in the blood

Radiologic features of simple CWP
1 Chest X-rays may be normal or minimally abnormal with mild disease documented at pathology
2 More extensive disease results in nodular or reticular opacities similar to silicosis, with upper lobe predominance
3 Calcification of parenchymal nodules or eggshell calcification of nodes is uncommon

Radiologic features of PMF
1 Unilateral or bilateral upper lobe opacities varying from 1 cm to an entire lobe, typically occurring in the upper lung
2 The solid masses begin in the lung periphery and migrate to the perihilar regions with intervening areas of emphysema developing
3 The lesions can cross fissures
4 Cavitation can develop
5 The conglomerate lesions may only develop radiologically or can progress only after dust exposure has been ceased

The **CT appearance** of CWP is similar to that of silicosis (see p. 398)

Caplan's Syndrome
Refers to rapidly enlarging lung nodules, 0.5–5.0 cm in diameter, in patients with underlying rheumatoid arthritis, originally described by Caplan in Welsh Coal Miners

- Subsequently described in coal miners with positive rheumatoid factor without associated arthritis, as well as in other dust exposures
- Rare in North America
- Microscopically, the lesions are classic rheumatoid nodules except for rings of coal dust at their periphery
- Patients often have associated subcutaneous nodules

Silicosis

Diagnosis of silicosis in coal workers is made by microscopic exam which reveals silicotic nodules

- Seen in approximately 10–15% of underground coal miners, usually against a background of simple CWP

Diffuse Interstitial Fibrosis

Reported in approximately 15% of autopsies of coal miners

- The etiology is unclear ? coal dust ? silica ? other

Chronic Bronchitis and Emphysema

Seen both in smokers and non-smokers where patients present with cough, sputum and variable airways obstruction

FARM WORKERS LUNG DISEASES

Organic Dust Toxic Syndrome

Agricultural dusts are a mixture of plant particles, insect parts, animal particles, bacteria, fungi, etc.

- Pathogenesis is unclear, but exposure to high concentrations whether or not overtly moldy, results in a flu-like illness with fever or facial warmth, chills, myalgias, anthralgias and headache
- Upper respiratory and airway symptoms may be present in the absence of clinical, radiologic or functional evidence of alveolitis
- Symptoms typically develop hours after exposure but may develop immediately and lack the selectivity seen in hypersensitivity pneumonitis

- The course of disease is benign with no long-term sequelae and no mortality, unlike hypersensitivity pneumonitis

Hypersensitivity Pneumonitis (see p. 368)

Grain Dust-Induced Lung Disease

A flu-like illness, upper respiratory symptoms and features of airways obstruction (cough, wheezing, chest tightness) can occur immediately or hours after a large exposure

- A late asthmatic reaction can occur hours following a large or small exposure
- Symptoms are more common in smokers and seen with exposures to many grains, most often Durum wheat and barley dust
- Chronic effects of exposure are similar to and additive to smoking

Silo-Filler's Disease

Acute lung injury caused by the inhalation of nitrogen dioxide in or near an agricultural silo

Clinical course varies from mild and self-limiting to fatal, including

1 Transient upper respiratory symptoms
2 Acute bronchitis and bronchiolitis
3 Pulmonary edema
4 Bronchiolitis obliterans developing weeks after the exposure
5 Nitrate-induced systemic hypotension, metabolic acidosis or methemoglobinemia
6 Rapid death from laryngospasm, bronchospasm or asphyxia

Follow-up studies vary from complete recovery to obstructive impairment of pulmonary function

Radiologic studies can be normal, reveal evidence of diffuse airspace edema or the multiple nodules of bronchiolitis

Pesticide-Induced Lung Disease

Multiple agents used including fungicides, insecticides, rodenticides, herbicides, with effects varying from respiratory irritation to bronchospasm, pulmonary edema or pulmonary fibrosis, depending on the exposure

Infections

1 Bacterial, e.g. brucellosis, pasteurellosis, tularemia
2 Fungal, e.g. histoplasmosis
3 Rickettsial, e.g. Q-fever
4 Chlamydia, e.g. psittacosis

HARD METAL PNEUMOCONIOSIS – GIANT CELL INTERSTITIAL PNEUMONITIS

Definition: Rare lung disease secondary to hard metal, an alloy composed mainly of tungsten carbide and cobalt and characterized by high temperature resistance and a hardness approaching that of diamond

- Defined **histologically** by large numbers of giant cells filling the airspaces, in addition to a mononuclear interstitial infiltrate and airspace macrophages
- Seen in workers involved in the manufacture or use of the metal, with cobalt thought to be primarily responsible as an identical disease is seen in diamond polishers exposed to high concentrations of cobalt alone

Clinical manifestations

1 Occupational asthma, thought to develop on an allergic basis with at least a 6 month latency before sensitization and asthma symptoms develop
   - Subjects with asthma can also develop features of hypersensitivity pneumonitis
2 Interstitial lung disease, which presents with acute or subacute episodes of fever, anorexia and dyspnea, improving when exposure is terminated but recurring on renewed exposure
   - The clinical and radiologic features are those of hypersensitivity pneumonitis
   - Over time, there is a transition to the picture of inter-

stitial fibrosis clinically and radiologically, with features of chronic cough, dyspnea, rales and clubbing

Chest X-rays vary from normal early in the disease to a non-specific reticular, reticulo-nodular or nodular pattern, eventually leading to the features of interstitial fibrosis

Diagnostic criteria

1. Cobalt exposure by history or analysis of sputum, BAL, blood, urine, hair and lung tissue for cobalt or tungsten content
2. History of repeated episodes of 'pneumonia'
3. Features of occupational asthma with
   - Progressive decline in flow rates during the day, but absent when exposure does not occur
   - Improvement or disappearance of asthma on removal from exposure with recurrence when exposure resumes
   - Improvement of asthma symptoms when work place exhaust ventilation is installed
   - Positive challenge test
   - Compatible radiologic findings
   - Giant cells on BAL or lung biopsy although late stages are characterized by fibrosis and little alveolitis

SILICOSIS

Definition: The occupational lung disease due to inhalation of crystalline silica, usually in the form of quartz

Pathologically, the typical lesion is the silicotic nodule which gradually enlarges to become visible on chest X-ray and can then coalesce to form mass-like lesions

- Birefringent silica crystals can be seen in the center of the nodules

Clinically, in **chronic simple silicosis**, patients are often asymptomatic with radiologic abnormalities present after 10–20 years of exposure

- Typical exposures include hard rock mining, ceramic and pottery industries, foundries, granite quarries, sand blasting, others
- Symptoms are usually non-specific but cavitation of conglomerate masses can result in jet-black sputum being coughed up
- Rales and wheezes are common on auscultation when patients are symptomatic
- The natural history of the disease is variable, depending on the severity of exposure
- Superimposed tuberculosis or atypical mycobacterial infection can result in both systemic as well as increasing pulmonary symptoms
- Fibrosis and disability are often progressive, even after removal from the dust exposure, with the potential development of respiratory failure and cor pulmonale

Complications include

1 Superinfection with tuberculosis, atypicals, anaerobes
2 Altered immunity with ⊕ RF, ⊕ ANA, immune complexes, hypergammaglobulinema, kidney disease, increased incidence of scleroderma
3 Broncholithiasis
4 Airway narrowing on bronchoscopy simulating carcinoma
5 Respiratory failure and cor pulmonale
6 Lymphohematogenous dissemination of silica with thoracic and extrathoracic adenopathy as well as silicotic nodules in the liver, spleen and bone marrow, in addition to the lungs
7 Increased risk of lung cancer as well as difficulty in diagnosing the early stage of malignancy

PFTS are normal early in the disease with restriction, obstruction or a combination common as silicosis progresses, accompanied by a reduction in diffusing capacity

Diagnosis is usually made from the history of an occupational exposure to high concentrations of silica, a compatible chest

X-ray and no likely alternative explanation for the clinical-radiologic findings

- Diagnosis can be confirmed by pathology (transbronchial, transthoracic or open biopsy) but occasionally requires specialized testing such as the ash content

Accelerated silicosis is a variant of classic silicosis where symptoms develop within 5–10 years of exposure with more rapid progression but similar radiologic findings

Acute silicosis is a rapidly progressive form of the disease, developing within months to a few years, and usually fatal

- Described in sand blasters, tunnellers, rock drillers and others where there is exposure to high concentrations of freshly fractured silica
- Infection with typical or atypical mycobacteria may complicate the underlying disease which is characterized by a lipid-rich proteinaceous material in the airspaces

Chest X-ray findings

1 Upper lobe predominance of nodular opacities <1 cm in diameter ('simple' silicosis) which can calcify
2 A reticular pattern, with or without nodules, may predominate with Kerley A + B lines
3 Hilar adenopathy ± eggshell calcifications
4 Areas of homogeneous consolidation can develop as nodules become confluent and form conglomerate or 'complicated' silicosis (progressive massive fibrosis)
   - The densities are non-segmental in distribution and vary from 1–2 cm in diameter to the size of a lobe, with the individual nodular densities becoming less apparent
5 'Masses' of nodules migrate from the midzone and lung periphery to the hila, leaving emphysematous spaces or bullae between the pleura and areas of consolidation centrally, the bullae potentially rupturing and causing a pneumothorax
6 Conglomerate lesions can cavitate from TB, atypical TB, ischemia or anaerobes – R/O bronchogenic cancer
7 Aspergillus colonization of the above cavities

8 Radiologic progression of the above abnormalities can occur after removal from the exposure
9 Development of pulmonary hypertension and cor pulmonale

CT scan findings

1 2–5 mm nodules, centrilobular and subpleural in location (confluent subpleural nodules can simulate pleural plaques)
2 Upper lobe predominance but diffusely distributed
3 Conglomerate masses which may reveal necrotic areas
4 Demonstrable lymphadenopathy in ~40% of patients

Role of CT scan

- May detect abnormalities when chest X-rays are normal
- May clarify the presence or absence of conglomerate lesions
- Can distinguish silicosis from sarcoid by
  - More bilateral, symmetric and uniform distribution of nodules
  - Very few reticular abnormalities
  - Absence of bronchovascular distribution of nodules
  - Absence of beaded septae

Variants

1 Acute silicosis is manifest by diffuse bilateral airspace disease similar to alveolar proteinosis
2 Caplan's syndrome is a manifestation of rheumatoid lung disease and characterized by rapidly evolving lung nodules

SMOKE INHALATION

Fire Environment

Exposure to a fire environment causes damage by

1 Smoke, defined as a suspension of visible particles in air and toxic gases, with particulates causing mechanical

irritation, traumatic injury or even anatomical airway obstruction

2 Toxic gases, chemicals and fumes are generated depending upon what is burning and will therefore differ in each fire setting but can include CO, hydrogen cyanide, aldehydes, hydrogen chloride, isocyanates, ammonia, hydrogen fluoride, hydrogen bromide, sulfur dioxide, etc.
   - The above and smoke are the main causes of respiratory morbidity and mortality in fire victims
3 Thermal injury, usually confined to the upper airway but lesions of the lower airway or parenchyma can be seen with steam or massive heat exposure
4 Decreased inspired oxygen concentration due to oxygen consumption by the fire, the F_iO_2 potentially falling to 10–15% during the flashover phase of a fire, when a room bursts into flames

Assessment of Respiratory Involvement

General history

- Patient location and duration of exposure
- Presence or absence of entrapment
- Level of consciousness
- Questioning fire personnel about the types of combustion and the specific gas/chemical exposures

Respiratory history

- Hoarseness, stridor or painful swallowing indicative of upper airway injury
- Cough, copious black sputum, dyspnea or chest pains from lower airway injury

Physical findings

- Facial burns, singed nasal hairs, hoarseness, stridor
- Tachypnea, rales, wheezes

Associated issues

- Traumatic injuries
- Skin burns

- Alcohol intoxication
- Drug abuse

Clinical Problems

1 **Upper airways obstruction**
   - Thermal exposure can acutely result in pharyngeal and laryngeal edema
   - Obstruction may be delayed, occurring only after fluid resuscitation and is occasionally caused by mucosal sloughing which occurs most often 3–4 days following exposure

2 **Lower airways obstruction**
   - Irritant gases, especially the aldehydes, (e.g. formaldehyde, acetaldehyde), and acrolein, cause inflammation with protein-rich exudates and sloughing of the respiratory tract epithelium, forming tracheobronchial casts as well as areas of atelectasis
   - Acute bronchitis, bronchiolitis and bronchospasm with resultant airways obstruction
   - Exacerbation of pre-existing asthma/COPD
   - Long term sequelae including bronchiectasis, bronchiolitis obliterans, endobronchial polyposis, airways hyperactivity and tracheal stenosis

3 **Parenchymal injury**
   - Early pulmonary edema from altered microcirculation permeability or hypoxemic cardiac injury
   - Delayed-onset injury, i.e. >7 days, with pulmonary edema or ARDS secondary to irritant gases, sepsis, hypotension
   - Pulmonary contusion from trauma
   - Residual pulmonary fibrosis may result

4 **Post-traumatic injuries** including pneumothorax, hemothorax, fractures of the ribs, spine or sternum

5 **Systemic diseases** including
   - Carbon monoxide poisoning (see p. 388)

  - Leading cause of death at the fire scene and in the first 24 hours following the fire
- Hydrogen cyanide poisoning
  - Produced from the combustion of polyurethanes and nylon
  - Interferes with oxygen utilization at the mitochondrial level with resulting anaerobic metabolism and lactic acidosis
  - Clinical manifestations reflect the blood cyanide levels with initial tachycardia and flushing followed by hypotension, respiratory depression, obtundation, dilated pupils and pulmonary edema
- Traumatic and/or crush injuries
- Alcohol and/or drug intoxication
- Cutaneous burns
- Neurologic disease
  - Alveolar hypoventilation
  - Altered sensorium progressing to coma
  - Loss of gag reflex and subsequent aspiration
- Peripheral thrombophlebitis and pulmonary emboli in immobilized patients

Investigations

1 **Chest X-ray**
   - Usually normal at presentation but multiple abnormalities are described including atelectasis as well as patchy or diffuse interstitial/airspace infiltrates, reflecting mucus plugs, edema or pneumonia
   - Signs of thoracic trauma can include lung contusion, hemothorax, pneumothorax or bony fractures

2 **ABGs**

3 **Blood levels** of CO, cyanide, and occasionally alcohol and drug toxicology screen

4 With serious burns, **laryngoscopy** for evaluation of the upper airway and **bronchoscopy** for the lower airway
   - Airway findings vary from mild erythema to soot, hemorrhage, ulcerations, blisters and bronchial casts, the

latter potentially causing life-threatening airways obstruction when dislodged

5 **Monitoring** airways obstruction with expiratory flow rates and flow-volume curves

TALCOSIS – INHALATIONAL

Talc is a hydrated magnesium silicate that can cause disease in isolation or more often in association with other minerals, e.g. often contaminated with asbestos, silica, etc.

- Disease is seen in mining, milling, industrial use, e.g. rubber industry, high doses of personal use

Clinically, patients present with non-specific respiratory symptoms accompanied by rales and clubbing

- Progressive disease can occur after exposure has stopped, leading to increasing dyspnea, hypoxemia and cor pulmonale

Radiologic findings

1 Pleural plaques, similar to asbestos plaques, often involving the diaphragm and occasionally the pericardium
2 Interstitial disease, reticular or nodular in pattern and similar to asbestosis
3 Confluent mass(es)

TOXIC INHALATION

Seen with inhalation of gases, fumes, vapors, aerosols and smoke, (e.g. ammonia, chlorine, sulfur dioxide, nitrogen oxides, phosgene) and the pulmonary effects include

1 Upper airway irritation including pharangeal, laryngeal and tracheal edema as well as laryngospasm
2 Lower airway inflammation with acute bronchitis, bronchiolitis, mucosal sloughing
3 Acute chemical pneumonitis with edema and hemorrhage which can progress to ARDS
4 Secondary superimposed bronchopneumonia

5 Sequelae can include
  - Bronchiectasis
  - Bronchiolitis obliterans
  - BOOP
  - RADS
  - COPD

Fraser R.S., Muller N.L., Colman N., Paré P.D. (1999) Diagnosis of Diseases of the Chest 4th Edn., WB Saunders.

Moss, A., Gamsu, Genant (1992) Thorax and neck. In: *Computed Tomography of the Body with Magnetic Resonance Imaging*, 2nd edn, vol. 1.: W.B. Saunders.

Webb, R., Muller, N.L., Naidich, D.P. (1996) *High Resolution CT of the Lung*, 2nd edn.: Lippincott-Raven.

Thurlbeck, W., Churg, A. (eds) (1995) *Pathology of the Lung*, 2nd edn.: Thieme Medical Publishers.

Baum, G.L., Crapo, J.D., Celli, B.R., Karlinsky, J.B. (eds) (1997) *Textbook of Pulmonary Diseases*, 6th edn.: Lippincott-Raven.

Fishman, A.P., Elias, J.A., Fishman, J.A., Grippi, M.A., Kaiser, L.R., Senior, R.N. (1998) *Fishman's Pulmonary Diseases and Disorders*, 3rd edn.: McGraw-Hill.

Remy-Jardin, M., Remy, J., Wallaert, B. *et al.* (1993) Subacute and chronic bird breeder hypersensitivity pneumonitis. Sequential evaluation with CT and correlation with lung function tests and BAL. *Radiology* **189**: 111–118.

Cormier, Y., Desmeules, M. (1994) Treatment of hypersensitivity pneumonitis – contact avoidance vs. corticosteroid treatment. *Can. Res. J.* **1**: 223–228.

Rose, C., King, T. (1992) Controversies in hypersensitivity pneumonitis. *ARRD* **145**: 1–2.

Richerson, H.B. *et al.* (1989) Guidelines for the clinical evaluation of hypersensitivity pneumonitis. *J. Allergy Clin. Immunol.* **84**: 839–844.

Adler, B.D., Padley, S., Muller, N. *et al.* (1992) Chronic hypersensitivity pneumonitis. *Radiology* **185**: 91–95.

Harris, M., Terrio, J., Mijer, W. *et al.* (1998) High-altitude medicine. *Am. Family Phys.* **57**: 1907–1914.

Nishimura, S., Broaddus, C. (1998) Asbestos-induced pleural disease. *Clinics in Chest Medicine* **19**: 311–329.

Begin, R., Dufresne, A., Plante, F. *et al.* (1994) Asbestos-related disorders. *Can. Res. J.* **1**: 167–185.

Kriebel, D., Brain, J., Sprince, N. *et al.* (1988) The pulmonary toxicity of beryllium. *ARRD* **137**: 464–473.

Meyer, K. (1994) Beryllium and lung disease. *Chest* **106**: 942–946.

Menzies, D., Bourbeau, J. (1971) Building-related illnesses. *NEJM* **337**: 1524–1530.

Dolan, M. (1985) Carbon monoxide poisoning. *CMAJ* **133**: 342–346.

Pico, G. (1992) Hazardous exposure and lung disease among farm workers. *Clinics in Chest Medicine* **13**: 311–328.

Douglas, W., Hepper, N., Colby, T. (1989) Silo-filler's disease. *Mayo Clinic Proc.* **64**: 291–304.

Cugell, D. (1992) The hard metal diseases. *Clinics in Chest Medicine* **13**: 269–279.

Loke, J. (1998) Thermal lung injury and acute smoke inhalation. In: Fishman, A.P., Elias J.A., Fishman, J.A., Grippi, M.A., Kaiser, L.R., Senior, R.N. *Fishman's Pulmonary Diseases and Disorders*. McGraw–Hill, ch. 65, pp. 989–1000.

49 Interstitial Lung Disease (ILD)

ETIOLOGIES

Anatomic Considerations

Definition: ILD is characterized radiologically by diffuse bilateral infiltrates of inhomogeneous radiologic density and can be seen in disorders **primarily** involving the

1 **Fiber skeleton**
   - *Central* or axial fibers extending from the hilar bronchi and pulmonary arteries to the centrilobular bronchioles and arterioles
   - *Peripheral* fibers marginating the secondary pulmonary lobule
   - *Septal* fibers joining the central and peripheral fibers

2 **Vessels**
   - Arterioles, capillaries, venules, lymphatics

3 **Bronchioles/bronchi**

4 **Air spaces**

The term ILD is misleading as extensive involvement of airspaces, airways and vessels may occur as well

The Following (Table 49.1) Can All Cause ILD

Allergic alveolitis	Edema
Alveolar proteinosis	Eosinophilic lung disease
Alveolar hemorrhage	Eosinophilic granuloma
Amyloid	Foreign body reactions
ARDS	Fungal infections
Aspiration	Gaucher's
Beryliiosis	Hamman-Rich
Bronchiolitis	Hemosiderosis
BOOP	Hermansky Pudlak
Bronchiectasis	i.v. drug abuse
Collagen diseases	Infections
DIP	
Drugs	
Inhalation injury	Neoplasms
– Organic dusts	Niemann Pick
– Inorganic dusts	Occupational
– Fumes	Pneumoconioses
– Gases	Poisons
– Vapors	Post-ARDS
LAM	Pulmonary granulomatoses
LIP	Pulmonary venous hypertension
Lymphangitic cancer	Sarcoid
Lymphomas	Tuberculosis
Lymphoproliferative diseases	Tuberous sclerosis
Metastatic cancer	UIP or variants
Miliary disease	Vasculitides

Table 49.1

Most common causes in clinical practice are

- Cardiac pulmonary edema
- Infections
- Usual interstitial pneumonitis
- Sarcoid
- Neoplasms
- Pneumoconiosis
- Hypersensitivity pneumonitis

CLUES TO DIAGNOSIS OF ILD

I. Determine if there is **isolated** pulmonary disease, e.g. allergic alveolitis, *vs.* associated **extrapulmonary** disease (clubbing or other organ system involvement) by
- History
- Physical exam
- Labs
- Radiologic (extrapulmonary)

II. **Chest X-ray/HRCT**
1. Mode of onset
2. Disease distribution on chest X-ray
3. Disease distribution on HRCT
4. Pattern of infiltrates on chest X-ray
5. Pattern of infiltrates on HRCT
6. Associated radiologic abnormalities involving the airways, parenchyma, pleura or mediastinum
7. Expiratory HRCT scan

III. **PFTs**

IV. Localize the probable **anatomic** site of involvement, i.e.: fiber skeleton, vessels, bronchioles, or airspaces – by history, physical, labs, physiologic and radiologic studies

V. **Invasive** procedures

(*Each is discussed below*)

I. Isolated Pulmonary *vs.* Extrapulmonary Disease

1 **Pulmonary history**
- Duration of symptoms, e.g. acute (weeks) *vs.* chronic (months, years) as well as rate of disease progression
- Age at presentation, e.g. sarcoid, LAM and eosinophilic granuloma present between 20–40

- Gender, e.g. LAM in premenopausal women
- Familial, e.g. UIP, tuberous sclerosis, cystic fibrosis, alveolar microlithiasis, Kartagener's, storage diseases, neurofibromatosis
- Occupations (past and present), hobbies, occupational
- history of family members, e.g. asbestosis from clothing
- Wheezing (see p. 51)
- Hemoptysis e.g. alveolar hemorrage syndromes, vasculitis, complicating carcinoma, any cause of pulmonary venous hypertension
- Fever, e.g. BOOP, vasculitis, drug reaction, hypersensitivity, collagen disease, infection
- Drug use including prescriptions, over-the-counter, oily nose drops, remote chemotherapy, e.g. carmustine
- Recurrent aspiration
- Smoking, e.g. eosinophilic granuloma, DIP, UIP, RB–ILD or nonsmoking, e.g. allergic alveolitis
- Prior neoplasms or radiation
- HIV risk factors – infections/Kaposi's sarcoma
- Exposure to birds, animals, woods, chemicals, water sources (hot tubs, air conditioner, humidifiers, water damage to walls and carpets) or agriculture to suggest allergic alveolitis
- Little or no symptomatology with extensive disease on X-ray suggests sarcoid, silicosis, eosinophilic granuloma, RB–ILD

Extrapulmonary history re thorough review of systems for extrapulmonary disease

2 **Physical findings**
- Rales are common but non-specific
- Inspiratory squeaks are common with bronchiolitis
- Cyanosis, pulmonary hypertension and cor pulmonale are manifestations of advanced disease
- Clubbing, e.g. asbestosis, IPF, bronchiectasis, cystic fibrosis, bronchogenic cancer with lymphangitic spread

Wheezing
- CHF or other causes of pulmonary venous hypertension
- Sarcoid
- Bronchiectasis
- Bronchiolitis
- Tropical eosinophilia
- Inhalational diseases – acute or chronic
- Allergic alveolitis
- Wegener's
- Any ILD on top of underlying airways disease

Skin lesions
- Erythema nodosum, e.g. sarcoid
- Subcutaneous nodules, e.g. rheumatoid arthritis, neurofibromatosis, lung cancer
- Telangiectasis, Raynauds, e.g. scleroderma
- Cutaneous vasculitis, e.g. systemic vasculitis, collagen vascular disease

Enlarged salivary glands
- e.g. Sarcoid, LIP

Lymphadenopathy/hepatosplenomegaly
- e.g. Sarcoid, neoplasms, eosinophilic granuloma

Pericarditis
- e.g. Collagen diseases/vasculitis, radiation, neoplasm, asbestosis

Arthritis
- e.g. Sarcoid, collagen diseases/vasculitis

3 **Lab studies** will depend upon clinical suspicions and might include
- Bloods
  - CBC, WBC and differential
  - Eosinophil count (± antifilarial AB, IgE)
  - Autoantibodies including ANCA, anti-GBM, ANA, LE, anti-RNP, RF
  - Anti-Jo-1 (a serum antibody against the cellular enzyme histidyl-trna-synthetase) is seen in up to ⅔

of patients with polymyositis/dermato-myositis and interstitial lung disease, and its presence should prompt a search for subclinical myositis
  - Precipitins for allergic alveolitis
  - HIV serology
  - CPK, BUN, Cr
- Sputum – cytology, mycology, AFB, pneumocystis
- Echocardiogram to R/O a cardiac etiology
- Urinalysis for nephrotic syndrome (e.g. SLE, amyloid), glomerulonephritis (e.g. vasculitis, collagen disease)
- Findings of diabetes insipidus (e.g. sarcoid, eosinophilic granuloma)

4 **Radiologic studies might include**
- Barium swallow for aspiration
- Skeletal survey/bone scan for metastases, sarcoid, eosinophilic granuloma
- Mammography, pelvic-abdominal CT/US if lymphangitic cancer is suspected

II. Chest X-ray/HRCT

1 **Mode of onset**

	Acute – Subacute
Fiber skeleton	• Infection – bacterial, mycoplasma, viral, fungal, parasitic • Drugs • Acute interstitial pneumonia (Hamman-Rich) • Allergic alveolitis • Granulomatous – sarcoid, tuberculosis, atypicals
Vessels	• Vasculitides • Miliary disease • Pulmonary venous hypertension – cardiac/non-cardiac • Lymphangitic cancer
Bronchioles	• Acute bronchiolitis • BOOP
Airspaces	• Aspiration • ARDS • Alveolar hemorrhage syndrome • Eosinophilic lung disease

Table 49.2

	Subacute – Chronic
Fiber skeleton	• Radiation pneumonitis • Drugs (also acute) • Eosinophilic granuloma • UIP, DIP, NSIP • Pneumoconioses • Allergic alveolitis (also acute) • Sarcoid (also acute) • Foreign body reactions • Deposits, e.g. amyloid • Collagen diseases
Vessels	• Any cause of pulmonary venous hypertension (also acute) • Lymphomas • Lymphangitic cancer • LAM • Tuberous sclerosis • Vasculitides
Bronchioles	• Bronchiolitis, e.g. RBILD, constrictive • BOOP
Airspaces	• Aspiration (also acute) • i.v. drug abuse • Alveolar proteinosis • Alveolar hemorrhage syndromes • Eosinophilic lung disease

Table 49.3

2 Disease distribution – chest X-ray

Upper lobe predominance

- Chronic eosinophilic pneumonia
- Pneumocystis
- Cystic fibrosis
- Ankylosing spondylitis
- Silicosis
- Sarcoid
- Eosinophilic granuloma
- TB, atypicals
- ABPA
- Fibro-bullous disease – RA
- Berylliosis
- Allergic alveolitis

Peripheral predominance

- Drug reaction, e.g. amiodarone
- BOOP (usually airspace)
- BOOP + eosinophilic pneumonia
- Eosinophilic pneumonia (usually airspace)
- Sarcoid (uncommon)
- UIP, primary or secondary
- Lymphangitic cancer (occasionally)

Lower lobe predominance

- Lipoid pneumonia
- Asbestosis
- UIP
- Collagen diseases

3 **Disease distribution – HRCT**

Overall distribution

- Central or peribronchovascular, e.g. sarcoid
- Central or peripheral, e.g. lymphangitic cancer
- Peripheral and subpleural
  - UIP
  - DIP (occasionally)
  - Drug-induced lung disease
  - Connective tissue diseases, e.g. RA, scleroderma
  - Asbestosis
  - Chronic aspiration
  - Sarcoid (uncommonly)
  - Lymphangitic cancer (occasionally)

Zonal distribution

- Upper, lower or random distribution is better appreciated

Secondary lobular abnormalities

- The secondary pulmonary nodule is a polyhedral unit with pulmonary veins and lymphatics at the periphery *vs.* the bronchiole and pulmonary arteriole at the center
- Centrilobular diseases involve the bronchiole, (e.g. bronchiolitis) or arterioles
- Involvement of the walls of lobules, i.e. interlobular

disease, is seen in pulmonary edema, lymphantitic cancer, UIP, sarcoid

- Intralobular disease is seen in many disorders including fibrosis, edema, lymphangitic cancer
- Lobular architecture may be maintained, (e.g. lymphangitic cancer) or lost, (e.g. UIP)

4 Pattern of infiltrates – chest X-ray

	Definition	Examples
'Ground glass'	Hazy increase in lung density without loss of vascular definition	Allergic alveolitis, BOOP, etc.
Reticular	Linear or curvilinear opacities	UIP, asbestosis
Reticulo-nodular	Combination of reticular and nodular	Sarcoid, lymphangitic cancer
Nodular	2–10 mm in diameter	Sarcoid, silicosis, CWP, hematogenous metastases, eosinophilic granuloma
Micro-nodular	<2 mm in diameter	Miliary disease, i.v. talcosis, silicosis, sarcoid, alveolar microlithiasis, hematogenous metastases
Cystic	Thin-walled spaces	LAM, eosinophilic granuloma
Honeycombing	Cystic spaces several mm to 1 cm in diameter, in close proximity to each other, with thick, clearly defined walls	Eosinophilic granuloma, UIP, others (see p. 180)
Normal		Seen in <10% of cases e.g. sarcoid, DIP, asbestosis, allergic alveolitis
Airspace infiltrates	• Interstitial lung disease producing an alveolar filling pattern	LIP
	• Diseases that are predominantly airspace but can have an interstitial component as well	Mineral oil aspiration, hypersensitivity pneumonitis, alveolar cell carcinoma, lymphoma, alveolar hemorrhage, others

Table 49.4

5 **Pattern of infiltrates – HRCT**

Reticular abnormalities may be caused by **fibrosis**, **edema** or **cellular infiltrates**

The location of changes can be peribronchovascular, centrilobular, intralobular, interlobular, sub-pleural or due to airway thickening

The findings of fibrosis (*vs.* edema or cellular infiltrates) include

- Architectural distortion
- Honeycombing
- Traction bronchiectasis
- Conglomerate masses

Nodular opacities

Interstitial nodules are well-defined and seen in the centrilobular or interlobular septa as well as sub-pleural and peribronchovascular in distribution

Airspace nodules are often ill-defined and seen in the centrilobular area

'Ground glass' opacity

Density is less than soft tissues but greater than normal parenchyma – may be a reflection of

- Interlobular septal thickening
- Alveolar wall thickening
- Airspace disease

Often patchy in distribution, affecting some lobules and sparing others, making the abnormal areas stand out on HRCT

Cystic

- Thin-walled (<3 mm) air-containing spaces >1 cm in diameter
- May have bizarre shapes due to fusion of cysts
- Cysts may not be obvious on chest X-ray

Honeycombing

- Often peripheral in location
- May be associated with other signs of fibrosis
- Seen in both interstitial fibrosis and bronchiectasis

Normal

Seen in a small percent of cases depending upon the underlying etiology, e.g. approximately 10% of sarcoid

6 **Associated radiologic abnormalities**

Airways – associated **hyperinflation** seen with

- LAM
- Eosinophilic granuloma
- Tuberous sclerosis
- Bronchiolitis
- Bronchiectasis
- Silicosis
- Asthma or COPD and superimposed interstitial lung disease
- Cystic fibrosis

Parenchyma

- Associated Kerley B lines
  - Lymphoma
  - Lymphangitic cancer
  - LAM
  - LV failure
  - Mitral valve disease
  - Pulmonary venous obstruction
  - Sarcoid
  - Silicosis
- Honeycomb lung
  - fibrosing alveolitis
  - eosinophilic granuloma
  - collagen diseases
  - rheumatoid lung
  - scleroderma
  - LAM
  - end stage sarcoid

Pleural disease

- Pleural effusion or thickening (CCRAIDLLSS)
  - **C**HF
  - **C**onnective tissue disease

- **R**adiation pneumonitis
- **A**sbestos exposure
- **I**nfection
- **D**rugs
- **L**AM
- **L**ymphangitic cancer
- **S**arcoid
- **S**arcoma – Kaposi's

- Recurrent pneumothoraces
  - Eosinophilic granuloma
  - LAM
  - Tuberous sclerosis
  - Pneumocystis
  - Any disease with honeycombing

Mediastinal disease

- Adenopathy
  - tuberculosis
  - fungus
  - sarcoid
  - berylliosis
  - lymphoma
  - lymphangitic cancer
  - Kaposi's sarcoma
  - silicosis
  - dilantin
  - amyloid
  - Although not seen on chest X-ray, enlarged nodes can be seen on CT scan in patients with UIP, collagen diseases, BOOP and allergic alveolitis
  - The nodes are usually <15 mm in diameter and few in number
- 'Eggshell' calcification
  - Silicosis
  - Sarcoid
  - Radiation
- Cardiomegaly
  - Pulmonary edema secondary to CHF
  - Lymphangitic cancer and a malignant pericardial effusion
- Esophageal disease
  - Air esophagogram with scleroderma
  - Functional or structural esophageal obstruction leading to recurrent aspiration

- Neurofibroma
  - Posterior mediastinal tumors associated with UIP of neurofibromatosis

7 **Expiratory HRCT scan**
- Bronchiolitis can present with a diffuse nodular pattern on HRCT
- An expiratory scan will show gas trapping to support the diagnosis of airways obstruction, with accentuation of the pattern of mosaic perfusion

III. Pulmonary Function Tests

Restrictive abnormality is usually present but an **obstructive** picture can be seen with

- Eosinophilic granuloma
- LAM/tuberous sclerosis
- Bronchiolitis
- Allergic alveolitis (associated bronchiolitis)
- Silicosis (associated bronchiolitis)
- Bronchiectasis
- Sarcoid
- Wegener's
- Underlying COPD or asthma with associated interstitial lung disease

IV. Probable Anatomic Site of Involvement from History, Physical, Labs, PFTs, X-rays

Fiber skeleton

1 Inflammatory cells +/or fibrous tissue: '**A RIDE UP**' mnemonic
- **A**spiration
- **R**adiation
- **I**nfection
- **D**rugs, e.g. nitrofurantoin, ASA, amiodarone, bleomycin, cyclophosphamide, methotrexate, drug-induced SLE
- **E**osinophilic granuloma
- **U**IP + UIP-DIP, LIP, GIP, AIP (Hamman-Rich), RB-ILD
- **P**neumoconiosis, e.g. asbestosis

2 Neoplastic cells – alveolar cell carcinoma, lymphangitic cancer
3 Ag–Ab deposits – allergic alveolitides
4 Granulomas – granulomatous vasculitides, bronchocentric granulomatosis, sarcoid, tuberculosis, atypicals, fungi, berylliosis, foreign body reaction, eosinophilic granuloma
5 Acellular deposits – amyloid, Gaucher's, Niemann Pick

Vessels
1 Arterioles (centrilobular) – vasculitides, e.g. Wegener's, i.v. talcosis
2 Capillary (alveolar walls) – miliary disease, e.g. tuberculosis, fungal, nocardia, salmonella
3 Venules (interlobular septa) – pulmonary venous hypertension, e.g. mitral stenosis CHF, veno-occlusive disease
4 Lymphatics (interlobular septa) – LAM, tuberous sclerosis, lymphangitic cancer, lymphoproliferative disorders

Bronchioles/bronchi – bronchiolitis, BOOP, bronchiectasis

Air space diseases which can give an interstitial pattern – alveolar hemorrhage, alveolar proteinosis, inhalational disorders, pulmonary edema, BOOP, vasculitides, collagen diseases

V. Invasive Procedures

Following the history, physical, lab tests, pulmonary function, chest X-ray and HRCT, patients fall into one of three categories
1 Features are **highly suggestive** of a specific diagnosis and no further investigations are required
2 Features are **suggestive** of a diagnosis and the decision to proceed with invasive studies must be individualized e.g. young age, rapidly progressive disease, absent steroid response

3 The above work-up is **non-specific** and definitive diagnosis requires BAL or biopsy
   - relative or absolute contraindications include end-stage honeycomb lung, advanced age, hypercapneic respiratory failure, end-stage cardiac or other organ disease

BAL of diagnostic value with
1 Infections – pneumocystis, tuberculosis, fungal
2 Neoplasms
3 Eosinophilic granuloma (Langerhan's cells)
4 Alveolar proteinosis
5 Asbestos bodies in asbestosis
6 Hemosiderin-laden macrophages with alveolar hemorrhage (multiple etiologies)
7 Lipid-laden macrophages in lipoid pneumonia
8 Berylliosis and a positive lymphocyte transformation test

Transbronchial biopsy of diagnostic value with
1 Infections
2 Lymphangitic cancer
3 Lymphoma
4 Eosinophilic granuloma
5 Alveolar proteinosis
6 Asbestosis
7 Amyloid
8 Sarcoid (endobronchial biopsy as well)
9 Eosinophilic pneumonia

Thoracoscopic/open lung biopsy required for
1 Idiopathic interstitial pneumonitis including
   - Usual interstitial pneumonitis
   - Non-specific interstitial pneumonitis
   - Acute interstitial pneumonitis
   - Respiratory bronchiolitis – interstitial lung disease
   - Desquamative interstitial pneumonitis
2 Lymphangioleiomyomatosis
3 Hypersensitivity pneumonitis

IDIOPATHIC INTERSTITIAL PNEUMONITIS (IIP)

IIP comprises a group of disorders with
1 ***Clinical** symptoms of cough and dyspnea, acute to chronic in presentation, with extrapulmonary disease usually absent
2 ***Radiologic** features of bilateral infiltrates
3 **PFTs** varying from normal to restrictive, obstructive or a combination
4 **ABGs** with hypoxemia at rest or only on exertion
5 **Transbronchial biopsy** demonstrating variable degrees of inflammation/fibrosis and therefore rarely able to give an accurate diagnosis

*usual presenting features

Clinical-Pathologic-Radiologic Syndromes

- Usual interstitial pneumonitis – (UIP)
- Non-specific interstitial pneumonitis (NSIP)
- Acute interstitial pneumonitis (AIP)
- Respiratory bronchiolitis – interstitial lung disease (RB-ILD)
- Desquamative interstitial pneumonitis (DIP)

USUAL INTERSTITIAL PNEUMONIA (UIP)

Also known as Idiopathic Pulmonary Fibrosis and Cryptogenic Fibrosing Alveolitis

UIP is defined pathologically
1 Temporal heterogeneity characterized by active fibroblastic foci, fibroblasts and myofibroblasts, relatively acellular collagen bundles, and areas of honeycombing, where discrete areas of lung appear to be damaged recurrently over time
2 Disease distribution is patchy with alternating zones of fibrosis, honeycombing (scarring and architectural restructuring), inflammation and normal lung, seen in different

low magnification fields, resulting in a non-uniform distribution of changes i.e. spatial heterogeneity
3 Mild degrees of inflammation without evidence of fibrosis early in the disease course e.g. asymptomatic relatives of patients with familial IPF
4 Grossly, the disease is preferentially peripheral and subpleural in distribution with relative sparing of the central lung

Pathophysiologically, an unknown stimulus triggers an inflammatory reaction in a susceptible person, the process then perpetuating itself with inflammation and fibrosis seen at various stages
* The clinical correlate of the recurrent lung injury histologically is disease progression over time

Clinical features

- Most patients between 40–65 with average age in the mid 50s and male to female ratio of 2:1
- Insidious onset of cough and dyspnea with initial presentation usually late in the disease and fibrosis established
- Systemic symptoms of malaise, weight loss, anthralgias, fever (approximately 15%)
- Clubbing and 'velcro' rales on exam with eventual development of pulmonary hypertension, cor pulmonale, right heart failure and cyanosis

Clinical course can include

- *Slow progression with an annual 10% mortality from respiratory failure or cardiac disease
- Acute exacerbation of symptoms with features of superimposed acute interstitial pneumonia histologically (diffuse alveolar damage)
- Steroid-induced complications of pneumonia, tuberculosis, myopathy
- Lung cancer typically occurring in the lung periphery where the greatest degree of fibrosis is present
- Stability, without disease progression, reflecting remote injury
- complicating pneumothorax

Lab abnormalities are non-specific and can include positive ANA and RF, cryoglobulins, increased ESR, immune complexes (circulating or lung bound)

'**Disease activity**' is reflected by

- Recurrent or worsening clinical symptoms
- Deterioration on serial radiologic studies
- Deterioration on serial PFTs
- Areas of 'ground glass' opacification on HRCT
- Significance of gallium scans is controversial
- ? interleukin-8 levels in serum and BAL fluid

Positive prognostic features

- Younger age
- Female > male
- Earlier stage of disease, i.e. less severe lung dysfunction at time of diagnosis (mild reductions in VC, TLC, DCO) and less dyspnea
- Earlier initiation of therapy relative to symptoms
- Lymphocytic predominance on BAL
- 'Ground glass' opacities on HRCT in the absence of the fibrotic findings of honeycombing and architectural distortion
- Absence of advanced fibrosis and honeycombing on biopsy
- Positive initial response to steroid treatment
- Controversial whether 'cellular' biopsies improve prognosis

Negative prognostic features

- Male gender
- More advanced disease with severe lung dysfunction and moderate to severe dyspnea
- Neutrophilia or eosinophilia on BAL
- Prominent reticular disease or honeycombing on HRCT
- Advanced fibrosis and honeycombing on biopsy
- Poor response to three months of high dose steroids

Deterioration on therapy – etiologies

1 Disease exacerbation, with superimposed acute interstitial pneumonia (DAD) histologically

2 Opportunistic infection in patients on immunosuppressives e.g. TB
3 Superimposed component of heart failure
4 Drug-induced lung disease secondary to cyclophosphamide or azathioprine
5 Lung cancer ('scar cancer')
6 Steroid myopathy with respiratory muscle involvement
7 Panic attacks/depression
8 Pneumothorax
9 Complications of transtracheal oxygen catheters

PFTs usually reveal a reduced DCO, followed by reductions in vital capacity, subdivisions of lung volume and supernormal flow rates, but there is poor correlation between symptoms, PFTs and chest X-ray abnormalities

Chest X-ray stages

I Normal (rarely seen clinically)
II 'Ground glass' opacities (uncommonly seen clinically)
III Fine reticular pattern with lower lobe predominance (common presentation)
IV Coarse reticular pattern with progressive volume loss (common presentation)
V Diffuse honeycombing (common presentation) with peripheral predominance and lower lobe distribution which then progresses to diffuse lung involvement

HRCT findings

1 **Increased reticular markings** due to fibrosis and/or inflammation with
   - Irregular interfaces with the pleura, bronchi, fissures and vessels
   - Interlobular septal thickening
   - Intralobular interstitial thickening manifest as a fine reticular pattern (net-like appearance of fine lines), peripheral in distribution and reflecting thickening of the distal peribronchiolar interstitial tissues, alveolar wall thickening, small honeycomb cysts or bronchiolectasis
   - Sub-pleural lines

2 Findings of **fibrosis**
   - Distortion of lobular architecture
   - Traction bronchiectasis and bronchiolectasis
   - Honeycombing – sub-pleural and concentric in distribution
3 **'Ground glass' opacities** (seen with inflammation or fibrosis) often represent areas of active alveolitis which can resolve or progress to fibrosis
4 **Peripheral subpleural** distribution of disease is a consistent feature and its absence should suggest another diagnosis
5 **Lower lobe predominance** is seen in ~70%, all lobes equally involved in ~20% and mainly upper lobe in ~10%
6 **Lymphadenopathy** is rarely seen on chest X-ray but seen in a majority of patients on CT with nodes usually <15 mm and involving only one or two nodal stations, most often the right lower paratracheal
   - Usually reactive histology but neoplasia should be ruled out, particularly if transplant is being considered
7 Rarely **normal**

Diagnostic workup
The combination of history, physical, labs, chest X-rays, HRCT scan and PFTs are often very suggestive of the diagnosis

'Secondary' UIP should be ruled out as UIP is an idiopathic disorder, but the identical pathologic and radiologic features can be seen in a variety of diseases including
1 **Inherited disorders**
   - Familial fibrocystic pulmonary dysplasia (familial IPF)
   - Neurofibromatosis
   - Hermansky-Pudlak syndrome
2 **Inhalational**
   - Asbestosis
   - End-stage allergic alveolitis (usually upper lobe predominance)

3 **Collagen vascular diseases**
   - * Rheumatoid arthritis
   - * Scleroderma
   - Sjogren's
   - Mixed connective tissue disease
   - Dermato/polymyositis
   - SLE
4 **Drugs**
   - Nitrofurantoin (chronic form), bleomycin, cyclophosphamide, busulfan, others
5 **Chronic aspiration**

Biopsy is indicated if atypical features are present, with thoracotomy or thoracoscopy required, as transbronchial biopsy cannot provide adequate tissue
Significant co-morbidity or advanced end-stage honeycomb lung would be contraindications to biopsy

NON-SPECIFIC INTERSTITIAL PNEUMONITIS (NSIP)

Definition: Pathologically defined by alveolar wall thickening due to a combination of inflammation (lymphocytes and plasma cells) and fibrosis, but distinct on biopsy from UIP, DIP or AIP

1 50% are mainly inflammatory with little fibrosis
2 40% are equal mixtures of inflammation and fibrosis
3 10% are mainly fibrotic

- Disease distribution is patchy or diffuse but differs from UIP histologically by the lack of 'active' fibrosis, little honeycombing, and temporal homogeneity, i.e. the injury appears to have occurred over a single narrow time span
- Focal areas of BOOP or DIP may be present and therefore NSIP is not histologically distinct
- NSIP appears to be a response to multiple insults as similar findings are seen in a diverse group of disorders
  – Immunocompetent patients

- — Connective tissue diseases, e.g. polymyositis, RA
  - — Hypersensitivity pneumonitis/inhalation injury
  - — Drugs
  - — Recent or recurrent ARDS
- – Immunosuppressed patients
  - — HIV
  - — Bone-marrow transplants
  - — Chemotherapy
  - — Post-radiotherapy
- NSIP should be termed idiopathic after known causes are ruled out, including environmental or occupational exposures, organic exposures, collagen vascular diseases, drugs, infection, or other resolving acute lung injury

Clinical features

- All age ranges but most often in middle-aged adults
- Slight female predominance
- Subacute > insidious onset of cough and dyspnea
- Fever may be present (~ ⅓ of cases)
- Rales (approximately 80%) and clubbing (approximately 20%) on exam

Prognosis is good with stability, improvement or complete recovery reported in the majority of cases, particularly when inflammation dominates the lung biopsy

- Steroid responsiveness is not as dramatic as is found in BOOP and relapses can occur with progressive fibrosis in those with a "fibrotic" pattern

Chest X-ray findings

1 Areas of 'ground glass' opacification or consolidation involving mainly the lower lung fields
2 Bilateral interstitial infiltrates or combined interstitial and airspace disease
3 Lack of the peripheral subpleural distribution of UIP
4 Normal X-rays occasionally reported

HRCT features

1 Areas of 'ground glass' opacity and patchy areas of alveolar consolidation

2 Bilateral interstitial thickening with patchy lower lobe predominance or diffuse distribution
3 Findings of fibrosis (much less common than in UIP)

ACUTE INTERSTITIAL PNEUMONITIS (AIP)

Definition: Pathologically defined by
1 Diffuse interstitial 'active' fibrosis with proliferating fibroblasts and myofibroblasts but minimal collagen deposition
2 Biopsies resemble the organizing stage of diffuse alveolar damage (DAD), a pattern of acute lung injury and repair following multiple types of insult
3 Changes are diffuse, massive, temporally uniform and appear relatively acute, occurring during a single period of time

Clinically, AIP was originally described by Hamman and Rich in four patients presenting with cough, dyspnea and death in 1–6 months

- All age groups are affected, but most patients are in their late 40s without sex predilection and previously healthy
- Viral-like prodrome is common, followed by the acute onset of dyspnea and cough accompanied by fever in approximately 50% of cases
- Dyspnea is progressive with the clinical picture that of fulminating pneumonia, progressing to respiratory failure and features of ARDS
- Mortality rates are approximately 50% at 6 months, but the prognosis of individual cases is difficult to predict, even with histology
- Survivors may stabilize and not show disease progression or present with recurrent acute exacerbations

AIP should be considered in the **differential diagnosis** of rapidly progressive community-acquired airspace disease, including
1 Acute and fulminating pneumonia
2 Acute eosinophilic pneumonia

3 Vasculitis
4 Diffuse alveolar hemorrhage syndrome
5 Collagen disease, e.g. polymyositis, SLE, RA
6 Drug reaction
7 Pulmonary edema
8 Allergic alveolitis
9 Idiopathic BOOP
10 Acute exacerbation of UIP
11 ARDS with a known etiology

Chest X-rays reveal diffuse bilateral airspace disease

HRCT findings

1 Diffuse disease, occasionally basal in distribution, but usually showing no lobar predominance
2 Airspace consolidation and 'ground glass' opacities acutely
3 Fibrotic stage with honeycombing and bronchiectasis developing in survivors

Routine **labs** are not helpful and the **diagnosis** can be made only on open lung biopsy with

1 Clinical presentation of idiopathic ARDS
2 Pathologic findings of DAD
3 Exclusion of infection or other known disorders

RESPIRATORY BRONCHIOLITIS – INTERSTITIAL LUNG DISEASE (RB-ILD)

Definition: Pathologically defined by inflammation of the membranous and respiratory bronchioles with intralumenal pigmented macrophages, as well as accompanying inflammation in the surrounding peribronchiolar parenchyma

- Thought to be an exaggerated form of the respiratory bronchiolitis of smokers (pigmented macrophages within respiratory bronchioles without accompanying interstitial disease) and an early stage in the development of DIP (?same entity)

Clinical features

- Mean age of 36 with a slight male predominance
- All patients are current or former smokers

- Symptoms are usually mild with the insidious onset of cough and dyspnea
- Coarse inspiratory and expiratory rales are frequent in the absence of clubbing

Prognosis is good with complete resolution on stopping smoking and progression to diffuse fibrosis not described

PFTs are usually restrictive with reduced lung volumes and DCO, but a mixed restrictive and obstructive picture may be present

Chest X-ray findings
1 Normal X-rays
2 'Dirty' lungs with bronchial wall thickening
3 An interstitial reticular or reticulonodular pattern similar to early UIP

HRCT features
1 Patchy 'ground glass' opacities in 50–90% of cases
2 Centrilobular nodules (50–90%) similar to hypersensitivity pneumonitis, (the latter disease rarely seen in smokers)
3 Diffuse or patchy in distribution
4 Some reticulation in 20–50% (not prominent)
5 Absence of honeycombing (unlike UIP)

DESQUAMATIVE INTERSTITIAL PNEUMONITIS (DIP)

Definition: Pathologically defined as a reaction pattern with
1 Filling of the airspaces with pigment-containing macrophages
2 Uniformity of the histopathologic changes from one field to another
3 Sparse interstitial cellular infiltrate with little fibrosis and minimal or absent honeycombing

- It is thought to be a more advanced stage of respiratory bronchiolitis interstitial lung disease (RBILD), the latter characterized by the accumulation of macrophages which are confined to the peribronchiolar areas, sparing the more distal airspaces

- DIP is often described as an early stage of UIP, but the pathologic, clinical and radiologic features are quite different with DIP not progressing to UIP
- DIP is an idiopathic disorder, although a 'DIP pattern' has been described in association with inorganic dust inhalation, e.g. asbestos, drugs, eosinophilic granuloma, smokers with UIP, etc.

Clinical features

- Average age in mid 40s
- Male to female ratio approximately 2:1
- Smoking history in 90% of cases
- Insidious onset of cough and dyspnea developing over weeks to months
- Clubbing in approximately 50% of patients

The course of disease is variable and can include

- Remission, either spontaneous or steroid-induced
- Remissions and relapses
- Progression to end stage fibrosis with the typical honeycombing of UIP

PFTs reveal a restrictive picture

Chest X-ray features

1 'Ground glass' lower lobe opacities in ~25% of cases (classic picture)
2 Reticular or reticulonodular lower lobe shadows
3 Normal X-ray in up to 10–20% of patients with biopsy proven disease

HRCT findings overlap those of UIP

1 Predominant middle and lower lobe distribution occasionally with mainly peripheral involvement
2 Areas of 'ground glass' opacity and airspace consolidation in 100% of cases
3 Mild fibrosis and focal honeycombing
4 Patchy or diffuse in distribution

HONEYCOMB LUNG – END-STAGE ILD

Clinically, patients are symptomatic and sequelae include

1 Hypoxemia
2 Pulmonary hypertension
3 Cor pulmonale
4 Pneumothorax

Chest X-ray findings of diffusely increased interstitial markings usually lack specificity and include one or more of the following

1 Honeycombing
2 Cystic spaces
3 Conglomerate fibrosis

The non-specific findings of **fibrosis** on **HRCT** include

- Interlobular septal thickening
- Intralobular interstitial thickening
- Honeycombing
- Traction bronchiectasis
- Visible intralobular bronchioles
- Architectural distortion
- Conglomerate masses

Biopsies are often non-specific, with varying degrees of fibrosis, inflammation and bronchiectasis

Etiologies include

1 Usual interstitial pneumonia
2 Survivors of acute interstitial pneumonitis
3 Non-specific interstitial pneumonitis (uncommon)
4 Neurofibromatosis
5 Eosinophilic granuloma
6 Drugs, e.g. nitrofurantoin, bleomycin, cyclophosphamide
7 Bronchiectasis, e.g. cystic fibrosis
8 Pneumoconiosis, e.g. asbestosis
9 Allergic alveolitis
10 Sarcoid
11 Collagen diseases, e.g. rheumatoid arthritis, scleroderma

Diagnostic Clues to Specific Etiology

1 **History and physical**

2 **Obstructive picture** on PFTs (see p. 168)

3 **Associated radiologic findings**

- Volume changes
  - Volume loss, e.g. UIP, asbestosis
  - Normal or increased volumes, e.g. LAM, eosinophilic granuloma
- Disease distribution
  - Upper lobe, e.g. silicosis, sarcoid, allergic alveolitis
  - Lower lobe, e.g. UIP, asbestosis
  - Subpleural, e.g. UIP, asbestosis
  - Peribronchovascular, e.g. sarcoid, silicosis
- Parenchymal abnormalities in addition to fibrosis
  - Nodules, e.g. silicosis, eosinophilic granuloma, sarcoid, allergic alveolitis
  - 'Ground glass' opacities, e.g. allergic alveolitis, sarcoid, asbestosis, UIP occasionally
  - Conglomerate masses, e.g. sarcoid, silicosis, talcosis
  - Cystic spaces, e.g. LAM, eosinophilic granuloma
- Pleural thickening or effusion
  - e.g. asbestosis, rarely sarcoid
- Lymphadenopathy
  - e.g. LAM, sarcoid

4 **Radiologic clues** to specific disorders

UIP

- Lower lung zones preferentially involved
- Peripheral subpleural disease distribution
- Lung volumes reduced

Sarcoid

- Upper lung zones preferentially involved
- Lung volumes maintained
- Peribronchovascular (central) distribution of the fibrosis and conglomerate masses with bronchi visible within the mass lesions
- Central cystic changes secondary to ectatic bronchi

- Subpleural honeycombing
- Small, well-defined nodules may be present

Eosinophilic granuloma

- Upper lobes preferentially involved
- Cystic spaces occasionally with bizarre shapes, sparing the lung bases and costophrenic angles
- Small nodules <5 mm in diameter
- Normal or increased lung volumes

LAM

- Diffuse distribution of lung cysts with no zonal predominance
- Unilateral or bilateral pleural effusions
- Normal or increased lung volumes
- Lymphadenopathy

Asbestosis

- Parenchymal findings are those of UIP
- Pleural thickening or plaques which may calcify
- Focal fibrotic masses representing subpleural fibrosis, fissural pleural plaques or round atelectasis

Allergic alveolitis

- End-stage fibrosis can be diffuse or preferentially involve the upper lung zones
- Nodular opacities
- Unilateral or bilateral 'ground glass' opacities

Silicosis

- Diffuse disease with upper lobe predominance
- Nodules, centrilobular and subpleural in location
- Conglomerate masses which can cavitate
- Bronchi splayed around the above masses
- Lymphadenopathy which may display egg-shell calcifications

INTERSTITIAL LUNG DISEASE – UNILATERAL

Uncommon clinically compared to bilateral ILD, the causes including

1 **Infections**
 - Acute infections, e.g. viral, mycoplasma
 - Post-infectious fibrosis
2 **Aspiration**
 - Recurrent, e.g. Zenker's
 - Lipoid pneumonia
3 **Bronchiectasis**
4 **Unilateral pulmonary edema**
 - Cardiac
 - Non-cardiac, e.g. pulmonary venous obstruction from fibrosing mediastinitis
5 **Amyloid**
6 **Post-radiation**
7 **Neoplastic disease**
 - Lymphangitic cancer
 - Lymphoma
 - Alveolar cell cancer

'STEROID-RESPONSIVE' ILD

1 BOOP
2 Acute bronchiolitis
3 Vasculitis
4 Collagen diseases
5 Sarcoid
6 Drug-induced
7 Allergic alveolitis
8 Idiopathic interstitial pneumonitis including AIP, DIP, LIP, NSIP, RBILD

Fraser R.S., Muller N.L., Colman N., Paré P.D. (1999) *Diagnosis of Diseases of the Chest* 4th Edn., WB Saunders.
Naidich, D.P., Zerhouni, E.A., Siegelman, S.S. (1998) *Computed Tomography and Magnetic Resonance of the Thorax*, 3rd edn. New York: Raven Press.
Moss, A., Gamsu, Genant (1992) Thorax and neck. In: *Computed Tomography of the Body with Magnetic Resonance Imaging*, 2nd edn, vol. 1.: W.B. Saunders.

Webb, R., Muller, N.L., Naidich, D.P. (1996) *High Resolution CT of the Lung*, 2nd edn.: Lippincott-Raven.

Thurlbeck, W., Churg, A. (eds) (1995) *Pathology of the Lung*, 2nd edn.: Thieme Medical Publishers.

Baum, G.L., Crapo, J.D., Celli, B.R., Karlinsky, J.B. (eds) (1997) *Textbook of Pulmonary Diseases*, 6th edn.: Lippincott-Raven.

Fishman, A.P., Elias, J.A., Fishman, J.A., Grippi, M.A., Kaiser, L.R., Senior, R.N. (1998) *Fishman's Pulmonary Diseases and Disorders*, 3rd edn.: McGraw-Hill.

Katzenstein, A., Myers, J. (1998) Idiopathic pulmonary fibrosis. Clinical relevance of pathologic classification. *Am. J. Resp. Crit. Care Med.* **157**: 1301–1315.

Reynolds, H. (1998) Diagnostic and management strategies for diffuse interstitial lung disease. *Chest* **113**: 192–202.

Leung, A., Miller, R., Muller, N. (1993) Parenchymal opacification in chronic infiltrative lung diseases: CT-pathologic correlation. *Radiology* **188**: 209–214.

Akira, M., Sakatani, M., Ueda, E. (1993) Idiopathic pulmonary fibrosis: progression of honeycombing at thin-section CT. *Radiology* **189**: 687–691.

Johkoh, T., Muller, N., Cartier, Y. *et al.* (1999) Idiopathic interstitial pneumonias. Diagnostic accuracy of thin-section CT in 129 patients. *Radiology* **211**: 555–560.

Johkoh, T., Muller, N., Cartier, Y. *et al.* (1999) Idiopathic interstitial pneumonias. *Radiology* **211**: 555–559.

Muller, N., Miller, R. (1990) Computed tomography of chronic diffuse infiltrative lung disease. *ARRD* **142**: 1206–1215, 1440–1448.

Niimi, H., Eun-Young Kang, J.S., Kwong *et al.* (1996) CT of chronic infiltrate lung disease: prevalence of mediastinal lymphadenopathy. *JCAT* **20**: 305–308.

Raghu, G. (1987) Idiopathic pulmonary fibrosis – a rational clinical approach. *Chest* **92**: 148–154.

Primack, S., Hartman, T., Ikezoe, J. *et al.* (1993) Acute interstitial pneumonia: radiographic and CT findings in nine patients. *Radiology* **188**: 817–820.

Primack, S., Hartman, T., Hansell, D., Muller, N. (1993) End-stage lung disease: CT findings in 61 patients. *Radiology* **189**: 681–686.

Wade, J., King, T. (1993) Infiltrative and interstitial lung disease in the elderly patient. *Clinics in Chest Medicine* **14**: 501–517.

King, T. (1993) Respiratory bronchiolitis interstitial lung disease. *Clinics in Chest Medicine* **14**: 693–698.

50 Lung Resection – Complications

Airways

1 **Secretions** and mucus plugs

2 **Acute bronchitis**

3 **Bronchospasm**

4 **Bronchopleural fistula**

5 **Post-right pneumonectomy syndrome**
   - Rare complication caused by rotation of the heart and great vessels, most often described with pneumonectomy in childhood or early adulthood, symptoms developing months to many years post-op
   - The trachea and left mainstem bronchus are compressed between the aorta and pulmonary artery, resulting in dyspnea, recurrent left-sided pneumonia, tracheobronchomalacia and postobstructive bronchiectasis, with eventual respiratory failure and death
   - Narrowing of the trachea and left mainstem bronchus can be demonstrated on CT scan or bronchoscopy
   - Diagnosis should be suspected in a post-pneumonectomy patient developing the above symptoms with a picture of airflow obstruction on PFTs

6 **Bronchial stump aspergillosis**
   - Secondary infection of silk (*vs.* nylon) suture material can result in cough, purulent sputum, hemoptysis, expectorated sutures and fungal material
   - Usually seen 6–12 months post-op but described several years later
   - Bronchoscopy reveals endobronchial silk thread, contiguous inflammation and positive cultures for

aspergillus while biopsy reveals necrosis and hyphae
- A similar syndrome is described at the anastomotic site post-lung transplant

Parenchyma

1 **Atelectasis/failure to expand**

2 **Pulmonary edema**

3 **ARDS** – likelihood of development increases with one of the following including sepsis, hypotension, gastric aspiration, lung contusion, multiple transfusions, multiple fractures, pancreatitis

4 **Pneumonia**
   - Bacteria causing community-acquired pneumonia, e.g. *Strep. pneumoniae*, hemophilus, anaerobes, legionella
   - 'KEEAPPS', i.e. klebsiella, enterobacter, *E. coli*, acinetobacter, proteus, pseudomonas, serratia, *Staph. aureus*

Pleura

The ipsilateral pleural space normally begins to fill with fluid 24 hours post-pneumonectomy

- Serosanguinous fluid accumulates at the rate of approximately two rib spaces daily and therefore rapid accumulation of fluid immediately post-op should suggest hemothorax or chylothorax
- The hemithorax is completely fluid filled in 90% of patients by 2 weeks and in all patients by 2–4 months
- There is simultaneous ipsilateral mediastinal shift, elevation of the ipsilateral hemidiaphragm and compensatory overinflation of the contralateral lung

Abnormal accumulations of fluid include

1 **Transudate** from CHF

2 **Exudate** from pulmonary infarct, subdiaphragmatic infection, pneumonia

3 **Empyema** post-pneumonectomy can occur immediately or many years post-op and etiologies include

  - Primary contamination of the pleural space (early)
  - Hematogenous dissemination from a distant infected source (late)
  - Bronchopleural or esophago-pleural fistula (early or late)
- Fever is common in the immediate post-op period and may be accompanied by the expectoration of serosanguinous or purulent fluid if there is an associated bronchopleural fistula
- Late onset empyema may present with non-specific flu-like symptoms of low grade fever, anorexia, weakness and weight loss
- Diagnosis is confirmed by the finding of pus in the post-pneumonectomy space and radiologic clues to the diagnosis include
  - Failure of the mediastinum to shift to the post-pneumonectomy space or mediastinal shift to the opposite side
  - A new air–fluid level
  - Sudden increase or decrease in a pre-existing air–fluid level

4 **Hemothorax** presents within the first 24 hours post-op with
- Hypotension
- Excessive drainage of blood from the chest tube
- Rapid filling of the post-pneumonectomy space with fluid

5 **Chylothorax** is a rare condition described after extrapleural pneumonectomy or following dissection of the ipsilateral or subcarinal nodes
- Most cases occur within 2 weeks of surgery with diagnosis confirmed on thoracocentesis
- Clinical presentation ranges from little symptomatology to rapidly progressive dyspnea and hypotension
- Radiologically there is rapid opacification of the post-op space with mediastinal shift to the non-operative side

6 **Extrapleural hematoma**

7 **Poor positioning** of the drainage tube with abnormal accumulation of post-op fluid

8 **Increasing air** in the post-pneumonectomy space
- Poor positioning of the chest tube
- Leakage of air from around the chest tube
- Bronchopleural fistula from the stump
- Leakage from the lung parenchyma following segmental or wedge resection
- Gas-forming organisms in the pleural space

9 **Bronchopleural fistula (BPF)** is seen in 1–4% of pneumonectomies, more often right-sided, the majority developing within 2 weeks post-op and presenting with:
- Persistent airleak from the chest tube
- Cough productive of bloody or purulent sputum
- Dyspnea
- Fever
- Increasing subcutaneous emphysema
- Accompanying empyema may or may not be present
- Massive hemoptysis or hemothorax from erosion of the bronchial stump into the pulmonary artery

Diagnostic clues include
- Increasing mediastinal and/or subcutaneous emphysema
- Drop in the air–fluid level with mediastinal shift to the remaining lung or
- A new air–fluid level in a previously opacified hemithorax or
- Multiple air–fluid levels plus
- Appearance of methylene blue in sputum after its injection into the post-pneumonectomy space
- Bronchoscopic visualization of larger fistulas

10 **Esophago-pleural fistula** is a rare complication, typically occurring one to several years post-pneumonectomy

- Usually right-sided and most commonly from mediastinal recurrence of tumor eroding into the esophagus or a mediastinal inflammatory process

Diagnostic clues and **workup** include
- Post-pneumonectomy empyema
- Undiagnosed fever
- Food or gastric contents in the pleural fluid
- New air–fluid level or decrease in a pre-existing air–fluid level on chest X-ray
- Contrast agent in the pleural fluid post-swallow
- Esophagoscopy

Neuromuscular

1. **CNS depression** from narcotics
2. **Neuromuscular blockade** from antibiotics
3. Rare case reports of **paralysis** due to interference with the blood supply to the spinal cord

Cardiac

1. **Arrythmias**
2. **Myocardial infarction**
3. **Cardiac herniation** is a rare and often fatal complication of pneumonectomy (either right or left-sided) and can occur when the pericardium has been opened
   - The heart moves though the pericardial defect and becomes twisted in the post-pneumonectomy space, with obstruction of the great vessels
   - Clinically, it usually occurs within 24 hours of surgery with the acute onset of hypotension, cyanosis, chest pain, often an acute superior vena cava syndrome, and a high mortality rate
   - Radiologically the heart can be seen in the post-pneumonectomy space and is a surgical emergency
4. **Postpericardiotomy syndrome**
5. **Intracardiac right-to-left shunt** is a rare complication of pneumonectomy and occurs at the atrial level, through a

patent foramen ovale or previously asymptomatic atrial septal defect

- Patients present with dyspnea, platypnea and cyanosis days to months post-pneumonectomy and a shunt can be documented by
  - Breathing 100% O_2
  - Perfusion lung scan with imaging over the brain and kidneys
  - Contrast echocardiography
  - Cardiac catheterization

Vasculature

1 **Post-pneumonectomy pulmonary edema** may occur secondary to
- Fluid overload
- Cardiac dysfunction
- Aspiration
- Pneumonia
- Sepsis
- Idiopathic
  - The idiopathic category is a diagnosis of exclusion, usually following right-sided and rarely described with left pneumonectomy
  - Uncommon disorder, ?permeability problem, typically occurring 1–4 days post-op and carrying a high mortality

2 **Thromboembolism**
- Risk factors include immobilization, underlying cancer and age > 60 years
- In addition to the usual potential sites of thrombosis, thrombi can develop in the pulmonary artery stump post-pneumonectomy and embolize to the remaining lung

3 **Systemic hypotension** may be present due to
- Respiratory, e.g. tension pneumothorax, massive pulmonary embolus

- Cardiac, e.g. arrythmias, acute ischemia, pericardial tamponade, cardiac herniation
- Anaphylactic, e.g. drugs, reaction to talc on surgical gloves
- Addisonian, e.g. iatrogenic
- Infectious, e.g. bacteremic, toxin-induced
- Hypovolemic
- Neurogenic, e.g. vasovagal
- Drug-induced

4 **Vascular infection – central line**
- Bacteremia/fungemia usually follow catheter colonization
  - Blood cultures reflect organisms cultured from the catheter or purulent material from the insertion site
- Septic thrombosis of the central veins or pulmonary artery manifest by
  - Bacteremia or fungemia progressing to sepsis
  - Signs of venous occlusions, e.g. neck, facial, or arm edema
  - Infection at the insertion site
  - Metastatic abscesses
  - Endocarditis
- Infective endocarditis may involve the right atrium, right ventricle, tricuspid or pulmonary valves
- Mycotic aneurysm of pulmonary artery
- Septic pulmonary emboli

Mediastinum

1 **Acute mediastinitis** post-median sternotomy is defined as suppurative inflammation of the anterior mediastinal space
- Multiple risk factors are described in the literature but unclear which are most important
- Clinically, the diagnosis should be suspected by the combination of wound drainage, sternal instability, fever, tachycardia and leucocytosis
- Chest wall edema and Hamman's sign may be present

- Presentation can be acute or subacute with signs of wound infection and bacteremia preceding or following the recognition of acute mediastinitis
- Usually presents within 2 weeks of surgery with the incubation period ranging from a few days to >1 year
- Chest X-rays may show a new alignment of the sternal sutures but mediastinal air, air–fluid levels or mediastinal widening are rarely seen
- CT scans reveal mediastinal air and/or a mediastinal fluid collection which can be complicated by a sternal osteomyelitis
- Mediastinal air and fluid can normally be present up to 21 days post-op in the absence of mediastinitis, whereas after this period of time the above findings are abnormal
- CT-guided retrosternal needle aspiration can confirm the diagnosis
- A wide range of organisms is responsible, with gram positives and gram negative each responsible for about half (other agents rarely described)

2 **Ipsilateral mediastinal displacement** is normal but temporary post-lobectomy, disappearing as the remainder of the lung undergoes compensatory overinflation
   - Post-pneumonectomy, ipsilateral mediastinal displacement is progressive and permanent, reaching its maximum in approximately 6 months, accompanied by compensatory overinflation of the contralateral lung
   - The absence of mediastinal shift post-op should suggest
     - Increasing intrapleural air
     - Empyema
     - Hemothorax
     - Chylothorax
     - Atelectasis in the contralateral lung
     - Return of the mediastinum and tracheal air column to the midline indicates an expanding process in the post-pneumonectomy space including recurrent

tumor, bronchopleural fistula, empyema, hemorrhage or chylothorax

3 **Cardiac herniation** through a pericardial defect

Diaphragm

1 **Phrenic nerve resection** with hemidiaphragmatic paralysis and elevation

2 **Phrenic nerve dysfunction** post-cardiac surgery is statistically associated with the use of ice slush for myocardial preservation
   - Vast majority of cases are left-sided
   - An elevated hemidiaphragm is not synonymous with phrenic nerve injury post-op and other causes must be ruled out, e.g. subdiaphragmatic process, atelectasis, pleural disease or a poor inspiratory effort
   - Post-op, these patients may require prolonged ventilatory support and have an increased length of stay
   - On discharge they may be asymptomatic or complain of dyspnea on excretion, the underlying pulmonary reserve being the critical determining factor

Fraser R.S., Muller N.L., Colman N., Paré P.D. (1999) *Diagnosis of Diseases of the Chest* 4th Edn., WB Saunders.

Baum, G.L., Crapo, J.D., Celli, B.R., Karlinsky, J.B. (eds) (1997) *Textbook of Pulmonary Diseases*, 6th edn.: Lippincott-Raven.

Fishman, A.P., Elias, J.A., Fishman, J.A., Grippi, M.A., Kaiser, L.R., Senior, R.N. (1998) *Fishman's Pulmonary Diseases and Disorders*, 3rd edn.: McGraw-Hill.

Kopec, S., Irwin, R., Umali-Torres, C. *et al.* (1998) The post-pneumonectomy state. *Chest* **114**:1158–1184.

Spirn, P.W. *et al.* (1988) Radiology of the chest after thoracic surgery. *Semin. Roent.* **23**:9–31.

51 Masses – Nodules; Opacities

SOLITARY LUNG MASS >3 CM DIAMETER

Airways

1 *Bronchogenic cancer
2 Bronchoalveolar cell cancer
3 Hamartoma
4 Bronchial adenomas or other tumors, benign/malignant
5 Bronchogenic cyst
6 BOOP
7 Bronchopulmonary sequestration
8 Pseudo-sequestration
9 Mucoid impaction in association with
   A. Asthma, allergic bronchopulmonary aspergillosis
   B. Bronchocentric granulomatosis, bronchiectasis, bronchial atresia, bronchogenic cancer
   C. Cystic fibrosis, COPD

Parenchyma

1 *Neoplasms, benign or malignant – primary/secondary
2 Infections
   - Bacterial – abscess, spherical pneumonia, anaerobic lung infection, legionella, tuberculosis, atypical mycobacteria, nocardia, actinomycosis, melioidosis
   - Parasitic – hydatid
   - Fungal – aspergillus, cryptococcus, coccidioidomycosis, blastomycosis
3 Inflammatory pseudotumor
4 Aspiration – lipoid pneumonia, foreign body granuloma
5 Amyloid
6 Pseudolymphoma
7 Progressive massive fibrosis – silicosis, CWP, talcosis, asbestosis
8 Round atelectasis

Vasculature

1 Pulmonary artery
   - Aneurysms, pulmonary artery hypertension, pulmonary artery neoplasms, e.g. hemangioma, sarcoma
2 Pulmonary capillary
   - Septic or bland infarcts, hematoma
3 Pulmonary vein varix
4 AV malformations
5 Vasculitis, e.g. Wegener's

Pleural

1 Mesothelial cyst
2 Pseudotumor – loculated fluid
3 Primary or secondary neoplasm
4 Round atelectasis
5 Pleural plaque in an interlobar fissure

Clues to Etiology

Statistically, about 75% of lung lesions more than 3 cm in diameter are neoplastic

- About 15% will be infectious and the remaining etiologies are individually uncommon

1 **Historical features**
- Previous films
- Smoking history
- Infectious symptoms and epidemiologic features
- Oil ingestion
- Occupational history
- i.v. drug abuse
- Known extrapulmonary neoplasm
- Systemic disease

2 **Isolated lung disease *vs.* extrapulmonary disease**
- History
- Physical, e.g. lymphadenopathy, hepatosplenomegaly
- Radiologically, e.g. pelvic/abdominal U/S or CT, testicular ultrasound

3 **Density of the mass**
- Fat-containing, e.g. hamartoma, lipoid pneumonia
- Cystic, e.g. bronchogenic, hydatid
- Vascular, e.g. aneurysm, varix, AV malformation
- Calcification, e.g. hamartoma

4 **Margins**
- Sharp borders, e.g. radiation pneumonitis
- Violation of anatomic boundaries, e.g. neoplasms, some infections
- Angle with the pleura, e.g. parenchymal *vs.* 'extrapleural'
- Spiculated margins, e.g. neoplastic

5 **Growth rate**

6 **Associated pleuropulmonary abnormalities**
- Airways disease, e.g. obstructed bronchus
- Parenchymal disease, e.g. silicotic nodules
- Pleural disease, e.g. rounded atelectasis
- Vascular disease, e.g. anomalous vessel, AV malformation

7 **Associated mediastinal lympadenopathy**
- *Neoplastic, e.g. carcinoma, carcinoid, lymphoma, melanoma, germ cell tumors, others

- Tuberculosis
- Fungal, e.g. histoplasmosis, coccidioidomycosis, sporotrichosis
- Progressive massive fibrosis, e.g. silicosis, CWP
- Sarcoid
- Amyloid
- Lymphomatoid granulomatosis

BILATERAL LUNG MASSES

1 **Neoplastic** – carcinoma, sarcoma, lymphoma, melanoma, myeloma, germ-cell tumors
2 **Infectious** – tuberculosis, atypical mycobacteria, coccidioidomycosis, echinococcus
3 **Vascular** – Wegener's granulomatosis, multiple infarcts (septic/bland), AV malformations
4 **Inflammatory** – sarcoid, lipoid pneumonia
5 **Inhalational** – silicosis, coal workers pneumoconiosis
6 **i.v. drugs** – talcosis
7 **Traumatic** – multiple hematomas

SOLITARY PULMONARY NODULE (SPN)

Definition: A round or oval circumscribed opacity less than 3 cm in diameter
Statistically the majority of SPNs are due to bronchogenic cancer, metastases and infectious granulomas, e.g., tuberculosis, histoplasmosis, coccidiodomycosis

Most important historical factors in determining etiologies are
1 Age
2 Smoking history
3 Exposure to asbestos (or other carcinogens)
4 Area of residence and travel re granulomatous lesions
5 History of an intrathoracic or extrathoracic malignancy

Solitary Pulmonary Nodule – Malignant

1 **Primary lung cancer** ~80%
- All histologic types can present as a SPN, most commonly adenocarcinoma and bronchioloalveolar cancer

2 **Metastatic cancer** ~20%
- Primary lesions include carcinomas, sarcomas, melanomas, lymphomas, germ cell tumors

3 **Carcinoid tumors** <1%
- 20% arise peripherally

Solitary Pulmonary Nodule – Benign

1 **Granulomas** – 80% of benign lesions
- *Tuberculoma* is a manifestation of primary or reinfection tuberculosis
  - Well-defined spherical or oval lesion, occasionally lobulated, usually upper lobe
  - Satellite lesions are common
  - Cavitation unusual
  - May calcify
  - May persist unchanged for years
- *Histoplasmoma* presents as a solitary nodule more often than multiple nodules, with areas of endemicity
  - Usually lower lobe, often with satellite lesions
  - May calcify with pathognomonic 'target' lesion
  - Rarely cavitates
  - May stabilize or enlarge on serial X-rays
- *Coccidioidomas* have a geographic distribution and present as a single, or less often, multiple nodules
  - Upper and mid lungs in distribution
  - May cavitate or calcify and have associated satellite lesions
- *Hyalinizing* granulomas are rare and can be single or multiple
  - Can cavitate, calcify and grow slowly resembling metastases
  - Etiology unclear ? end stage infection

2 **Hamartomas** – 10–15% of benign lesions
Defined as a lesion composed of normal tissues in the lung, mainly cartilage and fat, but arranged in a disorderly pattern
- Located either within the lung parenchyma (90%) or endobronchially (10%)
- Most common benign tumor of the lungs

Clinically, the parenchymal variety is usually asymptomatic with hemoptysis as the most common symptom
- Endobronchial lesions present with features of airways obstruction
- Radiologic studies (see below) may establish the diagnosis of peripheral lesions and make invasive testing unnecessary, although their appearance may be that of an indeterminate lung nodule which can be diagnosed by TTNA in many cases
- Lesions are usually benign with cure following surgical excision, although there are rare reports of malignancy developing

Radiologic features of the parenchymal variety
- *CT findings of fat > fat and calcium > calcium alone
- *'Popcorn' calcifications
- Solitary well-circumscribed peripheral nodule, rarely multiple
- Can enlarge over time, simulating a malignancy

Radiologic features of an endobronchial lesion are nonspecific and include signs of atelectasis and obstructive pneumonitis

3 The remaining 5–10% of **benign** causes include

Airways
- Bronchogenic cyst
- Bronchopulmonary sequestration
- BOOP
- Bronchiectasis

Pleura
- Round atelectasis
- Pleural plaque
- Localized fibrous tumor

- Mucoid impaction
- Tracheobronchial papilloma
- Tumors e.g. lipoma, fibroma

Parenchyma
- Lipoid pneumonia
- Foreign body granuloma
- Infectious (see below)
- Rheumatoid nodule
- Sclerosing hemangioma
- Intrapulmonary lymph node
- Amyloid

Vasculature
- Varix
- AV malformation
- Infarct
- Vasculitis, e.g. Wegener's
- Hematoma, e.g. post-traumatic

INFECTIOUS CAUSES OF A SPN

A — actinomycosis, aspergillosis (mucoid impaction, aspergilloma)
B — blastomycosis
C — cryptococcosis, coccidioidomycosis
D — dirofilaria
E — echinococcosis
H — histoplasmosis
L — lung abscess, legionella
M — mycetomas
N — nocardia
P — pseudallescheriasis, pneumocystis
S — sporotrichosis, septic emboli, spherical pneumonia
T — tuberculosis (typical/atypical)

SOLITARY NODULE – DIAGNOSTIC WORK-UP: 14 ISSUES

1 Investigations should be **delayed** at least 2–3 weeks as some nodules may resolve spontaneously, e.g. pneumonia, hematoma, infarcts

2 Determine the likely **anatomic** origin of the SPN, i.e. **parenchyma** and not

- Pleural, e.g. fluid, round atelectasis
- Airways, e.g. bronchogenic cyst
- Vascular, e.g. AV malformation
- Chest wall, e.g. rib
- Skin, e.g. nipple

3 **Benignity criteria** on chest X-ray or CT
- Lesion present for >2 years without change
- Lesion that has doubled in size in 3 weeks (exception is hemorrhage into a carcinoma) or newly appeared during that time is unlikely malignant
- Calcification
  - Diffuse, laminated, central, popcorn
  - Lesions may only reveal calcium on CT and not on chest X-ray
- Fat, e.g. hamartoma
- Cystic, e.g. bronchogenic cyst, fluid-filled bulla
- Vascular enhancement, e.g., AV malformation, hemangioma, varix

Often benign with
- Age <40
- High incidence of granulomas in the geographic area; history of tuberculosis exposure
- Branching, tubular or linear shape relates the nodule to the bronchial tree (e.g. mucus plug) or the vasculature
- A 'comet-tail' proximally and pleural thickening contiguous to an area of 'round atelectasis'
- Associated eosinophilia which may suggest a parasitic infection, e.g. dirofilaria
- Nodular density surrounded by an air crescent, suggesting a mycetoma

4 If benignity is not established, the nodule is **indeterminate** and often **malignant** with
- Age >45
- Smoking history

- Family history of lung cancer
- Asbestos exposure
- Nodule diameter >3 cm
- Enlargement on serial films
- Irregular margins
  - Smooth – 20% malignant
  - Scalloped – 60% malignant
  - Spiculated – 80% malignant
  - Corona radiata – 95% malignant
- Satellite lesions +/or cavitation are not helpful etiologically

5 **CT scan contribution**
- Densitometry
- Establish the presence of other nodules, e.g. metastases, synchronous cancers, combined granulomas and cancer
- Clarify the relation between the nodule and adjacent airways (positive bronchus sign)
- Identify mediastinal adenopathy
- Contrast enhancement of SPN, enhancement as an indication of vasculary and malignancy with an increase of >20 HU being very sensitive for malignancy but only ~75% specific (further studies needed)

6 **Positron emission tomography** – FDG (see Lung neoplasms p. 52)
- 95% of malignant SPNs will be positive on PET scan with ~75% specificity
- False positives can be seen with acute inflammation or infectious disorders, e.g. granulomas

7 **Remote** or **currently known** extrapulmonary cancer
- Extrathoracic squamous cell carcinoma
  - Probable independent lung lesion
- Extrathoracic adenocarcinoma
  - 50% metastatic
  - 50% primary lung

- Extrathoracic sarcoma, melanoma, lymphoma
  – Probably metastatic

8 **Systemic disease** which may be associated with a SPN, e.g. rheumatoid arthritis, Wegener's

9 **Operative risks**
- Patient age
- Lung function – PFTs, ABGs
- Cardiac function
- Other serious organ dysfunction

10 **Attitude** of patient re surgery

11 ± **Bronchoscopy**
- Bronchial brushing, BAL and transbronchial biopsy yield all increase with
  – Lesion >2 cm in diameter
  – Location in middle or inner third of lung
  – Positive bronchus sign, i.e. patent bronchus leading to or extending into the nodule
- Bronchoscopy may reveal endobronchial metastases pre-op in patients going for resection of metastases
- The yield for an unsuspected lesion in patients with a SPN is almost 0%

12 ± **TTNA**
- Diagnostic yields can reach 90% with larger nodules but as low as 25% with smaller ones
- A 'definitive' benign diagnosis is often not made

13 ± **Mediastinoscopy**

14 ± **Metastatic work-up**

APICAL MASS

Definition: An opacity of that part of the lung above the first rib, with the differential diagnosis including

Pleural

1 Pleural cap of aging (pleural scars and subpleural fibrosis)
2 Pleural tumor, primary, or metastatic
3 Pleural scarring from chronic or necrotizing upper lobe disease

Parenchymal

4 Infectious – tuberculosis, nocardia, actinomycosis, fungal, echinococcus
5 *Neoplasms – primary (Pancoast tumor) or metastatic
6 Radiation fibrosis

Vascular

7 Hematoma, AV fistula, aortic coarctation, subclavian artery aneurysm

Nerves

8 Neoplasms (intraspinal, intercostal, phrenic, vagus, sympathetic trunk)

Mediastinum

9 Soft tissue lesion of the esophagus, thyroid, lymph nodes

Neck

10 Neoplasms, pharyngeal diverticulum, abscess

Rib or spine

11 Hematoma, infections, neoplasm, degenerative disease of spine

Diagnostic Work-Up

1 Bone destruction, e.g. neoplasms, tuberculosis, nocardia, actinomycosis
2 'Extrapleural' configuration and involvement of contiguous structures, e.g. neck, mediastinum, chest wall
3 Vascular nature of the opacity on contrast CT or angiography
4 Cavitation e.g. infection, lung neoplasm
5 Esophageal disease on barium swallow

6 Chest wall invasion on CT
7 MRI better demonstrating invasion of the chest wall (coronal sections) and brachial plexus

'MASS-LIKE' OPACITY – ACUTE

Definition: Refers to a 'mass' developing in days to a few weeks

Airways

1 Mucoid impaction
2 BOOP

Parenchyma

3 Aspiration – lipoid pneumonia, foreign body granuloma
4 Infections
   - Bacterial – abscess, anaerobic lung infections, spherical pneumonia, legionella, tuberculosis, atypical mycobacteria, actinomycosis, nocardia, melioidosis
   - Fungal – aspergillus, cryptococcus, blastomycosis, coccidioiodomycosis
   - Parasitic – hydatid
5 Neoplastic – lymphomas developing post-immunosuppression
6 Atelectasis

Vascular

7 Vasculitis – Wegener's, lymphomatoid granulomatosis
8 Collagen disease – rheumatoid nodules
9 Pulmonary infarcts – septic or bland

INTRATHORACIC MASS – CHANGING POSITION

1 **Lung torsion**
   - Rare disorder described with the following
     – Surgical or non-surgical trauma

  - Pneumothorax
  - Spontaneously
- Clinically, patients present with non-specific respiratory symptoms which can progress to lung gangrene with sepsis and hypotension
- Bronchoscopy reveals distortion and narrowing or obstruction of the involved bronchi with venous engorgement
- Radiologic clues to diagnosis include
  - Changing position of an opacified lobe or mass
  - Rapid opacification of a lobe post-trauma
  - An opacified lobe in an unusual position

2 **Localized fibrous tumor** of the pleura
3 **Loculations of pleural fluid**

'PARATRACHEAL MASS'

1 Airway lesion, e.g. tracheal neoplasm
2 Parenchymal airspace disease
3 Pleural lesion, e.g. loculated paramediastinal effusion
4 Aneurysm
5 Chest wall mass
6 Mediastinal soft tissue lesion, e.g. thyroid, thymus, germ cell, other
7 Lymphadenopathy (see p. 497)
8 'Benign' lesions
- Azygous lobe
  - Seen in ~1% of the population, situated between the mediastinum and the pleural fissure
  - Caused by the descent of the azygous vein
  - The lobe may appear denser than the adjacent lung and simulate a true paratracheal mass
- Tortuous or ectatic innominate artery
  - Typically extends from the aortic arch to the thoracic inlet
- Paravertebral osteophyte

NODULES – MULTIPLE AND >1 CM DIAMETER

Distinguished from multifocal infiltrates by their round shape, homogeneous internal opacity, well-defined borders and usual absence of air bronchograms

Airways

- Multiple hamartomas
- Mucoid impactions
- Bronchopulmonary aspergillosis
- BOOP
- Broncho-alveolar cancer
- Tracheobronchial papillomatosis

Parenchyma

- *Neoplasms, including metastatic carcinoma (kidney, GI tract, breast, thyroid), germ cell tumors, sarcoma, lymphoma, melanoma
- Foreign body granulomas
- Granulomatous – nocardia, tuberculosis, hyalinizing granulomas, blastomycosis, coccidioidomycosis, cryptococcus, histoplasmosis
- Parasites – hydatid, dirofilaria, paragonimiasis
- Benign metastasizing leiomyomas
- Sarcoid or necrotizing sarcoid granulomatosis
- Amyloid
- Collagen diseases, e.g. rheumatoid nodules, SLE (rare)
- Caplan's syndrome

Vasculature

- Vasculitis, e.g. Wegener's, lymphomatoid granulomatosis, Churg-Strauss
- Infarcts, septic or bland
- Hematomas
- AV malformations
- Pyemic abscesses (cavitation common)
- Neoplasms, e.g. Kaposi's sarcoma, epithelioid hemangioendothelioma

Pleura

- Pleural plaques
- Pleural metastases

MICRONODULAR OPACITIES

Miliary Pattern or Multiple Small Nodules

Definition: Discrete lung opacities, <2 mm in diameter, with bilateral diffuse distribution, +/– uniform in size

1. **Airways**
   - bronchiolitis
   - Laryngotracheobronchial papillomatosis
2. **Vessels**
   - Arterial, e.g. intravenous talcosis, vasculitis
   - Capillary – miliary disease, e.g. tuberculosis, nocardia, salmonella, fungal
   - Venous, e.g. pulmonary hemosiderosis, mitral stenosis
   - Arteriovenous, e.g. fistulas
3. **Pleura**, e.g. metastatic nodules
4. **Parenchyma** – interstitial or airspace
   - Inhalational, e.g. silicosis, siderosis, CWP, berylliosis, allergic alveolitis
   - Inflammatory, e.g. sarcoid, eosinophilic granuloma
   - Infiltrative, e.g. amyloid
   - Neoplastic, e.g. alveolar cell cancer, metastatic cancer, lymphoma, melanoma
   - Infections, e.g. remote histoplasmosis or varicella
   - Aspiration, e.g. miliary granulomatosis
   - Alveolar microlithiasis

PIN-POINT OPACITIES

1. Alveolar microlithiasis
2. Post-lymphangiogram

3 Calcium inhalation – marble and limestone workers
4 Intravenous talcosis
5 Thesaurosis (hairspray inhalation)
6 Early stage of pneumoconioses e.g. silicosis, CWP, talcosis

SEGMENTAL OPACITIES

1 **Obstructive**, e.g. intralumenal, endobronchial or peribronchial

2 **Non-obstructive**
- Infectious, with a bronchopneumonia pattern which can be acute/chronic
  - Bacterial – *Staph. aureus*, tuberculosis, anaerobes, hemophilus
  - Mycoplasma
  - Viral
  - Fungal
- Lipoid pneumonia
- Pulmonary infarct
- Bronchiectasis
- 'RML syndrome'

BRANCHING OR TUBULAR OPACITIES

1 **Vascular disease**
- AV malformations
- Pulmonary venous varix
- Partial anomalous pulmonary venous return

2 **Mucoid impaction**
- *Generalized airways disease*
  - Bronchial asthma
  - COPD
  - Cystic fibrosis
  - Allergic bronchopulmonary aspergillosis
  - Bronchocentric granulomatosis

- *Localized airways disease*
  - Obstructed bronchus, e.g. adenoma, carcinoma, congenital bronchial atresia, bronchiolithiasis
  - Intralobar sequestration
  - Bronchogenic cyst

Fraser R.S., Muller N.L., Colman N., Paré P.D. (1999) *Diagnosis of Diseases of the Chest* 4th Edn., WB Saunders.

Naidich, D.P., Zerhouni, E.A., Siegelman, S.S. (1998) *Computed Tomography and Magnetic Resonance of the Thorax*, 3rd edn. New York: Raven Press.

Moss, A., Gamsu, Genant (1992) Thorax and neck. In: *Computed Tomography of the Body with Magnetic Resonance Imaging*, 2nd edn., vol. 1.: W.B. Saunders.

Baum, G.L., Crapo, J.D., Celli, B.R., Karlinsky, J.B. (eds) (1997) *Textbook of Pulmonary Diseases*, 6th edn.: Lippincott-Raven.

Fishman, A.P., Elias, J.A., Fishman, J.A., Grippi, M.A., Kaiser, L.R., Senior, R.N. (1998) *Fishman's Pulmonary Diseases and Disorders*, 3rd edn.: McGraw-Hill.

Ray, J.F., Lawton, B., Magnin, G. *et al.* (1976) The coin lesion story: update 1976. Twenty year's experience with thoracotomy for 179 suspected malignant coin lesions. *Chest* **70**:332–336.

Toomes, H., Delphendahl, A., Manke, H.G. *et al.* (1983) The coin lesion of the lung: a review of 955 resected coin lesions. *Cancer* **51**:534–537.

52 Mediastinum

MASS WIDENING – DIAGNOSTIC CLUES TO ETIOLOGY

I **Radiologic**
  1 Density features
  2 Location
  3 Benign/malignant features
  4 MRI features
  5 Extramediastinal disease

II **Blood tests**

III **Associated disorders – pulmonary or systemic**

Radiologic

1 **Density features**
- Air, e.g. bowel hernia
- Fat
- Cystic/necrotic
- Vascular (enhancing) on angiography, contrast CT, MRI
- Solid (LITHO)
  - **L**ymphadenopathy
  - **I**nfectious/**I**nflammatory
  - **T**umors
  - **H**ernias of the diaphragm
  - **O**rganomegaly
- I^{131} uptake (thyroid)
- Calcifications – bone, tooth, calcified tumors, granulomatous mediastinitis, calcified nodes

*The presence of extensive calcifications within the mass does not rule out malignancy

2 **Location**
- Diseases involving the airways, parenchyma, pleura, vasculature or chest wall contiguous to the mediastinum can **simulate** mediastinal widening
- Determine the **epicenter** of the mass and subsequently its likely origin as being mediastinal in origin
- The **division** of the mediastinum in which the lesion is present, i.e. anterior, posterior, middle, suggests certain pathologies as well as their likelihood of being benign or malignant, but **location does not predict malignancy of individual lesions*

Anterior mediastinum

Contents
- thymus
- lymph nodes
- connective tissue
- internal mammary art/vein
- ectopic thyroid/parathyroid

Typical lesions
- Thymic
- Germ cell tumors
- Lymphoma
- Thyroid/parathyroid

Middle mediastinum

Contents
- Heart/pericardium
- Lymph nodes
- Connective tissue
- SVC/IVC
- Aorta/brachiocephalic vessels
- Pulmonary arteries/veins
- Trachea
- Proximal mainstem bronchi
- Nerves
  - Phrenics
  - Upper vagus

Typical lesions
- Lymphoma
- Vascular
- Metastatic neoplasms
- Morgagni hernia
- Cysts
  - Bronchogenic
  - Pleuropericardial

Posterior mediastinum

Contents
- Spine/paraspinal zones
- Lymph nodes
- Connective tissue
- Esophagus
- Aorta
- Pulmonary arteries/veins
- Thoracic duct
- Nerves
  - Lower vagus
  - Sympathetic NS
  - Peripheral

Typical lesions
- Lymphoma
- Vascular
- Neurogenic
- Spine related
- Hernias
  - Hiatus
  - Bochdalek
- Cysts
  - Neurenteric
  - Gastroenteric
  - Thoracic duct

A mediastinal lesion occupying **more than one** compartment would include
- Neoplasms, e.g. lymphoma, metastatic cancer, connective tissue tumors
- Lymphadenopathy
- Aneurysms

- Esophageal lesions, e.g. achalasia
- Mediastinitis, e.g. granulomatous

3 **Benign/malignant features**

- Encapsulation (= benign lesion)
- The time course and subsequent growth rate of the mass
- Respiratory system involvement
  - Tracheobronchial displacement, compression, obstruction or encasement
  - Parenchymal lesions re nodule, mass, infiltration, granulomas
  - Pleural effusion
- Cardiovascular system disease looking for displacement, compression, obstruction or encasement of SVC, aorta, main pulmonary arteries or veins, heart
- Esophageal involvement
- Chest wall disease with invasion, erosion or bony destruction
- Hilar/mediastinal lymphadenopathy
- Mediastinal invasion with fatty infiltration and loss of the fascial planes

*The absence of demonstration of mediastinal, vascular or chest wall invasion on CT does not rule out malignancy

4 **MRI features** – advantages include

- Identification of fatty or cystic tissue when CT is not diagnostic
- Vessels, e.g. the aorta or superior vena cava, may be imaged without contrast
- Substernal thyroid or parathyroid hyperplasia may be identified easier than on CT
- Several neoplasms may be preferentially imaged including
  - Neurofibromas (precise delineation of neural foramen involvement with paravertebral tumors)
  - Pancoast's tumor with better detection of invasion of contiguous structures such as the chest wall

- Bronchogenic cancer with clearer demonstration of chest wall and mediastinal invasion (often indeterminate on CT)
- Detection of parathyroid adenomas or carcinoma
- Occasionally helpful in distinguishing scarring from residual tumor in lymphoma patients who are asymptomatic but have residual densities post-treatment

5 **Extra mediastinal lesions**

- Parenchymal lung mass
  - Neoplastic, e.g. carcinoma, carcinoid, melanoma, lymphoma, germ cell
  - Fungal, e.g. histoplasmosis, coccidioidomycosis, sporotrichosis
  - Progressive massive fibrosis, e.g. silicosis, CWP
  - Sarcoid
  - Amyloid
  - Lymphomatoid granulomatosis
- CT of neck, abdomen, and pelvis for lymphadenopathy, GI, GU or retroperitoneal disease
- Ultrasound of the scrotum for a testicular neoplasm

Blood Tests

1. α-fetoprotein or HCG in non-seminomatous germ cell tumors
2. Antibodies against acetylcholine receptors in myasthenia gravis with a thymoma
3. Hypogammaglobulinemia, anemia or red blood cell aplasia with thymomas
4. Calcium, phosphate, parathormone levels
5. T_3, T_4, TSH
6. Plasma catecholamines for pheochromocytoma

Associated Disorders – Pulmonary or Systemic

Mediastinal lesion	Pulmonary/systemic disorder
• Lipomatosis	• Hyperadrenalism – endogenous/exogenous
• Thymic hyperplasia	• Post-chemotherapy, myasthenia gravis, thyrotoxicosis
• Thymic cyst	• Post-radiation for Hodgkin's, post-thoracotomy
• Thymoma	• Myasthenia gravis, RBC aplasia
• Intrathoracic goitre	• Goitre, hyperthyroidism
• Parathyroid adenoma	• Hypercalcemia
• Germ cell tumor	• Trichoptysis, Klinefelter's syndrome, malignant histiocytosis, testicular mass
• Granulomatous mediastinitis	• Histoplasmosis or tuberculosis – recent or remote
• Posterior mediastinal neural tumor	• Neurofibromatosis
• Paraganglionoma	• Excess catecholamine secretion
• Lymphoma	• Peripheral lymphadenopathy, Pel-Ebstein fever

Table 52.1

*The absence of pulmonary or systemic symptoms does not rule out malignancy

MEDIASTINAL AIR – DIFFERENTIAL DIAGNOSIS

1 Esophagus, e.g. diverticula, tracheoesophageal fistula, megaesophagus from achalasia or stenosis, scleroderma, carcinoma
2 GI hernias, e.g. hiatus hernia, Bochdalek, Morgagni
3 Colonic interposition post-esophageal resection
4 Mediastinal abscess
5 Bronchogenic cyst
6 Cavitary lymph nodes secondary to TB
7 Pneumomediastinum, i.e. free gas in the mediastinal space, with potential sources including
   - Lung parenchyma

- Most common cause is alveolar rupture with air dissecting along the interstitial tissues
- Seen where there is a sudden rise in alveolar pressure, e.g. vomiting, coughing, sneezing, valsalva, exercise, chest trauma, mechanical ventilation, childbirth
- Clinically the patient may be asymptomatic but usually presents with retrosternal chest pain, often pleuritic
- Significant physical findings include subcutaneous emphysema and Hamman's sign
- Rarely a picture of mediastinal tamponade can develop with elevated venous pressures and systemic hypotension
- Radiologically on a PA film, air is best seen on the left side with the mediastinal pleura displaced laterally and gas between the heart and a line running parallel to it
- Air may be seen around the thoracic aorta and pulmonary artery as well as within the interstitial lung tissue
- The 'continuous' diaphragm sign is the visualization of the central part of the diaphragm, especially in supine patients, due to air under the heart
- Subcutaneous air can be seen extending into the neck and subcutaneous soft tissues of the chest wall, outlining the fibers of the pectoral muscles

- Tracheobronchial tree
  - Rupture of intramediastinal airways, e.g. post-trauma, asthma
- Esophagus
  - Rupture is seen with the associated findings of acute mediastinitis including pneumothorax, hydropneumothorax
- Fascial planes of the neck
- Abdominal cavity
  - Intraperitoneal or retroperitoneal air tracking upward following perforation of a hollow viscus

MEDIASTINAL FAT – DIFFERENTIAL DIAGNOSIS

1 **Diffuse – mediastinal lipomatosis**
  - Most prominent in the superior mediastinum without associated tracheal compression or displacement
  - Cardiophrenic angles and paraspinal areas are less often involved
  - The superior mediastinal and paraspinal widening on chest X-ray are diagnostic on CT as convexly bulging areas of fat
  - Seen with obesity, steroid treatment and Cushing's

2 **Localized fatty mass**
  - Pericardial fat pads
  - Herniation from the abdomen
    - Morgagni hernia (cardiophrenic angle mass)
    - Bochdalek hernia
    - Para-esophageal or omental hernia

3 **Fatty tumors**
  - Lipoma (2% of mediastinal tumors)
  - Thymolipomas
  - Liposarcoma
  - Fatty degeneration of other tumors, e.g. germ cell tumors
  - Neurofibroma
  - Hamartoma

MEDIASTINAL CALCIFICATIONS – DIFFERENTIAL DIAGNOSIS

1 Cysts – bronchogenic
2 Vascular – dissections, aneurysms, tortuous vessels, congenital anomalies, hematoma
3 Lymph nodes
  - Tuberculosis, fungal, pneumocystis
  - Sarcoid

- Silicosis, CWP
- Hodgkin's, metastatic colon cancer, osteogenic sarcoma

4 Infections – chronic granulomatous mediastinitis
5 Neoplasms – thyroid, parathyroid, germ cell, thymoma, lymphoma, neurogenic
6 Organomegaly – goitre

MEDIASTINAL CYSTS – DIFFERENTIAL DIAGNOSIS

1 **Pericardial or pleuropericardial (mesothelial) cysts**
- Congenital cysts which are usually asymptomatic and spherical or teardrop shaped
- Most often found in the right cardiophrenic angle and less often in the left or other paracardiac location
- The cyst contents are usually clear and described as 'clear water' or 'spring water' cysts
- Rare complications include infection or communication with the pericardial sac

2 **Bronchogenic cysts**
- Congenital cysts lined by respiratory epithelium, typically discovered in children or young adults and represent approximately 50% of all mediastinal cysts
- Clinical features
  - Asymptomatic finding
  - Superinfection and rupture
  - Hemorrhage
  - Increasing size with compression of adjacent airways (cough, wheezing, dyspnea and recurrent respiratory tract infections), esophagus and hilar vessels
  - Communication with the tracheobronchial tree
  - Spontaneous disappearance
- Radiologically present as a solitary, spherical, non-enhancing lesions of variable size and attenuation with rare calcifications and enhancement of the wall

- Usually located in the right paratracheal or carinal region but can occur in any mediastinal compartment
- Diagnosis can be confirmed by needle drainage of non-bloody fluid containing mucus and bronchial epithelial cells

3 **Enteric cysts**
- Usually present in infancy with compressive symptoms relating to the esophagus or tracheobronchial tree
- Lined by alimentary epithelium and may contain gastric or pancreatic tissue
- Esophageal duplication cysts are adherent to or present in the esophageal wall
- Gastroenteric cysts present in the posterior mediastinum as a lobulated opacity, usually paravertebral in location
- May be connected by a strand to the meninges or esophagus and rarely communicate with the infradiaphragmatic GI tract
- Neurenteric cysts may be associated with congenital spinal defects

4 **Thymic cysts**

5 **Pancreatic pseudocyst** (posterior mediastinum)

6 **Cystic lymphangioma**
- 90% diagnosed before age 2 and rarely present in adults
- 95% involve the neck or axilla with only about 10% extending into the upper anterior mediastinum
- radiologically manifest as a lobulated, multicystic tumor which can infiltrate into the mediastinum, making surgical removal difficult

7 **Secondary cystic degeneration of tumors**
- Thymoma, lymphoma, germ cell tumors (anterior mediastinum)

8 **Necrotic lymph nodes**
- Tuberculosis (may be cavitary), fungal, metastases, lymphoma

9 **Infections**
- Echinococcal

10 **Chronic mediastinal abscess**

11 **Old hematoma**

12 **GI hernias**, e.g. Bochdalek, Morgagni, hiatus hernia

Note: In exceptional cases, MRI may detect the cystic nature of a lesion when CT cannot

AORTIC LESIONS

Thoracic Aortic Aneurysms

75% occur in the descending thoracic aorta, are fusiform in shape and secondary to atherosclerosis
- Often seen in elderly hypertensives, males > females
- Associated abdominal aneurysms are common
- Usually asymptomatic although local compressive symptoms can result in cough, stridor, hoarseness, dysphagia as well as rupture

Other **etiologies** include
1 Traumatic (distal to the take-off of the left subclavian artery)
2 Mycotic
3 Aortic coarctation
4 Connective tissue diseases, e.g. Marfan's, Ehlers-Danlos, rheumatoid arthritis, ankylosing spondylitis

CT manifestations
1 The absolute diameter of the aorta is variable, but the descending aorta is always smaller than the ascending aorta
- <5 cm – 2% likelihood of rupture
- >10 cm – >50% likelihood of rupture

2 Intralumenal thrombi which are often crescentic in shape and may be calcified
3 Displacement, compression or erosion of adjacent structures
4 Features of rupture e.g. pleuropericardial effusions, perianeurysmal hemorrhage, mediastinal hematoma

Aortic Dissection

Predispositions

1 Male to female ratio 3:1
2 Hypertension (present in most patients)
3 Pregnancy, most often in third trimester
4 Marfan's syndrome
5 Congenital valve abnormalities, e.g. coarctation

Type A (Stanford classification)

Internal tear within a few centimeters of the aortic valve

- High mortality secondary to aortic insufficiency and pericardial hemorrhage
- Occlusion of major aortic branches and rupture can occur
- Requires surgical intervention

Type B

Involves the descending aorta distal to the origin of the left subclavian artery

- Tend not to extend proximally and therefore treated medically, although occlusion of major aortic branches and rupture can occur

CT findings

1 Detection of an intimal flap (linear structure separating true and false lumens)
2 Differential contrast enhancement of true and false lumens with compression of the true lumen by an unopacified or partially opacified false lumen
3 Displaced intimal calcification pre-contrast
4 Detection of intramural hematoma pre-contrast

CT limitations

1 Small percentage of false negative scans *vs*. angiography
2 Distinguishing a thrombosed false lumen of dissection with a thrombosed aneurysm
3 Reliance on intravenous contrast in patients with iodine allergy, renal or cardiac disease
4 Inability to detect or quantify aortic insufficiency

Intramural Hematoma

Defined as blood within the aortic wall and may occur without intimal disruption ? early stage of aortic dissection ? rupture of vasa vasorum ? unrecognized intimal tear

- Clinical presentation is indistinguishable from aortic dissection

CT findings include

- Crescentic area of high attenuation in the aortic wall which can be obscured by the use of contrast
- Distinguished from the false lumen of aortic dissection by lack of enhancement post-contrast although there are reports of aortic dissection following intramural hematoma

Penetrating Aortic Atherosclerotic Ulcer

Usually involves the descending aorta in elderly hypertensive patients where the presentation is that of aortic dissection

- The ulcer results in an intramural hematoma, which can then lead to a pseudoaneurysm, rupture, acute dissection or spontaneous healing
- CT findings include an intramural hematoma seen on pre-contrast with the penetrating ulcer visualized post-contrast

MESENCHYMAL TUMORS

Primary mediastinal masses of mesenchymal origin represent ~5% of mediastinal masses – can arise from any mediastinal compartment and numerous tissues including

1 Adipose tissue, e.g. lipoma (most common)
2 Muscle

3 Vessels, e.g. hemangioma, lymphangioma, angiosarcoma, hemangiopericytoma
4 Fibrous tissue
5 Other

MEDIASTINAL-ENHANCING LESIONS – DIFFERENTIAL

1 **Vascular**
- *Vascular tumors* (rare and usually anterior mediastinal)
  - Lymphangioma (cystic hygroma)
  - Hemangioma
    - May occur as an isolated tumor or part of the Osler-Weber-Rendu syndrome
    - Phleboliths are characteristic on CT
  - Angiosarcoma
  - Hemangiopericytoma
- *Normal or aberrant vessels*
  - Congenital aortic anomalies
  - Aberrant subclavian artery
  - Enlarged pulmonary artery
- *Aneurysms*
  - Aortocoronary by-pass graft aneurysm
  - Aortic aneurysm, dissection
  - Internal mammary artery aneurysm
  - Innominate artery aneurysm
- *Venous structures*
  - Dilatation of SVC, IVC
  - Persistent left SVC
  - Dilatation of azygous/hemiazygous veins
  - Dilatation of left superior intercostal vein
  - SVC syndrome
  - Pulmonary vein varix
  - Portal hypertension and varices
- *Mediastinal hematoma*
  - Traumatic: surgical, non-surgical

- Venous/arterial tears: dissection, catheterization
- Bleeding diathesis: uremia, dialysis, hemophilia, i.v. heparin, coumadin, streptokinase
- GI sources: pancreatitis, pancreatic pseudocyst, esophageal source

2 **Lymph nodes**
- Castleman's Disease
- Metastases – kidney, lung, carcinoid, thyroid
- Angioimmunoblastic lymphadenopathy
- Bacillary angiomatosis

3 **Neoplasms**
- Parathyroid adenoma
- Paraganglionoma

4 **Organomegaly**
- Goitre

ANTERIOR MEDIASTINUM

Definition: The space from the sternum anteriorly to the anterior pericardium and great vessels posteriorly (but the anterior margins of the aorta and brachiocephalic vessels are usually difficult to visualize on chest X-ray and anterior mediastinal masses often project over the heart)

Mass Widening – Differential Diagnosis

Density	Disorders
Air	• Morgagni hernia
Fat	• Mediastinal lipomatosis • Morgagni hernia • Cardiophrenic fat pad
Cyst (water density)	• Lymphangioma • Cysts: thymic, mesothelial, bronchogenic (may be solid) • Post-op fluid collection • Abscess • Cystic degeneration of tumors

Density	Disorders
Vascular (enhancing)	• Internal mammary artery aneurysm or tortuosity • Ascending aortic aneurysm • Hematoma
Solid	• Any cause of lymphadenopathy • Acute/chronic mediastinitis • Abscess • Tumors: *lymphoma, *thymoma, *germ cell, thyroid, parathyroid, connective tissue (fibrous, smooth muscle, vascular), sternal tumors (primary or metastatic) • Morgagni hernia • Thymic hyperplasia • Goitre
I^{131} uptake	• Thyroid (anterosuperior mediastinum)
Calcifications	• Bronchogenic cyst • Vessels • Chronic mediastinitis • Tumors of thymus, thyroid, parathyroid, germ cells (bone, tooth) • Lymph nodes

Table 52.2

Anterior Cardiophrenic Angle Mass*

1 Cardiovascular
- Cardiac aneurysm
- Pericardial fat pad or cyst
- Varices secondary to portal hypertension

2 Mediastinum
- Any anterior mediastinal tumor, e.g. thymoma, teratoma

3 Nodes
- Diaphragmatic adenopathy

4 Lung parenchyma
- any cause of a lung mass

5 Pleura
- mass, fluid, mesothelial cyst

6 Diaphragm
- Morgagni hernia

- Neoplastic: primary lipoma, sarcoma or metastases
- Eventration

*may present radiologically as 'cardiomegaly'

Anterior Mediastinal Mass – Solid and Large

1. Lymphoma
   - Nodular sclerosing Hodgkins
     - May present as a discrete mass
     - Look for adjacent adenopathy
   - Lymphoblastic lymphoma
     - Rapidly enlarging mass presenting with features of local invasion
   - Primary mediastinal B cell lymphoma with sclerosis
2. Thymoma or other thymic tumors
3. Germ cell tumors
4. Thyroid tumor or goitre
5. Metastatic cancer
   - Likely primary sites include breast, lung, melanoma, kidney, germ cell, colon, head and neck, including thyroid
6. Castleman's Disease
7. Chronic mediastinitis

THYMUS

Normal Thymus – Radiologically

Stage I Birth → age 12

- Bilobed anterosuperior mediastinal soft tissue mass

Stage II Age 12 → age 24

- Increasing fat radiologically with thymus being triangular or bilobar in shape
- Lies anterior to the great vessels below the level of the horizontal portion of the left brachiocephalic vein

Stage III Age 24 → age 40

- Increasing fat and decreasing soft tissue with concave outer borders and progressive inability to detect a distinct thymus

Stage IV >Age 40

- Fat only usually

Thymic Enlargement – Differential Diagnosis

1 Enlarged gland, but **normal histologically**
- Children recovering from burns
- Endocrine disorders – hyperthyroidism, Addison's, acromegaly

2 **Thymic hyperplasia**
- 50% of cases manifest thymic enlargement on CT
  - Isolated
  - Association with myasthenia gravis, thyrotoxicosis
  - Rebound hyperplasia following cessation of chemotherapy

3 **Thymic cysts**
- Congenital
- Post-inflammatory
- Post-thoracotomy
- Post-radiotherapy for Hodgkin's disease

4 **Thymic neoplasms**
- *Thymoma*
  - Most common primary tumor of the anterior mediastinum
  - Typically occur in patients > age 40
  - Tumors are usually solid, average 5–10cm in diameter, but vary considerably and can have foci of calcification, cystic degeneration and hemorrhage
  - Histologic subtypes include lymphocytic, epithelial or spindle cell tumors but they do not predict response to therapy

- Electron microscopy can distinguish thymomas from other thymic neoplasms, e.g. lymphoma, carcinoids
- Irrespective of histology, the following staging system is used

  Stage I — intact capsule
  Stage II — tumor extends through the capsule into the surrounding fat, pleura, pericardium
  Stage III — intrathoracic metastases
  Stage IV — extrathoracic metastases

Clinically, the majority of patients are asymptomatic
- Features of compression and invasion of local structures are seen in approximately 30% of cases
- Paraneoplastic mainfestations include
  — Myasthenia gravis – approximately 30%
  — Hypogammaglobulinemia – approximately 10%
  — RBC aplasia – approximately 5%
  — Other autoimmune diseases
- The best criteria for distinguishing benignity from malignancy is the presence or absence of local invasion at thoracotomy supported by the histologic occurrence of tumor outside the capsule
- 70% of tumors are benign and encapsulated with absence of local invasion, although they may be adherent to local structures
- 30% are malignant with invasion of the capsule and mediastinal fat
- Local invasion involves the pleura, pericardium, trachea, great vessels, lung and chest wall
- Droplet spread can occur through the pleura with circumferential encasement of the lung simulating a mesothelioma
- Transdiaphragmatic extension can occur into the abdomen and retroperitoneum
- Lymph node and hematogenous metastases are rare

- Regular radiologic follow-up is indicated, as a small percent of resected encapsulated thymomas can recur months to years after excision

Radiologically, the usual presentation is that of a well-defined, rounded or lobulated mass usually in the upper anterior mediastinum and typically growing toward one side of the midline, less common bilaterally
- CT may reveal cystic areas as well as calcifications
- Vascular compromise, infiltration of the mediastinum or an irregular interface with lung suggest malignancy

- **Thymic carcinoma**
  - Usually squamous cell or lymphoepithelioma-like aggressive tumors with malignant histology (unlike thymoma), local invasion, as well as metastases to regional nodes and distant sites
  - Metastatic involvement from other sites, e.g. lung, must be ruled out
  - Radiologically, they present as an infiltrating anterior mediastinal mass with pleuropericardial involvement
  - Prognosis is determined by histologic grade

- **Thymolipoma**
  - Benign and slow growing tumor, most often affecting young adults
  - Asymptomatic (50%) or presents with non-specific respiratory symptoms
  - Tumors are encapsulated, can weigh several pounds and tend to sink into the anterior inferior mediastinum
  - Can conform to adjacent structures and thus simulate cardiomegaly or diaphragmatic elevation
  - CT scan reveals a combination of fat and soft tissue elements

- **Thymic carcinoids**
  - Rare tumor identical to carcinoids occurring at other sites

- Patients can be asymptomatic, present with non-specific respiratory symptoms or endocrine abnormalities, most often Cushing's syndrome
- Usually presents as an invasive anterior mediastinal mass which can include regional as well as distant metastases

- **Thymic lymphoma**
  - Seen in approximately 30% of patients with Hodgkin's disease
  - Associated mediastinal adenopathy is typical

GERM CELL TUMORS

Majority are located in the anterior mediastinum, rarely posteriorly, with about 80% benign and 20% malignant

- Patients are usually young adults with >70% of malignant lesions occurring in males

1 **Teratoma** is the most common type and by definition composed of tissues that arise from more than one of the three primitive germ cell layers: ectoderm, endoderm and mesoderm
   - Ectodermal elements dominate with this component seen in about 90% of tumors

     Mature teratoma
     - Most common type of teratoma, containing only mature elements and lacking immature elements or poor differentiation
     - Benign and occurring equally in women and men
     - Often asymptomatic, but can present with non-specific respiratory symptoms due to compression or encompassment of surrounding structures
     - Local erosion by the tumor or digestive enzymes secreted by intestinal or pancreatic tissue can result in rupture and communication with surrounding tissues including

Mediastinal tissue	→ mediastinitis
Pleura	→ empyema
Pericardium	→ tamponade
Tracheobronchial tree	→ trichoptysis (pathognomonic)
Great vessels	→ hemorrhage

- CT reveals an encapsulated multiloculated cystic lesion whose diagnostic features include
  - Fat–fluid level
  - Bone
  - Tooth
  - Combination of fat, calcium and soft tissue

Immature teratoma

- Teratoma containing fetal tissue
- Local recurrence or distant metastases can occur

Malignant teratoma

- Uncommon solid tumor containing mature and immature elements as well as foci of malignancy, most commonly adenocarcinoma
- Local and distant spread result in a poor prognosis

2 **Dermoid cyst**

- Benign encapsulated lesion containing only ectodermal elements, e.g. tooth, skin, hair

3 **Seminoma**

- Most common malignant germ cell tumor, occurring almost exclusively in males 20–40 years old and located in the anterior mediastinum
- Lesions are either asymptomatic (30%) or present with non-specific respiratory symptoms
- 5–10% of patients have elevated β-HCG levels
- Can present with local spread, regional or distant metastases, e.g. bones
- All patients should have a careful testicular exam and ultrasound as well as evaluation of the retroperitoneum for nodes, to rule out a primary gonadal lesion

4 **Non-seminomatous**
- Includes embryonal carcinoma, choriocarcinoma, endodermal sinus tumor, mixed tumors with multiple malignant cell types
- Seen in young males who present with compressive or invasive symptoms
- Radiologically manifest as a large anterior mediastinal mass with local, regional and often distant spread and prognosis is poor
- Described in association with Klinefelter's syndrome, thrombocytopenia and hematologic malignancies including acute megakaryocytic leukemia, acute myelogenous leukemia, malignant histiocytosis, myelodysplasia
- Elevated β-HCG levels seen with choriocarcinoma and embryonal carcinoma (causing gynecomastia), while elevated α-fetoprotein is seen with embryonal carcinoma or endodermal sinus tumors
- 10% of patients will have normal serum levels of both markers

MEDIASTINAL GOITER

Usual etiology is a multinodular goiter which grows slowly over many years
- Rarely acute or chronic thyroiditis or thyroid carcinoma can present as an anterior mediastinal mass
- 20% of cervical goiters extend intrathoracically of which 80% are anterior to the trachea in the anterior superior mediastinum and 20% posterior to the trachea
- Primary intrathoracic goiter without a cervical component is rare and there is often a history of previous thyroid surgery

Clinically, they are often asymptomatic with a palpable cervical goiter frequent, but compressive symptoms can develop insidiously and include

- Recurrent laryngeal nerve(s) → hoarseness, stridor
- Esophagus → dysphagia
- SVC → SVC syndrome
- Trachea → stridor, dyspnea, occasionally being positional
- Thoracic duct obstruction → chylothorax
- Acute life-threatening airways obstruction from hemorrhage into the goiter
- Phrenic nerve → diaphragmatic paralysis
- Cervical sympathetic chain → Horner's syndrome

Tracheal symptoms (or other compressive features) can relate to a benign goiter, thyroiditis, carcinoma or fibrosing mediastinitis associated with Riedel's thyroiditis

Diagnostic Features and Work-Up

1 Goiter on **physical exam** may be accompanied by tracheal deviation with subclinical hyperthyroidism more common than clinical

2 **Levels of TSH** and **thyroid hormones**

3 **I^{131} scan**
- Uptake is diagnostic when positive, but they are seldom functioning
- Must be done before a contrast CT or iodine uptake will not be demonstrated for approximately 1 month

4 Documentation of **upper airways obstruction** on flow–volume curves

5 **Chest X-ray findings**
- Most often an anterior mediastinal mass with lateral and posterior tracheal displacement +/– compression
- Differential diagnosis involves other anterior mediastinal masses including aneurysms
- Uncommonly a posterior mediastinal mass with anterior tracheal displacement and esophageal compression
- Calcification is common
- May compress and displace the brachiocephalic vessels

6 **CT features**
- Communication with the cervical thyroid
- Heterogenous densities including calcifications, cysts and high density areas due to iodine
- Intense and prolonged contrast enhancement
- Displacement, compression or obstruction of contiguous structures, e.g. SVC, aorta, trachea, esophagus
- Adenopathy and loss of fascial planes with malignant lesions

7 **MRI** demonstrates the extent of intrathoracic disease

PARATHYROIDS

Parathyroid tumors are rarely large enough to widen the mediastinal silhouette

Primary hyperparathyroidism is usually caused by a parathyroid adenoma more often than primary parathyroid hyperplasia and rarely by a cyst or carcinoma

- Diagnosis is entertained by finding an elevated serum calcium

Diagnostic tests include

1 Ultrasound
2 Thallium scan
3 CT scan for detection of an anterior mediastinal mass
4 Selective arteriography and venous catheterization
5 MRI

MIDDLE MEDIASTINUM

Definition: The space between the anterior pericardium and brachiocephalic vessels anteriorly, the pericardium and trachea posteriorly, the thoracic inlet and the diaphragm

Mass Widening – Differential Diagnosis

Density	Disorders
Air	
Fat	• Pericardial fat pad • Mediastinal lipomatosis
Cysts (water density)	• Cysts: *pericardial, *bronchogenic (may be solid) • Abscess • Post-op collection • Cystic degeneration of a tumor
Vascular (enhancing)	• Aortic aneurysm/dissection • Congenital vascular abnormalities, e.g. right aortic arch, aberrant right subclavian artery, aortic coarctation • Enlarged pulmonary artery • Pulmonary venous varix • SVC syndrome • Left SVC draining into left atrium or coronary sinus • Azygous or hemiazygous vein enlargement • Aortocoronary by-pass graft aneurysm
Solid	• *Any cause of lymphadenopathy, e.g. lymphoma, carcinoma, TB, histoplasmosis, sarcoid, Castleman's disease • Acute or chronic mediastinitis • Tumors, i.e. tracheobronchial, pericardial, mesothelioma, neurofibroma of phrenic nerve, thymic or germ cell tumors (usually seen anteriorly) • Thoracic kidney
Calcifications	• Bronchogenic cysts • Vessels • Chronic mediastinitis • Lymph nodes • Thymic, germ cell tumors

Table 52.3

Aorto-pulmonary Window

Normal anatomy

1 Boundaries defined
   - Superiorly by aortic arch
   - Inferiorly by left pulmonary artery
   - Medially by left mainstem bronchus
   - Laterally by mediastinal pleura and left lung visceral pleura
   - Anteriorly by ascending aorta
   - Posteriorly by descending aorta

2 Contents include
   - Fat
   - Lymph nodes
   - Ductus arteriosus ligament
   - Left recurrent laryngeal nerve
   - Paraganglia

Lesions

1 Solid
   - Any cause of lymphadenopathy (see p. 497)
   - Bronchogenic cancer
   - Neurofibroma
   - Aorticopulmonary paraganglionoma (R/O Carney's triad)
   - Mediastinitis

2 Fat
   - Mediastinal lipomatosis

3 Cystic
   - Pleuropericardial (mesothelial) cyst
   - Bronchogenic cyst

4 Calcifications
   - Nodes
   - Granulomatous or fibrosing mediastinitis

5 Vascular
   - Aortic or pulmonary artery lesions

POSTERIOR MEDIASTINUM

Definition: The space from the posterior tracheal wall and posterior pericardium to the posterior border of the vertebral bodies and from the first rib to the diaphragm

Mass Widening – Differential Diagnosis

1 Spine

Vascular	• Hematoma post-fracture
Inflammatory	• Eosinophilic granuloma
Infectious	• Tuberculosis, acute osteomyelitis
Neoplastic	• Primary, e.g. myeloma, lymphoma, sarcoma • Metastases
Degenerative	• Osteophytes

2 Paraspinal soft tissues

Density	Disorders
Air	• Bochdalek hernia, esophageal diseases
Fat	• Mediastinal lipomatosis, Bochdalek hernia, liposarcoma, component of neural tumors
Cystic	• *Enteric cysts, *bronchogenic cysts, thoracic duct cysts • Meningocele/meningomyelocele • Pancreatic pseudocyst • Dilated esophagus • Abscess • Post-op fluid collection
Vascular	• Aneurysm/dissection • Azygous continuation of IVC • Portal hypertension and varices • Hematoma

Continued

Density	Disorders
Solid	• *Tumors, e.g. neurogenic • Lymphadenopathy – any cause • Acute or chronic mediastinitis • Hernias, e.g. Bochdalek, hiatal, paraesophageal • Extramedullary hematopoiesis • Esophageal disorders, e.g. diverticula, achalasia, fistulas, benign/malignant tumors • Thoracic kidney

Table 52.4

3 Distinguish from **pleural disease** contiguous to the paraspinal shadows including
- Tumors – primary or metastatic
- Pleural thickening
- Loculated pleural fluid

4 Distinguish from **pulmonary disease** contiguous to the paraspinal shadows including
- Tumors – primary or secondary
- Atelectasis
- Consolidation

RETROCARDIAC MASS – DIFFERENTIAL DIAGNOSIS

1 **Hiatus hernia**

2 **Mediastinal neoplasms**
- Neurogenic
- Lymphoma

3 **Vascular**
- Aortic aneurysm
- Para-esophageal varices

4 **Cysts**
- Bronchogenic
- Enteric

5 **Pancreatic pseudocyst**

- Rare lesions with usual extension through the esophageal foramen but occasional extension through the foramen of Morgagni into the anterior mediastinum or diaphragmatic erosion into the middle mediastinum
- Typically seen with a history of alcoholism, chronic pancreatitis or trauma
- Presentation is that of non-specific GI and respiratory symptoms
- CT scan demonstrates a cystic lesion with extension from the pancreas into the mediastinum
- Clinical course varies from spontaneous resolution to infection, rupture, hemorrhage or other intra-abdominal complications

6 **Psoas abscess**

- Presents as a unilateral or bilateral posterior mediastinal mass with obliteration of the paraspinal line and medial border of the hemidiaphragm
- Etiologies include
  - Primary pyogenic abscess, hematogenous and usually due to *Staph. aureus*
  - Secondary pyogenic abscess from contiguous spread, often Crohn's disease
  - Tuberculous psoas abscess
    - Arises by direct extension from tuberculosis osteomyelitis
    - Characteristic features include narrowing of the intervertebral disk space, loss of cortical vertebral outline and calcifications within the abscess

7 **Thoracic kidney**

- Rare disorder, usually asymptomatic and left > right-sided
- Seen as a congenital disorder or in association with diaphragmatic eventration, hernias or traumatic rupture

- Chest X-ray shows a mass extending into the chest in a medial location on posteroanterior films and along the posterior diaphragm on lateral
- Diagnosis can be made with ultrasound or CT

NEUROGENIC TUMORS

90% occur in the posterior mediastinum and they are the most common cause of a posterior mediastinal mass
80% are benign and 50% are asymptomatic

1 **Benign peripheral nerve tumors** – Neurofibroma and Neurilemoma (Schwannoma)
Clinically, these are benign, slow growing tumors and usually asymptomatic with an excellent prognosis, although manifestations can include
   - Intercostal nerve compression with chest pains, paresthesias
   - Airways compression and dyspnea
   - 10% extend through the intervertebral foramen with spinal compression and leg weakness
   - Von-Recklinghausen's neurofibromatosis is seen in approximately ⅓ of patients

   Radiologic features
   - Rounded, lobulated mass in the paravertebral region
   - Bony abnormalities include an expanded intervertebral foramen as well as erosion of ribs and the vertebral pedicles
   - CT scan reveals a homogenous or heterogenous mass (from cystic changes, fat, hemorrhage) with occasional punctate calcification and enhancement following i.v. contrast
   - A 'dumbell' or hourglass configuration is seen with extension through the intervertebral foramen and into the spinal cord
   - MRI can exclude intraspinal tumor extension

2 **Malignant peripheral nerve tumors**

Malignant schwannoma or neurofibrosarcoma comprise about 10% of peripheral nerve tumors

- 50% of patients have neurofibromatosis
- May arise from a simple or plexiform neurofibroma

Clinically, patients are usually symptomatic from local growth as well as mediastinal invasion, chest wall invasion and hematogenous metastases (often to the lungs)

- Recurrence is frequent with incomplete excision and prognosis is poor

Radiologic manifestations include a mass lesion with local invasion of the mediastinum and chest wall

3 **Sympathetic ganglia tumors – Ganglioneuroma**

Clinically rare tumors, seen from childhood to young adulthood with 50% asymptomatic

- Can extend through the intervertebral foramen with symptoms of spinal cord compression
- Good progress with surgical resection

Radiological features

- A broad-based, encapsulated oblong mass along the anterolateral aspect of the vertebral column
- Scoliosis
- Erosions of surrounding bony structures
- Homogeneous or heterogeneous elongated mass on CT
- Intraspinal extension can occasionally be seen

4 **Sympathetic ganglia tumors – Ganglioneuroblastoma**

Clinically seen in patients under 10 years of age and vary from benign to malignant

- Symptoms relate to large tumor size, local invasion including intraspinal extension, as well as to metastases
- Prognosis depends upon the extent of local and distant spread

Radiologic manifestations vary from an oblong paraspinal mass to signs of local invasion and disseminated disease

5 **Sympathetic ganglia tumor – Neuroblastoma**
Clinically a malignant tumor of young children, most of whom present with symptoms of local invasion or distant metastases

6 **Paraganglionoma**
Clinically rare tumors that arise in either the middle mediastinum (aortopulmonary paraganglia) or the posterior mediastinum (aortosympathetic paraganglia)
- 50% are asymptomatic while others present with nonspecific respiratory symptoms or features of excess catecholamine production

7 **Meningocele and meningomyelocele**
Rare posterior mediastinal lesions due to the leptomeninges ballooning through the intervertebral foramen
- Most patients have neurofibromatosis but the lesions are often asymptomatic
- Radiologically they are similar to other neurogenic tumors and present as a paraspinal mass with enlargement of the foramen and bony erosions
- CSF continuity can be seen on CT or MRI

EXTRAMEDULLARY HEMATOPOIESIS (EH) – THORACIC

Definition: Compensatory production of blood cells outside the bone marrow due to marrow dysfunction

Clinically, the liver, spleen and lymph nodes are the most common sites of EH, but several other sites, including the chest, can be involved
- Asymptomatic masses seen most often in congenital hemolytic anemias, e.g. thalassemia, congenital spherocytosis, congenital hemolytic anemia and occasionally in sickle cell disease
- Other causes of bone marrow insufficiency can rarely give a similar picture

- Course is one of slow or no growth over time
- Origin of the hematopoietic tissue is unclear ? bone ? heterotopic cells

Radiologic features

1. Unilateral or bilateral, smooth, sharply defined, often lobulated paraspinal masses
2. Usually located below T6
3. May be accompanied by paracostal masses
4. Lacy architecture of vertebrae as well as widening of the vertebral ends of ribs with periosteal elevation is seen on CT as a manifestation of marrow hyperplasia
5. No erosions seen in vertebrae or ribs
6. Adipose tissue may be detected within the mass on MRI
7. Bone marrow scans may reveal intense uptake by the mass(es)

MEDIASTINAL LYMPHADENOPATHY

General Features

- Normal nodes <1 cm in the short axis
- Round or oval soft tissue densities contrast with the surrounding mediastinal fat
- Neoplastic or non-neoplastic nodal disease can result in
  - Enlargement
  - Coalescence with fusion of adjacent nodes into a mass
  - Invasion of local fat and connective tissue with no recognizable node identified

CT Shortcomings

1. Can only detect abnormal nodes by size
2. Cannot distinguish hyperplastic from neoplastic adenopathy
3. May miss significant adenopathy found at thoracotomy
4. Vessels may be confused with nodes

Classification

1 **Parietal nodes** drain the thoracic well and extrathoracic structures
  - Anterior
    - Internal mammary nodes
  - Posterior
    - Intercostal nodes (costo-vertebral junction)
    - Juxtavertebral nodes
  - Diaphragmatic
    - Paracardiac nodes (pericardial attachment to diaphragm)
    - Juxtaphrenic nodes (phrenic nerves meet the diaphragm)
    - Retrocrural nodes

2 **Visceral nodes** drain the intrathoracic structures
  - Prevascular nodes
  - Posterior mediastinal nodes
    - Peri-esophageal
    - Peri-aortic
  - Tracheobronchial nodes
    - Paratracheal
    - Azygous
    - Aortopulmonary
    - Bronchopulmonary
    - Subcarinal

Sequelae of Lymphadenopathy

- Paratracheal nodes
  - SVC syndrome
- Hilar nodes
  - Pulmonary artery compression/obstruction
- Sub-carinal nodes
  - Esophageal compression/obstruction
  - Pulmonary artery or vein compression/obstruction

*all can cause tracheobronchial compression, obstruction, broncholithiasis

Etiology of Mediastinal Lymphadenopathy

1 ***Infectious**
- Bacterial (BBATT)
  - **B**ubonic plague
  - ***B**ordetella pertussis*
  - **A**nthrax
  - **T**ularemia
  - **T**uberculosis
- Mycoplasma
- Viral
  - Epstein-Barr
- Fungal
  - Histoplasmosis
  - Coccidioidomycosis
  - Sporotrichosis
- Parasitic
  - Toxoplasmosis
- Chlamydia
  - Psittacosis

2 ***Inflammatory**, e.g. sarcoid, Castleman's disease, Kikuchi's syndrome

3 ***Inhalational**, e.g. silicosis, berylliosis, coalworkers' pneumoconiosis

4 ***Neoplastic**
- Lymphoma
- Metastatic – lung, breast, melanoma, colon, kidney, germ cell, head and neck (including thyroid)

5 **Angioimmunoblastic lymphadenopathy**

6 **Lymphomatoid granulomatosis**

7 **LAM**

8 **Dilantin**

9 **Amyloid**

10 **Septic emboli**

11 **Whipple's disease**

12 **Normal**

13 **Pseudoadenopathy**, i.e. enlarged nodes diagnosed radiologically but not seen pathologically

14 **Pathologic diagnoses without specific etiology**, e.g. hyperplastic, edematous, fibrous capsular thickening

Diagnostic Clues and Investigation

1 **Density features**

- **Non-specific calcifications**
  - Tuberculosis
  - Fungal (histoplasmosis)
  - Sarcoid
  - Silicosis
  - CWP
  - Hodgkin's (post RT)
  - Pneumocystis (rare)
  - Metastatic colonic adenocarcinoma (rare)
  - Castleman's disease (rare)
  - Amyloid (rare)
  - Scleroderma (rare)
- **Eggshell calcifications** where the periphery of nodes are calcified with the central portions sometimes showing additional calcifications

  Silicosis
  - Seen in approximately 5% of cases
  - Hilar nodes most ofen involved but can also be seen in the mediastinal, cervical and intraperitoneal nodes

  CWP
  - Seen in approximately 1% of cases

  Sarcoid
  - Seen in a few percent of patients, typically those with advanced parenchymal disease

  Lymphoma
  - Post-radiotherapy
  - Develops one to several years post-treatment

  Rarely seen with tuberculosis, histoplasmosis, amyloid, scleroderma

- **Necrotic** (low density) – tuberculosis, fungal, lung cancer, lymphoma, seminoma
- **Cavitary** (hilar nodes) – tuberculosis
- **Vascular** (enhancing)
  - Metastatic cancer, kidney, lung, thyroid, carcinoid
  - Castleman's disease
  - Angioimmunoblastic lymphadenopathy
  - Bacillary angiomatosis

2 **Location**

- Bilaternal hilar, paratracheal and aortopulmonary nodes are typical of sarcoid
- Anterior and posterior mediastinal nodes are common in lymphoma but uncommon in sarcoid
- Paracardiac nodes are almost always malignant and secondary to non-Hodgkin's lymphoma, metastatic cancer
- Internal mammary nodes are usually secondary to metastatic breast cancer or Hodgkin's lymphoma and rare in lung cancer or granulomatous diseases, e.g. tuberculosis
- Posterior mediastinal nodes are usually due to non-Hodgkin's lymphoma and rare in Hodgkin's disease

3 **Associated radiologic abnormalities**

- Airways, e.g. endobronchial neoplasm
- Parenchyma, e.g. silicosis, tuberculosis, sarcoid, pneumonia, neoplasm
- Pleura, e.g. nodular or diffuse pleural thickening and/or pleural effusion from mesothelioma or metastatic neoplasm
- Mediastinum, e.g. primary mediastinal neoplasm
- Chest wall, e.g. axillary nodes, breast cancer, metastatic bone disease

4 **Extrathoracic disease**

- Known extrapulmonary malignancy or other systemic disease which might have associated mediastinal lymphadenopathy

- Hepatosplenomegaly or lymphadenopathy involving the pelvis, abdomen, neck or axilla

5 **Asymptomatic lymphadenopathy** – suspect the following
- Tuberculosis
- Fungal infection
- Sarcoid
- Castleman's disease (localized hyaline vascular type)
- Lymphoma
- Metastatic cancer
- Dilantin
- Amyloid

CASTLEMAN'S DISEASE

Also known as **Angiofollicular Hyperplasia; Giant Lymph Node Hyperplasia**

Definition: Group of rare lymphoproliferative disorders of unknown etiology, classified into localized and disseminated disease

Localized Castleman's Disease

Disease confined to one mediastinal component (radiologically or surgically) without clinical or radiologic evidence of extrathoracic disease

Pathologically, there are hypervascular masses with large feeding vessels histologically characterized by the hyaline vascular variant on lymph node biopsy with
- Nodal hyperplasia and atrophic follicles surrounded by concentric rings of small lymphocytes
- Capillary proliferation with hyalinized vessels entering the follicles
- Plasma cell variant is rare (see below)

Clinically, it is seen in all age groups with a peak in the fourth decade and female predominance, presentations including

- Asymptomatic radiologic finding
- Non-specific respiratory symptoms due to compression or invasion of contiguous structures
- Systemic symptoms (uncommon)

Diagnosis usually requires mediastinoscopy or open biopsy as fine needle aspirates are usually non-diagnostic

- Prognosis is good, particularly if complete excision can be performed

Radiologic features

1 A soft tissue mass in the hilum or any mediastinal compartment, most commonly the middle mediastinum
2 Intense tumor blush on angiography with large feeding vessels arising from the intercostals, internal mammary and bronchial arteries
3 CT findings
   - *Solitary mass which may be encapsulated, without associated disease
   - Solitary mass with local compression/invasion of contiguous structures, e.g. bronchi, or associated lymphadenopathy in the same mediastinal compartment
   - Multiple enlarged nodes in the same mediastinal compartment in the absence of a dominant mass
   - Enhancement is universal but the degree is variable
   - Calcifications in 5–10% of cases

Disseminated Castleman's Disease

Disease in more than one mediastinal compartment or the presence of extrathoracic disease clinically or radiologically

Histologically, it is characterized by the plasma cell variant (rarely hyaline vascular), manifest by a paucity of follicular hyalinized vessels and an accumulation of plasma cells in the interfollicular areas

Clinically, it is seen in all age groups, peaks in the fifth decade, has a female predominance and can present with

- Non-specific respiratory symptoms
- Systemic symptoms of fevers, night sweats, weight loss
- Anemia, polyclonal gammopathy
- Extrathoracic manifestations of neuropathy, splenomegaly, ascites, lymphadenopathy (peripheral, retroperitoneal)
- Associated diseases including AIDS, Kaposi's, POEMS
- Rarely asymptomatic
- Prognosis is poor with behavior that of malignant lymphoma

Radiologic features

1 Bilateral mediastinal widening often involving the anterior compartment, a solitary mass rarely seen on chest X-ray
2 CT findings
   - Multiple enlarged nodes in several different areas without a dominant mass
   - Variable enhancement post-contrast
   - Rare parenchymal reticulo-nodular densities

Diagnosis can be made by biopsy of thoracic or extrathoracic disease

KIKUCHI'S DISEASE

Definition: Self-limited disease of unknown etiology ? viral, usually described in Japanese or other Asians but now reported in other racial and ethnic groups in other countries

- Patients present as an acute illness of 2–3 weeks duration with cervical adenopathy, fever, weight loss, GI complaints, skin rash
- Nodal involvement is usually unifocal although multifocal involvement of all nodal areas including mediastinal lymphadenopathy has been described, as has hepatosplenomegaly
- Usually seen in young adults with a 4:1 ratio of females to males

- Leucopenia, atypical lymphocytes and increased ESR are the common hematologic features
- Diagnosis is based on histology which shows necrotizing lymphadenitis
- The clinical differential includes tuberculosis, fungal infections, sarcoid, lymphoma, HIV, CMV, toxoplasmosis, cat-scratch fever

MEDIASTINAL LYMPHOMAS

Primary Mediastinal Lymphoma

1 Hodgkin's – usually nodular sclerosing
2 Non-Hodgkin's
  - Lymphoblastic lymphoma comprises ~60% of cases of primary non-Hodgkin's mediastinal lymphoma, the majority of patients being children or adolescents
    - Patients present with chest symptoms related to invasion of the tracheobronchial tree, pleura, pericardium as well as involvement of extrathoracic sites, e.g. nodes, CNS, leukemic phase
  - Primary mediastinal B cell lymphoma with sclerosis
    - A non-Hodgkin's lymphoma of B cell origin, clinically seen in young adults and presenting subacutely with symptoms of a rapidly enlarging intrathoracic mass
    - SVC syndrome is common in association with non-specific respiratory symptoms as well as systemic features of fevers, night sweats and weight loss
    - 90% of cases are confined to the chest with kidneys the most common extrathoracic organ involved
    - Radiologically usually presents as an anterior superior mediastinal mass
    - The mediastinal lesion may occur in isolation, spread directly to adjacent nodes in the hilar/supraclavicular region and/or invade contiguous intrathoracic organs

- Differential diagnosis includes
  - Hodgkin's lymphoma
  - Other non-Hodgkin's lymphomas
  - Malignant thymoma
  - Germ cell tumor
  - Metastatic cancer

Features Common to Hodgkin's (HD) and Non-Hodgkin's Lymphoma (NHL)

Mediastinal adenopathy is the most common intrathoracic manifestation of disease and can occur in isolation or as part of generalized lymphoma, with 5–10% of patients presenting as a primary mediastinal lesion

Radiologic findings

1 Discrete mass, usually lobulated and located in the anterior-superior mediastinum
   - Middle mediastinal lesions are less common and a posterior mediastinal presentation is rare

2 Multiple rounded soft tissue masses, i.e. lymph nodes

3 Thymic mass

4 Extension of mediastinal nodal disease
   - Respiratory system
     - Tracheobronchial narrowing
     - Peribronchial spread into the lungs
     - Pleural invasion
     - Chest wall invasion
   - CVS
     - SVC syndrome
     - Compression or obstruction of other vascular structures
     - Pericardial or myocardial invasion
   - Esophagus
   - Mediastinal soft tissues
   - Axillary adenopathy

5 Residual masses may remain after radiotherapy with difficulty distinguishing 'sterile' from active disease, MRI and gallium scans potentially of value

6 Recurrent nodal lymphoma must be distinguished from
   - Spontaneous mediastinal hemorrhage secondary to radiotherapy/chemotherapy
   - Rebound thymic hyperplasia
   - Thymic cyst post-radiotherapy
   - Thymic lymphoma
7 Chest X-rays may underdiagnose diseases involving the internal mammary, subcarinal and hilar nodes
8 CT may reveal masses of soft tissue attenuation which are heterogeneous in density due to hemorrhage, cystic degeneration or necrosis

Differential Features of HD and NHL

Clinically	HD	NHL
Frequency	• 30% of lymphomas	• 70% of lymphomas
Distribution	• Supradiaphragmatic disease, usually with cervical or supraclavicular adenopathy	• Generalized disease is common
Systemic features	• 25% have constitutional symptoms of fever, night sweats, weight loss; only 5% have extranodal disease	• Majority have constitutional symptoms; extranodal disease is common
Presentation	• Often asymptomatic, occasional non-specific respiratory symptoms, rarely invasive symptoms	• non-specific respiratory or invasive symptoms are common
Isolated mediastinal disease	• <10% (superficial or retroperitoneal node involvement is typical)	• <10% but typical of primary mediastinal B cell lymphoma with sclerosis

Table 52.5

Radiologically	HD	NHL
Mediastinal disease at presentation	• 65% (most commonly nodular sclerosing)	• <20% and seen with lymphoblastic lymphoma or primary mediastinal B cell lymphoma with sclerosis
Tumor origin	• Unifocal	• Multifocal
Spread to other nodal regions	• Contiguous	• Often non-contiguous
Nodal density	• May be necrotic or may calcify post-Rx	• Same
Nodal distribution	• Anterior mediastinal and paratracheal are most common although any nodal group can be involved	• Same
Disease extension	• May extend into the mediastinum with compressive/invasive symptoms	• Same
Pleuropulmonary disease Presentation: Subsequently:	• 10–15% • Up to 40% • Recurrent disease post-radiation most often manifest as a parenchymal mass (+/or upper mediastinal adenopathy) • Other malignancies developing post-treatment include acute leukemia, non-Hodgkin's lymphoma, lung cancer	• 5% • Up to 30%

Table 52.6

MEDIASTINITIS

Acute Mediastinitis – Etiology

1 Esophageal rupture
- Spontaneous (Boerhaave's syndrome)
- Carcinoma
- Perforated esophageal ulcer
- Foreign body
- Instrumentation

2 Post-surgical (see Lung Injuries p. 442), e.g. cardiac surgery, colon interposition
3 Suppurative head and neck infections spreading via the retropharyngeal space
4 Tracheobronchial rupture
5 Retroperitoneal abscess
6 Vertebral osteomyelitis
7 Anthrax
8 Penetrating trauma
9 Hematogenous dissemination

Esophageal Perforation

Clinical presentation is that of acute pleuritic retrosternal chest pain, usually in conjunction with vomiting, but occasionally seen with acute asthma, exercise or labor

- The patient appears acutely ill with subcutaneous emphysema in the soft tissues of the neck, positive Haman's sign and fever
- Often a rapid downhill course with hypotension and death
- If the patient survives the initial insult, the sequelae include mediastinal abscess with fistula formation

Chest X-ray findings

1 Mediastinal widening
2 Gas within the mediastinum, subcutaneous soft tissues, and pleura
3 Mediastinal air–fluid level
4 Pleural effusion, left (distal esophageal perforation) or right (mid-esophageal perforation)

CT scan findings
1 Soft tissue attenuation in mediastinal fat
2 Mediastinal gas or abscess
3 Obliteration of the mediastinal fat planes
4 Displacement or compression of mediastinal structures

Diagnostic studies include
1 Oral contrast study revealing extravasation from the esophagus
2 Pleural tap revealing a low pH, high salivary amylase, food particles, squamous epithelial cells, +/– positive cultures

Chronic Mediastinitis – Fibrosing or Granulomatous

Definition: Inflammation and fibrosis, often progressive, of the mediastinal soft tissues with pathology being granulomatous or fibrosing

- Granulomatous
  - Histoplasmosis, tuberculosis, other fungi
  - More benign process than the fibrosing variant and usually presents as a mediastinal mass
- Fibrosing
  - End-stage infection, most often histoplasmosis, where an agent is not identified
  - Non-infectious and associated with fibrosis in the retroperitoneum orbit, thyroid or cecum
  - Case reports following radiation, other fungal infections

The mediastinal reaction can be focal or diffuse
- Focal – due to tuberculosis or fungi, with local invasion in tuberculosis, but a hypersensivity reaction to histoplasma antigen in histoplasmosis
- Diffuse – involving the entire mediastinum but mainly the paratracheal and perihilar regions

The **clinical** spectrum ranges from an asymptomatic widening of the mediastinum, usually paratracheal in location, to SVC syndrome (common clinical presentation), to a multitude of chest symptoms depending upon the **site** of involvement as well as the **specific structures** involved (see below)

- Isolated hilar involvement can present with bronchial compression/obstruction simulating neoplastic disease as well as pulmonary artery occlusion with resulting oligemia resembling thromboembolic disease

Areas of involvement	Structures	Complications
Hilar nodes	• Main stem bronchi	• Narrowing or obstruction • Obstructive pneumonitis • Broncholithiasis • Hemoptysis
	• Pulmonary arteries	• PA narrowing/occlusion • PA thrombosis • Pulmonary hypertension • Pulmonary infarction
	• Recurrent laryngeal n.	• Hoarseness
Subcarinal nodes	• Main stem bronchi	• As above
	• Pulmonary arteries	• As above
	• Pulmonary veins	• Venous hypertension and transudative effusions • Hemoptysis
	• Esophagus	• Esophageal narrowing • Tracheo-esophageal fistula
	• Pericardium	• Constrictive pericarditis
Paratracheal nodes	• SVC	• SVC syndrome
	• Azygous vein	• Venous obstruction
	• Trachea	• Tracheal narrowing
	• Thoracic duct	• Chylothorax

Table 52.7

Chest X-ray findings

May be normal in patients with extensive disease but radiologic findings can include

1 **Airways**
  - Tracheobroncheal narrowing

2 **Parenchyma**
  - Pulmonary edema
  - Pulmonary infarction

- Granulomatous lesions
- Obstructive pneumonitis

3 **Pleura**

- Pleural effusions

4 **Vasculature**

- Pulmonary artery hypertension
- Pulmonary artery compression/occlusion
- Oligemia
- Signs of pulmonary venous hypertension and edema

5 **Mediastinum/hilum**

- Lobulated paratracheal mass, right > left (most common radiologic manifestation)
- Calcifications
- Hilar mass or lymphadenopathy which often calcifies
- Esophageal narrowing or tracheo-esophageal fistula formation

CT findings

1 Infiltrative mediastinal process with obliteration of fat planes
   - +/– mass lesion
   - +/– calcifications
   - +/– lymph node calcifications
   - +/– splenic calcifications
2 Visualization of the above chest X-ray findings, particularly tracheobronchial narrowing
3 Evidence of collateral blood flow
4 Thrombosis of SVC

Diagnosis can be suspected from the clinical presentation and the above radiologic abnormalities
Definitive diagnosis requires tissue confirmation from mediastinoscopy or thoracotomy

Prognosis is generally poor but the natural history of disease can vary
Deaths are often secondary to cor pulmonale, bronchial obstruction, bronchial infection and hemoptysis, the latter

potentially arising from the bronchial tree, pulmonary arteries or pulmonary vein invasion by fibrotic tissue

Fraser R.S., Muller N.L., Colman N., Paré P.D. (1999) *Diagnosis of Diseases of the Chest* 4th Edn., WB Saunders.

Naidich, D.P., Zerhouni, E.A., Siegelman, S.S. (1998) *Computed Tomography and Magnetic Resonance of the Thorax*, 3rd edn. New York: Raven Press.

Moss, A., Gamsu, Genant (1992) Thorax and neck. In: *Computed Tomography of the Body with Magnetic Resonance Imaging*, 2nd edn., vol. 1.: W.B. Saunders.

Baum, G.L., Crapo, J.D., Celli, B.R., Karlinsky, J.B. (eds) (1997) *Textbook of Pulmonary Diseases*, 6th edn.: Lippincott-Raven.

Fishman, A.P., Elias, J.A., Fishman, J.A., Grippi, M.A., Kaiser, L.R., Senior, R.N. (1998) *Fishman's Pulmonary Diseases and Disorders*, 3rd edn.: McGraw-Hill.

Strollo, D., Rosado-de-Christenson, L., Jett, J. *et al.* (1997) Primary mediastinal tumors. *Chest* **112**: 511–522, 1344–1357.

Lazzarino, M., Orlandi, E., Paulli, M. *et al.* (1993) Primary mediastinal B-cell lymphoma with sclerosis. *J. Clin. Oncol.* **11**: 2306–2313.

Quintanilla-Martinez, L., Wilkins, E., Choi, N. *et al.* (1994) Thymoma. *Cancer* **74**: 606–616.

Jolles, H., Henry, D., Robertson, J. *et al.* (1996) Mediastinitis following median sternotomy: CT findings. *Radiology* **201**: 463–466.

Norris, A., Krasinskas, A., Shalhaney, K. *et al.* (1996) Kikuchi-Fujimoto disease – a benign case of fever and lymphadenopathy. *AJM* **171**: 401–405.

Unger, P., Rappaport, K., Strauchen, J. (1987) Necrotizing lymphadenitis. *Arch. Pathol. Lab. Med.* **111**: 1031–1034.

Rosado-de-Chirstenson, M., Pugatch, R., Moran, C. *et al.* (1994) Thymoplioma: analysis of 27 cases. *Radiology* **193**: 121–126.

Lewis, J.E., Wick, M.R., Scheithauer, B.W. *et al.* (1987) Thymoma: a clinicopathologic review. *Cancer* **60**: 2727–2743.

Casson, A.G., Incubt, R. (1990) Pancreatic pseudocyst – an uncommon mediastinal mass. *Chest* **98**: 717–718.

Verley, J., Hollmann, K. (1985) Thymoma: a comparative study of clinical stages, histologic features and survival in 200 cases. *Cancer* **55**: 1074–1086.

Onik, G., Goodman, P.C. (1983) CT of Castleman's disease. *AJR* **140**: 691–692.

Loyd, J. E., Tilman, B., Atkinson, J. *et al.* (1988) Mediastinal fibrosis complicating histoplasmosis. *Medicine* **67**: 295–310.

Goodwin, R.A., Nickell, J., Roger M., Des Prez. (1972) Mediastinal fibrosis complicating healed primary histoplasmosis and tuberculosis. *Medicine* **52**: 227–246.

Pescarmong, E. *et al.* (1990) Analysis of prognostic factors and clinicopathologic staging of thymoma. *Ann. Thor. Surg.* **50**: 534–538.

53 Neoplasms

LUNG CANCER – CLINICAL PRESENTATIONS

Pulmonary

1 Asymptomatic radiologic finding (in ~10% of patients)
2 Airways invasion
    - e.g. cough (most common presenting symptom), hemoptysis, dyspnea, stridor, post-obstructive pneumonia, wheezing
3 Parenchymal disease
    - e.g. cough, hemoptysis, dyspnea, bronchorrhea, post-

obstructive pneumonitis, abscess, reactivation of tuberculosis

4 Wheezing
- e.g. associated COPD or asthma, vocal cord paralysis, endotracheal/endobronchial tumor, peribronchial tumor/lymph nodes, lymphangitic cancer, carcinoid syndrome, pulmonary edema from pulmonary vein or myocardial invasion by cancer

5 Vascular invasion
- Pulmonary artery, e.g. pulmonary infarction
- Pulmonary veins, e.g. pulmonary edema

Extrapulmonary Intrathoracic

1 Chest wall invasion
- Thoracic inlet, e.g. Pancoast's
- Sternum, ribs, vertebral column, e.g. chest or back pains, spinal cord symptoms

2 Pleural
- e.g. pleural pain from invasion or pneumothorax

3 Cardiac disease
- Pericardial
  - Most frequent cardiac manifestation clinically
  - Secondary to tumor infiltration or radiotherapy
  - Sequelae include effusion, tamponade and constrictive pericarditis
- Myocardial
  - Secondary to tumor infiltration or drugs, e.g. adriamycin
  - Sequelae include arrythmias, failure
- Endocardial
  - May be secondary to marantic endocarditis, bacterial endocarditis, tumor invasion of the valves or mural endocardium, radiation
  - Sequelae include ventricular outflow obstruction, valvular insufficiency, vegetations with emboli
- Coronary vessels
  - Coronary narrowing may be secondary to tumor compression of vessels, tumor emboli, thromboemboli or *in situ* thrombosis due to coagulopathy

- Sequelae include angina, arrythmias, CHF, conduction blocks

4 Vascular invasion
- Superior vena cava, e.g. superior vena cava syndrome

5 Esophageal invasion
- e.g. dysphagia, tracheo-esophageal or broncho-esophageal fistula, recurrent aspiration pneumonia

6 Other mediastinal invasion
- e.g. retrosternal pain or fullness
- e.g. nerve invasion with
  - Hoarseness (recurrent laryngeal)
  - Dyspnea (phrenic)
  - Horner's syndrome (sympathetic chain)

Extrathoracic Metastases

(⅓ of patients will present with distant metastases)

1 Scalene, supraclavicular, or anterior cervical lymphadenopathy
2 Liver, e.g. abdominal pains, jaundice, ascites
3 Bone, e.g. hypercalcemia, pathologic fracture, bone pain, swelling
4 CNS, e.g. brain (presenting feature in ~10% of patients), spinal cord, meninges
5 Skin, e.g. nodules
6 Eye, e.g. proptosis
7 GI metastases, e.g. obstruction, ulceration, perforation, bleeding, anemia
8 Adrenals, e.g. flank or abdominal pain, Addison's disease

Extrathoracic Non-Metastatic

(Seen in ~10% of patients)

1 **Non-specific systemic symptoms** of anorexia, fatigue, weight loss and weakness

2 **Neuromuscular disorders**
- Neurologic, with involvement of any component of the nervous system from cerebral hemispheres (encephalopathy) to the peripheral nerves (neuropathies)
- Muscular – dermatomyositis, polymyositis
- Neuromuscular – Lambert-Eaton syndrome

  - Normally, a depolarizing action potentially promotes the flow of calcium into the presynaptic terminal via the voltage-gated calcium channels which are embedded in the presynaptic membrane
  - In the presence of calcium, the presynaptic acetylcholine-containing vesicles release their contents into the synaptic cleft, activating post-synaptic receptors, resulting in depolarization and subsequent muscle-fiber contraction
  - Small cell lung cancer antibodies are thought to cross-react and destroy the pre-synaptic voltage-gated calcium channels, resulting in the neurologic symptoms described below
  - Seen with small cell carcinoma where patients present with slowly developing leg weakness and fatigue
  - Autonomic dysfunction, particularly a dry mouth, is common, as well as constipation, impotence and blurred vision
  - Diplopia and ptosis are the major cranial nerve manifestations with dysparthria, dysphagia and impaired chewing also occurring

3 **Cutaneous**

- Clubbing
- Hypertrophic pulmonary osteoarthropathy
  - 90% are secondary to bronchogenic cancer, squamous > adenocarcinoma, but not seen with small cell cancers
  - Can also be seen with localized fibrous tumors of the pleura and rarely in mesothelioma, tuberculosis or metastatic disease
  - Clinically presents with warm, swollen, tender hands, feet and lower legs as well as small joint effusions
  - Bone scan is pathognomonic with superiosteal bone formation at the distal end of the long bones
- Multiple other cutaneous syndromes described

4 **Hematologic**

- Anemia/polycythemia

- Hypercoagulopathy
- Leucocytosis/eosinophilia/leucoerythroblastic smear
- Migratory thrombophlebitis
- Non-bacterial thrombotic endocarditis
  - Characterized by the development of fibrinous vegetations on any heart valves, usually left-sided
  - Seen with adenocarcinomas, e.g. lung, pancreas and may be a manifestation of a hypercoagulable state with an abnormal coagulation profile often demonstrated
  - Clinical features are those of peripheral emboli including
    - Renal and splenic (most common) infarcts
    - Cardiac with infarction
    - Cerebral with stroke or encephalopathy
    - Limb occlusions
    - Mesenteric artery occlusions
    - Subungual hemorrhages
  - Diagnostic features
    - Heart murmur (often absent)
    - Underlying neoplasm
    - Evidence of peripheral emboli
    - Negative blood cultures
    - Vegetations on echocardiography

5 **Endocrine**

- Hyponatremia, hypercalcemia, multiple others described

6 **Renal**

- Glomerulonephritis, others

LUNG CANCER – RADIOLOGIC MANIFESTATIONS

Radiologic manifestations reflect the histologic type, size and location of the primary tumor as well as local, regional and distant spread

'Normal' chest X-ray

1 Endotracheal/endobronchial lesion
2 Small peripheral lesion
3 Lesion hidden by ribs
4 Lesion seen but misinterpreted as overlapping shadow or calcified first costal cartilage
5 Perihilar tumor

Airways

1 Tracheal narrowing – intrinsic/extrinsic
2 Bronchial narrowing/obstruction – intrinsic/extrinsic
3 Mucoid impaction (distal to an obstructing lesion)
4 Bronchial wall thickening – 'cuff sign' (cuff of soft tissue surrounding a bronchus)

Parenchyma

1 Atelectasis/volume loss
2 Obstructive pneumonitis
3 Solitary nodule ('coin' lesion)
4 Multiple nodules
5 Mass lesion including an apical or superior sulcus mass
6 'Pneumonia-like' consolidation (bronchioloalveolar cancer)
7 Unilateral or bilateral infiltrates
8 Cavitation (squamous > large cell > adeno but absent with small cell)
9 Eccentric calcifications
10 Expiratory air trapping
11 Localized hyperlucency (rare)
12 Localized hyperinflation (rare)

Vascular

1 Pulmonary infarction (central pulmonary artery occlusion)
2 Localized pulmonary edema (pulmonary vein obstruction)
3 Lymphangitic spread with reticulo-nodular disease (localized/generalized)

Pleura

1 Effusion
2 Thickening, nodules, masses
3 Apical cap
4 Pneumothorax

Hilum

1 Enlargement secondary to adenopathy or primary tumor
2 Increased hilar density

Chest wall

1 Hemidiaphragm paralysis
2 Diaphragmatic invasion
3 Bone destruction
4 Chest wall mass

Mediastinum (secondary to nodal metastases or local invasion)

1 Lymphadenopathy/mass (hilar/mediastinal nodes are most common extrapulmonary metastatic site)
 - Widened superior mediastinum with lobulated contours
 - Thickened right paratracheal line
 - Convexity of the aorto-pulmonary window
 - Widened carina with increased subcarinal density
 - Posterior mediastinal nodes
2 Interdigitation of tumor with mediastinal fat
3 Compression, displacement, obstruction or encasement of mediastinal structures
4 Cardiomegaly secondary to pericardial effusion

Distant metastases

1 Adrenal enlargement
2 Liver masses
3 Brain masses
4 Bony lesions
5 Kidney mass
6 Contralateral lung
7 Any other organ

CT Utility

1 Diagnosis of a **benign** peripheral lesion
   - Calcification (e.g. granuloma)
   - Fat (hamartoma)
   - Enhancing (AV malformation)
2 **Confirmation** that a nodule on chest X-ray is a parenchymal opacity versus a focal scar, a pleural or a chest wall lesion
3 Diagnosis of possible **metastatic** disease from an extra-pulmonary site based on the presence of two or more nodules
4 Diagnosis of **non-resectable** lung cancer
   - T_4 disease
   - N_3 disease, i.e. contralateral hilar or mediastinal adenopathy
   - M_1 disease
5 **Strongly suspect** but not prove peripheral lung cancer
   - Spiculated or lobulated margins
   - Size >3 cm diameter (less than 5% are benign)
   - Air bronchogram with a cut-off, ectatic or tortuous bronchus
6 **Stage** a known lung cancer i.e. TNM, including evaluation of the adrenals and liver

CT shortcomings

1 Lymphadenopathy
   - Cancer within normal sized nodes
   - Enlarged hyperplastic nodes without cancer, particularly with obstructive pneumonitis
   - Undetected enlarged nodes, the sensitivity and specificity for evaluation of mediastinal nodes >1 cm in diameter being ~65%
2 Subtle mediastinal invasion with
   - Abutment of the tumor on the mediastinum, or
   - Loss of the fat plane between the tumor and adjacent mediastinal structures
   - Resectability is often only determined at surgery
3 Distinguishing neoplastic contiguity with the pleural surface from pleural or chest wall invasion, the latter only

being definitive with visualization of a chest wall mass or rib destruction

4 Submucosal bronchial extension of cancer
5 Undetected pleural/pericardial tumor nodules

MRI utility

1 Evaluation of superior sulcus tumors
2 Determining the presence of chest wall, vertebral, spinal canal or diaphragmatic invasion
3 Perihilar pulmonary artery or vein invasion
4 Pericardial invasion e.g. bronchogenic cancer, mesothelioma
5 Mediastinal invasion
6 MRI shortcomings are similar to CT shortcomings

Positron emission tomography (PET)

PET scan with ^{18}F-fluoro-2-deoxyglucose (FDG) is used as a 'metabolic' imager to complement the anatomic information from CT scan

- Rationale for its use is the increased activity of cell membrane glucose transporters and intracellular hexokinase in malignant cells with the accumulation of FDG and its subsequent detection

There is still controversy as to its role but the uses postulated for PET scanning include

1 Separation of malignant from benign nodules (sensitivity ~95% and specificity ~75%), with granulomas or active infection mainly responsible for false positive results
    - False negatives can result from small tumor size, low tumor metabolic activity (carcinoids, alveolar cell cancer) or uncontrolled hyperglycemia
2 Detection of mediastinal metastases with sensitivity ~70–90% (false negatives usually secondary to micrometastases) and specificity ~95% (usually secondary to granulomas)
    - More sensitive and specific in detection of metastases in normal-sized nodes and differentiating enlarged benign from malignant nodes

3 Detection of distant metastases where it is said to have 95% accuracy for bone metastases (better than that of bone scans) but is insensitive for brain metastases
   - High sensitivity (~100%) and specificity (~80%) for detection of adrenal metastases

4 Differentiating recurrent cancer from scar tissue post-surgically

CENTRAL CANCER – DIFFERENTIAL OF PERIPHERAL INFILTRATES

Airways disease (obstructed bronchus on CT scan or bronchoscopy)
- Mucoid impaction
- Atelectasis
- Obstructive pneumonitis

Vascular disease
- Pulmonary infarct secondary to central artery invasion or thromboemboli
- Localized pulmonary edema secondary to pulmonary venous obstruction
- Lymphangitic carcinoma (HRCT)

Parenchymal disease
- Subacute necrotizing pulmonary aspergillosis
- Bacterial pneumonia
- Tuberculosis
- Tumor spread – bronchogenic/hematogenous
- Radiation pneumonitis (diagnosis of exclusion)
- Chemotherapy-induced pneumonitis (diffuse and bilateral)
- Generalized pulmonary edema post-radiation myocarditis

CLASSIFICATIONS AND STAGING

TNM Classification (non-small cell carcinoma)
- The TNM staging is initially a clinical stage, i.e. cTNM, based upon clinical, radiologic and invasive studies, while

following surgery, a pathologic, i.e. pTNM classification will more accurately indicate prognosis

T

Tx – Malignant cells in bronchopulmonary secretions without radiologic or bronchoscopic visualization of cancer

TIS – Carcinoma *in situ*

T_1 – ≤3 cm in diameter
- Surrounded by lung or intact visceral pleura
- Involvement of a lobar or more distal bronchus

T_2 – >3 cm in diameter
- Invasion of the visceral pleura
- Atelectasis or obstructive pneumonitis extending to the hilum but not involving an entire lung
- ≥2 cm from the carina

T_3 – Tumor of any size with invasion of chest wall (including superior sulcus tumors), diaphragm, mediastinal pleura or parietal pericardium
- <2 cm from the carina without carinal invasion
- Atelectasis or obstructive pneumonitis of an entire lung

T_4 – Tumor of any size with
- *Respiratory*
  - Malignant pleural effusion +/or pleural metastases, tracheal or carinal invasion, satellite tumor nodule(s) within the primary-tumor lobe
- *CVS*
  - Heart, superior vena cava, aorta, pulmonary artery or pulmonary vein invasion
- *GI*
  - Esophageal invasion
- *Mediastinal invasion*
  - Interdigitation of tumor with fat
  - Phrenic or recurrent laryngeal nerve invasion

- Compression, displacement, obstruction or encasement of mediastinal structures
- *Musculoskeletal*
  - Vertebral column invasion
  - Extensive chest wall invasion

N

N_x – Regional nodes cannot be assessed

N_0 – No regional node metastases

N_1 – Metastases to N_1 nodes which are distal to the mediastinal pleural reflection and within the visceral pleura, i.e. intrapulmonary

- #10: hilar nodes (hilar enlargement)
- #11: interlobar nodes (hilar enlargement)
- #12: lobar nodes
- #13: segmental nodes
- #14: subsegmental nodes

N_2 – Metastases to N_2 nodes which lie within the ipsilateral mediastinal pleura (ipsilateral mediastinal and subcarinal nodes)

- *Superior mediastinal nodes*
  - #1: highest mediastinal nodes
  - #2: upper paratracheal nodes
  - #3: prevascular and retrotracheal nodes
  - #4: lower paratracheal nodes
- *Aortic nodes*
  - #5: subaortic nodes (aortopulmonary window)
  - #6: para-aortic nodes (ascending aorta or phrenic)
- *Inferior mediastinal nodes*
  - #7: subcarinal nodes
  - #8: paraesophageal nodes (below carina)
  - #9: pulmonary ligament nodes

N_3 – Metastases to contralateral mediastinal or hilar nodes
– Metastases to ipsilateral or contralateral scalene or supraclavicular nodes

M

M_0 – No distant metastases

M_1 – Distant metastases

- Intrathoracic
  - Ipsilateral or contralateral lymphangitic or hematogenous metastases
  - Ipsilateral or contralateral pleural metastases
- Extrathoracic
  - Adrenal, liver, brain, bone, kidney, other

International Staging System – TNM Subsets*

Staging is used to (1) predict prognosis (2) decide therapeutic options

Stage (clinical)	TNM	5 yr survival of resected patients	
0	$T_{is}N_0M_0$	Very high	
1A	$cT_1N_0M_0$	61% (*p stage 67%*)	
1B	$cT_2N_0M_0$	38% (*p stage 57%*)	
IIA	$cT_1N_1M_0$	34% (*p stage 55%*)	Squamous > adeno
IIB	$cT_2N_1M_0$	24% (*p stage 39%*)	$T_1 > T_3$
	$cT_3N_0M_0$	22% (*p stage 38%*)	Single nodal site > multiple
IIIA	$cT_3N_1M_0$ $cT_1N_2M_0$ $cT_2N_2M_0$ $cT_3N_2M_0$	13% overall but 15%–30% when N_2 disease requires thoracotomy for diagnosis *vs.* <5% when bulky nodes are diagnosed radiologically and confirmed on mediastinoscopy or transbronchial needle biopsy	
IIIB	T_4, any N, M_0 Any T, N_3 M_0	<5%	
IV	Any T, any N, M_1	1%	

Table 53.1

Note: 1–2% risk/patient/year incidence of developing a second lung cancer after surgical cure of a non-small cell cancer *vs.* 6% risk/patient/year following small cell cancer.

* Mountain C.F. (1997) *Chest* **111**: 1710–1717.

ROLE OF BRONCHOSCOPY

1 Evaluate vocal cord function/paralysis
2 Endobronchial 'T' staging
   - T_1: lobar or more distal bronchus
   - T_2: ≥2 cm from carina
   - T_3: <2 cm from carina without invasion
   - T_4: tracheal or carinal invasion
3 Identify carinal widening or other evidence of adenopathy with subsequent Wang needle biopsy
   - Sensitivity of TBNA for mediastinal staging is ~50% and improved with prebiopsy CT scan, cytologist on site, skilled bronchoscopist
4 Identification of second primary lesions (rare)
5 ? Fluoroscopic localization of peripheral lesions with bronchial washings, brushing, transbronchial biopsy, TBNA

MEDIASTINAL NODE STAGING

1 **Mediastinoscopy**
   - *Sampling enlarged mediastinal nodes from the right paratracheal area and often subcarinal nodes
     - Reduces the rate of non-therapeutic thoracotomy e.g. multilevel nodal involvement
     - Identifies patients with 'false positive' mediastinal adenopathy
     - Identifies a subset of patients with lowest station, solitary, intracapsular spread without fixation and a good response to resection (~10% of patients with N_2 disease)
   - Controversial areas include the absence of enlarged nodes radiologically plus
     - Lesions within the medial third of the lung
     - T_2 or T_3 tumors
     - Adenocarcinoma or large cell undifferentiated tumors on pre-op biopsy

  - Vocal cord paralysis with left upper lobe lesions
  - Stage I small cell cancer
- Shortcoming of mediastinoscopy is the inability to assess several nodal groups including the posterior subcarinal, aorto-pulmonary, para-aortic, subaortic, periesophageal and pulmonary ligament nodes

2 **Mediastinotomy** for left-sided nodes
3 **Thoracotomy** for left-sided nodes
4 **Transbronchial nodal aspiration** for right paratracheal or subcarinal nodes
5 **Transesophageal ultrasound** can detect/Bx nodes >4 mm in diameter including the aortopulmonary, subcarinal and paraesophageal
6 **CT-guided transthoracic needle aspiration**

WORK-UP FOR RESECTABILITY – 10 STEPS

I **Patient willingness**

II **Age**

III **Bloods**, including CBC, WBC and differential, lytes, BUN, Cr, albumen, liver profile (usually abnormal with extensive metastases), calcium, alkaline phosphatase
- Serum tumor markers are not of value for screening or staging

IV Adequate **pulmonary function** and gas exchange on ABGs

V Adequate **cardiac function** without evidence of recent infarction within three months, refractory failure or refractory ventricular arrythmias

VI **Absence** of marked constitutional symptoms, e.g. weight loss or severe extrathoracic organ dysfunction – neurologic, renal, GI, hepatic, hematologic, musculoskeletal

VII **Absence of T_4 Disease** (CT scan, PET scan)

- Respiratory
  - Tracheal or carinal invasion
  - Pleural mass or malignant effusion
- CVS
  - Endocardial or myocardial invasion, malignant pericardial effusion
  - Invasion of superior vena cava, aorta, major pulmonary artery or veins
- GI
  - Esophageal invasion
- Musculoskeletal
  - Vertebral column or extensive chest wall invasion
- Mediastinum
  - Infiltration of fat
  - Phrenic or recurrent laryngeal nerve invasion
  - Compression, obstruction, encasement, displacement of mediastinal structures

VIII **Absence of N_3 Disease** (CT scan, PET scan)

- Contralateral mediastinal or hilar nodes
- Ipsilateral or contralateral scalene or supraclavicular nodes

IX **Absence of multilevel nodal disease (N_2) and/or extracapsular lymph node metastases**

X **Absence of M_1 disease**

- Ipsilateral or contralateral lymphangitic or hematogenous metastases
- Ispilateral or contralateral pleural metastases
- *Cerebral metastases*
  - 'Silent' metastases in 5–10% of patients
  - Brain CT should be done with signs/symptoms of CNS disease, when the cell type is adenocarcinoma or large cell carcinoma, or when metastatic disease is suspected by marked constitutional symptoms

- False positive scans are reported in up to 10% of patients and solitary lesions may require biopsy before calling the patient unresectable

- *Bone involvement*
  - Results from direct extension or metastatic spread
  - Bone scan should be done with bone pain/tenderness, hypercalcemia, elevated alkaline phosphatase, bone mets described in 10–40% of all patients at the time of death
  - Lesions are usually osteolytic but can be osteoblastic, with the vertabrae, pelvis and femurs most often involved (hematogenously)
- *Liver metastases*
- *Adrenal metastases*
  - Frequent site of spread and may be the only site of metastases
  - Manifest as unilateral or bilateral adrenal enlargement although a normal size adrenal does not rule out metastases
  - Adrenal adenomas/nodular hyperplasia account for ~$^2/_3$ of adrenal masses with metastases <$^1/_3$
  - The gold standard is adrenal biopsy but noninvasive tests include
    - Low attenuation coefficient of adenomas on CT due to their fatty content
    - Size, with lesions <1 cm usually adenomas while >3 cm are usually neoplastic
    - MRI
    - PET scan

a. *Unilateral adrenal enlargement – differential*
   - Primary adrenal tumors with adenoma most common (found in up to 5% of the population) but a wide range of benign or malignant lesions, cortical or medullary, hormonally active or inactive, may be responsible

- Metastatic tumors, most often from lung, breast or colon
- Infections, e.g. tuberculosis, fungal
- Hemorrhage
- Compensatory hypertrophy

b. *Bilateral adrenal enlargement – differential*
- ACTH-dependent Cushing's syndrome
- Phaeochromocytoma
- Bilateral metastases
- Infection – tuberculosis, fungal
- Amyloid
- Hemorrhage
- Hematologic malignancies
- Idiopathic hyperplasia, hypertrophy
- Congenital adrenal hyperplasia

STAGE I – PROGNOSTIC FEATURES

1 Lesion Diameter – decreasing survival as size increases

2 Histologic Features
- Lymphatic invasion has poorer prognosis
- Squamous and adenocarcinoma are similar but in subtypes alveolar cell has the best while solid mucin adenocarcinoma has the worst prognosis

3 Segmental/wedge resection increases the risk of local recurrence (versus lobectomy)

4 Adequate mediastinal sampling to rule out a higher stage

5 Molecular biology eg proto-oncogenes, tumor suppressor genes, etc.

PRIMARY LUNG NEOPLASMS – ADOLESCENTS/YOUNG ADULTS < 20

Rare lesions which can be either endobronchial or parenchymal

- Presentation is that of non-specific respiratory symptoms and rarely asymptomatic compared to about 25% of older patients being symptom-free
- Malignant lesions outnumber benign causes by about 2 to 1 with the following etiologies

Benign

1 *Inflammatory pseudotumor responsible for about 50% of the benign lesions with parenchymal lesions being more common than endobronchial
2 Hamartomas comprise about 20% of benign lesions
3 Others

Malignant

1 *Bronchial adenomas are most common with carcinoid tumors being the most frequent type, followed by mucoepidermoid and finally adenoid cystic tumors
2 Bronchogenic cancer, most often adenocarcinoma and small cell
3 Blastoma
4 Sarcomas
5 Others

PLEURAL EFFUSIONS IN MALIGNANCY – ETIOLOGY

Most common effusion is an exudate

- RBC count varies from low to that of a hemothorax
- Lymphocytic predominance with neutrophils less than 25%

- pH less than 7.3 and low glucose in about $^1/_3$ of cases
- 10% have high salivary amylase
- Eosinophilia is uncommon

Clinically, dyspnea, cough and chest pains are typical

- Pleural tap results in an improvement in TLC equal to about $^1/_3$ and in FVC to about $^1/_6$ of the volume of fluid removed
- Dyspnea may be little relieved following thoracocentesis if atelectasis, obstructive pneumonitis or infiltrating parenchymal disease are present
- A malignant effusion is defined by positive cytology or positive pleural biopsy but thoracoscopy may be required if the preceeding are negative and resectability has not been ruled out

Transudates

1 Obstructed bronchial lumen and secondary atelectasis
2 Hypoalbumenemia
3 Constrictive pericarditis secondary to radiation
4 Early mediastinal node invasion

Exudates

5 *Mediastinal node invasion (most common cause)
6 Pleural metastases
7 Parapneumonic effusion secondary to post-obstructive infection
8 Pulmonary emboli secondary to a hypercoagulable state
9 Radiation pleuritis, occurring weeks to months post-radiotherapy or developing as a late complication of constrictive pericarditis or fibrosing mediastinitis
10 Drug induced (chemotherapy)
11 Trapped lung

Bloody

12 Pleural metastases

Pus

13 Empyema secondary to post-obstructive infection

Chylous

14 Thoracic duct disruption

PLEURAL METASTASES – RADIOLOGIC MANIFESTATIONS

1 Pleural effusion, e.g. metastatic breast cancer
2 Diffuse pleural thickening, often nodular in appearance
3 Discrete areas of thickening with pleural nodules(s) or mass(es), e.g. pleural implants from malignant thymoma
4 Combination of the above, e.g. diffuse pleural thickening and effusion with mesothelioma

LYMPHANGITIC CARCINOMA

Lymphatic invasion can occur in retrograde fashion from hilar nodes or hematogenously with tumor extension into the interstitium

- Resultant interstitial lung disease reflects intralymphatic tumor, edema from obstructed lymphatics and fibrosis, with the most common primaries being adenocarcinomas of lung, breast, prostate, pancreas, stomach or of unknown origin

Chest X-ray

1 Normal in up to 50% of cases
2 Increased bronchovascular markings, reticular to reticulonodular, simulating pulmonary edema, with reduced lung volumes
3 Kerley B lines
4 Bilateral > unilateral distribution
5 Associated hilar/mediastinal adenopathy
6 Associated pleural effusion(s)
7 Evidence of a primary (or previous) lung tumor or prior mastectomy

HRCT

1 Smooth or nodular thickening of the peribronchovascular interstitium, fissures and interlobular septae
2 Absence of architectural distortion of the lobules
3 Associated lymphadenopathy which is usually asymmetric
4 Associated pleural effusion(s)
5 Distribution can be unilateral or bilateral and focal or diffuse
6 Evidence of a primary tumor elsewhere, e.g. lung lesion, breast mass, prosthesis or mastectomy
7 Associated lung nodules representing hematogenous metastases

SUPERIOR VENA CAVA (SVC) SYNDROME

Etiologically, 90% are neoplastic and include

1 Bronchogenic cancer responsible for ~80% of all cases, with small cell being the most frequent histologic subtype
2 Lymphomas in ~10% of cases and usually non-Hodgkin's
3 Metastatic cancer, most often from breast
4 Other mediastinal neoplasms, e.g. germ cell
5 Benign e.g. organomegaly (goiter, aortic aneurysm), radiation, mediastinitis (fibrosing/granulomatous), thrombosis (catheters, 1°)

Clinical features include

- *Dyspnea and tachypnea
- *Facial and neck edema with plethora
- Arm and hand edema
- Jugular venous distension without hepatojugular reflux
- Telangectasias of the chest and upper back
- Stridor
- Cyanosis
- Signs of increased intracranial pressure varying from changes in mental status to seizures and coma

Severity of the superior vena cava syndrome is influenced by

- Etiology
- Site and extent of obstruction

- Rapidity of obstruction
- Collateral vessels
- Concurrent superior vena cava thrombosis

Mortality is caused by tracheal obstruction, elevated intracranial pressure and systemic hypotension

Radiologically, there is usually a superior mediastinal and/or right hilar mass (tumor +/– dilated veins)
- An associated parenchymal mass or right pleural effusion is occasionally present
- Chest X-rays are normal in ~10% of cases
- Intravascular filling defects, opacification of collateral veins, non-opacification of veins downstream of obstruction

Investigations include
1 CT with infusion/MRI
2 Venography
3 Nuclear scan
4 Sputum cytology/Bronchoscopy
5 Biopsy
    - Mediastinoscopy
    - TTNA
    - Palpable neck nodes
    - Bone marrow biopsy may be positive with small cell carcinoma or lymphoma

PANCOAST'S SYNDROME

Definition: An apical lung lesion in association with
- Shoulder and arm pains in the distribution of C8 and T1
- Horner's syndrome
- Weakness and atrophy of the hand muscles

- The vast majority of cases are caused by bronchogenic cancer occurring at the lung apex (superior sulcus tumor) with local extension
- Squamous cell and adenocarcinoma are the most common cell types described (<5% one small cell), although rare causes of the syndrome include

- Infections: bacterial, tuberculosis, fungal, hydatid
- Other neoplasms: primary thoracic, metastases from extrathoracic sites, lymphoma, plasmacytoma
- Cervical rib
- Amyloid
- Subclavian artery aneurysm

• Tissue diagnosis is therefore indicated prior to therapy

Clinical presentations

1 ***Shoulder/arm pains** due to invasion of the brachial plexus, parietal pleura, ribs or vertebral column
2 ***Horner's syndrome**, i.e. miosis, ptosis, anhidrosis due to invasion of the sympathetic chain and stellate ganglion
3 ***Weakness and atrophy** of the intrinsic hand muscles due to C8 and T1 nerve root invasion
4 Spinal cord compression and paraplegia
5 Recurrent laryngeal nerve invasion and hoarseness
6 Phrenic nerve paralysis
7 Superior vena cava syndrome
8 Supraclavicular lymphadenopathy
9 Weakness/swelling of the upper extremity from compression of the subclavian artery/veins

Staging

Superior sulcus tumors are **staged** as T3, with invasion of the mediastinum, brachial plexus or vertebral bodies defining a T_4 lesion

• The staging of lymph nodes and distant metastases is the same as bronchogenic cancer elsewhere
• Prognosis is positive in ~30% of patients with T_3 N_0 lesions but poor with T_4, T_3 N_1or T_3 N_2 lesions
• A complete metastatic workup should be done including
  - Chest and upper abdominal CT
  - Bone scan
  - Brain CT
• For patients who are potential surgical candidates, mediastinoscopy is recommended following tissue confirmation prior to thoracotomy as CT and MRI are often not definitive in ruling out mediastinal invasion

Radiologic features

1 Apical mass [or]
2 Apical cap >5 mm [or]
3 Asymmetry of both apical caps of >5 mm
4 Chest wall invasion with destruction of the upper ribs and vertebral column, more clearly defined on CT than chest X-ray as is distinguishing a tumor mass from pleural thickening
5 ± Mediastinal invasion/adenopathy
6 ± Encasement of the subclavian artery
7 MRI may be more accurate than CT in detecting chest wall, vascular, neurologic and vertebral body invasion

CARNEY'S TRIAD

Definition: Rare syndrome, most often described in females between ages 10–30, and characterized by at least 2 of the following uncommon tumors

1 Gastric leiomyosarcoma
   - Usually multicentric, often relatively slow growing, and can demonstrate indolent progression, even in the presence of metastases to the liver or other organs
   - Often presents with a GI bleed and anemia
2 Extra-adrenal paraganglionoma
   - Multicentric tumors, catecholamine-producing with resultant hypertension, often slow growing and rarely associated with pheochromocytoma (adrenal medullary paraganglionoma)
3 Pulmonary chondroma
   - Usually asymptomatic and manifest radiologically as a cartilaginous mass which can be calcified or ossified

Intrathoracic radiologic manifestations include

- Chondromas
- Metastatic leiomyosarcoma
- Posterior mediastinal or aorticopulmonary paraganglionoma

ENDOBRONCHIAL METASTASES

Usually seen in association with a known primary lesion and radiologic evidence of pulmonary metastases, although they may be the sole manifestation

- Common primary neoplasms responsible include breast, melanoma, colon/rectal, kidney and uterus
- Presentation ranges from asymptomatic to features of airways obstruction with cough, wheezing, hemoptysis and expectoration of tumor fragments

Radiologic manifestations

1 Atelectasis and obstructive pneumonitis when complete airways obstruction is present
2 Oligemia and hyperinflation with partial airways obstruction

CELL TYPES

Squamous Cell Carcinoma (SCC)

Accounts for about 30% of lung cancers, characterized histologically by keratin, squamous pearls and cellular bridges

- Classified as well, moderately and poorly differentiated types which influence their growth
- Most often located in a segmental or lobar bronchus, with sequential progression from dysplasia to carcinoma *in situ*, and finally invasive carcinoma, accepted only for squamous cell carcinoma
- Carcinoma *in situ* is rarely diagnosed clinically, although it can be seen bronchoscopically in smokers presenting with a normal chest X-ray and, e.g. hemoptysis, as well as on screening sputum cytologies
- Tends to be slow growing with an estimate of 3 years required from an *in situ* carcinoma to be a clinically apparent tumor
- Narrowing or obstruction of the bronchial lumen is frequently accompanied by invasion of submucosal and peribronchial connective tissue

- SCC spreads centrally involving lymph nodes and invades blood vessels/lymphatics with resultant distant metastases

Radiologic features

1. A hilar mass is the most common manifestation (>65% arise in central bronchi) with atelectasis and post-obstructive pneumonitis typical, atelectasis varying from segmental to an entire lung
   - Post-obstructive pneumonitis results from an inflammatory infiltrate in the lung, preventing total collapse as occurs in simple atelectasis, with air bronchograms usually absent
   - The combination of a proximal hilar mass (convex) with an elevated minor fissure (concave) results in the S-sign of Golden (right hilar cancer)
2. Although usually central in origin, squamous cell carcinoma can present as a peripheral mass with central cavitation (most often in an upper lobe) and a thick irregular wall
   - Peripheral squamous cancers are often the largest of all types of bronchogenic cancers
3. Signs of mediastinal invasion
4. Most common cell type to cause Pancoast's tumor
5. Distant metastases in ~25% of cases

Adenocarcinoma

Most common histologic subtype of lung cancer, responsible for 30+%

- Several histologic subtypes are described including acinar, papillary, solid with mucus formation and bronchioalveolar
- Majority are located in the lung periphery (~70%), represents ~⅓ of peripheral lung tumors, often subpleural in location, and cavitation is rare
- Early vascular invasion is typical with diagnosis often made at the time of pleural, chest wall, diaphragmatic invasion or with distant metastases
- Most common cell type associated with peripheral scar cancers

- Uncommonly arises in a central airway, presenting with features of obstructive pneumonitis
- Difficulties arise in some patients distinguishing a lung primary from either metastatic adenocarcinoma or mesothelioma

Radiologic features

1. Round or oval peripheral nodule with malignancy suggested by a corona radiata, lobulation or a poorly defined border
   - May demonstrate eccentric calcification
   - May be slow growing with only slight increase on serial films over a few years
2. Changing or enlarging lesion in association with a long standing granuloma or parenchymal scarring
3. Central mass simulating squamous cell cancer
4. Associated hilar/mediastinal adenopathy which can occur concurrent with only a small nodule
5. Distant metastases

Bronchioloalveolar Carcinoma (BACA)

Definition: A subset of pulmonary adenocarcinoma with malignant cells growing along intact alveolar septae and spreading via the airways

- A peripheral pulmonary neoplasm, arising either in distal bronchioles or alveolar walls

BACA can be subdivided into sclerosing, mucinous and non-mucinous varieties on the basis of gross appearance, light microscopic and ultrastructural features

- Responsible for ~10% of primary lung cancers and has the weakest association with smoking
- Described in patients with underlying interstitial inflammation/fibrosis, e.g. scleroderma as well as in younger individuals compared to other cell types

Histologically, must be distinguished from

1. Metastatic adenocarcinoma, e.g. breast, colon, prostate, pancreas, thyroid, stomach, ovary

2 Reactive hyperplasia
3 Peripheral component of a primary lung adenocarcinoma

Two distinct clinical entities are described with the same histologic features

Solitary or focal disease

Clinically, this is usually asymptomatic, although non-specific respiratory symptoms can be present

- Controversial how often the solitary form evolves into diffuse disease (see below)
- Prognosis is good following surgery, although even the solitary nodule may spread to the hilum, mediastinum and pleura, particularly with size > 3 cm in diameter

Radiologic features

1. Peripheral nodule or mass with an air bronchogram/bronchiologram often present
2. A 'tail sign' is described, i.e. linear streaks extending from the nodule to the lung periphery, but is seen in other tumors, e.g. adenocarcinoma as well as in granulomatous disease
3. Serial X-rays typically show slow progressive growth over months to years
4. Can rarely cavitate or calcify

Diffuse disease

Clinically, usually symptomatic with non-specific respiratory and systemic complaints which may be accompanied by bronchorrhea

- Severe bronchorrhea can result in fluid and electrolyte abnormalities
- With extensive tumor and secretions, ventilation is compromised but perfusion preserved, resulting in right-to-left shunting and refractory hypoxemia
- The airways proximal to the tumor may be filled with secretions making BAL and transbronchial biopsies falsely negative
- Diffuse multifocal disease has a poor prognosis with intrathoracic as well as systemic metastases occurring

Radiologic features

1 Multiple nodules resembling metastatic tumor
2 Pneumonic (airspace) disease involving one or several lobes, unilateral or bilateral
3 Combination of the above
4 Air bronchograms
5 Rarely a diffuse interstitial pattern
6 May be accompanied by pleural effusions, hilar/mediastinal lymphadenopathy

Differential diagnosis of the **diffuse** form of bronchioalveolar carcinoma includes

1 Alveolar proteinosis
2 Infections, e.g. tuberculosis, atypicals, fungi including pneumocystis
3 Chronic eosinophilic pneumonia
4 Lipoid pneumonia
5 Lymphomatoid granulomatosis
6 Wegener's granulomatosis
7 Lymphoma – Hodgkin's or non-Hodgkin's
8 Alveolar hemorrhage
9 Allergic bronchopulmonary aspergillosis
10 Bronchocentric granulomatosis
11 BOOP
12 Sarcoid

Small Cell Carcinoma

Responsible for 20% of lung cancers, with ~95% of patients being smokers

- Typically disseminated at presentation with local and systemic signs/symptoms reflecting early invasion of lymphatics and vessels
- More paraneoplastic syndromes seen than with other cancers, most commonly SIADA, Cushing's syndrome or neurologic disorders

Radiologically, lesions are central (rarely peripheral) and present with endobronchial obstruction and associated lymphadenopathy which is often extensive

- The adenopathy is bulky and usually involves the hilum and mediastinum
- With progression the mediastinal nodes coalesce, infiltrating the entire mediastinum with compression, obstruction and invasion of structures
- Low attenuation centers of necrosis with an enhancing rim can be seen on contract CT

The TNM staging system is generally not used as surgery is rarely an option (exception is the rare patient with a peripheral nodule)

Two-staging systems are used with **limited** disease defined as confined to a single radiation port, i.e. one hemithorax including mediastinal/hilar nodes/supraclavicular nodes, whereas **extensive** disease is involvement of sites outside the above

- A small number of patients with limited disease are cured, but a second lung primary is seen in about 4% of patients per year, after being cancer-free for two years
- An increased incidence of other smoking-related cancers is reported including head and neck as well as esophageal primaries

Large Cell Carcinoma

Responsible for about 10% of lung cancers with histologic variants giant cell and clear cell carcinoma, both rare

- Poorly differentiated non-small cell lung cancer and diagnosis of exclusion after eliminating squamous or adenocarcinoma at the light microscopic level
- Incidence of this subtype declines when electron microscopy is used or the amount of tissue available for examination increases
- Presents as a large peripheral lesion which grows rapidly and demonstrates early invasion of lymphatics and blood vessels, resulting in nodal and distant metastases

Adenoid Cystic Carcinoma

Second most common malignant tumor of the trachea and main bronchi (squamous cell is most common) and unrelated to cigarette smoking, with most tumors diagnosed between ages 40–50

- Clinically, presents with non-specific symptoms of airways disease or 'asthma' refractory to treatment
- Resection can result in cure, although local extension into the mediastinum or lung as well as distant metastases can occur, occasionally many years after initial diagnosis, due to the tumor's slow growth

Radiologic features

1 Tracheal narrowing
2 Bronchial narrowing or obstruction
3 Uncommonly as a peripheral lesion

Mucoepidermoid Carcinoma

Rare neoplasm of the tracheobronchial glands, usually arising within the mainstem or lobar bronchi, rarely from the trachea, and thought to arise from the minor salivary glands lining the tracheobronchial tree

- Pathologically they are mainly endoluminal while histologically composed of mucus-secreting cells, squamous cells and undifferentiated intermediate cells

Clinically, described in all age groups with ~$^1/_2$ of patients under age 30

- Patients can be asymptomatic or present with non-specific airway symptoms of cough, dyspnea, wheezing and hemoptysis
- Tumors are classified as high or low grade malignancy
- Low grade tumors are slow growing, have a good prognosis and tend to remain endoluminal, without local, regional or distant spread
- High grade tumors are unpredictable, have a poor prognosis with greater tendency to pulmonary parenchymal invasion, nodal involvement or distant spread

Radiologic features

1 Mass (>3 cm) or nodule (<3 cm)
2 Post-obstructive signs including atelectasis, post-obstructive pneumonitis, mucoid impaction, distal air trapping

3 Endobronchial localization on CT
4 Punctated calcifications on CT

Carcinosarcoma

Clinically, a rare aggressive, smoking-related neoplasm composed of a mixture of malignant epithelial, (usually squamous cell), and sarcomatous tissues (usually spindle-cell type)

- Patients present with features or endobronchial or parenchymal disease without any pathognomonic clinical or radiologic features
- Metastatic spread can be epithelial, sarcomatous or both with intra and extrathoracic spread, prognosis being poor with survival often ~6 months

Radiologic features

1 Endobronchial narrowing with atelectasis and obstructive pneumonitis
2 Peripheral nodule/mass lesion

Carcinoid Tumors

Uncommon low grade malignant neoplasms, unrelated to cigarette smoking or asbestos exposure

- Seen in all age groups with the mean age of diagnosis ~50 years
- Responsible for 90% of 'bronchial adenomas' with 3 types described

1 **Central carcinoid**
   - Typical carcinoid and responsible for ~80% of all tumors
   - Arise centrally with its origin varying from the trachea (uncommon) to the subsegmental bronchi, usually with well-defined margins
   - Usually extend from the lumen to the outside wall as well as the surrounding lung parenchyma and may invade the mediastinum
   - Most of the tumor may be extralumenal with only slight intralumenal disease – 'iceberg tumor'

- Histologically may be misdiagnosed as small cell carcinoma on small biopsy fragments and should be particularly suspected when the latter presents as a solitary lung nodule or absence of hilar/mediastinal adenopathy
- Neurosecretory granules are seen on electron microscopy
- Multiple neuroendocrine products may be detected on immunohistochemistry

2 **Peripheral carcinoid**
- Typical carcinoid, usually solitary but can be multiple and associated with tumorlets
- May be histologically identical to central lesions or have a 'spindle cell' appearance

3 **Atypical carcinoid**
- Comprises 10% of all carcinoid tumors and can be central or peripheral in location
- Resembles the above types but have histologic features suggestive of more aggressive lesion
- Spreads earlier than typical carcinoids with a poorer prognosis

Clinically, 25% are asymptomatic, particularly the peripheral carcinoids
- Central lesions present with symptoms of bronchial obstruction, often hemoptysis, as well as obstructive pneumonitis and can simulate asthma
- Hormone production can result in
  - Carcinoid syndrome
    - Rarely seen and then only with extensive metastases present
    - Symptoms include flushing, nausea, vomiting, diarrhea, wheezing, dyspnea and hypotension
    - Elevated levels of 5-HIAA and serotonin in the urine
  - Others including *Cushing's syndrome (elevated ACTH levels), acromegaly, Zollinger-Ellison syndrome, SIADH, hyperinsulinemia, multiple endocrine neoplastic syndrome

- Diagnosis of central lesions is usually made on bronchoscopy with peripheral lesions at surgery ? role of somatostatin receptor scintigraphy using ^{123}I-octreotide, a somatostatin analogue, to identify primary and metastatic tumor
- Prognosis of 'typical' carcinoid is good, particularly when nodes are uninvolved
- Regional nodes are involved in ~5% of patients while distant metastases are rare and may be slow growing with prolonged survival
- Slow tumor growth can result in tumor recurrence years after 'curative' resection and therefore regular follow-up is indicated
- Unpredictable which 'typical' neoplasm will metastasize
- Bony metastases can be osteolytic or osteoblastic
- Atypicals have a much poorer prognosis with distant spread often seen at the time of diagnosis

Radiologic features depend on the location and type of tumor

- *Central carcinoids*
  - Atelectasis and obstructive pneumonitis +/– central mass
  - Central mass
  - Volume loss and oligemia
  - Bronchiectasis and lung abscesses
  - Mucoid impaction unaccompanied by atelectasis
  - Normal chest X-ray

- *Peripheral carcinoids*
  - Peripheral nodule or mass

- *Atypical carcinoids*
  - Peripheral nodule or mass with smooth, lobulated or spiculated margins
  - Central mass
  - Mediastinal or hilar lymphadenopathy

CT contribution

1 Tumor enhancement post-contrast
2 Endobronchial disease (rarely ossified)

3 Ossification or calcifications (reflecting bone seen on pathology), usually with central tumors
4 Assessment of local invasion

Large Cell Neuroendocrine Carcinoma

Rare tumor, defined histologically and previously classified as atypical carcinoid or small cell carcinoma

- Prognosis is between that of the above two neoplasms
- Strongly related to cigarette smoking
- May be central or peripheral in local
- Ectopic hormone production is not a feature

Pulmonary Tumorlets

Definition: Microscopic to 3 mm foci of proliferating neuroendocrine cells

- Generally multiple, rarely visible radiologically, and usually discovered at autopsy or surgical removal of an unrelated lesion
- Electron microscopy and immunochemistry findings are similar to those of carcinoid tumors with neurosecretory granules and peptide hormones
- May be seen in association with
  - Bronchiectasis
  - Foci of parenchymal fibrosis
  - Normal lung
  - Carcinoid tumors
- They are clinically asymptomatic, seen in older patients, show a female predominance, and behave in a benign fashion

Epitheloid Hemangioendothelioma

Uncommon vascular tumor of endothelial cell origin, usually occurring in women, with 50% of cases under age 40

- Multifocal neoplasms, originally termed intravascular bronchioloalveolar tumors
- May be confined to the lungs or occur in other organs, e.g. liver, and represent either metastatic spread from the lungs or a multicentric origin

Clinical features
1 Asymptomatic radiologic finding (most common)
2 Non-specific respiratory or systemic symptoms
3 Variable course from slow growth and prolonged survival to progressive disease with respiratory failure or complications of extrathoracic tumor

Definitive diagnosis requires thoracoscopic or open biopsy

Radiologic features
1 Multiple nodules which resemble metastases or infarcts
2 Growth rates are variable
3 Pleural effusion and/or adenopathy in ~10% of cases

Moss, A., Gamsu, Genant (1992) Thorax and neck. In: *Computed Tomography of the Body with Magnetic Resonance Imaging*, 2nd edn., vol. 1.: W.B. Saunders.

Thurlbeck W., Churg A. (eds) (1995) *Pathology of the Lung*. 2nd edn.: Thieme Medical Publishers.

Baum, G.L., Crapo, J.D., Celli, B.R., Karlinsky, J.B. (eds) (1997) *Textbook of Pulmonary Diseases*, 6th edn.: Lippincott-Raven.

Fishman, A.P., Elias, J.A., Fishman, J.A., Grippi, M.A., Kaiser, L.R., Senior, R.N. (1998) *Fishman's Pulmonary Diseases and Disorders*, 3rd edn.: McGraw-Hill.

Staples, C.A., Muller N., Miller, R. *et al.* (1988) Mediastinal nodes in bronchogenic carcinoma: Comparison between CT and mediastinoscopy. *Radiology* **167** (Suppl): 367–372.

Epstein, D. (1990) Bronchioloalveolar carcinoma. *Semin. Roent.* **xxv**: 105–111.

Herman, S., Winton, T., Weisbrod, G. (1994) Mediastinal invasion by bronchogenic carcinoma: CT signs. *Radiology* **190**: 841–846.

White, C., Templeton, P. (1993) Radiologic manifestations of bronchogenic cancer. *Clinics in Chest Medicine* **14**: 55–67.

Kulke, M., Mayer, R. (1999) Carcinoid tumors. *NEJM* **340**: 858–866.

Coates, G., Skehaw, S. (1999) Emerging role of PET in the diagnosis and staging of lung cancer. (Journal title) **6**: 145–152.

Sahn, S. (1993) Pleural effusion in lung cancer. *Clinics in Chest Medicine* **14**: 189–198.

Leong, S., Lima, C., Sherman, C. *et al.* (1999) The 1997 international staging system for non-small cell cancer. *Chest* **115**: 242.

Mountain, C.F. (1997) Revisions in the international system for staging lung cancer. *Chest* **111**: 1710–1717.

Lababede, Meziane, M., Rice, T. (1999) TNM staging of lung cancer. *Chest* **115**: 233–235.

Arcasoy, S., Jeh, S. (1997) Superior pulmonary sulcus tumors and Pancoast's syndrome. *NEJM* **337**: 1370–1375.

Knight, S., Delbeke, D., Stewart, J. *et al.* (1996) Evaluation of pulmonary lesions with FDG-PET. *Chest* **109**: 982–988.

Margulies, K., Sheps, S. (1988) Carney's triad: guidelines for management. *Mayo Clinic Proc.* **63**: 496–502.

American Thoracic Society/European Respiratory Society (1997) Pre-treatment evaluation of non-small cell lung cancer. *Am. J. Resp. Crit. Care Med* **156**: 320–332.

Colice, G. (1994) Chest CT for known or suspected lung cancer. *Chest* **106**: 1538–1550.

Mountain, C.F., Dressler, C.M. (1997) Regional lymph node classification for lung cancer staging. *Chest* **111**: 1718–1723.

Tae Sung Kim, Kyung Soo Lee, Joungho Han. *et al.* (1999) Mucoepidermoid carcinoma of the tracheobronchial tree: radiographic and CT findings in 12 patients. *Radiology* **212**: 643–648.

54 Neuromuscular Disorders

DIAGNOSTIC WORK-UP

Lung disease is an important cause of morbidity and mortality in patients with neuromuscular disease leading to the complications of

- Hypoxemia with cor pulmonale and right heart failure
- Hypercapneic respiratory failure
- Restrictive PFTs
- Sleep-related breathing disorders
- Aspiration and difficulty clearing secretions with secondary atelectasis and pneumonia
- Positional upper airway obstruction from the tongue

1 **History**
   - Dyspnea and fatigue, initially on exertion, progressing to symptoms at rest, although uncommonly the first manifestation of neuromuscular disease can be ventilatory failure
   - Orthopnea seen with severe diaphragmatic involvement and may be more marked than dyspnea on exertion
   - Abnormal sleep patterns with clinical features of obstructive sleep apnea, e.g. early morning headaches from hypercapnia, daytime somnolence

- Cough and difficulty clearing secretions
- Associated bulbar findings of dysphagia, aspiration and difficulty with speech
- Associated limb weakness is often present but does not correlate with the extent of respiratory muscle weakness
- Family history of neuromuscular disease, e.g. muscular dystrophies
- History of trauma or poisoning, e.g. botulism, organophosphates
- Acute onset of neuromuscular disease, e.g. Guillain-Barré, myasthenia, toxic agents, *vs.* chronic onset of disease, e.g. myopathies, ALS, muscular dystrophies
- Clinical course may be progressive, e.g. ALS, reversible, e.g. Guillain-Barré, relapsing, e.g. multiple sclerosis
- Acute deterioration in symptoms may be seen with infection, e.g. myasthenia
- Thromboembolic complications should be sought in poorly mobile patients

2 **Physical exam**
- Resting tachypnea with shallow breathing
- Nasal quality to the speech with frequent cough
- Diaphragmatic weakness manifest as reduced or absent diaphragmatic excursions, dullness to percussion with decreased breath sounds at the lung bases
- Absence of outward movement of the abdomen on inspiration or paradoxical abdominal movement with bilateral diaphragmatic paralysis
- Use of accessory muscles including the inspiratory neck muscles, e.g. scalenes, sternomastoids as well as the abdominal muscles on expiration
- Ineffective cough and absence of a gag reflex
- Signs of pulmonary hypertension and cor pulmonale
- Signs of upper airway dysfunction, e.g. drooling, dysarthia, tongue obstructing the upper airway, difficulty swallowing

3 **Chest X-ray** evidence of poor inspiration manifest as low lung volumes and bibasilar plate atelectasis

4 **Fluoroscopic** demonstration of diaphragmatic dysfunction

5 **ABG findings**

	PO_2	PCO_2	pH
Mild weakness	N→↓	N→↓	N→↑
Marked weakness	↓	↑	↓

(↑PCO_2 with respiratory muscle strength <30% N)

6 **PFTs**
- Spirometry
  - VC falls when respiratory muscle strength is <50% normal
  - Reductions in VC from upright to the supine position
  - Restrictive picture with supernormal flow rates
- Flow–volume curve abnormalities including
  - Delay reaching peak expiratory flow
  - Truncation of expiratory flows
  - Rapid drop in expiratory flows at the end of expiration
  - Truncation of peak inspiratory flows
- Lung volumes
  - Normal to increased FRC
  - Reduced TLC in proportion to the inspiratory muscle weakness
  - Increased RV in proportion to the expiratory muscle weakness
- Respiratory muscle strength
  - Reductions in Pi_{max}, Pe_{max} and transdiaphragmatic pressures not correlating with the degree of limb weakness

7 **Phrenic nerve stimulation** to assess phrenic function and diaphragmatic contractility by monitoring
- Phrenic nerve latency
- Diaphragmatic contractility fluoroscopically
- Twitch Pdi

8 **Nerve/muscle biopsy**

9 **Sleep study** to assess
- Nocturnal hypoxemia/hypoventilation
- Sleep apneas
- Upper airways obstruction
- Daytime abnormalities in ABGs

10 **Differential diagnosis** including diseases of
- Spinal cord
  - Cervical trauma
  - Multiple sclerosis
  - Tumors
  - Transverse myelitis
  - Degenerative disk disease
  - ALS
  - Syringomyelia
- Anterior horn cells
  - ALS
  - Polio
  - Post-polio syndrome
    - New neuromuscular symptoms developing many years, usually 30–40, after recovery from acute paralytic polio
    - Thought to represent dysfunction of the surviving motorneurons *vs.* recent or reactivation infection
    - The syndrome of progressive post-polio muscular atrophy is a slowly progressive disease with inter-patient variability as well as long periods of stability within the same patient
    - Patients present with increasing weakness, dyspnea on exertion, sleep disturbances and respiratory muscle involvement can result in respiratory failure
- Peripheral nerves
  - Guillain-Barré
- Myoneural junction
  - Myasthenia gravis

- Myasthenia-like syndromes
- Botulism
  - Due to a neurotoxin inhibiting acetylcholine release with features of slurred speech, visual disturbances, dry mouth, dysphagia, nausea, vomiting, diarrhea, extraocular muscle paresis, muscle weakness leading to dyspnea and respiratory failure
- Organophosphate poisoning
  - Agents inhibiting acetylcholinesterase reflecting muscarinic and nicotinic effects, respiratory manifestations including laryngospasm, bronchospasm and respiratory center depression

- Muscle
  - Muscular dystrophies
  - SLE
  - Inflammatory myopathies e.g. polymyositis, dermatomyositis, inclusion-body myositis
  - Endocrine, e.g. hyperthyroidism, hypothyroidism, hyperadrenalism
  - Steroid myopathy
    - Characterized by bilateral, symmetric, proximal muscle involvement with non-tender muscles, normal CPK and normal or minimal changes on EMG
  - Electrolyte disorders, e.g. ↓potassium, ↓phosphate
  - Rhabdomyolysis
  - Nutritional
  - Metabolic, e.g. acid maltase deficiency or other glycogen storage diseases, mitochondrial myopathies, disorders of lipid metabolism
  - Periodic paralysis

MYASTHENIA GRAVIS

Skeletal muscle weakness and fatigue are due to an antibody-mediated attack on the nicotinic acetylcholine receptors of the neuromuscular junction, with serum antibodies to the acetylcholine receptor present in ~90% of patients

- Muscle biopsy specimens reveal only ~⅓ the normal number of acetylcholine receptors compared to normal controls
- Muscle weakness is increased with repeated activity but improves with rest or the administration of an anticholinesterase

Clinical features include

1 Involvement of the extraocular and eyelid muscles early in the course of disease with ptosis and diplopia
  - Disease remains localized to these muscles in ~15% of patients

2 Bulbar and facial muscle disease with difficulty chewing, swallowing and resultant aspiration

3 Generalized limb and trunk weakness, including the diaphragm, are seen in ~85% of cases

Pulmonary complications include

Airways

1 Bulbar dysfunction manifest as difficulty swallowing, speaking, handling oral secretions, aspiration and stridor

2 Direct evidence of vocal cord dysfunction and upper airways obstruction on laryngoscopy as well as demonstration of variable extrathoracic airways obstruction with an inspiratory plateau on flow volume curves

3 Increased airways resistance and obstruction in patients with underlying airways disease treated with anticholinesterases

4 Increased airways secretions from cholinesterase inhibitors

Parenchyma

5 Plate atelectasis with V/Q mismatch and hypoxemia

6 Aspiration pneumonia

7 Opportunistic infection complicating immunosuppressive therapy

Chest wall

8 Orthopnea and paradoxic abdominal wall motion on inspiration reflecting diaphragmatic weakness
9 Impaired cough from expiratory muscle weakness
10 Respiratory muscle weakness may be more severely affected than that of the limb muscles and progress to respiratory failure
- May develop gradually or present acutely as a myasthenic or cholinergic crisis
- A crisis occurs when (a) respiratory muscle weakness impairs ventilation or (b) bulbar dysfunction results in laryngeal muscle weakness, stridor and upper airways obstruction
- A myasthenic crisis occurs from disease progression or inadequate anticholinesterase therapy and can occur spontaneously or be secondary to infection, surgery (e.g. post thymectomy), emotional upsets, others
- A cholinergic crisis occurs with an excess of acetyl-cholinesterase inhibitors and is characterized by muscarinic and nicotinic side-effects as well as muscle weakness, with worsening of symptoms following tensilon
- Reductions in maximal inspiratory and expiratory mouth pressures, transdiaphragmatic pressure (Pdi_{max} or sniff *P*di), and vital capacity (exacerbated when supine) improve post-tensilon
- Reduced vital capacity with normal to elevated residual volume

Mediastinum

11 Thymic abnormalities are seen in about 75% of patients with 15% of these having a thymoma and 85% displaying hyperplasia

Associated autoimmune disease which can affect the lungs, e.g. polymyositis

AMYOTROPHIC LATERAL SCLEROSIS

Definition: Progressive degenerative disease of the upper and lower motor neuron with all patients eventually developing respiratory muscle involvement, the latter monitored by mouth pressures and vital capacity

Pulmonary complications include

1 Normal gas exchange when awake but sleep desaturation early in the course of disease
2 Impaired swallowing and resultant aspiration with bulbar involvement
3 Impaired cough and resultant pneumonia
4 Eventual respiratory failure and death due to involvement of the diaphragm and the intercostal muscles
   - Hypoventilation typically occurs in the setting of established limb and bulbar involvement but can rarely be the initial manifestation of disease

MULTIPLE SCLEROSIS

Definition: Inflammatory demyelinating disease of the CNS white matter, the incidence of respiratory failure being low and an uncommon cause of death

Case reports of respiratory involvement describe

1 Diaphragmatic weakness/failure in patients with lesions of the cervical cord
   - There is associated upper limb weakness with reductions in maximal inspiratory and expiratory mouth pressures
2 Disorders of respiratory control including Ondine's curse, loss of voluntary control, hyperventilation
3 Acute respiratory failure from extensive bulbar or cervical cord involvement
4 Neurogenic pulmonary edema
5 Obstructive sleep apnea

6 Impaired cough with aspiration and pneumonia as common terminal events

PARKINSON'S DISEASE

Pulmonary complications include

1 Aspiration pneumonia (the commonest cause of death)
2 Upper airways obstruction secondary to muscle dysfunction is seen in 5–10% of patients
3 Restrictive picture on PFTs secondary to reduced chest wall compliance and neuromuscular disease
4 L-dopa induced dyspnea ? secondary to dyskinesia of the respiratory muscles
5 Central hypoventilation

GUILLAIN-BARRÉ SYNDROME

Definition: An acute, progressive, symmetric demyelinating polyneuropathy and the most common peripheral neuropathy to cause respiratory failure

- The ascending nature of paralysis involves the chest wall and abdominal muscles before the laryngeal and pharyngeal muscles

Respiratory and bulbar musculature involvement can result in

1 Inability to swallow with subsequent aspiration
2 Upper airways obstruction
3 Impaired cough, retention of secretions and pneumonia
4 Atelectasis and resultant hypoxemia
5 Tachypnea and dyspnea, progressing to respiratory failure with hypercapnia secondary to progressive reductions in vital capacity
    - Vital capacity and maximal mouth pressures should be monitored q4h, with VC values <15 ml/kg requiring intubation

6 Cardiovascular lability during intubation due to dysautonomia present early in disease
7 Complications of tracheostomy
8 Pulmonary emboli complicating prolonged inactivity

SPINAL CORD TRAUMA

Respiratory signs and symptoms reflect the level of disease, with lesions above C2 having the more severe effects on the respiratory musculature due to phrenic nerve involvement (C2,3,4)

High cervical lesions result in

1 Phrenic nerve involvement
2 Absent cough
3 Marked use of the inspiratory neck muscles
4 Severe dyspnea and tachypnea with ventilatory support required
5 Abdominal paradox
6 Poor chest expansion with predominant upward chest motion

Mid-lower cervical lesions result in

1 Sparing of the phrenic nerve
2 A preserved but weak cough due to loss of the expiratory intercostals and the abdominal muscles
3 Mild use of the inspiratory neck muscles
4 Mild dyspnea and tachypnea
5 No abdominal paradox
6 Chest expansion maintained

Complications include

1 Spinal shock and acute hypotension
2 Pulmonary infections from retained secretions and atelectasis due to expiratory muscle weakness with impaired cough, bronchial mucus hypersecretion, failure to sigh
3 Deep vein thrombosis and pulmonary emboli from prolonged stasis

4 Associated injuries
5 Impaired consciousness and resultant aspiration
6 Neurogenic pulmonary edema
7 ARDS from aspiration, trauma, sepsis

Fraser R.S., Muller N.L., Colman N., Paré P.D. (1999) *Diagnosis of Diseases of the Chest* 4th Edn., WB Saunders.
Baum, G.L., Crapo, J.D., Celli, B.R., Karlinsky, J.B. (eds) *Textbook of Pulmonary Diseases*, 6th edn.: Lippincott-Raven.
Fishman, A.P., Elias, J.A., Fishman, J.A., Grippi, M.A., Kaiser, L.R., Senior. R.N. *Fishman's Pulmonary Diseases and Disorders*, 3rd edn. (Place of publication): McGraw-Hill.
Rochester, D., Esau, S. (1994) Assessment of ventilatory function in patients with neuromuscular disease. *Clinics in Chest Medicine* **15**: 751–761.

55 Pleura – Mass, Thickening, Effusion

PLEURAL DISEASE – FOCAL

1 **Healed pleuritis**
- Usually secondary to remote pneumonia, but can be seen with a remote hemothorax, empyema, sarcoid, rheumatoid arthritis, systemic lupus
- Typically basal in location with blunting or obliteration of the posterior and/or lateral costophrenic angles
- Appearance is similar to that of a small pleural effusion with lateral decubitus films or ultrasound needed to rule out the above

2 **'Apical cap'**
- Curved shadows in the apices of one or both hemithoraces
- Etiology unclear with pathology showing a combination of pleural and parenchymal fibrosis, without granulomatous inflammation

3 **Pleural plaques**

- Localized collections of dense collagenous tissue and the most common manifestation of asbestos exposure
- Typically involve the parietal pleura postero-laterally with sparing of the apices and costophrenic angles
- Latency period approximately 15 years between asbestos exposure and development of pleural plaques
- Unilateral in 25% of cases and often asymptomatic even when bilateral
- HRCT is more sensitive than chest X-ray in the diagnosis of plaques

4 **Calcified fibrous pseudotumor**

- Manifest radiologically as a solitary pleural mass or multiple well circumscribed masses with calcification seen on CT scan
- Histologically, it is similar to the inflammatory pseudotumor of lung except for extensive calcifications

5 **Pleural neoplasms**

- *Localized fibrous tumor of the pleura*
  - Rare pleural tumor, unrelated to asbestos exposure
  - 60% of tumors are benign and often attached to the visceral pleura by a pedicle
  - 40% of tumors are malignant, usually arise from the parietal pleura and are associated with chest wall invasion and pleural effusion

  Clinical presentations
  - Asymptomatic intrathoracic mass
  - Non-specific respiratory symptoms
  - Extrathoracic manifestations including hypoglycemia and hypertrophic osteoarthropathy

  Radiologic features
  - Round or lobulated mass that can grow to a very large size with eventual difficulty determining the pleural origin
  - Change in position of the mass with posture or breathing

- Vascular enhancement on CT occasionally with central areas of necrosis

- *Pleural lipoma/liposarcoma*
  - Rare tumors revealing fat attenuation on CT, homogeneous for lipoma but heterogeneous for liposarcoma
  - Often asymptomatic and discovered on routine chest X-ray, location being intrathoracic with occasional extension to the chest wall

- *Malignant mesothelioma* – usually diffuse

- *Metastatic cancer* – usually diffuse and reflecting spread from lung, breast, lymphoma or other extra-pulmonary site
  - Direct seeding of the pleura can occur with, e.g. malignant thymoma, resulting in discrete pleural nodules or masses

6 **Loculated pleural effusion**

7 **Pleural hematoma**

PLEURAL DISEASE – DIFFUSE

Definition: An uninterrupted pleural opacity involving >25% of the chest wall, with the differential diagnosis including

1 **Pleural fibrosis** (fibrothorax)
- Healed tuberculosis
- Empyema
- Asbestos pleuritis
- Old hemothorax

2 **Chronic infection**
- Tuberculosis
- Chronic aspergillosis

3 **Neoplasm**
   - Malignant mesothelioma
   - Metastatic cancer from lung, breast, lymphoma, ovary, stomach or another extrathoracic site

4 **Rheumatoid arthritis** (rare)

5 **Sarcoid** (rare)

Clues to Diagnosis

1 Extensive calcifications occur with tuberculosis or empyema but rarely in asbestos exposure
2 Bilateral pleural fibrosis suggests an asbestos etiology *vs.* the other causes of a fibrothorax
3 Mediastinal pleural involvement is often malignant
4 Nodular and mass-like pleural thickening suggests malignancy
5 Associated intrathoracic disease, e.g. adenopathy, parenchymal involvement or endobronchial disease may suggest a specific etiology

PLEURAL EFFUSION – RADIOLOGIC FEATURES

1 Pleural effusions most frequently present with blunting of the posterior, then lateral, and finally the anterior costophrenic angles with a meniscus-like arc at the interface between the fluid and the chest wall
   - Less common patterns of free fluid can simulate lobar consolidation or cardiomegaly when arranged around an individual lobe or the heart respectively

   CT demonstrates a sickle-shaped opacity posteriorly in the most dependent part of the thorax with free-flowing pleural fluid

2 Subpulmonic effusions lie beneath the lung base without extension into the costophrenic angles and are characterized by

- Displacement of the apex of the diaphragm lateral to the midclavicular line
- No vessels are seen below the diaphragmatic dome
- Increased distance between the gastric air bubble and the apparent left hemidiaphragm
- Frequent extension of fluid into the major fissure

3 Encapsulated or loculated pleural fluid results from adhesions between the perietal and visceral pleura
- Chest X-rays reveal no change in the location of the fluid with positional changes
- Rounded or lenticular fixed opacities are seen in a dependent or non-dependent location on CT when fluid is loculated

4 Interlobar fluid collections occur most often in the right minor fissure and have biconvex contours (pseudotumor) giving them a 'cigar-shape'
- Major fissure encapsulation results in a concave kidney-shaped density
- Minor and major fissure encapsulation result in the 'double-bubble' sign

5 Effusions on supine films often display a diffuse increase in opacity of the hemithorax and little else but enough fluid may separate the lung from the chest wall laterally

RADIOLOGIC CLUES TO ETIOLOGY

Chest X-Ray

1 **Cardiac abnormalities**
- Enlarged cardiac silhouette, e.g. CHF, pericardial effusion
- Pericardial calcifications, e.g. constrictive pericarditis

2 **Associated pleural disease**
- Pneumothorax, e.g. external trauma, esophageal rupture, lung abscess, ruptured bulla, necrotizing pneumonia, gas-forming organisms, BPF

- Pleural plaques, e.g. asbestos exposure
- Foreign body

3 **'Chest wall' abnormalities**
- Bone pathology, e.g. fracture, neoplasm, infection
- Absent breast shadow, e.g. metastatic breast cancer
- Subdiaphragmatic air–fluid level, e.g. subphrenic abscess
- Pancreatic calcifications, e.g. pancreatitis

4 **Mediastinal widening**, e.g. adenopathy, aortic dissection, mediastinitis, neoplasms

5 **Absence of mediastinal shift** is seen with
- Small to moderate effusions
- Ipsilateral endobronchial obstructing lesion
- Mesothelioma with lung encasement and compression of the ipsilateral bronchi medially
- 'Frozen' mediastinum from metastatic nodes with inability to shift

6 **Duration of effusion**
- Pulmonary infarction – 10–14 days
- Uncomplicated parapneumonic effusion – 1–2 weeks
- Post-pericardiotomy – several weeks
- Benign asbestos effusion – weeks–months
- Radiation – weeks–months
- Tuberculosis – 1–4 months
- Yellow-nail, trapped lung, chylothorax, rheumatoid – years

CT Contribution to Undiagnosed Effusion

1 Empyema typically reveals loculation of fluid and enhancement of the surrounding pleura following contrast
- An associated pneumonia or cavity may be seen

2 Fluid–fluid level or areas of increased attenuation in a hemothorax

3 Tuberculosis may demonstrate an underlying parenchymal infiltrate (+/– cavitation), lymphadenopathy or a bony lesion
4 Associated pleuroparenchymal findings of asbestos exposure in an asbestos-related effusion
5 Nodular pleural thickening or a thick pleural rind with mesothelioma or metastatic cancer
   - Small metastatic nodules may be present on the pleura and pericardium at surgery but not seen on CT scan
6 Demonstration of an endobronchial obstructing lesions +/– mediastinal adenopathy
7 Sub-diaphragmatic abnormalities, e.g. subphrenic fluid collection, pancreatic calcifications or pseudocyst
8 Underlying parenchymal disease, e.g. neoplasm, abscess, pneumonia
9 Differentiate the causes of mediastinal widening
   - Adenopathy, e.g. neoplasm, TB
   - Calcifications, e.g. granulomatous mediastinitis
   - Primary mediastinal tumor, e.g. germ cell
   - Dissecting aneurysm
10 Identify an associated pericardial effusion (see Pleuropericarditis, p. 578)

PLEURAL EFFUSION – TYPES

Transudate

- Clear, LDH <200, protein <3 gm/dL
- $\frac{\text{Pleural fluid}}{\text{Serum}}$ LDH <0.6
- $\frac{\text{Pleural fluid}}{\text{Serum}}$ protein <0.5
- WBC <1000/mm^3 with 80% mononuclear cells
- RBC <5000/mm^3
- Cholesterol <60 mg/dL
- Some patients who clinically have a transudate but biochemically an exudate can be accurately classified as a

transudate by the serum to pleural fluid albumin gradient >1.2 mg/dL
- pH equal to or > blood pH

Exudate
- Clear, cloudy or bloody, LDH <200, protein <3 gm/dL
- $\frac{\text{Pleural fluid}}{\text{Serum}}$ LDH <0.6
- $\frac{\text{Pleural fluid}}{\text{Serum}}$ protein <0.5
- WBC >1000/mm^3
- RBC count is variable
- Cholesterol >60 mg/dL

Hemothorax
- Fluid Ht >50% of blood Ht

Empyema
- Grossly purulent
- and/or ⊕ culture
- and/or ⊕ grain stain

Chylothorax
- ± milky
- Triglycerides >110 mg/dL
- Chylomicra on lipoprotein electrophoresis
- pH > 7.20

TRANSUDATES – ETIOLOGIES

1 **Cardiac** – CHF, constrictive pericarditis
  - Constrictive pericarditis
    - Pleural effusions seen in approximately 50% of cases and may be the presenting feature
    - Unilateral (right > left) or bilateral and usually a transudate with lymphocytic predominance
    - Etiologies include *post-cardiac surgery, *mediastinal radiation, *uremia, *idiopathic, tuberculosis,

RA, SLE, malignancy, sarcoid, fibrosing mediastinitis
– The clue on chest X-ray is an enlarged 'cardiac silhouette' with associated pericardial calcifications

2 **Renal** – nephrotic syndrome, peritoneal dialysis, urinothorax

3 **Hepatic cirrhosis**
- May be unaccompanied by ascites as all the fluid can be intrapleural

4 **Pulmonary venous obstruction and hypertension**
- Mediastinal disease compressing the pulmonary veins, e.g. fibrosis, tumor

5 **Pulmonary emboli** (10–20% are transudates)

6 **Malignancy** (5–10% are transudates)

7 **Meig's syndrome**
- Originally described as the combination of a pleural effusion and ascites occurring in women with an ovarian fibroma
- Typically occurs with large tumors which secrete fluid into the peritoneal cavity and subsequent transfer of the fluid into the pleural space via diaphragmatic defects
- Most often seen at menopause, although described at all ages
- A similar syndrome was subsequently described with other pelvic tumors, both benign and malignant, in the absence of metastatic disease
- Radiologic features are those of right-sided (most common) > bilateral > left-sided effusions in the absence of associated abnormalities
- Diagnostic criteria
  – Pleural effusion and ascites in a female with an ovarian or other pelvic tumor
  – Absence of liver disease

   - Straw-colored fluid (occasionally blood containing) with no etiology determined
   - Resolution of the fluid within a few weeks post-tumor resection

8 **Ovarian hyperstimulation syndrome** (transudate or exudate)
- Seen in patients receiving gonadotrophins for induction of ovulation with
   - Bilateral ovarian enlargement on ultrasound
   - Shift of intravascular fluid into the third space with abdominal distension, ascites, pleural effusions and dyspnea
   - Less commonly pulmonary edema, ARDS, pericardial effusion

9 **Transdiaphragmatic spread of transudative ascites**

10 **Myxedema**

EXUDATES – COMMON CAUSES (Table 55.1)

Cause	Diagnostic criteria
1 ***Traumatic***	
Esophageal rupture	• Sterile exudate → empyema • pH ~6 • ↑ Salivary amylase • Food particles • Squamous epithelial cells
External trauma – open/closed	• History of trauma, fractured ribs, grossly bloody effusion
Post-thoracotomy	• Diagnosis of exclusion
2 ***Vascular***	
Post-cardiac injury syndrome	• Diagnosis of exclusion, ± bloody
Aortic dissection	• Grossly bloody in setting of dissection
Pulmonary infarct	• Varies from serous to bloody, no diagnostic features, 20% transudates
Vasculitis	
Churg-Strauss syndrome	• Eosinophilia
Wegener's	• No diagnostic features

Continued

Cause	Diagnostic criteria
3 ***Infectious***	
BACTERIAL	
Acute	• ⊕ Gram stain and culture
Tuberculosis	• Lymphocytic predominance, paucity of mesothelial cells, ⊕ AFB smears in approximately 10%, ⊕ culture approximately 25%, ↑ adenosine deaminase, ↑γ interferon, positive PCR
Nocardia	• ⊕ Culture
MYCOPLASMA	• Non-diagnostic
VIRAL	• May demonstrate intranuclear inclusions or multinucleated giant cells but usually non-diagnostic
FUNGAL	
Histoplasmosis	• Cultures rarely ⊕, rare eosinophilia
Blastomycosis	• Budding yeasts, ⊕ culture
Coccidioidomycosis	• ⊕ Cultures approximately 20%
Aspergillus	• Clumps of fungal hyphae, ⊕ cultures
Cryptococcus	• ⊕ Culture, cryptococcal Ag
PARASITIC	
Paragonimiasis	• ± Eosinophilia
Amebiasis	• Anchovy-colored
Echinococcus	• Eosinophilia, scolices
RICKETTSIAL	
Q fever	• Non-diagnostic
CHLAMYDIAL	• Non-diagnostic
4 ***Neoplastic***	*Radiologic clues to the malignant nature* • A rind of thick nodular pleura encompassing the lung • Areas of nodular pleural thickening
Mesothelioma	• High viscosity due to hyaluronic acid • Cytology may be ⊕
Metastatic (carcinoma of lung, breast, stomach, ovary as well as other carcinomas, sarcoma, melanoma, myeloma, leukemia, germ cell, mediastinal and chest wall tumors)	• Cytology ⊕ in approximately 60% of cases

Cause	Diagnostic criteria
Lymphoma	• Monoclonal cells in lymphoma or ⊕ pleural biopsy; lymphomatous invasion is an uncommon and late finding in Hodgkin's disease, but may be present early on with non-Hodgkin's lymphoma, even in the absence of intrathoracic lymphadenopathy
Non-metastatic Meig's syndrome	• Non-diagnostic findings
5 ***Collagen diseases***	
SLE	• Mononuclear cells or polys • LE cells • Low complement • ANA ≥1/160 • $\frac{\text{Pleural fluid}}{\text{Serum}}$ – ANA > 1
Rheumatoid arthritis	• Serous to turbid • May be yellow-green in color • Mainly mononuclear cells • Low complement • RF ≥1/320 • $\frac{\text{Pleural fluid}}{\text{Serum}}$ – RF > 1 • ± Glucose < 20 mg % • ± High cholesterol level • ± pH < 7.2
Progressive systemic sclerosis, mixed connective tissue disease	• Non-diagnostic
6 ***Pneumoconiosis***	
Asbestos-related	• History of asbestos exposure • Serous to bloody • Eosinophilia common • Diagnosis of exclusion after a 3 year follow-up where no neoplasm develops
7 ***Sub-diaphragmatic***	
Pancreatitis-related	• Elevated amylase
Hepatic, splenic or subphrenic abscess	• Varies from non-diagnostic to empyema • Brown or anchovy-colored fluid with amebiasis • Scolices may be seen in echinococcosis • Look for CT or U/S evidence of a subphrenic abscess

Continued

Cause	Diagnostic criteria
Splenic hematoma	• Non-diagnostic
Splenic infarct	• Non-diagnostic fluid but suspect with underlying endocarditis, hemoglobinopathy, chronic myeloid leukemia

Table 55.1

EXUDATES – UNCOMMON CAUSES

'TRUDDYS BEHAALF'

T – Trapped lung
R – Radiation
U – Uremia
D – Drugs
D – Dialysis
Y – Yellow nail syndrome
S – Sarcoid
B – BOOP
E – Eosinophilic pneumonia (acute)
H – Hypothyroidism
A – Ascites (exudative)
A – Amyloid
L – LAM
F – Familial Mediterranean fever

TRAPPED LUNG

The visceral pleura becomes encased with tumor, (e.g. mesothelioma, lung, breast), or a fibrous peel, (e.g. uremic pleurisy, rheumatoid effusion, TB, hemothorax, post-surgical, post pneumonic)

- Lung expansion is inhibited and creates a more negative pleural space, resulting in altered pleural fluid dynamics and an effusion

Diagnostic features

1 Hemithorax on the side of the effusion is smaller than the normal side
2 R/O an endobronchial obstruction
3 Failure of the lung to expand post-thoracocentesis with rapid recurrence of the effusion
4 With nonmalignant causes, the effusion may remain little changed for months to years, often with a history of one of the above disorders
5 Thoracoscopic visualization

EXUDATES – DIAGNOSTIC STUDIES

Gross features

1 Smell
   - Putrid – anaerobes
   - Urine – urinothorax
2 Color
   - Yellow-green – rheumatoid arthritis
   - Bloody – trauma, neoplasms, infarction
   - Brown – amebic abscess
   - Black – aspergillus
   - White – chyle, cholesterol effusion
   - Green – empyema
3 High viscosity – mesothelioma
4 Cloudy
   - Remains post-centrifugation – chylothorax, pseudo-chylothorax
   - Clears post-centrifugation – cells or debris

Microscopic features

1 >10% eosinophilis
   - Any cause of air or blood in pleural space, Churg-Strauss, drug reaction (nitrofurantoin, dantrolene, bromocryptine) benign asbestos effusion, paragonimiasis, hydatid cyst
   - Unlikely TB or cancer but not R/O
   - Often undiagnosed
2 >75% small lymphocytes
   - R/O tuberculosis, tumor, post CABG (delayed)
3 >50% neutrophils
   - Acute inflammation or infection
   - Typical of a parapneumonic effusion but seen in other disorders including pulmonary emboli, drugs, RA, SLE, lung cancer, early TB, pancreatic disease, intra-abdominal infection, viral infection, Dressler's
4 Monoclonal lymphocytes
   - Lymphoma

5 ⊕ Cytology
   - Seen in approximately 60% of malignant effusions
6 >100 000 RBC/mm^3
   - Trauma, tumor, infarction
7 >5% mesothelial cells
   - Unlikely tuberculosis

Biochemistry

1 Elevated amylase – acute or chronic pancreatitis, pancreatic pseudocyst or abscess, pancreatico-pleural fistula, esophageal rupture, neoplastic disease (most commonly lung)
2 Low glucose – multiple conditions
3 Low pH – multiple conditions
   pH > 7.4 – unlikely tuberculosis
4 Triglycerides >110 mg/dL – chylothorax
5 Elevated adenosine deaminase – tuberculosis

Immunology

1 ⊕ ANA ≥ 1:160 or $\frac{\text{Pleural fluid}}{\text{Serum}} \geq 1$ – SLE
2 ⊕ LE cells – SLE
3 ⊕ RF ≥ 1:320 or $\frac{\text{Pleural fluid}}{\text{Serum}} \geq 1$ – RA
4 Immunochemistry – malignancy
5 PCR – tuberculosis

Microbiology

1 ⊕ Gram stain, culture
2 ⊕ Fungal smears, cultures
3 ⊕ AFB smears, cultures

HEMOTHORAX

Definition: A pleural fluid hematocrit >50% of the venous blood value

*Traumatic

1 External, e.g. post-op, rib fractures, closed chest trauma
   - Often accompanied by a pneumothorax, although an effusion may not be seen immediately post-trauma and therefore follow-up X-rays should be done 3–6 hours later

2 Internal, e.g. spontaneous pneumothorax (5% of cases), aortic dissection and rupture

Non-traumatic

1 Neoplastic, e.g. mesothelioma, metastatic disease
2 Anticoagulation for pulmonary embolism
3 Infections, e.g. necrotizing bacteria, aspergillus, mucor
4 Thoracic endometriosis
   - Occurs 1–2 days after the onset of menstruation and 85% are right-sided
   - Most common presentation after pneumothorax

5 Pulmonary AV malformations, e.g. Osler-Rendu-Weber syndrome
6 Rupture of other major vessels
7 Coagulopathy
8 Others

PLEURAL EFFUSION AND FEVERS >10 DAYS

1 Esophageal rupture
2 Dressler's syndrome
3 Vasculitis, e.g. Wegener's, Churg-Strauss
4 Empyema – acute bacterial, tuberculosis, fungal, parasitic
5 Lymphoma
6 Collagen disease, e.g. SLE, rheumatoid
7 Subdiaphragmatic, e.g. pancreatitis, abdominal abscess
8 Drug-induced lupus
9 Sarcoid
10 BOOP
11 Familial Mediterranean fever

PLEUROPERICARDITIS

1 **Traumatic**
- Penetrating/non-penetrating

2 **Vascular**
- Dressler's syndrome
- Aortic aneurysm
- Pulmonary infarction with a hemopericardium complicating anticoagulation therapy

3 **Inflammatory**
- Bacterial
  - Acute, e.g. *Strep. pneumoniae*
  - Chronic, e.g. tuberculosis, actinomycosis
- Viral
- Fungal

4 **Neoplastic**
- Mesothelioma
- Metastatic – carcinoma, sarcoma, melanoma, leukemia, lymphoma, germ cell, mediastinal tumor

5 **Collagen diseases**
- SLE, RA

6 **Pneumoconiosis**
- Asbestosis

7 **Radiation**

8 **Uremia**

9 **Drugs**
- Hydralazine, pronestyl

10 **Sarcoid**

11 **Hypothyroidism**

12 **Familial Mediterranean fever**

13 **Fibrosing/granulomatous mediastinitis (transudative effusion)**

14 **Congestive heart failure (transudative effusion)**

15 **Constrictive pericarditis (transudate or exudate)**

Fraser R.S., Muller N.L., Colman N., Paré P.D. (1999) *Diagnosis of Diseases of the Chest* 4th Edn., WB Saunders.

Naidich, D.P., Zerhouni, E.A., Siegelman, S.S. (1998) *Computed Tomography and Magnetic Resonance of the Thorax*, 3rd edn. New York: Raven Press.

Moss, A., Gamsu, Genant (1992) Thorax and neck. In: *Computed Tomography of the Body with Magnetic Resonance Imaging*, 2nd edn, vol. 1.: W.B. Saunders.

Felson, B. (1973) *Chest Roentgenology*.: W.B. Saunders.

McLoud, T.C., Isler, R., Noveline, R. *et al.* (1981) Review. The apical CAP. *AJR* **137**: 299–306.

Muller, N. (1993) Imaging of the pleura. *Radiology* **186**: 297–307.

McLoud, T.C. (1998) CT and MR in pleural disease. *Clinics in Chest Medicine* **19**: 261–275.

Hiller, E., Rosenow, E., Olsen, A. (1972) Pulmonary manifestations of the yellow nail syndrome. *Chest* **61**: 452–458.

Sahn, S. (1998) Malignancy metastatic to the pleura. *Clinics in Chest Medicine* **19**: 351–361.

Light, R. (1992) Disease-a-month. *Pleural Diseases* **xxxviii**: 266–331.

Robison, L., Reilly, R. (1994) Localized pleural mesothelioma. The clinical spectrum. *Chest* **106**: 1611–1615.

Antman, K.H. (1991) Clinical and natural history of benign and malignant mesothelioma. *Semin. Oncol.* **8**: 313–320.

56 Pleuritic Chest Pain – R/O Pulmonary Embolus

Vascular disorders

1 Pulmonary thrombo-embolus
2 Septic embolus
3 Pulmonary vasculitis
4 Aspergillosis or other angioinvasive fungus in an immunocompromised patient
5 Dressler's syndrome
   - ECG evidence of a recent MI
   - Associated pericarditis on clinical exam or on echocardiography
6 Pericarditis of other etiologies
   - Pericardial rub
   - ECG changes
   - Pericardial fluid on ECHO
7 Aortic aneurysm – rupture/dissection
   - Hemothorax
   - New onset aortic insufficiency
   - Echocardiographic findings
   - Documentation on aortogram or contrast CT
8 Myocardial infarction

Parenchymal disease

9 Pneumonia
   - Clinical features of cough, fever, purulent sputum, recent family history, leucocytosis
   - Parenchymal disease on chest X-ray

Pleural disease

10 Tuberculous pleurisy
11 Empyema
   - Defined by gross pus, positive culture or positive gram stain of pleural fluid

12 Viral pleuritis
  - Personal or family history of URI
  - Symptoms of a lower RTI
  - Small pleural effusion or normal X-rays
  - Negative W/U for pulmonary embolus
  - Diagnosis of exclusion

13 Pneumothorax
  - Pathognomonic X-ray findings but may require an expiratory film

14 Asbestos pleuritis
  - Exposure history
  - Pleural plaques on X-ray

15 Collagen disease – SLE, RA
  - Known connective tissue disorder
  - X-rays may be normal, reveal pleural thickening or an effusion

16 Neoplastic disease (usually subacute – chronic presentation), primary or metastatic

Chest wall

17 Musculoskeletal pains with a history of trauma, chest wall tenderness, rib fracture

Mediastinum

18 Esophageal rupture, spasm, reflux
19 Pleuropericardial fat pad necrosis
20 Fibrosing/granulomatous mediastinitis

Subdiaphragmatic causes

21 Perforated viscus with free air under the diaphragm
22 Infarction – splenic, renal, bowel
23 Inflammatory – pancreatitis, cholecystitis
24 Infectious
  - Splenic, pancreatic or subdiaphragmatic abscess, manifest as a soft tissue mass ± gas, with displacement of intra-abdominal viscera
  - May be seen on plain films, abdominal CT, ultrasound or gallium scan

57A Pneumonia

COMMUNITY-ACQUIRED PNEUMONIA DIAGNOSTIC APPROACH

STEP I **History, Physical, X-rays**
(Severity, Etiologic clues)
↓

STEP II **Bloods** +/– other **Fluid** studies

STEP III Determine **Underlying Etiology** of Pneumonia

STEP IV R/O **Non-Infectious** diseases simulating pneumonia

STEP V **Risk Assessment** → Home / → Hospitalize

STEP VI **Pathogen-directed *vs.* Empiric Therapy**

Clues from History, Physical and Chest X-rays

History

1. Age
   - Elderly patients may not have a 'classic' presentation and can present with isolated fever, hypothermia, altered mentation, tachypnea or combination of the above
   - Relative frequency of 'atypical' pneumonia becomes less

2. Presentation
   - Onset re acute, subacute or chronic
   - Upper respiratory symptoms including sinus, nasal, pharyngeal or dental problems
   - Pleuritic pain, rusty sputum and dyspnea are more common with bacteria *vs.* 'atypical' agents

3. Personal factors
   - Smoking
   - Alcohol/drug abuse
   - HIV risk factors
   - Occupational history
   - Allergic history
   - Hobbies
   - Mineral oil use
   - Social factors, e.g. no care-giver

4. Epidemiology
   - Nursing home patients e.g. *Strep. pneumoniae*, *Staph. aureus*, gram negatives
   - Recent hospital discharge, e.g. *Staph. aureus* (including MRSA), gram negatives
   - Place of birth and travel history
   - Exposures to
     - Birds, e.g. psittacosis or other pets
     - Soil enriched with bird or bat droppings, e.g. histoplasmosis, cryptococcosis
     - Rabbits, e.g. tularemia
     - Farm animals, e.g. Q-fever

  - Family members with a RTI, e.g. viral, mycoplasma, chlamydia
  - Influenza outbreak, e.g. influenza, *Strep. pneumoniae*, *Staph. aureus*, hemophilus
  - Legionella outbreak
  - Tuberculosis
  - Rats, e.g. hantavirus, leptospirosis, plague

5 Underlying cardiopulmonary disease, e.g. COPD (*Strep. pneumonia*, hemophilus, moraxella, legionella), reserve and functional status
- Known congenital or acquired pulmonary diseases

6 Other co-morbidity including
- Risk factors for aspiration
  - Alcoholism, e.g. *Strep. pneumoniae*, anaerobes, gram negatives
  - Poor oral hygiene, e.g. anaerobes
  - Dysphagia
  - Recent dental work
  - Recent general anesthesia
- i.v. drug use, e.g. anaerobes, tuberculosis, *Staph. aureus*
- Pregnancy, e.g. aspiration, HIV-related, viral, fungal
- Underlying diseases which can result in immunosuppression

7 Drugs
- Allergies
- i.v. abuse
- Drug-induced lung disease
- Immunosuppressives predisposing to opportunistic infection

Physical findings

1 Vital signs
- RR > 30
- Requirement for mechanical ventilation

- Severe brady/tachycardia
- Hypotension

2 Extensive pleuropulmonary disease on exam
3 Cyanosis
4 Altered sensorium with inability to clear secretions
5 Oliguria
6 Extrapulmonary disease
- Upper respiratory findings, e.g. abscess, gingivitis, decaying tooth
- Septic focus with meningitis, brain abscess, arthritis, pericarditis, endocarditis, peritonitis, empyema
- Bullous myringitis, e.g. mycoplasma
- Erythema nodosum, e.g. 1° tuberculosis
- Erythema multiforme, e.g. mycoplasma
- Splenomegaly, e.g. psittacosis
- Retinitis, e.g. CMV, toxoplasmosis
- Skin rash, e.g. measles, atypical measles, chicken pox
- Skin nodules, e.g. blastomycosis, coccidioidomycosis, sporotrichosis

Radiologic studies

1 Suggest etiologies depending upon **pattern recognition**
- *Interstitial*
  - Miliary, e.g. TB, nocardia, salmonella, coccidio, crypto, blastomycosis
  - Reticular, e.g. viral, pneumocystis, mycoplasma, chlamydia
- *Interstitial and air space*
  - e.g. mycoplasma, viral, pneumocystis
- *Airspace*
  - Homogenous with air bronchograms, unifocal/multifocal, e.g. *Strep. pneumoniae*, legionella
  - Non-homogenous patchy airspace disease, e.g. *Staph. aureus*, viral, mycoplasma
  - Mass-like: single or multiple
    - Bacterial, e.g. *Strep. pneumoniae*, anaerobes, abscess, legionella, tuberculosis, atypical mycobacteria

— Fungal, e.g. aspergillus, cryptococcus, blastomycosis, coccidioidomycosis
- diffuse bilateral 'white-out', e.g. influenza, *Staph. aureus*, *Strep. pneumoniae*, legionella

- *Nodular pattern*: interstitial and/or airspace, e.g. tuberculosis, varicella, atypical measles, mycoplasma, psittacosis, histoplasmosis, coccidioidomycosis, cryptococcus
- *Normal*, e.g. dehydration, severe neutropenia, pneumocystis, early disease, difficulty in film interpretation due to baseline abnormalities

Limitations of pattern recognition

- A given organism, e.g. mycoplasma, can cause different patterns, e.g. unifocal airspace disease, multifocal airspace disease, interstitial, interstitial and airspace disease or nodular pattern
- Mixed patterns occur
- Airspace disease obscures underlying interstitial disease
- Underlying abnormal lung, e.g. emphysema or interstitial disease, will distort the radiologic picture

2 **Demonstrate complications**

- Cavitation, e.g. abscess formation, gangrene (necrotic lung in an abscess cavity)
- Adenopathy
- Pleural effusion
- Pneumatoceles, e.g. *Staph. aureus* in children, *P. carinii* in AIDS

3 **Evaluate severity**

- Extent of disease – number of lobes involved
- Rapidity of spread

4 **CT scan contribution**

- Detection of early airspace disease when chest X-ray is normal, e.g. aspergillus
- Detection of early interstitial disease, e.g. pneumocystis
- Demonstration of cavities, lymphadenopathy, pleural

effusion or empyema which are not apparent on chest X-ray
- Detection of multifocal disease

5 Identify a **co-existing predisposition** to pneumonia, e.g. obstructed bronchus

6 **R/O pneumonia** and suggest an alternative diagnosis, e.g. bronchitis

7 Suggest a **non-infectious disorder** simulating pneumonia

History, Physical and X-rays will determine which Blood Tests or other Fluid Studies are Indicated

Bloods

1 ABGs/pulse oximetry
2 Blood cultures: ~10% of hospitalized patients with CAP will have positive blood cultures
3 CBC, WBC and diff.
- WBC >30 000 or <4000 – severe infection
- neutrophils <1000 – severe infection
- lymphopenia <1000 or CD_4 <200 – advanced HIV infection
- WBC >15 000 suggests a bacterial etiology

4 INR, PT, PTT, platelets, fibrin split products
5 Multisystem involvement with abnormal renal and hepatic function
6 Lytes (for hyponatremia) + glucose
7 Cold agglutinins
8 HIV testing where clinically indicated
9 PCR for pneumococcal DNA, legionella, mycoplasma (availability restricted at present)
10 Serology for legionella, mycoplasma, viruses, fungi, chlamydia – used for epidemiologic studies but not useful acutely when therapeutic decisions must be made
- Single positive serum is diagnostic of HIV or HANTA virus – otherwise paired sera are necessary

11 Fungal antigens, e.g. cryptococcal Ag

Sputum (experienced observer important)

1 Gram stain showing >25 neutrophils and <10 squamous epithelial cells per lower power field
   - Large numbers of bacteria with features of a likely pulmonary pathogen will suggest antibiotic choice and often correlates with organism identified on subsequent culture
   - Absence of *Staph. aureus* or gram negatives on culture makes these unlikely causes of the pneumonia
   - Standard smears and cultures will not detect many important pathogens including legionella, viruses, mycoplasma, chlamydia, anaerobes
   - Patient may have non-productive cough or have received prior antibiotics
2 Acid-fast stains for tuberculosis, atypicals, nocardia, legionella, rhodococcus
3 Fluorescent antibody for legionella, viruses, parasites
4 PCR for legionella, chlamydia, ? mycoplasma, ? viral, ? viruses, ? parasites (no FDA approved kits)
5 KOH for fungi
6 Giemsa for parasites
7 Rapid 'membrane' enzyme immunoassay for influenza A, B and RSV (nasopharyngeal swab)

Bronchoscopy

- Telescoping plugged catheter +/– BAL

TTNA (considered in non-responding patient)

1 Gram stain, C/S
2 Acid-fast stains and cultures
3 Fungal smears and cultures
4 Fluorescent antibody for legionella

Pleural effusion

- Parapneumonic effusion should always be tapped if possible to
  – Positively identify the responsible organism
  – R/O empyema
  – Guide therapy re drainage *vs.* antibiotics alone

Metastatic site

- Aspiration of an extrapulmonary septic focus

Urine

1. Detection of legionella antigen, limited to *L. pneumophilia* serogroup I, which is responsible for approximately 80% of cases and has an 85% sensitivity
2. Histoplasma polysaccharide antigen
3. Cryptococcal antigen (usually detected in serum)
4. Pneumococcal soluble antigen

Attempt to Determine the Presence of an Underlying Disease

Initial pneumonia or **recurrent pneumonia in the same lobe** may be secondary to

1. Obstructing bronchial lesion
   - Intralumenal, e.g. foreign body, broncholith
   - Intramural, e.g. neoplasm
   - Extramural, e.g. mediastinitis
2. Localized bronchiectasis
3. Broncho-esophageal fistula, e.g. neoplasm
4. Bronchopulmonary sequestration
5. Bronchogenic cyst

Initial pneumonia or **recurrent pneumonia in different lobes** may be secondary to

1. Respiratory disease, e.g. COPD, bronchiectasis, chronic sinusitis
2. Esophageal disease, structural or functional, e.g. achalasia, scleroderma, Zenker's diverticulum
3. Other disorders predisposing to aspiration
4. Cardiac disease, e.g. CHF
5. Other organ diseases including liver disease (e.g. alcoholism, cirrhosis), renal failure, diabetes, hematologic disease (e.g. leucopenia/hypo/agammaglobulinemia, myeloma, leukemia, lymphoma)
6. Drugs, e.g. steroids/immunosuppressives

R/O Non-infectious Disease Simulating Pneumonia

Airways diseases

- BOOP
- ABPA
- Bronchiectasis
- Bronchopulmonary sequestration
- Bronchocentric granulomatosis

Vascular diseases

- Alveolar hemorrhage syndromes, e.g. Goodpasture's syndrome, capillaritis
- Eosinophilic lung diseases, e.g. Loeffler's, acute or chronic eosinophilic pneumonia
- Infarcts, septic or bland
- Fat emboli
- Vasculitis, e.g. Wegener's, Churg-Strauss, microscopic polyarteritis
- Collagen diseases, e.g. SLE
- Vascular tumors
- Acute chest syndrome in sickle cell crisis
- Pulmonary leukoagglutinin transfusion reaction

Parenchymal diseases

- Allergic alveolitis
- Drug reaction, e.g. methotrexate, nitrofurantoin
- Transfusion reaction
- Alveolar proteinosis
- Sarcoid
- Lipoid pneumonia
- Pulmonary edema
- Neoplasms, e.g. lymphoma, alveolar cell carcinoma
- ARDS
- Radiation pneumonitis
- Plasma cell granuloma (inflammatory pseudotumor)
- Aspiration
- AIP, UIP, DIP, LIP

The following should be particularly sought as they are all potentially responsive to steroid treatment and include

'Steroid treatable diseases' simulating acute pneumonia

- BOOP
- ABPA
- Vasculitides
- Collagen diseases
- Eosinophilic pneumonia – acute
- Sarcoid
- Allergic alveolitis
- Drug reaction
- Hamman-Rich (AIP)

Risk Assessment with decision as to which patients can be sent Home *vs.* Hospitalized

Criteria for hospitalization

History

- Age > 65
- Comorbidity, acute or chronic
- Social factors

Physical findings

- RR > 30
- Severe brady or tachycardia
- Hypotension
- Extensive pleuropulmonary disease on exam
- Cyanosis
- Sepsis and end-organ dysfunction, e.g. altered sensorium, oliguria
- Extrapulmonary septic complications

Radiologic abnormalities

- Multilobar involvement
- Rapidly progressive disease
- Cavitation
- Pleural effusion

Bloods

- Neutropenia
- Severe leucocytosis
- Hematocrit <30
- Abnormal renal or hepatic function
- $PO_2 < 60$; $PCO_2 > 45$; acidemia

- Na < 130
- DIC picture

Clinical course

- Failure to respond to out-patient treatment in 48–72 hours

Pathogen-directed *vs.* Empiric Therapy

Pathogen-directed

The rationale for an etiologic determination of pneumonia is to

- Select an antibiotic with activity against a specific pathogen
- Limit the effects of antibiotic use in terms of cost, adverse reactions and drug resistance
- Evaluate the epidemiologic consequences of specific organisms

Confirmation of the diagnosis – usually will not be made during initial patient evaluation

1. Recovery of a likely agent from an **uncontaminated site** – blood, pleural fluid, TTNA, metastatic site, ? bronchoscopy using a protected specimen brush and BAL
2. Demonstration of an organism in **respiratory secretions** which is **not** present in the absence of disease
   - Bacterial, e.g. *M. tuberculosis*, legionella
   - Viral, e.g. influenza, respiratory syncytial
   - Fungal, e.g. histoplasmosis, blastomycosis, coccidioidomycosis, pneumocystis
   - Parasitic, e.g. stronglyloides, toxoplasma
3. **Antigen detection**
   - Blood, e.g. pneumococcal polysaccharide Ag
   - Urine, e.g. legionella Ag, histoplasma polysaccharide Ag, cryptococcal Ag, pneumococcal Ag
   - Respiratory secretions, e.g. DFA test for legionella, ? pneumococal polysaccharide Ag
4. **Antibody Detection**
   - Four-fold increase in antibody titers over several weeks
   - Increased levels of specific IgM antibody with legionella, mycoplasma, chlamydia

5 **Nucleic acid detection**, e.g. PCR

Possible – probable diagnosis

1 Compatible clinical-radiologic presentation with identification of a **likely** pulmonary pathogen in respiratory secretions (sputum or bronchoscopic sample) on gram stain +/– culture
2 Shortcomings include a 'poor' sample, prior antibiotic treatment, significance of *Strep. pneumoniae* on cultures, inability to diagnose anaerobes or atypical organisms

Possible diagnosis

Viral etiology of pneumonia suspected with

1 No organism recovered from sputum of other fluids studied
2 Non-improvement or progression of disease in spite of several days of antibiotic therapy for 'atypicals'
3 Epidemiologic factors, e.g. season, community epidemic

Empiric therapy – why?

- Wide range of potential organisms
- Extensive testing fails to identify an etiology in >50% of cases
- Two or more etiologies found in ~3% of cases
- 'Typical' and 'atypical' organisms merge in presentation in spite of clinical, radiologic and sputum studies
- Preceding work-up will give information on severity and need for hospitalization but will only suggest likely etiologies
- With the difficulties identifying a specific etiology, the American Thoracic Society has developed guidelines for the treatment of community-acquired pneumonia with stratification into four classes, and subsequent antibiotic recommendations

I Outpatient without co-morbidity and age <60
II Outpatient with co-morbidity and/or age >60
III Requiring hospitalization
IV Requiring ICU admission

PNEUMONIA MORTALITY

Patients under 50 years of age with stable vital signs and no co-morbidity, sent home on antibiotics, have a mortality of <1%

- Hospitalized patients have approximately 10–20% mortality
- *Strep. pneumoniae* is responsible for ~⅔ of all fatal cases of pneumonia
- Mortality rates increase with
  - Increasing age
  - Patients from nursing homes
  - Co-morbidity including alcoholism, malignancy, immuno-suppression, neurologic disease, congestive heart failure, diabetes
  - Respiratory failure/hypotension
  - High risk pathogens, e.g. legionella, gram negatives
  - Bacteremic *vs.* non-bacteremic cases

ETIOLOGY – CAP

The frequency with which the following agents are responsible will vary with

1 Geographic area
2 Co-morbidity in the community
3 Percentage of nursing home patients
4 Average age of the population
5 Primary *vs.* a referral center
6 Extent of testing

Group A – Most Common

Bacterial

- *Strep. pneumoniae* – responsible for ~⅔ of all cases of pneumonia where an etiologic diagnosis is made
- *Haemophilus influenzae*, gram negatives, *Staph. aureus*, anaerobes

Atypicals

- Mycoplasma, chlamydia pneumoniae, legionella

Viral

- Influenza

Mixed infections

Opportunistic

- Bacterial – any agent found in normal hosts in addition to *Staph. aureus*, gram negatives, acid-fast organisms including tuberculosis, atypical mycobacterial, *Legionella micdadei*, nocardia, *Rhodococcus equi*
- Viral – *Herpes simplex*, *Herpes zoster*, CMV
- Fungal – mucormycosis, aspergillus, candida, cryptococcus, systemic histoplasmosis, pneumocystis
- Parasitic – toxoplasmosis, strongyloides

Group B – Less Common to Uncommon

Bacterial

- Other streptococcal species, *Moraxella catarralis*, actinomycosis, nocardia, *M. tuberculosis*, atypical mycobacteria

Viral

- Para-influenza, respiratory syncytial, adenovirus, rhinovirus

Fungal (dependent on geographic location)

- Histoplasmosis, blastomycosis, coccidioidomycosis

Group C – Rarely Seen

Bacterial

- *Bordetella pertussis*, tularemia, bubonic plague, anthrax, brucellosis

Viral

- Hanta

Fungal

- Other than the above

Parasitic

Rickettsial

- *Coxiella burnetti*

Chlamydial

- *C. psittaci*

ATYPICAL PNEUMONIA

Definition: Confusing term and historically was used to describe cases of pneumonia that were 'atypical' for classic pneumococcal pneumonia

- Sub-acute onset
- Absence of pleuritic pain and rusty sputum
- X-rays often out of proportion to symptomatology, frequently with multifocal abnormalities
- No bacterial pathogen in the sputum
- Mild leucocytosis
- No response to sulfas
- Little mortality
- Slow resolution clinically

Patients presenting with the above were said to have '**atypical**' or '**primary atypical**' pneumonia (Table 57A.1)

	Typical	Atypical
X-ray	Single focus usually	Single or multiple foci
Gram stain	Often ⊕	Negative
Bloods	⊕ Cultures	⊕ Serology Negative cultures
WBC	>15 000	<15 000
Cell wall antibiotics	Effective	Ineffective
Pathophysiology	Aspiration	Inhalation
Person-to-person	Absent	⊕ Often
Clinically	• Abrupt onset • Productive cough • Pleuritic pain common	• Prodrome common • Often dry cough • Pleuritic pain rare

Table 57A.1

With sophistication of laboratory testing, more and more organisms were described to give this syndrome and the **etiologies** today include

- **Mycoplasma**: *up to 50% of cases
- **Viral**: influenza, parainfluenza, RSV, EBV, hanta
- **Chlamydial**: **Chlamydia pneumoniae*, *Chlamydia psittaci*
- **Rickettsial**: Q-fever
- **Bacterial**: primary TB, *legionella, *Francisella tularensis*
- **Fungal**: primary histoplasmosis. Blasto, coccidio
- **Parasitic**: toxoplasmosis

Infection with these agents ranges from asymptomatic to mild or life-threatening but infection rates are hard to determine

- Detection in respiratory secretions by culture or PCR is difficult
- Paired sera are usually required
- Some agents, e.g. mycoplasma, may be present in the healthy population
- Different studies have their own diagnostic criteria – a sensitive, specific and readily available 'gold standard' is absent
- Result of the above is the lack of contribution of testing for atypicals early in the course of disease when an antibiotic choice is being made

Difficulties distinguishing typical from atypicals include

1. A single organism, e.g. legionella (or even pneumococcus), can present clinically as a 'typical' or 'atypical' pneumonia, with the patients physiologic and immunologic status often contributing to the clinical presentation
2. The two syndromes, 'typical' and 'atypical' pneumonia, often overlap in presentation and patients with 'atypical' pneumonia cannot be reliably distinguished from 'typical'
3. Patients may have a mixed infection of typical, usually *Strep. pneumoniae*, with an atypical agent

*__Identification__ of a specific cause of pneumonia is generally **not helped** by classifying a patient as 'typical' or 'atypical' and initial therapy is usually empiric, covering a wide range of potential agents

CAP – REQUIRING ICU ADMISSION

Criteria for ICU Admission

Required in ~10% of hospitalized patients with CAP and due to

1 Respiratory failure with
 - RR > 30
 - Inability to clear secretions and protect the airway
 - Requirement for mechanical ventilation

2 Circulatory failure with
 - Systolic pressure <90 mmHg
 - Diastolic pressure <60 mmHg
 - Vasopressor requirement, e.g. septic shock
 - Oliguria, acute renal failure or requirement for dialysis

3 Clinical progression in spite of optimal ward therapy
 Radiologically there is usually
 - Bilateral disease
 - Multilobar involvement
 - Progressive infiltrates with clinical deterioration

Comorbidity and Mortality

A previously healthy individual is seen in ~⅓ of cases, underlying diseases most often being

1 *COPD
2 CHF
3 Alcoholism
4 Diabetes

Mortality rates vary from 20–50% in different series with death usually secondary to refractory hypoxemia, shock and/or multi-organ failure

Etiologies

1 *Strep. pneumoniae*
Hemophilus
Staph. aureus
Gram negatives
Legionella
Mycoplasma
— Responsible for 90% of cases where a pathogen is identified

2 Acid-fast organisms – TB, atypicals, nocardia, rhodococcus (specific host factors usually present)
3 Viral – influenza, parainfluenza, adeno, respiratory syncytial
4 Environmental exposures
- Q-fever from inhalation of contaminated dust particles from infected cattle, sheep, hides and milk, or attending the birth of livestock or cats
- *C. psittaci* from inhalation of infectious particles from birds which may be asymptomatic but more often ill with a diarrheal disease
- *F. tularensis* from skin contact or airbone transmission from infected rabbits or other animals, bites contaminated with feces of infected ticks or inanimate objects in contact with infected rabbits

5 Geographic history to suggest a specific fungal, bacterial or parasitic infection
6 Immunosuppression
- Bacteria, e.g. TB, atypicals, nocardia
- Viral, e.g. CMV, *Herpes simplex*, *Herpes zoster*
- Fungal, e.g. mucor, aspergillus, cryptococcus, candida, histo, pneumocystis
- Parasitic, e.g. strongyloides, toxoplasmosis

Diagnostic Work-up

1 Sputum microscopy and cultures for bacteria, acid-fast organisms, fungi, parasites as well as detection of legionella or pneumococcal antigen
2 Blood cultures
3 Pleural tap if effusion is present
4 Serum antigen testing for pneumococcus, histoplasma, cryptococcus

5 Urine antigen testing for legionella, histoplasma, cryptococcus, pneumococcus
6 Serology for
   - Bacteria – tularemia
   - Viruses, including HIV
   - Mycoplasma
   - Fungae
   - Chlamydia – *C. psittaci* or *pneumoniae*
   - Rickettsia – Q-fever
7 Bronchoscopy for endobronchial disease as well as protected specimen brush and BAL, with microscopy and cultures for bacteria, mycobacteria, legionella, viral agents, fungi and parasites
8 TTNA
9 Chest CT
10 Open lung biopsy

The extent of initial testing is controversial as most patients will not be diagnosed prior to institution of antibiotics (which is usually empiric)

Factors which would favor an invasive procedure include
- Progressive disease in spite of broad spectrum antibiotics
- Suspicion of opportunistic infection
- History of a specific environmental exposure, e.g. travel, hobbies, occupation
- Suspicion of non-infectious disease

NOSOCOMIAL PNEUMONIA (NON-ICU SETTING)

Definition: Present in a patient who has been in hospital at least 48 hours (excluding infection incubating at the time of admission) and has developed a new pulmonary infiltrate in association with fever, cough, purulent sputum, fever and leucocytosis
- Both overdiagnosis and underdiagnosis are common with controversies around diagnosis and treatment

Routes of Bacterial Entry

1 *Microaspiration of oropharyngeal secretions heavily colonized with pathogenic bacteria
2 Aspiration of esophageal/gastric contents
3 Hematogenous spread from a distant site
4 Direct airway inoculation, e.g. suctioning
5 Spread from a contiguous site, e.g. pleura

Shortcomings of Diagnosis

- Sputum, B-scope, BAL and PSB results are difficult to interpret as colonization does not equate with infection
- Gram stains are negative with legionella, chlamydia, viral infections
- The potential list of organisms is large
- Infections may be polymicrobial
- Purulent tracheobronchitis cannot be distinguished from pneumonia in patients with other reasons for pulmonary infiltrates, e.g. failure
- Non-infectious disorders can mimic or mask pneumonia
- Presentation may be atypical, particularly in the elderly

Etiologies

1 Organisms most commonly seen in community acquired pneumonias – *Strep. pneumoniae*, hemophilus, legionella, anaerobes, chlamydia
2 Gram negatives – 'KEEAPPS' – klebsiella, enterobacter, *E. coli*, acinetobacter, proteus, pseudomonas, serratia
3 *Staph. aureus* including MRSA
4 Polymicrobial
5 Others

The probability of a specific organism is influenced by

- Severity of the pneumonia
- Time of onset, i.e. early or late
- Specific risk factors

Risk Factors

1 Aging
2 Increased duration of hospitalization

3 Impaired host defenses from
   - 1° immunologic abnormalities – cellular/humoral
   - Diseases affecting immune status, e.g. alcoholism, malnutrition, DM, CRF, liver failure, steroids, immunosuppressives, malignancy
4 Factors favoring colonization by gram negatives, e.g. antibiotics, gastric acid neutralization
5 Factors favoring aspiration of large bacterial inocula, e.g. altered sensorium, dysphagia, increased gastric bacteria
6 Extrapulmonary septic focus leading to bacteremia
7 Factors favoring inhalational infection, e.g. contaminated aerosols, contacts with medical personnel
8 Breakdown of skin or mucosal boundaries, e.g. endobronchial intubation, central lines, nasogastric tubes
9 Impaired clearance of infections from the lung, e.g. COPD, CHF

PNEUMONIA – SLOWLY OR NON-RESOLVING

Definition: This is variable but refers to a **pulmonary infection** in the absence of other potential **non-infectious** causes, with (a) lack of a 'usual' response within 7 days of treatment, or (b) failure to completely clear by 4–6 weeks

1 **Organism-related**
   - Etiology, e.g. legionella may take several months to resolve radiologically, frequently with residual fibrosis
   - Severity of infection
   - Polymicrobial infection which has been incompletely diagnosed and treated
   - Unsuspected organisms
     - Bacterial, e.g. tuberculosis, atypical mycobacteria, anaerobes, legionella, nocardia, actinomycosis
     - Mycoplasma, viral, parasitic
     - Fungal, e.g. histoplasmosis, blastomycosis, coccidioidomycosis, aspergillus (sub-acute necrotizing)

2 **Antibiotic-related**
- Inadequate dose, penetration or absorption (if given p.o.)
- Antibiotic resistance

3 **Local factors**
- Obstructive lung disease, e.g. COPD, bronchiectasis
- Localized airway narrowing – intralumenal, endobronchial or extramural
- Congestive heart failure
- Bronchopulmonary sequestration
- Infected bronchogenic cyst

4 **Systemic factors**
- Aging (decreased immunity, underlying chronic diseases, atypical presentation, unusual organisms)
- Impaired cellular or humoral immunity, either primary (cellular/humoral) or in association with multiple disorders including diabetes mellitus, SLE, chronic renal failure, alcoholism, malnutrition, hematologic malignancy, steroids, immunosuppressives, HIV

5 **Recurrent aspiration**

6 **Pneumonia progression to**
- Abscess formation
- Empyema
- BOOP
- 'Organizing pneumonia' with persistent airspace consolidation and air bronchograms

7 **R/O diseases simulating pneumonia**

PNEUMONIA – WORSENING

1 **Organism-related**
- Virulent organism not responding to antibiotics
- Superinfection
- Unidentified agent not covered by antibiotics chosen –

bacterial, mycoplasma, viral, fungal, parasitic, rickettsial, chlamydial
- Initial natural progression of pneumonia prior to improvement

2 **Antibiotic-related**
- Antibiotic-induced lung disease
  - Allergic alveolitis
  - Loeffler's
  - BOOP
- Inadequate antibiotic dosage
- Resistance to antibiotic chosen
- Failure of antibiotic to penetrate the lung, e.g. aminoglycosides

3 **Local factors**
- Obstructed bronchus – intralumenal, intramural, peribronchial
- Bronchopulmonary sequestration

4 **Impaired immunity**
- Selective or diffuse reductions in gammaglobulin levels
- Lymphocytopenia or neutropenia
- Underlying hematologic diseases including lymphoma, leukemia, myeloma, myelodysplasia, myelofibrosis, Waldenstrom's, others
- Immunosuppressive agents
- HIV (and an unrecognized organism)

5 **Recurrent aspiration** secondary to impaired mentation, dysphagia, broncho-esophageal fistula
- Bacterial innocula
- Lipoid pneumonia
- Miliary granulomatosis

6 **Pneumonia progression** to
- Abscess formation
- Empyema
- BOOP
- 'Organizing pneumonia'
- ARDS

7 **R/O diseases simulating progressive pneumonia** including
- BOOP
- Alveolar hemorrhage
- Eosinophilic lung disease
- Pulmonary infarcts
- Vasculitis
- Neoplasms
- Pulmonary edema
- Acute interstitial pneumonia or variants, e.g. DIP, LIP, etc.

PNEUMONIA AND HILAR ADENOPATHY

Bacterial	
• Whooping cough	• Contact history, lymphocytosis
• Bubonic plague	• Travel history, rodent contact
• Anthrax	• Exposure to animals, hides, imported wool
• Tularemia	• Exposure to rabbits, muskrats or tick bite
• Tuberculosis – primary	• Exposure history, unilateral adenopathy (80%)
Mycoplasma (adenopathy rare in adults)	
Viral	
• Ebstein-Barr	• Other features of infectious mononucleosis
• Varicella, rubela	• Skin rash
Fungal	
• Histoplasmosis, coccidioidomycosis	• Geographic area
• Sporotrichosis	• Gardening history, alcoholism, skin lesions
Parasitic	
• Toxoplasmosis	• Infectious mono-like presentation
• Tropical eosinophilia	• Geographic history, diffuse interstitial disease

Rickettsial

- Q-fever
  - Occupational history, consumption of unpasteurized milk

Chlamydial

- *C. psittaci*
  - History of exposure to birds

Any post-obstructive pneumonia

- Concurrent hilar mass

PNEUMONIA – NON-PULMONARY CAUSES OF FEVER

1 Endocarditis
2 Bacteremia/fungemia
3 Thrombophlebitis
4 Mycotic aneurysm
5 Drug fever
6 Occult septic focus
7 Skin infection at the site of an i.v. or central line
8 Antibiotic-induced pseudomembranous colitis
9 Associated head and neck infection – sinusitis, meningitis

PNEUMONIA AND 'MONONUCLEOSIS-LIKE' SYNDROME

Clinically, patients present with fever, lymphadenopathy, pharyngitis and hepatosplenomegaly

Pulmonary involvement varying from common, (e.g. sarcoid), to rare, (e.g. brucellosis), and etiologies include

1 Ebstein-Barr virus
   - Heterophil positive
   - Pulmonary involvement is uncommon but manifestations can include
     – Hilar lymphadenopathy

  - Interstitial disease resembling viral or mycoplasma pneumonia
  - Upper airways obstruction from enlarged tonsils or adenoids
2. Heterophil negative agents, e.g. toxoplasma, CMV, herpes simplex, adenovirus
3. Primary HIV infection usually presents as a mononucleosis-like illness with the above described symptoms as well as headache and truncal rash
   - Elevated LFTs, leukopenia with atypical lymphocytes and thrombocytopenia are common
   - Clinical illness lasts about 3 weeks during which time tests for HIV antibody are negative but tests for HIV RNA or DNA are positive
4. Disseminated fungal infection, e.g. histoplasmosis, coccidioidomycosis
5. Disseminated tuberculosis
6. Other bacteria including typhoid, tularemia, brucella, bartonella (bacillary angiomatosis)
7. *Chlamydia psittaci*
8. Lymphoma
9. Sarcoid
10. Castleman's disease

PNEUMONIA AND 'FLU-LIKE' PRESENTATION

Patients present with pulmonary infiltrates in a normal host, multisystem involvement, negative routine cultures and fevers >3 weeks

1. Bacterial, e.g. legionella, tuberculosis, typhoid fever, tularemia, bartonella
2. Mycoplasma
3. Viral, e.g. EB, CMV, ?HIV
4. Fungal, e.g. histoplasmosis, coccidioidomycosis, cryptococcosis

5 Parasitic – toxoplasmosis
6 Rickettsial – Q-fever
7 Chlamydia – *C. psittaci*

PNEUMONIA AND CAVITARY DISEASE

Bacterial

- *Staph. aureus*
- gram negatives
- anaerobes
- rhodococcus
- legionella (~5%)
- actinomycosis
- nocardia
- *M. tuberculosis*
- atypical mycobacteria
- *Strep. pneumoniae* (rare)

Fungal

- *Coccidioidomycosis
- Histoplasmosis
- Cryptococcus (uncommon)
- Blastomycosis (uncommon)
- Sporotrichosis
- Aspergillus
- *Pneumocystis

Parasites

- *Echinococcus
- *Paragonimiasis
- Amebiasis

(*Cavities are often thin-walled)

57B Specific Pneumonias

ACTINOMYCOSIS – THORACIC

A chronic suppurative infection that can involve the chest wall, lungs, pleural space and mediastinum with most cases caused by *A. israelii*

- Pulmonary disease comprises approximately 25% of actinomycotic infections, the remainder being cervicofacial (55%) or abdominopelvic (20%)
- Pulmonary infection is usually secondary to aspiration of organisms from tonsillar crypts, dental caries or gingivitis
- Less commonly chest disease can develop from extension of cervicofacial suppuration into the mediastinum or transdiaphragmatic spread from abdominopelvic disease
- Actinomycosis usually exists as a mixed infection with associated anaerobes or aerobes

Clinically, it is a rare disorder with an insidious onset, chronic course, often non-specific respiratory symptoms and constitutional manifestations, simulating tuberculosis, neoplastic disease or fungal infection

- Chest wall invasion or sinus tract formation should suggest the diagnosis
- Extrathoracic manifestations include
  - Clubbing
  - Amyloid
  - Dissemination to the brain, heart valves, bones, muscles and subcutaneous tissues

Radiologic manifestations include

**Parenchyma*

1 Airspace consolidation resembling bacterial pneumonia or a 'mass-like' density simulating bronchogenic cancer
2 Single or multiple cavities are common
3 'Aspiration segments' typically involved, most often unilaterally
4 Infiltrate extends across lobar fissures unlike most bacterial infections
5 CT findings include
   - Airspace consolidation (less often a mass or nodule)

- Multiple central low attenuation areas with peripheral enhancement
- Frank cavitation within the consolidation with thickened irregular walls

Pleura

1. Pleural thickening is common overlying areas of parenchymal disease
2. Pleural effusions may occur secondary to pneumonia, esophageal abscess or extension from abdominopelvic disease in the absence of pulmonary disease
3. Effusions loculate early and may develop into an empyema

Airways

1. Infection of the bronchial mucosa can occur without parenchymal disease and present as endobronchial narrowing with subsequent atelectasis
2. Bronchocutaneous fistula can rarely develop

Chest wall

1. Chest wall mass secondary to pleuro-parenchymal disease with abscesses and draining sinuses
2. Periosteal rib involvement or bony destruction, (e.g. ribs, vertebral column), can occur and simulate neoplasm
3. Diaphragmatic invasion described

Mediastinum

1. Mediastinal infection presents as a mass lesion simulating a neoplasm with potential tracheo-esophageal fistula as well as invasion of the pericardium, pulmonary arteries or vena cava
2. Occasional lymphadenopathy

Diagnostic criteria

1. Positive culture from body fluids (ideally sterile sites) or tissues
2. Demonstration of thin, branching filaments which are silver stain positive
3. Sulfur granules in sputum, pleural fluid or exudates from

sinus tracts are very suggestive but not pathognomonic, the sulfur granules being composed mainly of immunoglobulins but containing a high concentration of organisms
4 Endobronchial biopsy (rare)
5 Radiologic features as above

AMEBIC PLEUROPULMONARY DISEASE

Clinically, pleuropulmonary disease develops in 15–20% of patients with liver disease, with the pathophysiology being either direct extension from a hepatic abscess into the right lower lobe, hematogenous spread to the lungs (rare) or lymphatic spread from the liver to the diaphragm

- There is a 15:1 ratio of male to female involvement

Intrathoracic complications

- Rupture into the pleural cavity with empyema formation
- Rupture into the lung with pneumonia, abscess or a hepatobronchial fistula with expectoration of 'chocolate-sauce' or 'anchovy-sauce' sputum
- Bronchobiliary fistula with bile expectoration
- Pericarditis and effusion
- Sympathetic effusion secondary to a liver abscess or subphrenic abscess

Radiologic features

1 Right pleural effusion and basal lung disease
2 RLL consolidation progressing to cavitation and abscess formation
3 Consolidation/cavitation remote from the diaphragm
4 Pericardial effusion

Diagnostic features

1 Expectoration of the characteristic sputum
2 Amebic serology is positive in >90% of patients
3 Trophozoites in sputum, pleural fluid or material from needle aspiration, the latter typically 'non-smelling' with absence of WBCs which have been lysed (histolytica)

4 Stools for cysts or trophozoites of *Entamoeba histolytica* (simultaneous organisms in stool are uncommon)
5 Leucocytosis and eosinophilia (uncommon)

ANAEROBIC INFECTIONS

The frequency with which anaerobes are responsible for CAP or nosocomial pneumonia is unknown as uncontaminated specimens which bypass the normal mouth flora are rarely taken

- The usual pathophysiology is aspiration – of oropharyngeal or paranasal sinus flora – and uncommonly bacteremic

Bacteriologically, anaerobic infections are usually polymicrobial with an average of three species of anaerobes, often in association with aerobes

- The most common organisms include bacteroides, fusobacterium, spirochetes, streptococcal species, and in some cases, clostridium and actinomyces
- Sputum gram stain slows a mixed flora with definitive diagnosis from cultures of pleural fluid, TTNA, blood or ? protected brush specimens, anaerobic specimen transport being crucial for recovery of organisms

Clinically, the predisposing conditions include

- Altered sensorium – structural, e.g. CVA, or functional, e.g. alcoholism, drug overdose, seizures
- An anaerobic upper respiratory infection, e.g. dental abscess, gingivitis, tonsillitis, sinusitis
- Any cause of dysphagia – structural, e.g. Zenker's, or functional, e.g. myasthenia gravis
- Endobronchial lung cancer
- Progressive massive fibrous of silicosis with cavitation
- Bacteremic spread, e.g. clostridia or bacteroides from a GI or GU source
- The ratio of infection in males to females is about four to one, with an onset that can vary from acute (hours) to chronic (months)

- The presentation ranges from asymptomatic to fulminant, but is most often insidious
- Symptoms are usually non-specific and indistinguishable from other bacterial pneumonias, but indolent symptoms, foul-smelling sputum, poor oral hygiene and clubbing (chronic infections) along with an above predisposing condition should suggest the diagnosis

Radiologically, the disease is in an 'aspiration segment,' i.e. posterior segments of upper lobes, superior segment or basal segments of lower lobes, right lung twice as often involved as the left

1 *Aspiration pneumonia
   - Segmental homogenous consolidation in an aspiration segment
2 *Necrotizing pneumonia
   - Areas of cavitation, often with air–fluid levels, developing in the preceding aspiration pneumonia
3 *Lung abscess
   - Dominant focus of cavitation
   - Air–fluid levels frequent
   - May be accompanied by a surrounding pneumonitis
   - Sequential X-rays may show the transition from 1 → 2 → 3
4 *Parapneumonic effusion/empyema
   - May be seen with or without associated parenchymal disease
   - Fluid tends to loculate, often posteriorly, with multiple pockets being typical

Rare radiologic manifestations include

5 Lung gangrene
6 Peripheral mass simulating cancer
7 Hilar/mediastinal adenopathy
8 Pyopneumothorax from gas-forming organisms, e.g. *B. fragilis*, *C. perfringens*

Lemierre's Syndrome

Describes the combination of an anaerobic pharyngitis/tonsillitis progressing to septic pulmonary emboli

Mouth anaerobes, e.g. *Fusobacterium necrophorum*, cause an oropharyngeal infection with sore throat for a few days

- There is secondary development of a suppurative thrombophlebitis of the internal jugular vein, the latter being either subclinical or manifest as fever, palpable induration, and a warm tender neck swelling
- 3–10 days later septic emboli develop, most often involving the lungs and simulating right-sided endocarditis

Diagnostic features

1. CT scan with contrast demonstrating thrombosis of the internal jugular vein
2. Anaerobic bacteremia
3. Characteristic chest X-ray features of septic emboli (see p. 238)

ASCARIASIS

Ascaris lumbricoides is commonly found in rural areas with poor sanitation where fecal contamination of soil or foodstuffs occurs

- In the intestine larvae hatch from the swallowed eggs as second-stage larvae and are carried hematogenously to the liver and lungs
- In the lungs the larvae penetrate the capillary bed, molt into third-stage larvae, ascend the tracheobronchial tree and are then swallowed where they mature into adult worms in the intestine, producing eggs

Lung disease is manifest as Loffler's syndrome during the transpulmonary passage, with cough, dyspnea, occasional hemoptysis, fever, and urticaria in ~10% of patients

- The disease is seen in the second week after ingestion of eggs and usually subsides spontaneously in 1–2 weeks

Diagnostic features

1. Ascaris larvae in pulmonary or gastric secretions
2. Elevated antibody titers
3. Peripheral and sputum eosinophilia (non-specific)
4. Elevated IgE (non-specific)

5 Eggs in stool are seen only 6 weeks following ascaris pneumonia

ASPERGILLOSIS

A fungus of worldwide distribution present in water, soil and decaying organic material

- Disease can be caused by about 300 different species of aspergillus, the most important being *A. fumigatus*
- No documented person-to-person transmission
- Infection usually occurs by inhalation of air-borne conidia from contaminated sources, intact macrophages inhibiting the germination of conidia into hyphae, with neutrophils directed against aspergillus hyphae

Clinical Syndromes

Saprophytic

- Aspergilloma
- Airways colonization, e.g. asthma, bronchiectasis, cystic fibrosis, chronic bronchitis
- Colonization of necrotic lung tissue
- Bronchial stump aspergillosis

Invasive

- Angioinvasive/bronchopneumonic
- Tracheobronchial aspergillosis
- Subacute necrotizing pulmonary aspergillosis

Allergic

- Loeffler's syndrome
- Allergic bronchopulmonary aspergillosis (ABPA)
- Extrinsic allergic alveolitis
- Bronchocentric granulomatosis (BCG)
- Asthma (IgE mediated response to aspergillus mold, e.g. bakers)
- ? Eosinophilic pneumonia

*Transformation from one syndrome to another may occur, e.g. ABPA can lead to an aspergilloma in a bronchiectatic cavity or may convert to invasive aspergillosis with steroids

Aspergilloma (Mycetoma, Fungus Ball)

Definition: A mass of fungal hyphae, fibrin, mucous and cellular debris in a lung cavity or bronchus

Pathologically, an aspergilloma can develop in
- Lung cavities – *tuberculosis, *sarcoid, abscess, cavitary cancer, sequestration, apical bullae of ankylosing spondylitis or rheumatoid arthritis, radiation fibrosis, emphysematous bullae
- Bronchi – bronchiectasis, bronchial stump, bronchogenic cyst, complication of ABPA
- Pleura – rarely

Clinical presentations
- Asymptomatic radiologic finding
- Cough, sputum and hemoptysis (50–90%), the latter occasionally being massive
- Development in association with asthma and ABPA
- Systemic symptoms of fever and malaise (uncommonly)
- Progressive lung disease, pleural invasion, vertebral invasion with cord compression, systemic dissemination (rarely) when host defenses become impaired

Radiologic findings
1. *Mass within a cavity, often in an upper lobe, surrounded by an air crescent
    - May be demonstrated on CT before its appearance on chest X-ray
2. Movement of the mass as patient changes position (often absent in bronchiectasis or when the cavity is completely filled by the mass)
3. Thickening of the cavity walls before a mass is visible
4. Pleural thickening contiguous to the cavity
5. Solitary lung nodule (if air crescent is absent)

Radiologic course
1. Stability over time
2. Lysis of the aspergilloma, either spontaneously or secondary to pyogenic infection in 5–10% of cases
3. Pleuropulmonary invasion

4 Calcification of the mass
5 Enlarging pulmonary nodule

Radiologic differential diagnosis

1 Necrotic cancer, e.g. squamous cell carcinoma
2 Gangrenous lung
3 Blood clot
4 Hydatid cyst
5 Invasive aspergillosis
6 Other fungi
7 Wegener's granulomatosis
8 Lung abscess

Diagnostic features

1 Radiologic appearance
2 Aspergillus precipitins – present in almost 100% of patients
3 Positive culture/smear of aspergillus from bronchial washings or TTNA

Invasive Aspergillosis (IA) – Angioinvasive/Bronchopneumonic

Definition: The extension of aspergillus organisms into viable tissue with tissue destruction

- Pathologically, inhaled spores set up a nidus of infection which locally invade vessels
- *In situ* thrombosis is followed by lung infarction and invasion by aspergillus hyphae

Clinically, seen in immunocompromised patients, typically with lymphoreticular or hematologic malignancies, (e.g. acute myelogenous leukemia), post-transplant, post-influenza or other viral infection, diabetes, renal or hepatic failure, AIDS, others

- Patients are often on immunosuppressive therapy, antineoplastic drugs and/or antibiotics for gram negative infection
- Granulocytopenia is usual, with the risk of developing IA increasing with the duration of the neutropenic phase

- The lungs are involved in approximately 50% of patients, followed by local invasion of the pleura, pericardium, mediastinal vessels (e.g. SVC), chest wall, esophagus, trachea and finally systemic dissemination to the GI tract, brain, liver, kidneys
- Rare case reports of invasive aspergillosis occurring in normal hosts
- Mortality varies from 50 to 80%

Clinical presentations

1 Unremitting fever and/or progressive pulmonary infiltrates despite broad spectrum antibiotics in neutropenic patients
2 Initial response to antibacterials followed by a relapse, representing superinfection with aspergillus
3 'Hemorrhagic infarction' picture with acute pleuritic pain and hemoptysis (in association with a nodular or wedge-shaped opacity on X-ray – see below)
4 'Bacterial pneumonia' presentation with acute onset of fever, cough, sputum and chest pain in the absence of positive sputum smears or cultures for bacteria
5 Rarely bronchiolitis, bronchiolitis obliterans, miliary disease may occur independently or accompany pneumonia

Radiologic features

1 Normal X-rays in approximately 25% of cases at the onset of symptoms
2 Patchy segmental airspace consolidation in a bronchopneumonia pattern, unilateral or bilateral
   - Individual areas can become confluent with homogenous consolidation involving a large area of lung (acute airspace pneumonia) and can cavitate
   - May become increasingly nodular +/– cavitation and resemble the angioinvasive variety
3 Single or multiple nodules which can cavitate and develop an air crescent sign (angioinvasive)
4 Peripheral wedge-shaped or mass-like infiltrates repre-

senting segmental consolidation due to hemorrhagic infarction (angioinvasive)

- Cavitation can develop as well as concurrent pleural effusion or pneumothorax

5 Invasion and fistula formation to the pleura (effusion, pneumothorax), chest wall or esophagus

CT scan may provide early clues to diagnosis

1 Detection of pulmonary lesions when chest X-rays are normal
2 Identification of cavitation with an air crescent sign, the latter representing air between retracted necrotic lung and adjacent lung parenchyma
   - The pulmonary 'sequestrum' radiologically resembles a mycetoma but pathologically and clinically is very different from the saprophytic fungus ball
3 Demonstration of the 'halo sign', i.e. a zone of 'ground glass' attenuation surrounding a non-specific pulmonary mass, pathologically representing hemorrhage surrounding a central necrotic nodule
   - Air crescents or cavitation may subsequently develop within days to weeks
   - Seen in other infections, e.g. mucor, candida as well as non-infectious disorders, e.g. Wegener's, Kaposi's sarcoma
4 May reveal the characteristic centrilobular nodules of an associated broncholitis in addition to areas of airspace or 'ground glass' consolidation

Diagnosis should be suspected with

1 Predisposing immunocompromised state
2 One of the above clinical presentations
3 Chest X-ray and CT abnormalities as defined above – suggestive but not specific
4 Evidence of extrapulmonary disease, (e.g. sinus tenderness, surveillance nasal cultures and epistaxis may be clues to an associated aspergillus sinusitis) although any organ can be potentially involved
5 Positive cultures from bronchial washings or BAL

- Definitive diagnosis by open lung biopsy, with histopathology showing septate acute branching hyphae and positive cultures
- Transbronchial biopsy is positive in approximately 50% of patients (varies from 20 to 80%)
- Sputum and blood cultures as well as serology are unreliable with positive cultures potentially reflecting colonization
- PCR presently being investigated

Invasive Aspergillosis – Tracheobronchitis

Pathologically, this is a pseudomembranous and necrotizing infection of the trachea and bronchi, associated with intralumenal mucous plugs and microscopic hyphal invasion of the tracheobronchial wall

Clinically, it is a variant of invasive aspergillosis, seen in the same group of immunocompromised patients but most often lung or heart transplants, and may or may not be accompanied by pneumonia

- Presentation is acute with fever, cough, wheezing, dyspnea and hemoptysis, the diagnosis often made only postmortem
- Chest X-rays may be normal or reveal airways narrowing with secondary atelectasis, obstructive pneumonitis and occasionally an associated necrotizing pneumonia
- Attempted bronchoscopic removal of the pseudomembrane has resulted in fatal hemorrhage

Diagnosis can be made on bronchoscopy and cultures while differential of the pseudomembrane includes

- *Corynebacterium diphtheria*
- Post-viral, hemophilus or *Staph. aureus* infection
- Other fungi

Invasive Aspergillosis – Subacute Necrotizing Pulmonary Aspergillosis

Definition: Indolent cavitary lung disease secondary to aspergillus species, usually developing over weeks to months

Clinically, it is a more chronic and localized form of invasive aspergillosis occurring as a complication of pre-existing lung disease, e.g. old tuberculosis, sarcoid, ankylosing spondylitis, prior radiotherapy, COPD, pneumoconiosis

- Patients may be mildly immunocompromised, e.g. diabetic, alcoholic, steroid-treated
- Presentation is that of non-specific respiratory complaints and systemic symptoms of fevers and weight loss developing over several months
- Differential diagnosis includes tuberculosis, atypical mycobacteria, anaerobes, nocardia, actinomycosis, other fungi, lung cancer

Radiological features

1 Typically begins as an upper lobe infiltrate which subsequently cavitates over weeks to months
2 Mycetomas are common in cavities that have been formed by fungal invasion and necrosis of lung tissue
3 Associated pleural thickening overlying the diseased lung is frequently seen

Diagnosis is definitively established by demonstration of septate hyphae in lung tissue with cultures demonstrating aspergillus

- In the absence of biopsy confirmation, diagnostic criteria include
  - Culture of aspergillus from lung tissue, BAL, bronchial washings or sputum
  - Radiologic features as above
  - Absence of tuberculosis, bacteria or other fungi on cultures
  - Positive serum precipitins (often present)
  - Absence of disseminated aspergillosis
  - Response to antifungal treatment

Allergic Bronchopulmonary Aspergillosis

Disease of patients with underlying asthma (in North America) where airway colonization with aspergillus is responsible for sensitization to the fungus

- This results in asthma exacerbations, mucus plugging in segmental bronchi, eosinophilia and serologic abnormalities in the absence of tissue invasion

Clinically, patients typically present with exacerbation of prior asthma or new acute asthma although the syndrome is well described in non-asthmatics from the United Kingdom

- Often an allergic history, i.e. rhinitis, conjunctivitis, eczema, anaphylaxis, food and drug allergies
- Expectoration of mucus plugs or copious secretions as well as recurrent respiratory infections are usual
- Exacerbations may be subclinical and manifest only by elevated IgE levels and radiologic abnormalities (see below)
- The long term prognosis in individual cases is variable with some patients developing extensive bronchiectasis (following the resolution of mucoid impactions), pulmonary fibrosis and respiratory failure
- Other patients follow a more benign course with asthma exacerbations but less deterioration in lung function

Clinical stages

Stage I – Acute

- Asthma
- Increased IgE levels
- Pulmonary infiltrates
- Proximal bronchiectasis
- Positive immediate skin test to aspergillus antigen

Stage II – Remission

- Asthma symptoms resolving
- Normal IgE levels
- Acute pulmonary infiltrates disappear

Stage III – Exacerbation

- Increasing asthma symptoms and/or elevated IgE and/or new pulmonary infiltrates

Stage IV – Steroid-dependent asthma

- Asthma requiring steroids for suppression
- IgE levels may remain elevated or normalize

Stage V – Fibrosis and bronchiectasis

Diagnostic criteria

Vary in different series and comprise a combination of features

1 Clinically there is a history of asthma and expectoration of plugs
2 Eosinophilia (blood and sputum), increased total IgE, increased IgG and IgE to aspergillus, precipitins to aspergillus
3 Positive sputum cultures for aspergillus
4 Positive immediate and delayed skin tests to aspergillus
5 Characteristic histology of the mucus plus composed of alternating layers of mucus and eosinophils with hyphae demonstrated in the mucus
   - Bronchial biopsies may demonstrate bronchocentric granulomatosis while eosinophilic pneumonia may be seen in the parenchyma
6 The radiologic findings are identical to those of mucoid impaction and include
   - Finger-like shadows, representing mucus filling of segmental bronchi, and manifest as
     - 'Gloved-finger' or tubular opacity
     - 'Y' or 'V' configuration
     - 'Cluster of grapes'
     - Solitary lung nodule
   - Bronchial wall-thickening – 'ring shadows' on cross section or 'tramlines' when seen longitudinally
   - Shadows may remain stable, enlarge, disappear or evolve into residual bronchiectasis
   - Dilated bronchiectatic areas may contain an air–fluid level or an aspergilloma
   - Patchy airspace consolidation
   - Segmental or lobar atelectasis
   - CT scan reveals proximal bronchiectasis with normal caliber of the bronchi distally and upper lobe predominance

Extrinsic allergic alveolitis

Rare disorder where inhalation of a large number of spores of aspergillus, often in enclosed spaces, can result in a biphasic response characterized clinically by

- Acute asthma within minutes of exposure, followed hours later by fever, hypoxemia and pulmonary infiltrates, with X-rays resembling pulmonary edema
- Aspergillus precipitins and elevated IgE levels seen in the serum
- Described initially in malt workers after exposure to the spores of *A. clavatus*

BLASTOMYCOSIS – NORTH AMERICAN

Epidemiologically, it is an uncommon disease that occurs as a sporadic or epidemic infection in a geographic distribution similar to histoplasmosis, but extending further north and east

- The fungus is prevalent in the moist soil of wooded areas along waterways while clinical infection has been associated with occupational and recreational outdoor activities, e.g. hunting, camping, canoe trips
- Lung infection results from spore inhalation with a marked male predominance although there are no reliable diagnostic tests to determine infection rates in high risk populations

	Blastomycosis	Histoplasmosis
Pathology	Pyogenic + granulomatous	Granulomatous
Incubation period	3–15 weeks (mean: 5 weeks)	2 weeks
Relative frequency of diagnosis	1	10
Lobar consolidation on chest X-ray	Common	Not seen
Dissemination	Skin, bone, meninges	Liver, spleen, lymph nodes, bone marrow

Table 57B.1

Clinically, disease presentation is highly variable in normal hosts, representing either primary infection or endogenous reactivation in the lungs or other organs, and includes

- Asymptomatic infection with the radiologic abnormalities as described below
- Acute presentation with pleuritic chest pain resembling pneumococcal pneumonia
- 'Flu-like' illness with fever, headache, myalgias, arthralgias, cough and an abnormal X-ray (see below)
- fulminating disease with ARDS
- Subacute to chronic presentation resembling tuberculosis with several weeks to months of fevers, night sweats, weight loss and non-specific respiratory symptoms
- Extrathoracic disease with skin lesions, osteomyelitis, intracranial abscess, prostatitis, with or without concurrent lung disease in ~¼ of cases

- Often, a self-limited disease, but treatment is required for advanced or disseminated infection
- In immunocompromised patients, the presentation is usually more acute and fulminating with frequent systemic dissemination

Radiologic features are quite variable and include

1. Localized airspace disease
2. Focal mass simulating malignancy
3. Diffuse interstitial pattern (in immunocompromised patients)
4. Cavitation (15%), pleural effusion (10%) and lymphadenopathy are uncommon in normal hosts
5. Other patterns

Diagnostic Clues

Symptoms of a RTI in an endemic area with

- Recent exposure to woods and streams
- Lack of antibiotic response in spite of X-rays resembling acute airspace pneumonia
- Mass-like lesion on chest X-ray where neoplastic disease is unlikely

- Extrapulmonary disease including ulcerated skin lesions, destructive bone lesions, prostatitis, meningitis

Diagnostic Criteria

1. Demonstration of organisms in sputum, BAL or tissue biopsy, appearing as thick-walled yeasts with a broad-based single bud, i.e. a broad neck of attachment
2. Cultures of sputum or extrapulmonary sites
3. Serologic tests are unreliable with complement fixation positive in <10% and immunodiffusion in <30% of cases
   - Enzyme immunoassay is more sensitive but lacks specificity

CANDIDA PNEUMONIA

Candidiasis is primarily a systemic and not a pulmonary infection complicating neutropenia, steroid therapy, in-dwelling vascular catheters or hyperalimentation

- Candida pneumonia is a rare nosocomial infection which occurs as a manifestation of hematogenous dissemination from bowel wall or skin and is seen in
  - Immunocompromised or debilitated hosts
  - Major trauma
  - Complicated GI surgery
- Respiratory symptoms are non-specific and may be accompanied by skin, eye and CNS involvement with microabscesses
- The radiologic features are non-specific
  - With hematogenous spread, often from the GI or GU tract, there is a diffuse miliary or nodular pattern with eventual coalescence and an ARDS pattern
  - With aspiration from the upper airway, there is bibasilar disease, often nodular in appearance

CHLAMYDIA

Chlamydia Psittaci Pneumonia

Uncommon human infection which is usually acquired from birds – parakeets, pigeons, budgerigars or poultry

- The bird may be overtly sick or a carrier with infection resulting from inhalation of dried, contaminated bird excreta
- Rare cases of pneumonia have been reported following contact with abortions in cattle, sheep or goats
- An exposure history is present in about 90% of cases with the disease mislabelled as 'viral' without a complete history and appropriate serology being performed
- Incubation period is 1–2 weeks with the clinical spectrum including
  - 'Flu-like' illness
  - Pneumonia, varying from atypical to fulminating
  - 'Typhoid-like' syndrome
  - Extrapulmonary disease including myocarditis, encephalitis, hemolytic anemia, hepatosplenomegaly, lymphadenopathy
- Pulmonary disease usually resolves clinically and radiologically over a few weeks

Radiologic features are non-specific and highly variable

Diagnostic criteria

1. Serology
2. Isolation of organisms from sputum, blood, spleen or liver in lab animals or tissue cultures

Chlamydia Pneumoniae – Twar Strain

Epidemiologically, about 50% of adults worldwide have been infected with primary infection resulting in

1. Rapid rise of genus-specific complement fixation antibodies, e.g. cross-reaction with *C. trachomatis*
2. Species-specific IgM antibodies within a few weeks
3. Species-specific IgG antibodies developing in 1–2 months and persisting for months to years

- Reinfection is common and characterized by elevation of IgG antibodies without the other 2 types
- Levels of IgG between 1:16 and 1:512 are taken as markers of prior infection
- Clinically responsible for about 10% of community-acquired pneumonias
- Persistently elevated antibody levels are described in patients with angiographically proven coronary artery disease and are associated with an increased risk of acute myocardial infarction
- Acute infection does not confer life long immunity with reinfection being common

Clinical spectrum is quite variable and includes

1 Asymptomatic infection
2 Pharyngitis-tracheobronchitis
3 Exacerbations of asthma, bronchitis, sinusitis
4 'Atypical' pneumonia syndrome, often accompanied by upper respiratory symptoms of sore throat, hoarseness and headache
5 Severe pneumonia – uncommon and seen with underlying pulmonary or systemic disease
6 Extrapulmonary disease, particularly rheumatologic, e.g. reactive arthritis, and cardiac, e.g. myocarditis, as well as meningoencephalitis and Guillain-Barré

Radiologic manifestations

1 Unilateral or bilateral interstitial/airspace opacities
2 Unilateral or bilateral pleural effusions
3 Cardiomegaly

Diagnostic criteria

1 Serologic diagnosis is controversial as there is no diagnostic gold standard
   - 4-fold antibody rise
   - ? single IgM $\geq$ 1: 16
2 BAL, sputum or pleural fluid culture, *but* – tissue culture is required, can take three to seven days, success rates are 50–75%, and the incidence of asymptomatic carrier rates is unclear

3 PCR detection in BAL, sputum, bronchial washings or pleural fluid – but no FDA-approved kits

COCCIDIOIDOMYCOSIS

Definition: Highly infectious mycotic disease caused by *Coccidioides immitis*, found mainly in the Southwestern United States, i.e. Arizona, California, Texas, New Mexico, Utah and Nevada, as well as in Northern Mexico and parts of Central and South America

- In soil, it grows as a mycelium of septate hyphae with arthroconidia which are dispersed by the wind and germinate in soil to form new hyphae and arthroconidia
- In tissues, the arthroconidia transform into spherules which undergo internal septation to produce endospores
- In the lungs, the spherules rupture and release the endospores which extend disease locally or disseminate via lymphatics
- The fungus exists as parasitic endospores in tissue with the exception of hyphae which can be found only in cavitary lesions
- Incidence of infection is very high in endemic areas with skin test conversion alone usually the only manifestation
- Infections occurring outside endemic areas are due to recent travel to an endemic area, less often reactivation of quiescent disease acquired earlier, and rarely infection by fomites from an endemic area
- Infection results from dust inhalation with an incubation period of 1–3 weeks and subsequent immunity to exogenous reinfection (like tuberculosis)

The **clinical** spectrum includes

1 Asymptomatic infection – seen in about 70% of patients
2 Acute pulmonary syndrome
3 Chronic pulmonary coccidioidomycosis
4 Disseminated coccidioidomycosis

Acute Pulmonary Syndrome

Most symptomatic cases present as a self-limited pneumonia (Valley Fever)

- Seen in ~30% of cases, lasts approximately 2 weeks and characterized by a flu-like illness with fatigue, malaise, headache, fever, cough, pleuritic chest pain, skin rash
- The rash can be non-specific or less commonly erythema nodosum or erythema multiforme, biopsies of which are culture negative but demonstrate a non-specific vasculitis with variable eosinophilic infiltrate
- Peripherally, eosinophilia is seen in ~25% of cases

Sequelae of symptomatic infection are

- Spontaneous resolution in >90% of patients within a few weeks
- ARDS resulting from intense dust exposure with a large innoculum of fungus, presenting with rapidly progressive pneumonia
- Chronic pulmonary disease (uncommon)
- Dissemination (rare)

Radiologic features of the acute pulmonary syndrome

1. *Single or multiple areas of consolidation (similar to community-acquired bacterial or viral pneumonia) which
    - Resolves over weeks to months
    - Can cavitate
    - Can resolve in one area and appear in another
    - Can be misdiagnosed as primary eosinophilic pneumonia when peripheral eosinophilia is present
2. Normal chest X-ray
3. Hilar or mediastinal adenopathy is seen in ~20% of cases and may occur without parenchymal disease
    - Adenopathy may be massive, slow to resolve and persist for years
    - May be associated with disease dissemination
4. Pleural effusions occur in up to 20% of patients and are often associated with peripheral eosinophilia and high complement fixation titers
    - The fluid is a lymphocytic exudate, granulomatous

histologically, with pleural fluid and pleural biopsies usually positive on culture

Chronic Pulmonary Coccidioidomycosis

Definition: Primary disease persisting for longer than 6–8 weeks or radiologic signs of nodular disease, cavitation or progressive pneumonia

- May be symptomatic or asymptomatic and seen in 5–10% of patients with acute pulmonary coccidioidomycosis

Solitary pulmonary nodule (SPN)

Approximately 5% of pneumonias evolve into a SPN

- Clinically, they are usually asymptomatic and the major problem is their differentiation from a neoplasm
- Serology is usually negative whereas TTNA may demonstrate granulomas as well as the diagnostic spherules
- Radiologically, most are located within 5 cm of the hila but cannot be distinguished from other causes of a SPN

Multiple pulmonary nodules

Less common than a SPN, often asymptomatic, resembling metastatic cancer

Cavitary nodule

Often asymptomatic lesions, 2–4 cm in diameter, with spherules and hyphae seen on biopsy

- Diabetics seem prone to cavitation
- Sputum cultures are often positive
- Cavities are often thin-walled and ~50% of cavitary nodules close spontaneously, the remainder developing complications which include
  - Continued coccidioidal infection
  - Secondary bacterial infection
  - Mycetoma from coccidioides or aspergillus
  - Rupture into the pleural space with pneumothorax or pyopneumothorax
  - Symptoms of fever, cough, hemoptysis which can be massive, in association with systemic features of fever, night sweats and weight loss

Persistent coccidioidal pneumonia

Pulmonary infiltrates fail to clear, may cavitate and develop the above complications of a cavitary nodule

- Patients are often symptomatic similar to the presentation with acute illness

Chronic progressive coccidioidomycosis

Clinically, seen in approximately 1% of patients who present with asymptomatic radiologic disease or an insidious onset of fever, weight loss, cough, hemoptysis and dyspnea, mimicking tuberculosis

- Presentation can very closely follow the primary infection or reactivate at a later time
- Insulin-dependent diabetics and non-white individuals are more often affected and dissemination rarely occurs
- The **radiologic** changes are also similar to tuberculosis with bilateral upper lobe cavitary or non-cavitary infiltrates

Disseminated Coccidioidomycosis

Clinically, this is a rare manifestation of infection (0.5%) with predisposition for males, pregnant females in the third trimester, immunocompromised and non-whites

- May occur as a complication of primary infection or reactivation of latent disease
- The presentation varies from acute and fulminating to chronic and insidious
- Extensive pulmonary disease is seen in association with other organ involvement including the skin (wart-like nodules), bones (osteomyelitis of skull, spine, hands, feet, tibia), joints (knees, ankles), kidneys, meninges
- The **radiologic** features include extensive airspace disease as well as a miliary pattern

Diagnostic clues

Symptoms of a RTI occurring in an endemic area with

1 Erythema nodosum or erythema multiforme and anthralgia

2 Radiologic progression of pneumonia to a nodule which then cavitates
3 Intrathoracic lymphadenopathy
4 Lack of antibiotic response
5 Extrapulmonary disease involving skin, bone, meninges

Diagnostic tests

1 Demonstration of the spherules in tissue specimens
2 Positive cultures of fungus from the clinical specimen, e.g. sputum or bronchial washings, usually in 2–5 days
3 Serologic tests for detection of anticoccidioidal antibody using immunodiffusion, complement fixation or enzyme immunoassay (ELISA)
4 Skin tests are of limited value as anergy can occur with progressive disease, whereas a positive test only reflects prior infection

CRYPTOCOCCOSIS

Epidemiologically, most cases are caused by *Cryptococcus neoformans*, a thin-walled non-mycelial budding yeast with a thick polysaccaride capsule, that is worldwide in distribution and exists in a yeast form in nature and in infected mammalian tissue

- Dried pigeon excreta is the most important natural habitat with infection acquired by inhalation of the organisms
- Cases are usually sporadic with outbreaks reported, but a history of pigeon exposure is often lacking
- Primary disease occurs in the lung with little inflammatory response and therefore few or absent respiratory symptoms

Clinically, cryptococcosis is predominantly a CNS infection preceded by a subclinical pulmonary infection, but can present with primary pulmonary disease

- Approximately 75% of cases occur in immunocompromised patients with impaired cell-mediated immunity, particularly AIDS, Hodgkin's disease, steroid-treated

- Colonization with positive cultures are occasionally seen, particularly in COPD or old tuberculosis, and therefore finding cryptococcus in sputum may not necessarily explain an associated mass lesion or nodule
- Manifestations include
  - Asymptomatic infection seen in approximately ⅓ of patients with isolated pulmonary disease
  - 'Flu-like' illness with fever, cough
  - A 'pneumonia-like' presentation with non-specific respiratory and systemic symptoms that can be acute, subacute or chronic
  - Disseminated disease involving the CNS, skin, bones, subcutaneous tissues and other sites which may occur in the absence of lung disease, clinically or radiologically
  - In immunocompromised hosts, clinical presentation may be similar, but fulminant as well as disseminated pulmonary and extrapulmonary disease are more common
- Pulmonary disease in normal hosts is usually isolated and self-limited but work-up at the time of diagnosis of lung disease should exclude evidence or dissemination or immunocompromised status, as the latter conditions require treatment

Radiologic features

1. Lung mass is the most common manifestation, usually solitary (cryptococcoma) simulating bronchogenic cancer, but can present with multiple masses simulating metastases
2. Single or multiple nodules are common
3. Pneumonia picture with airspace consolidation, unilateral or bilateral, segmental or non-segmental and air bronchograms may be seen
4. Miliary pattern is rare in normal hosts *vs.* immunocompromised patients
5. Cavitation, hilar or mediastinal lymphadenopathy and pleural effusion are uncommon in normal hosts but more common in the immunocompromised
6. Absence of a predilection for any specific lobe or lung region

Definitive diagnosis requires histopathologic identification of organisms in tissue, a unimorphic yeast with narrow-based budding, but suggestive criteria include

1 History of exposure to pigeon excreta (often absent)
2 Positive smears and culture of organisms from sputum, bronchial washings or lung tissue, with growth in 48–72 hours
3 Radiologic abnormalities as described above
4 Latex agglutination detection of capsular polysaccharide cryptococcal antigen in pleural fluid, bronchial lavage, TTNA specimen, serum
   - Suspect dissemination with a positive serum test and 'pure' pulmonary infection
5 CNS disease (meningitis and/or mass lesions)
   - Positive cryptococcal antigen in CSF
   - Positive CSF culture
   - Direct visualization of the organisms with 'India ink preparation'
6 Culture of the organism from blood, urine or bone marrow, indicating disseminated disease

CYTOMEGALOVIRUS (CMV)

Primary CMV Infection

Acquired from childhood through early adulthood with latent CMV infection usually persistent for life

- Viral transmission occurs through close interpersonal contact, sexual contact or direct inoculation with infected cells or body fluids
- Over half the adult population will show serologic evidence of infection
- In normal hosts, infection is usually asymptomatic, although fever or an infectious mononucleosis syndrome may develop
- Transplant patients, particularly lung and bone marrow recipients, can acquire infection from the donor organ, from transfusion of blood products from a seropositive donor or by reactivation of latent infection in a seropositive recipient

CMV infection can be defined by

1 Seroconversion via antibody measurements
2 Virus isolation in body fluids, e.g. blood, sputum, BAL, urine
3 Virus isolation in tissue, e.g. lung, in the absence of inflammation pathologically or disease clinically
4 CMV antigen detection in infected cells
5 ? PCR

CMV Pneumonia

Although immunocompromised patients may have asymptomatic infections, they often develop clinical disease involving the lung and other organs

- The respiratory presentation of patients with CMV pneumonia is completely non-specific
- The tendency for CMV to predispose to other opportunistic infections, e.g. gram negative, aspergillus, candida and pneumocystis, makes diagnosis even more difficult, with untreated CMV pneumonia mortality approaching 100%

Patients at risk for CMV pneumonia include

1 Transplant patients with *allogeneic stem cell > lung > liver/heart > renal > autologous stem cell
2 Advanced HIV
3 Other immunocompromised patients

In addition to pneumonia, other CMV manifestations include

- Esophagitis, gastroenteritis, colitis, proctitis
- Chorioretinitis
- Hepatosplenomegaly
- Fever and lymphocytosis
- Graft rejection and failure
- Bronchiolitis obliterans

Radiologically, several non-specific patterns are described including

1 Multiple small nodules
2 Interstitial reticular pattern
3 Airspace disease – 'ground glass' or consolidation
4 Combinations of 1, 2 and 3

- The above may be unilobar or diffuse and associated with small unilateral or bilateral effusions

Diagnostic gold standard for the diagnosis of CMV pneumonia is the histopathologic verification by lung biopsy or autopsy

- CMV is often shed in secretions (e.g. respiratory) during immunosuppression with positive cultures not necessarily reflecting disease

Although there is no clear concensus, less invasive **criteria for diagnosis** include

1 Clinical and radiologic evidence of pneumonia
2 BAL findings
    - Cytopathology revealing CMV inclusion bodies
    - Positive viral culture (1–4 weeks)
    - Detection of early CMV Ag (DeaFF) with fluorescent monoclonal antibody using the rapid shell-vial culture technique
    - Positive PCR
    - Absence of other pathogens in BAL
3 Viremia is usually seen with invasive CMV disease and manifests as
    - ⊕ Buffy coat culture (less sensitive)
    - Antigenemia (more sensitive)
    - PCR (too sensitive with quantification required)
4 Response to treatment with gancyclovir and CMV immunoglobulin
5 ? Histologic and cultural evidence of CMV at an extra-pulmonary site
6 Serology revealing a four-fold rise in titer but not of practical value due to the time delay as well as the potential elevation of titers by co-infections which stimulate lymphocytes
    - Serology is most useful with seroconversion from negative to positive

DIROFILARIA IMMITIS

Dirofilaria immits is a filarial heart worm of domestic and wild carnivorous animals

- Mosquitoes of the genera *Aedes*, *Culex* and *Anopheles* transmit the larvae from, e.g. infected dogs to humans during blood meal, with eventual larval migration into the venous system, right ventricle and finally the pulmonary vasculature
- A single worm in the branch of a pulmonary artery induces an inflammatory response with subsequent occlusion and a spherical infarct

Clinically, most patients are asymptomatic although non-specific respiratory symptoms can occur

Radiologic features are those of a rounded, non-calcified, well-circumscribed nodule, usually solitary, and may develop in an area of previous pneumonitis

Diagnosis is usually made by surgical resection for a suspected neoplasm but the diagnosis should be considered in areas of high canine prevalence

- A minority of patients have peripheral eosinophilia although eosinophilia is seen in pleural fluid if an effusion develops
- Filarial serology is usually positive

GRAM NEGATIVE PNEUMONIAS

Important cause of nosocomial pneumonia following colonization of the upper respiratory tract

- Rare cause of CAP and uncommon commensals in healthy persons
- Should be suspected in the elderly, nursing home patients, diabetics, malignancy, neutropenia, alcoholics, immunosuppression as well as in patients with underlying cardiorespiratory or renal disease
- Responsible organisms include 'KEEAPPS,' i.e. **K**lebsiella, **E**nterobacter, ***E***. *coli*, **A**cinetobacter, **P**roteus, **P**seudomonas, **S**erratia
- Definitive diagnosis can be made by:
  – Blood culture

– Pleural fluid culture
– TTNA

Klebsiella Pneumonia

Gram negative, encapsulated rod, the polysaccharide capsule seen on gram stain of expectorated sputum

- More than 75 capsular types have been identified with most pneumonias caused by serotypes 1 to 6

Epidemiologically, it is the most common cause of gram negative pneumonia in the community, typically in male alcoholics, and in nursing home patients (as well as nosocomial pneumonia)

Clinically, it is seen in debilitated patients, caused by aspiration of oropharyngeal secretions, and presents acutely similar to the classic form of streptococcal pneumonia, resulting in Friedlander's pneumonia

- The typical patient is a chronic alcoholic male with symptoms of acute pneumonia as well as a bloody and mucoid sputum often copious in amount, with a 'currant jelly' appearance
- Concurrent liver disease is common and accompanies signs of lobar consolidation
- Bacteremia occurs in 20–60% of cases
- Rapidly progressive pleuropulmonary disease including lung gangrene, as well as extrapulmonary disease, result in high mortality

Radiologic features

1 *Acute airspace consolidation, often RUL and lobar in distribution with air bronchograms
2 Less frequently a bilateral patchy bronchopneumonia pattern
3 Frequent occurrence of parapneumonic effusion or empyema
4 Bulging of interlobar fissures
5 Abscess formation and cavitation with rupture into the pleural space leading to bronchopleural fistula, empyema, pneumothorax, pyopneumothorax

6 Lung gangrene and formation of a pulmonary sequestrum
7 Evolution into a 'chronic pneumonia' resembling tuberculosis
8 Residual bronchiectasis, fibrosis and thickened pleura in patients who recover

Enterobacter

Rare cause of community-acquired pneumonia but described in nursing home patients and as a nosocomial pneumonia, often multiresistant

- Pathophysiology is aspiration or bacteremia in patients with serious underlying diseases
- Bronchopneumonia is common with reports of cavitation and empyema

Escherichia coli

Second most common gram negative organism to cause community-acquired pneumonia, typically in the middle-aged to elderly who have underlying disease

- Community and nosocomial infections occur as a result of bacteremia from the GI or GU tract as well as from aspiration following oropharyngeal colonization
- Clinically the onset is acute with radiologic features of bilateral often lower lobe bronchopneumonia being most common, although lobar consolidation is described
- Empyema, cavitation as well as progression to an ARDS picture can also occur

Acinetobacter

Rare infection acquired by aspiration from the oropharynx (seen in a small percent of normal patients) or by inhalation

- Community-acquired infection is seen with underlying disease, often alcoholism and pneumocomioses, whereas nosocomial infection occurs mainly in the ICU setting
- Clinically symptoms are non-specific and chest X-rays usually reveal lower lobe consolidation with frequent effusion and abscess formation

Proteus mirabilis

Uncommon cause of community or nosocomial pneumonia and typically seen in patients with chronic suppurative lung disease, tracheostomy, alcoholism

- Pathophysiology is aspiration following oropharyngeal colonization
- Airspace consolidation is often accompanied by abscesses but effusions are uncommon

Pseudomonas aeruginosa

Rare in the community (excluding cystic fibrosis patients) but seen with chemotherapy-treated cancer patients, neutropenia and occasionally COPD, pneumonia occurring by aspiration

- Commonest gram negative organism to cause nosocomial pneumonia, with the majority of cases occurring in an ICU in patients who are debilitated, on immunosuppressives, have underlying systemic diseases or are being ventilated
- Hospital-acquired infection is either aspiration or hematogenous in origin
- Clinical presentation is acute with non-specific respiratory symptoms
- Radiologically, the disease is bilateral, multifocal, with lower lobe predominance and features can include
  - Patchy or confluent airspace consolidation with a bronchopneumonia pattern resembling *Staph. aureus*
  - Bilateral nodular shadows, usually representing bacteremic spread
  - Coalescence of the above 2 features with rapidly progressive airspace disease leading to an ARDS picture
  - Cavitation, single or multiple, thick or thin-walled, rarely with pneumatocele formation
  - Effusions are common, empyema is rare

Serratia marcescens

Described in nursing home patients as well as in nosocomial pneumonia, often in a post-operative setting in patients with underlying diseases

- Clinical symptoms are non-specific with chest X-rays showing a patchy bronchopneumonia which may be accompanied by pleural effusions, but cavitation and lobar consolidation are rare

HANTAVIRUS PULMONARY SYNDROME (HPS)

Epidemiologically, originally described in rural areas of the Southwestern United States but now sporadically reported in multiple geographic areas with most cases from Arizona, Colorado, Utah and New Mexico

- Sin Nombre virus (SNV), a member of the genus *Hantavirus*, is the main cause of the HPS but other Hantaviruses may be responsible
- Typically seen in previously healthy young adults with a fatality rate of ~50%

Clinically, there is a history of contact with rodents or rodent droppings, aerosolization of virus from urine, stool or saliva being the mode of transmission

- Patients present with a 'flu-like' prodrome of fever, chills, myalgias, headache and GI symptoms following a 3 week incubation period
- The 3–6 day prodrome is followed by cough, progressive dyspnea, hypoxemia and either stable hemodynamics or respiratory failure and shock
- Peripheral blood smears reveal thrombocytopenia, left shift in the myeloid series and large immunoblastoid lymphocytes
- Chest X-rays initially are normal or demonstrate non-specific infiltrates which can progress to an ARDS picture

Diagnostic criteria

1. Detection of Hantavirus-specific IgM or IgG
2. PCR for detection of viral RNA
3. Detection of Hantavirus antigen by immunochemistry

HEMOPHILUS PNEUMONIA

Vast majority of cases are caused by *H. influenzae* and rarely *H. parainfluenzae*, gram negative coccobacilli

- Encapsulated strains are divided into types 'a' to 'f', depending upon antigenic differences in polysaccharide antigen, but both encapsulated and non-encapsulated strains can cause respiratory infections
- Can act as a primary pathogen or complicate viral infections, e.g. influenza

Clinically, patients can present with multiple respiratory disorders including otitis, epiglottitis, tracheobronchitis, bronchiolitis, pneumonia, pleural effusion, while non-respiratory complications include endocarditis, pericarditis, meningitis, septic arthritis

- Acute bronchitis is the most common pulmonary manifestation in normal hosts with pneumonia typically in COPD
- Pneumonia is also well described in normals as well as in patients with diabetes, alcoholism, asplenia, immunoglobulin deficiencies, myeloma, sickle-cell disease, HIV, drug addicts, elderly, and following viral infections, e.g. influenza
- Common cause of community-acquired pneumonia (15–20% of cases) as well as nosocomial pneumonia, but there are no pathognomonic features of clinical presentation
- Extrapulmonary complications include bacteremia, septic arthritis, endocarditis and pericarditis

Radiologic features

1 Bronchopneumonia pattern, typically involving one or both lower lobes
2 Airspace pattern similar to that of *Strep. pneumoniae* in up to 50% of cases
3 Interstitial pattern alone or associated with airspace disease in ~20% of cases
4 Pleural effusions are common but empyema is rare
5 Cavitation is uncommon
6 Rare manifestations include pneumatocele formation and bulging fissures

Definitive diagnosis requires culture of the organism from a normally sterile site, e.g. blood or pleural fluid, as positive sputum cultures may simply reflect colonization

HISTOPLASMOSIS

Histoplasmosis is caused by inhalation of the spores of the dimorphic fungus *Histoplasma capsulatum* which grows as a mold in soil, particularly that contaminated by bird or bat droppings

- Worldwide in distribution, but most reports are from the Ohio, Mississippi and St. Lawrence River valleys
- Approximately 80% of people are infected in the above endemic areas with outbreaks reported where soil is disturbed, e.g. demolition, caves explored, dead wood cut with a chainsaw, etc.
- Unlike tuberculosis, skin test positivity is not permanent and post-primary infection is exogenous
- Inhalation of spores is followed by conversion of the organism to the yeast phase, development of pneumonitis and dissemination to regional lymph nodes and to the reticuloendothelial organs throughout the body (pre-immune phase)
- The development of cell-mediated immunity is followed by granuloma formation and healing in the lungs, hilar lymph nodes, liver and spleen

Clinical-radiologic Presentations

1 **Asymptomatic** state in 90–95% of patients with a low inoculum exposure, normal immune status and no underlying lung disease

   Radiologic manifestations include
   - Normal chest X-rays with negative histoplasma-specific antibodies but positive skin test
   - Histoplasmoma
     - Solitary or multiple
     - May enlarge over time, simulating a neoplasm
     - Often calcifies with a pathognomonic 'target' lesion, i.e. central calcification surrounded by laminated layers of calcification
     - Rarely cavitates
   - Fibrocalcific scars

- Organizing pneumonia
- Hilar/mediastinal lymphadenopathy
  - May enlarge
  - May calcify ± eggshell pattern
- Multiple punctate pulmonary, splenic, hepatic and adrenal calcifications
- Broncholithiasis ± atelectasis

2 **Acute 'flu-like' illness** clinically which may be accompanied by a normal chest X-ray or airspace pneumonia
- With acute symptomatic cases the incubation period is typically 2 weeks
- This and pneumonia (see below) are seen in <5% of patients with low level exposure but more often following extensive exposure to heavily contaminated soil or droppings

3 **Acute pneumonia-type illness**, either 'bacterial' or 'atypical' in presentation with radiologic features of
- Air space consolidation which may clear in one area and appear in another
- Mediastinal lymphadenopathy
- Hilar adenopathy which can result in atelectasis, obstructive pneumonitis, broncholithiasis

4 **Acute 'epidemic' exposure**, varying from non-specific respiratory symptoms to fulminating disease, with respiratory failure, progressive extrapulmonary dissemination and radiologic features of
- Disseminated discrete nodules up to 4 mm in diameter which can resolve, fibrose or calcify
- Bilateral patchy areas of airspace disease
- Miliary pattern
- Residual diffuse fibrosis

5 **Localized extrapulmonary diseases** including hepatosplenomegaly, lymphadenopathy, erythema nodosum, erythema multiforme

6 **Chronic pulmonary disease** due to exogenous reinfection and occurring in patients with underlying centrilobular emphysema

- Symptoms are those of underlying COPD in addition to superimposed respiratory and systemic symptoms similar to post-primary tuberculosis

Radiologic features

- Upper lobe consolidation in non-cavitary chronic histoplasmosis
- Chronic cavitary disease resembling reactivation tuberculosis
  - Areas of consolidation in the lung apices surrounding centrilobular emphysematous spaces
  - Bronchogenic spread
  - Pleural thickening adjacent to cavities
  - Aspergillomas in cavities/chronic necrotizing pulmonary aspergillosis
  - Cavitary rupture and bronchopleural fistula
  - Disease progression with destruction and scarring of lung in ~⅓ of cases
  - R/O superimposed atypical mycobacteria or tuberculosis

7 **Granulomatous or fibrosing mediastinitis** (see p. 508) ? secondary to an atypical immunologic response to *H. capsulatum*, and manifest as

- Tracheobronchial narrowing
- Tracheo-esophageal fistula
- Dysphagia from esophageal compression
- Pericarditis which usually represents an immunologic response to histoplasma in adjacent nodes and rarely spread of organisms into the percardium
- Pulmonary artery or venous obstruction
- SVC syndrome

Radiologic findings include mediastinal widening and/or calcified hilar nodes on chest X-ray, while CT demonstrates an infiltrative mediastinal process

8 **Broncholithiasis** (see p. 114)

9 **Mediastinal granuloma** is defined as an enlarging mass of encapsulated, caseous mediastinal lymph nodes, with a necrotic central core occasionally present

- Clinical presentation is similar to that of granulomatous mediastinitis with compression of adjacent structures
- Radiologically the mass can be up to 10cm in diameter, compressing or obstructing adjacent structures, with a central lucency in nodes reflecting caseous necrosis

10 **Disseminated disease** with asymptomatic hematogenous dissemination is the norm during primary infection and manifest as calcifications in the liver, spleen and adrenals, histoplasmosis being the most common infectious cause of Addison's disease
   - Clinically apparent disseminated disease is rare except in immunocompromised patients, e.g. HIV and can be acute, subacute or chronic in presentation
   - Manifestations include fever, hepatosplenomegaly, lymphadenopathy, anemia, leucopenia or thrombocytopenia from bone marrow involvement, Addisons's disease, gastrointestinal ulcers, meningitis, endocarditis and oropharyngeal/laryngeal ulcers (the latter may be the presenting feature of disease)
   - Lung lesions can vary from localized to miliary
   - Biopsy reveals granulomas and yeasts but HIV patients may not demonstrate granulomatous inflammation

Diagnostic Clues for Acute Histoplasmosis

Symptoms of a RTI in an endemic area with

1. Diffuse micronodular pattern on X-ray following an intense exposure
2. Lymphadenopathy and a focal infiltrate, the latter evolving into a nodule
3. Focal infiltrate with erythema nodosum, arthralgias
4. Lack of antibiotic response

Diagnostic Criteria

1. **Smears and cultures** (may take 2–4 weeks to detect growth)

- Positive sputum smears are seen with thick-walled cavitary disease but uncommonly with asymptomatic or self-limited disease
- Positive blood and bone marrow smears are seen with severe and disseminated infections
- Positive sputum and BAL cultures in up to 80% of cases with chronic pulmonary histoplasmosis but only in about 10% of acute histoplasmosis
- Positive cultures of blood, bone marrow, liver and urine are seen with disseminated disease
- Tissue stains may demonstrate the organisms in addition to granulomas

2 **Antibody detection**

- Several tests available, but there is disagreement as to absolute levels of antibody required or the optimal method for their determination
- Both immunodiffusion and complement fixation only become positive about 4 weeks following infection and are therefore insensitive acutely when a patient with an acute febrile illness and pulmonary infiltrates has not responded to antibiotics
- The above tests are positive in
  - 80–100% of chronic pulmonary histoplasmosis
  - 90% of acute pulmonary histoplasmosis
  - 50–80% of disseminated histoplasmosis
  - 70% of immunocompromised patients
  - Antibody levels decline with time, e.g. 50% positive with granulomatous mediastinitis but usually negative with a coin lesion or broncholithiasis
  - Remote infection with persistent elevation of antibody titers
- False positive antibody levels are seen with other fungi, e.g. blastomycosis, coccidioidomycosis, aspergillus, candida
- Useful epidemiologically, but not in acute decision-making as both acute and convalescent titers are required (the patient has already recovered or died!)

3 **Histoplasma polysaccharide antigen**
- Can be detected in blood or urine and a sensitive indicator of disseminated disease (sensitivity related to the organism load), particularly in AIDS patients
- Also seen in ~75% of patients with diffuse micronodular disease but less often positive with focal infiltrates or cavitary disease
- Can cross-react with other fungi, e.g. blastomycosis, paracoccidioidomycosis

4 **Skin tests**
- Useful epidemiologically but not in individual cases

5 **PCR** – being developed

HYDATID DISEASE

Epidemiologically, most cases are caused by *Echinococcus granulosus* (less often *Echinococcus multilocularis*), and exist in a sylvatic and pastoral variety
- Humans (who may serve as intermediate hosts) are infected by ingestion of eggs (food contaminated with feces) produced by the adult worm which is present in the definitive host (dogs, wolves)
- Hydatid cysts form in the lung by trapping larvae which spread via the bloodstream after release in the intestine and occasionally by transdiaphragmatic spread following rupture of liver cysts

Sylvatic
– Mainly seen in Alaska and Northern Canada
– Intermediate hosts are herbivores, e.g. moose, caribou, with the definitive hosts being dogs, wolves, foxes or coyotes
– Incidence of lung cysts is greater than liver cysts

Pastoral
– Seen in sheep-raising Mediterranean areas as well as in rural areas of Australia, South America, Soviet Union, Africa

- Intermediate hosts are sheep, cows or pigs with dogs as the definitive host
- Incidence of lung and liver cysts is about equal

Pathologically, the hydatid cyst is composed of

- Pericyst
  - Outer layer derived from the host
- Exocyst
  - Parasite derived laminated larger
- Endocyst
  - Inner germinal layer giving rise to broad capsules containing protoscolices
  - Forms daughter cysts
  - Gives rise to additional hydatid cysts in the intermediate host when rupture occurs
  - Contains fluid and hydatid sand, i.e. hooklets, scolexes

Clinical presentations

1 Asymptomatic lung lesion
2 'Mass effect' with compression of adjacent structures and resultant hemoptysis, cough, chest pain
3 Rupture with bronchospasm, fever, cough, systemic allergic symptoms of urticaria, anaphylaxis, eosinophilia, as well as pleuropulmonary spread with new cysts
   - Rupture may be spontaneous or secondary to infection, trauma
4 Secondary infection of a ruptured cyst by bacteria or fungi

Radiologically, cysts can be single or multiple (approximately 30%) with a lower lobe predominance

1 Oval or spherical homogeneous mass, with smooth borders, surrounded by normal lung tissue
2 May have an irregular or lobulated shape which can change on inspiration, expiration, upright or supine films, reflecting its fluid contents
3 Pleural effusion or hydropneumothorax following rupture into the pleural space
4 'Meniscus' or 'crescent sign' following cyst rupture into the bronchial tree with air between the pericyst and exocyst

5 Cyst rupture and bronchial communication with the endocyst resulting in
   - Air–fluid level in the parenchyma
   - Pneumonic consolidation secondary to aspirated fluid
   - 'Water-lily sign' representing membranes floating on the fluid surface
   - Residual cavity which can become secondarily infected

6 Mediastinal involvement of
   - Anterior mediastinum with tracheal compression
   - Middle mediastinum with compression and erosion of the great vessels
   - Posterior mediastinum with rib and vertebral erosion as well as spinal cord compression

7 CT scan may demonstrate
   - Pathognomonic daughter cysts free within the hydatid cyst or attached to the germinal layer
   - Cystic nature of the mass
   - Enhancing thin-walled rim

Diagnostic features

1 Chest X-ray/CT findings as above
2 Post-rupture or TTNA appearance of protoscolices and hooklets in sputum or pleural fluid
3 Peripheral eosinophilia (suggests a leaking cyst)
4 ⊕ serology in approximately 50% of lung cysts and 90% of liver cysts with occasional false positives due to other helminthic infections
5 Very rare outside the typical epidemiological context

INFLUENZA PNEUMONIA

Epidemiologically, influenza viruses are divided into Groups *A, B and C

- Group A is sub-divided on the basis of surface glycoproteins hemagglutinin and neuraminidase, antibodies against which confer immunity to infection

- The virus changes the sturcture and antigenic nature of the glycoproteins unpredictably, resulting in sporadic cases, epidemics and pandemics

Clinically, influenza is very contagious with an incubation period of 24–48 hours and spread by respiratory droplets

- Infection ranges from asymptomatic to fulminating pneumonia, the latter occasionally occurring in previously healthy individuals (in about ⅓ of cases), but typically in COPD, pregnancy, mitral stenosis, immunocompromised hosts, the elderly and often in the institutionalized

Pulmonary complications

1. **Typical influenza** with back and leg pains, fever, chills, headache, conjunctivitis, dry cough, but little pharyngitis or rhinorrhea
   - Chest X-rays are normal but small airways obstruction can often be demonstrated e.g. reduced flows at low lung volumes and ↑A-a O_2 gradient
2. **Lower respiratory tract** infection with scattered rales and rhonchi, reflecting acute bronchitis and/or bronchiolitis
   - May exacerbate underlying lung disease, e.g. asthma, COPD, CF
   - Chest X-rays are normal
3. **Viral pneumonia** developing 12–36 hours after the onset of illness reflecting viral spread to the lung parenchyma
   - Patients are acutely ill and may have underlying conditions, e.g. mitral stenosis, chronic bronchitis, pregnancy
4. **Bacterial pneumonia** developing within days to 2 weeks of initial symptoms and secondary to superinfection e.g. *Staph. aureus*, hemophilus, streptococci, neisseria meningitidis, others
   - Patients acutely deteriorate with purulent sputum and can develop the pulmonary or systemic complications associated with these organisms
5. **Croup** (laryngotracheobronchitis) seen mainly in young children

6 BOOP
7 Residual pulmonary fibrosis
8 Secondary pulmonary complications from
   – myopericarditis
   – CNS disease e.g. seizures, Guillan-Barré, myelitis

Radiologic findings

1 Disease distribution ranging from unilateral and unifocal to bilateral and diffuse
2 Lower > upper lobes
3 Patchy to homogeneous consolidation of above

Diagnostic criteria

1 Viral culture
2 Immunofluorescent staining of nasopharyngeal aspirate, wash, swab or sputum
3 Rapid enzyme immunoassay of above
4 Serology

LARYNGEAL PAPILLOMATOSIS

Clinically, a disease of children between 18 months and 3 years of age, characterized by laryngeal papillomas which can spontaneously disappear or recur post-resection

- Majority of cases caused by the human papilloma virus
- 98% of cases are confined to the larynx with approximately 2% involving the lower airways, usually the trachea, but occasionally the bronchi, bronchioles and alveoli
- Often an interval of approximately 10 years between laryngeal and pulmonary lesions
- Rarely does lower airway involvement precede laryngeal involvement or occur in its absence
- Adults can present without a prior history of disease
- The typical adult with lung disease will present with a history of laryngeal papillomas, have a tracheostomy and present with cough, hemoptysis, obstructive pneumonitis or an asthma-like picture
- Squamous cell carcinoma is described as a complication

Radiologic features

1 Tracheostomy tube (usually present)
2 Atelectasis, obstructive pneumonitis, post-obstructive abscess, bronchiectasis
3 Nodules, which may cavitate
4 Bronchogenic cancer

LEGIONELLA INFECTION

Epidemiologically, most cases are due to *L. pneumophilia* serogroup I, although other subtypes as well as other species can cause disease

- Water sources, e.g. air conditioners, hot water tanks, are the major origins of infection with the pathophysiology being inhalation or microaspiration of contaminated water
- Infections can be sporadic or epidemic with outbreaks described in hotels, cruise ships or office buildings

Clinically responsible for 2–15% of community-acquired pneumonias requiring hospitalization, often in patients with increasing age, transplant recipients, COPD, malignancy, renal failure

- The reported frequency of nosocomial infection correlates with the availability of diagnostic tests as well as the presence of legionella in the local water supply
- No evidence of person-to-person transmission
- The clinical spectrum is quite variable and can include
  - Asymptomatic infection
  - Pontiac Fever
    - An acute flu-like illness where pneumonia does not develop
    - Incubation period is 1–2 days with fever, headaches, +/– arthralgias, cough, GI complaints
    - Disease is self-limited with recovery occurring in a few days without antibiotic treatment
    - Diagnosis can be confirmed serologically

- – 'Atypical' pneumonia syndrome
- – 'Bacterial pneumonia' picture
- – Septic shock
- – ARDS with multiorgan failure

- The most common clinical syndrome is that of pneumonia, beginning with a 'flu-like' illness of fever, headaches, myalgias and diarrhea, followed by dry cough, chest pains and occasional hemoptysis
- Physical findings are those of pneumonia with bradycardia relative to fever found in some patients
- Multisystem disease can occur, most frequently involving the heart, liver, kidneys, or CNS, but virtually all organ systems can be involved without pathognomonic features
- Mortality rate of pneumonia varies from 5–25%
- WBC counts range from normal to elevated with variable hyponatremia but lab findings are non-specific

Radiologic findings

1 *Airspace consolidation begins unilaterally, segmental or non-segmental in distribution, progresses to lobar consolidation (often despite appropriate antibiotics), then multilobar involvement either contiguous or non-contiguous, and finally bilateral disease
   - All other types of infiltrates have been reported

2 Pleural effusion occurs in approximately 40% of patients but adenopathy is rare

3 Bilateral nodular opacities, often pleural-based, and cavitation are uncommon in normal hosts but occur in immunocompromised patients

4 Resolution of pneumonia can take up to 8 weeks or more with organization occasionally occurring

Diagnostic tests

1 Positive sputum or pleural fluid culture is the gold standard for diagnosis but requires a lab with technical expertise

2 Fluorescent antibody staining of sputum or BAL fluid with variable sensitivity reported in culture-positive cases

3 Urinary antigen for *L. pneumophilia* serogroup I, with the test remaining positive for weeks in spite of antibiotics, maximal sensitivity being within the first week
4 Serology (not commonly available)
   - A four-fold increase in antibody titer to 1:128 or more
   - A single convalescent titer of >1:256 in some studies to >1:1024 in others
5 PCR in urine, serum or BAL – under development

MELIOIDOSIS

Disease caused by *Pseudomonas pseudomallei*, a gram negative non-encapsulated rod, occurring mainly in rodents, cats and dogs and endemic in Southeast Asia and Northern Australia

- **Acute septicemic illness** presents with fever, chills, acute dyspnea, chest pains and high mortality
  - Abscesses develop in the lungs and other tissues with disseminated nodules and cavitation seen on chest X-ray
- **Chronic illness** simulates tuberculosis clinically and radiologically with granulomatous lesions on biopsy of lungs or other tissues
- Definitive diagnosis requires culture of the organism from sputum, blood, urine, stool or CSF

MORAXELLA CATARRHALIS

Gram negative aerobic diplococcus which can be a normal inhabitant of the upper respiratory tract of children and adults, making recovery from sputum difficult to interpret

- Clinical disease spectrum includes otitis, sinusitis, laryngitis, tracheobronchitis and pneumonia
- The most important risk factor for tracheobronchitis or pneumonia is COPD, although the immunocompromised, alcoholics, as well as patients with CHF or malignancy are also at risk

- Characteristic clinical and radiologic features are absent with symptoms being non-specific for infection
  - Extrapulmonary disease is rare with pleural effusion, empyema and sepsis being uncommon although positive blood cultures are reported
  - X-rays show bronchopneumonia or alveolar consolidation
  - Diagnosis is suggested by gram stain of sputum showing gram negative diplococci in association with positive cultures
  - Pure growth from TTNA or transtracheal aspirate in the presence of pneumonia would confirm the diagnosis
- High frequency of β-lactamase production is seen on sensitivity testing

MUCORMYCOSIS

Definition: Infections caused primarily by the three genera, *Mucor*, *Absidia* and *Rhizopus* in the class Zygomycetes, manifest as sino-orbital, pulmonary or disseminated disease

Clinically, a rare disorder in healthy individuals with most case reports in diabetes mellitis, renal failure or hematologic malignancy in patients with accompanying neutropenia, steroids or other immunosuppressive therapy

- Pulmonary disease most often described in leukemia, with pneumonia resulting from spore inhalation or hematogenous dissemination from another infected site
- Lung disease develops acutely and is indistinguishable from that of bacterial pneumonia or pulmonary infarction due to the angioinvasive nature of the organisms
- Poorly controlled diabetics can also develop the above but more often have the clinical syndrome of rhinocerebral mucormycosis, with infection beginning in the nose then spreading to involve the sinuses, palate, periorbital area and finally the brain via the cavernous sinus

Radiologic patterns

1 Focal infiltrate or consolidation
2 Focal mass

3 Cavitation
4 Pulmonary gangrene
5 Pulmonary artery mycotic aneurysms (rapidly enlarging mass lesions)
6 'Halo sign' on chest CT

Diagnosis requires the demonstration of non-septate hyphae with right angle branching on biopsy along with positive cultures

- Sputum stains and cultures are rarely positive and serology is unreliable
- Diagnosis should be considered in immunocompromised patients developing progressive pulmonary disease in spite of antibiotics

MYCOPLASMA PNEUMONIAE

Most common cause of community-acquired non-bacterial pneumonia with person-to-person transmission occurring by droplet inhalation

- Most often seen in adolescents and young adults, but the very young and elderly are also affected
- Seen throughout the year in sporadic form or as local outbreaks
- The incubation period is 2–4 weeks with epidemics in closed populations evolving slowly

Clinically, *Mycoplasma pneumoniae* is responsible for approximately 50% of 'atypical' pneumonia, although presentations are quite variable and also include

1 Asymptomatic infection (approximately 20%)
2 Upper respiratory infection
3 Epiglotitis
4 Acute tracheobronchitis
5 Exacerbation of asthma and COPD
6 Acute bronchiolitis, bronchiolitis obliterans, BOOP
7 Fulminant pneumonia with ARDS

- Infections are usually mild and acute to subacute in onset
- Typically begins in the upper respiratory tract with

pharyngitis, otitis and hoarseness, progressing to cough with small amounts of yellow sputum, fever, headache, malaise

- Hemoptysis, pleuritic pain, and GI symptoms are uncommon
- Physical findings can include absence of acute toxicity ('walking pneumonia'), pharyngeal erythema, bullous myringitis (rare), and minimal rales often with a marked discrepancy between the chest X-ray and physical findings
- Uncomplicated infection is characterized by resolution of symptoms in 1–2 weeks, although shedding of organisms can occur for weeks after clinical recovery
- Severe disease has been reported in patients with sickle-cell or sickle-related hemoglobinopathies

Extrapulmonary complications include the following with potential long term sequelae

1 Cold agglutins with hemolysis, thrombophlebitis, Raynaud's phenomenon
2 Neurologic diseases including encephalitis, aseptic meningitis, Guillain-Barré, transverse myelitis, cranial nerve palsies
3 Bullous myringitis
4 Pericarditis, cardiomyopathy
5 Hepatosplenomegaly
6 Arthritis, arthralgias
7 Maculopapular skin rash, erythema multiforme, Stevens-Johnson syndrome

Labs include

1 Normal (85%) or mild elevation of WBC
2 Neutrophils but no organisms on sputum gram stain
3 Cold agglutinins in approximately 50% of patients are non-specific for mycoplasma with titers >1:64 more specific but less sensitive
   - IgM antibodies directed against an altered I antigen on the surface of red blood cells
   - They are present by 7–10 days, peak at 2–3 weeks, and persist for 2–3 months

Radiologic features

1 Unilateral or bilateral consolidation, usually lower lobe
   - Begins as a single focus or multiple foci of interstitial disease progressing to airspace disease
   - Segmental or subsegmental in distribution and inhomogeneous (unlike the classic homogeneous non-segmental consolidation of *Strep. pneumoniae*)

2 Less common patterns are diffuse reticular interstitial infiltrates or bilateral perihilar infiltrates

3 Small pleural effusions in approximately 20% of cases

4 Hilar adenopathy is uncommon in adults but seen in children

5 Case reports of pneumatocele formation, bronchiectasis, Swyer-James syndrome

Diagnostic criteria

1 Serology
   - Four-fold or greater rise of complement-fixing antibodies in paired acute and convalecent sera
     - They are present at 2–3 weeks of infection and persist for 2–3 months
   - single elevated mycoplasma specific IgM titer (takes at least one week) or a high titer of cold agglutinins is suggestive of a recent infection

2 Positive cultures from throat, sputum or BAL (may take ten days to four weeks)

3 PCR from BAL (no FDA-approved kits)

NOCARDIOSIS

N. asteroides is responsible for approximately 90% of cases, with *N. brasiliensis* in 8% (mainly skin and soft tissue infections) and *N. caviae* in 2%

- The organisms are gram positive, weakly acid-fast branching filamentous hyphae with pulmonary disease caused by inhalation of organisms from contaminated soil and rare reports of person-to-person transmission

Clinically, infections are rare in clinical practice with 85% of cases seen in patients with underlying diseases including

1. Immunocompromised patients, particularly transplants and hematologic malignancies
2. Chronic pulmonary disorders, e.g. alveolar proteinosis, COPD, tuberculosis
3. Chronic inflammatory disorders, e.g. SLE

- Nocardia can occasionally be cultured from sputum in the absence of clinical disease
- Presentation is variable and ranges from an asymptomatic radiologic finding to acute, subacute or chronic disease with non-specific respiratory and systemic symptoms
- Pulmonary diseases predominate in 90% of cases with local complications, e.g. empyema, rib osteomyelitis, SVC syndrome, purulent pericarditis as well as dissemination most often involving the CNS or skin

Radiologic features

1. Localized airspace consolidation ± cavitation (may mimic tuberculosis when upper lobe in distribution)
2. Mass-like lesion ± cavitation
3. Single or multiple nodules ± cavitation
4. Diffuse disease – alveolar, reticulonodular or miliary
5. Pleural effusion in approximately 50% of cases with empyema (~⅓) or bronchopleural fistula
6. Chest wall invasion
7. Rare hilar adenopathy

Diagnostically, sputa may be negative, with BAL, TTNA, transbronchial or open biopsy often required for positive smear and culture, the latter occasionally taking up to three weeks

- The disease should be suspected in patients with one of the above predisposing conditions who manifest progressive pulmonary infiltrates and abscess formation in spite of broad spectrum antibiotics

PARAGONIMIASIS

Caused by flukes of the genus *Paragonimus* with *P. westermani* responsible for most cases

- Most frequently seen in Southeast Asia although described in many other geographic locations, with humans infected by ingestion of undercooked crab or crayfish or water contaminated by them
- After human ingestion, metacercariae excyst in the duodenum, penetrating the intestinal wall, peritoneum and diaphragm to migrate in the pleura and lung parenchyma, the main site of localization

Clinically, the early phase occurs between infection and egg production (~2 months) and is manifest by

1. Unilateral or bilateral pleuritic pain
2. Pneumothorax
3. Pleural effusion with eosinophilia
4. Loeffler's-like syndrome with changing infiltrates and peripheral eosinophilia reflecting larval migration in the lung

Late phase disease is seen with mature flukes in the lung which can last for years

- Recurrent hemoptysis is typical and reflects rupture of the encapsulated flukes into a bronchiole
- There is little or no peripheral eosinophilia and radiologic findings include
  - Normal X-rays in approximately 20% of cases (eggs present in the sputum)
  - Features simulating post-primary tuberculosis
  - Multiple ring shadows resembling cystic bronchiectasis, reflecting the lucency of the cyst contents
  - Linear streaks reflecting burrowing tracts of the flukes
  - Resolution of the above and appearance of new lesions
  - Pleural thickening or effusion

Diagnosis is presumptive in the early phase before eggs are produced

- In the late phase diagnosis is based upon
  - Eggs in sputum (not seen on gram stain as it destroys the eggs), pleural fluid, stools or TTNA
  - Serology

PNEUMOCYSTIS

1 HIV patients (see p. 328)
2 Non-HIV patients
   - 90% are on steroids at the time of diagnosis, usually >15 mg daily for >8 weeks and are on treatment for malignancy, transplant rejection or an inflammatory condition
   - The presentation is more fulminent than in the HIV population with more severe hypoxemia, respiratory failure and mortality
   - BAL typically reveals fewer organisms but more neutrophils

PSEUDALLESCHERIASIS

Rare fungal disease caused by *Pseudallescheria boydii*, an organism present in soil, water and manure, with farmers particularly susceptible

- In immunocompetent patients, it usually presents with skin and subcutaneous infections which can progress to osteomyelitis

Clinical presentations

1 *Colonization of the respiratory tract in patients who are immunocompromised or who have underlying fibrotic disease, e.g. sarcoid, tuberculosis
2 Near drowning in dirty water
3 Mycetoma formation, asymptomatic or with recurrent hemoptysis
4 Primary pneumonia in immunocompromised and rarely normal hosts

- Multiple radiologic patterns are described
- Diagnosis is based upon culture of the organism

Q-FEVER

Rickettsial disease caused by *Coxiella burnetti*, with human infection secondary to

- Inhalation of organisms from laboratory cultures
- Contact with laboratory, farm or domestic animals, especially after parturition
- Contact with animal related materials, e.g. wool, straw, manure

Clinically, the disease should be suspected in farmers, abattoir workers, lab personnel, veterinarians and others working with animals

- Incubation period is 4 days to 4 weeks and the presentation is variable, including
  - 'Flu-like' illness, typically self-limited within 2 weeks
  - Pneumonia, varying from 'atypical' to severe
  - Extrapulmonary features include FUO, endocarditis, myocarditis, hepatitis, encephalitis, meningoencephalitis
- Resolution occurs in 2–3 weeks with fatalities being unusual

Radiologic manifestations are variable and non-specific

Diagnosis can be definitively established by serology ("phase II" Ab diagnostic of acute disease) or culture of the organism from blood, sputum, pleural fluid or urine (not readily available)

RESPIRATORY SYNCYTIAL VIRUS (RSV)

Major cause of severe bronchiolitis and bronchopneumonia in infants and small children

- In otherwise normal adults presentations include a URTI, tracheobronchitis and airway hyper-reactivity lasting several weeks

- Incubation period ranges from 2–8 days with symptoms of a RTI frequently present in family members
- In the elderly and those with underlying disease, an influenza-like illness, bronchitis and pneumonia are common manifestations
- Community-acquired and nosocomial pneumonia are increasingly described in immunocompromised patients, particularly recipients of a bone-marrow transplant
- RSV should be considered in the differential diagnosis of diffuse interstitial lung disease in this population although other radiologic presentations, e.g. lobar infiltrates, have been described

Diagnostic features

1. Rapid tests by immunofluorescence or enzyme immunoassary
2. Positive BAL cultures > sputum or throat cultures, with results in 2–5 days
3. Lung biopsy for virus isolation, histology and antigen identification
4. PCR is presently being investigated

SCHISTOSOMIASIS

Parasitic disease caused by flukes, the most important being

- *S. mansoni* and *S. hematobium* in the Middle East and Africa
- *S. mansoni* in the Caribbean with Puerto Ricans most often involved in Canada and the U.S.
- *S. japonicum* in Japan, China and the Philippines

Life Cycle

- Cercariae are liberated from snails in water, penetrate the skin, pass as schistosomules through the pulmonary capillaries, enter the systemic circulation, and develop as adult worms in the mesenteric venous plexus (*S. mansoni*, *S. japonicum*) or the vesical venous bed (*S. hematobium*)
- Female worms lay eggs in the venules of the bowel or bladder which either are extruded into the lumen or trans-

ported via the mesenteric venous system into the liver or via the vesicular veins directly to the lungs

Acute Pulmonary Schistosomiasis (Katayama Fever)

Clinical syndrome seen in persons not previously infected, e.g. visitors to an endemic area, and occurs with the migration of immature worms and later eggs to the lungs

- Fever, cough, dyspnea, diarrhea, arthralgias and eosinophilia develop 2–8 weeks after infection
- Radiologically, interstitial infiltrates or a Loeffler's syndrome may develop
- The acute syndrome is self-limited with resolution in 1–2 months without permanent sequelae

Diagnostic features

1 Egg detection in stool or rectal mucosa but not seen acutely as several weeks are required for worms to mature and shed eggs
2 Antischistosomal antibodies in serum

Chronic Pulmonary Schistosomiasis

Seen in patients after years of persistent infestation and characterized by pulmonary hypertension and interstitial lung disease

- Eggs, passing directly from the urinary bladder or indirectly from the mesentery (following the development of portal hypertension with bypass of the liver), become wedged in pulmonary arterioles and capillaries
- Extrusion of eggs into the surrounding perivascular tissues result in an obliterative arteriolitis as well as interstitial infiltrates
- Patients present with dyspnea while disease progression results in cor pulmonale

Radiologic features

1 Enlargement of the hilar arteries and right heart
2 Nodular interstitial infiltrates

Diagnostic features

1 Ova in sputum, BAL, urine, stools
2 Ova in bowel or bladder mucosa
3 Lung biopsy – transbronchial or open
4 Liver biopsy demonstrating Symmer's pipestem fibrosis

SPOROTRICHOSIS

Rare cause of lung infection due to the dimorphic fungus *Sporothrix schenckii*, a common saprophyte from soil, thorns, decaying vegetable material, other

Epidemiologically, it is found in the United States (states bordering the Mississippi and Missouri Rivers), South America, South Africa and Japan, with occupations at risk including gardeners, farmers, florists, ranchers, greenhouse and forestry workers

Lung disease occurs from inhalation of spores (no associated skin lesions) or spread from the skin (due to innoculation or bites)

- Presentation is that of a chronic respiratory infection, frequently with underlying systemic disease, e.g. alcoholism, diabetes or lung disease such as COPD
- Systemic symptoms of fever and weight loss are seen in ~50% of patients

Radiologic features include

1 Single or multiple cavities, usually thin-walled, unilateral > bilateral and an upper lobe predilection resembling post-primary TB
2 Multiple small non-cavitary nodules
3 Solitary lung nodule – sporotrichoma
4 Hilar/mediastinal adenopathy

Diagnosis should be suggested in patients with an occupational exposure to plants, soil, etc. in combination with a clinical and X-ray picture of tuberculosis but a negative work-up

Definitive diagnosis is established by

1 Serology
2 Positive cultures from sputum, BAL, lung, pleural fluid
3 Histology of caseating or non-caseating granulomas with demonstration of organisms by stains or direct fluorescent antibody (DFA)

STAPHYLOCOCCUS AUREUS PNEUMONIA

Epidemiologically, may be community-acquired (rare) or nosocomial and pathophysiologically can be

1 Aerogenous, causing a primary pneumonia, e.g. underlying lung disease, immunosuppression, risk for aspiration or secondary to, e.g. influenza
   - Positive blood cultures in approximately 30% of cases
2 Hematogenous and secondary to tricuspid endocarditis, i.v. catheters, hemodialysis, septic focus

Clinically, the presentation is variable and includes

- Minimally symptomatic state with the insidious onset of non-specific respiratory symptoms
- Acute fulminating pneumonia
- ARDS
- May follow typical influenza with acute deterioration within about 2 weeks postviral infection
- Underlying endocarditis or vascular infection may predominate when hematogenously acquired
- Complications include cavitation, parapneumonic effusion or empyema, ARDS, residual bronchiectasis, bronchopleural fistula, toxic shock syndrome, endocarditis, meningitis, metastatic abscesses, e.g. brain, kidney; in children – pneumothorax, pyopneumothorax and pneumatoceles

Radiologic features for the **aerogenous** route include

1 Segmental bronchopneumonia with patchy, homogeneous or mixed consolidation and rare air bronchograms
2 Unilateral or bilateral distribution, single or multiple lobes involved with lower lobe predominance

3 Abscess formation in approximately 20% of cases, single > multiple
4 Pleural effusion/empyema in up to 50% of cases
5 Pneumatoceles and pneumothoraces are common in children
6 Atelectasis or a bulging fissure are uncommonly described

Radiologic features for the **hematogenous** route include
1 Multiple bilateral nodular densities which can become confluent and resemble homogeneous consolidation
   - Erosion into the tracheobronchial tree results in cavitation and air–fluid levels
2 Wedge-shaped subpleural septic infarcts

Definitive diagnosis requires culture from an uncontaminated site, e.g. blood cultures, (positive in up to 50% of patients), pleural fluid, TTNA, metastatic site
- Sputum cultures are sensitive (~90%) but not specific as the organism can be a commensal

STREPTOCOCCUS PNEUMONIAE

Streptococcus pneumoniae is a gram positive encapsulated organism, colonizing the nasopharynx in approximately 20% of normals, with pneumonia caused by aspiration from the upper airway
- Multiple serotypes are identified on the basis of the polysaccharide composition of the capsule, with specific antigenic types, e.g. type 3, associated with bacteremia and high mortality
- May occur as primary pneumonia or complicate viral infections, e.g. influenza
- Responsible for about ⅔ of all pneumonias where an etiologic diagnosis is made
- Accounts for about ⅔ of all fatal pneumonias

Clinically, it is the most common community-acquired bacterial pneumonia

- Can occur in normal hosts, but predisposing conditions include alcoholic liver disease, renal failure, poorly controlled diabetics, COPD, CHF, lymphoma, leukemia, sickle cell disease, multiple myeloma, AIDS and the elderly
- Classic presentation is an acute onset with fever, shaking chills, pleuritic chest pain, cough which can be dry, rusty or purulent, dyspnea, ± preceding URI, but this presentation is relatively uncommon and more often seen in otherwise healthy young adults
- Disease in the majority of elderly patients is subacute or insidious in onset with altered sensorium or deteriorating functional status overshadowing the respiratory symptoms
- Mortality with pneumonia in one lobe is ~1% but increases with
  - Increasing age
  - Severe underlying illness
  - Multilobar involvement
  - Bacteremia which occurs in 10–40% of patients, usually in those with a co-morbid illness, and has 20% mortality unchanged since the 1920s
  - Leucopenia
- 40% of all deaths occur within 24 hours of hospitalization

Labs are non-specific with WBC counts typically >18 000/mm^3 but vary from leucopenia to a leukemoid reaction

- Mild hyperbilirubinemia may occur

Complications include

1. Parapneumonic effusion is seen in about 20% of cases and is usually small and sterile
2. Empyema
3. Lung abscess or gangrene (rare) – R/O concomitant aerobic or anaerobic infection
4. Superinfection with gram negatives
5. ALPS syndrome, i.e. alcoholism, leucopenia and pneumococcal sepsis with progression to thrombocytopenia, shock, ARDS and high mortality
6. Pericarditis (pericardial rub, hypotension, persistent fever, increasing precordial pain)

7 Delayed resolution with fever, rales and radiologic infiltrates persisting 4–6 weeks is uncommon but seen in the elderly, alcoholics or COPD patients
   - Diagnosis of exclusion after local airways obstruction or superinfection has been ruled out
8 Hyperbilirubinemia and transaminitis
9 Meningitis
10 Septic arthritis

Other clinical syndromes caused by *Strep. pneumoniae* include
1 Direct spread causing otitis media, sinusitis, meningitis, tracheitis, bronchitis
2 Hematogenous spread to heart valves, CNS, bones, joints, peritoneal cavity and DIC
   - Endocarditis may occur on normal or damaged heart valves and may present concurrent with or subsequent to the pneumonia
3 Primary bacteremia with no obvious source
4 Gangrene of the extremities usually in association with DIC

Classic radiologic features
1 Homogeneous non-segmental consolidation adjacent to a pleural surface with air bronchograms
2 Usually involve only part of a lobe although complete lobar consolidation as well as multilobar involvement can occur
3 Pleural effusion in approximately 10% of cases
4 Complete resolution, often within 2 weeks in community-acquired infection, although a delay is seen in the elderly, COPD, CHF and with bacteremia

Less common radiologic features
5 'Spherical' pneumonia
6 Segmental distribution
7 Inhomogenous consolidation, e.g. COPD patients
8 ARDS
9 Cavitation/lung gangrene (very rare)
10 Organization or carnification post-treatment (very rare)

Definitive diagnosis can be made by culture of the organism from blood, pleural fluid, TTNA or an extrapulmonary septic focus

- *Strep. pneumoniae* can be cultured from sputum in the absence of pneumonia and may be absent from the sputum even when bacteremia is documented, although gram stain of purulent sputum showing lancet-shaped diplococci in the absence of other flora is strongly suggestive of the diagnosis (in the appropriate clinical setting)

STREPTOCOCCUS PYOGENES

Group A β-hemolytic gram positive organism, commonly responsible for pneumonia in the pre-antibiotic era following measles, pertussis or influenza

- Uncommon today but occurs following pharyngitis/tonsillitis, measles, influenza, in epidemic form or in previously normal individuals

Clinically, there may be a preceeding sore throat but onset is abrupt and similar to that of *Strep. pneumoniae* with fevers, rigors, pleuritic pain, cough and purulent/bloody sputum

- Pleural complications are frequent, most often effusion or frank empyema
- Other intrathoracic complications include bronchopleural fistula, bronchiectasis, pericarditis and residual pleural thickening with a trapped lung
- Streptococcal toxic shock-like syndrome usually follows a soft tissue infection, e.g. necrotizing fasciitis, but can follow other local infections, e.g. pneumonia, where patients present with fever, hypotension, renal failure and ARDS

Radiologically, the picture is that of a bronchopneumonia similar to *staph. aureus*

- Lower lobes are preferentially involved, unilaterally or bilaterally, with abscess formation and pleural effusions, the latter often developing rapidly

Diagnosis can be confirmed from pleural fluid, blood cultures or TTNA

STRONGYLOIDIASIS

Most cases caused by *Strongyloides stercoralis*, endemic in tropical and subtropical regions where filariform larvae penetrate the skin and are brought by the blood to the lungs
- They migrate from capillaries into alveoli and subsequently the upper airway where they are then swallowed and develop into adult females in the small bowel, where they release their eggs
- The eggs develop into non-infectious rhaditiform larvae that (a) can be passed in the stool or (b) develop within the intestine into filariform larvae which can penetrate the bowel and migrate to the lungs (autoinfection)

Clinically, infection in normal hosts is often asymptomatic or results in mild symptoms, but immunocompromised patients (e.g. malignancy, steroid-treated), can develop a 'hyperinfection syndrome' with pulmonary disease caused by migration of larvae from capillaries into the airspaces and airways
- Respiratory symptoms can be non-specific but new onset or exacerbation of pre-existing asthma may occur as can GI complaints

Radiologic features
1 Non-segmental, patchy consolidation (? allergic)
2 Hyperinfection
   - Focal or diffuse airspace consolidation
   - Diffuse reticulonodular, nodular or miliary pattern
   - ARDS picture
3 Pleural effusion +/– associated parenchymal disease

Diagnostic clues and criteria
1 Immunocompromised patient with an appropriate geographic history and the above radiological abnormalities
2 History of a preceding skin rash
3 Peripheral eosinophilia (absence of exogenous steroids)

4 Asthma symptoms
5 Larvae in sputum, BAL, stool
6 ELISA test (in an immunocompetent patient)

TOXOPLASMOSIS

Caused by *Toxoplasma gondii*, an intracellular protozoan with humans infected by ingestion of (a) cysts from infected tissue such as undercooked lamb, or (b) food contaminated by oocysts from cat feces (cats are the definitive hosts)

Clinical findings in adults

- *Asymptomatic infection following ingestion of organisms, parasitemia and organ invasion
- Lymphadenopathy
  - May be asymptomatic and usually cervical but may present with an 'infectious mononucleosis' syndrome with fever and atypical lymphocytes
  - Mediastinal lymphadenopathy can also be present
- Chorioretinitis
- Rare dissemination in normal hosts
  - The above usually occurs in immunocompromised patients with encephalitis, CNS mass lesions, myocarditis, fever, pneumonia as well as other organ involvement

Radiologic features

1 Focal interstitial or airspace disease resembling viral pneumonia
2 Hilar or mediastinal lymphadenopathy
3 Miliary pattern in immunocompromised patients

Diagnostic criteria

1 Characteristic histology in lymph nodes
2 Serology but false positives and negatives can occur
3 Direct visualization of trophozoites in tissue
4 Isolation of organisms from blood or CSF by tissue cultures or mice injection
5 PCR

TULAREMIA

Caused by *Francisella tularensis*, a gram negative bacillus, most common in rodents and small animals, with humans infected by

1 Skin contact from rabbits, muskrats, hunting knives (described in Canada and Northern U.S.)
2 Inhalation from animals or culture materials in labs
3 Bites from ticks, deer flies, mosquitoes (most often reported from Arkansas, Oklahoma, Utah, Missouri)
4 Ingestion of contaminated meat or water

Clinically, six forms of the disease are described – glandular, ulceroglandular, occuloglandular, oropharyngeal, typhoidal, and pneumonic

- Pulmonary disease results from inhalation or hematogenous dissemination, the latter from typhoidal or ulceroglandular disease
- Exposure history can include visits to an endemic rural area, park/zoo, hunting trips or laboratory work
- Spectrum of pulmonary disease varies from asymptomatic infiltrates to an ARDS picture
- Usually presentation is of a flu-like illness, 1–14 days post-exposure, with skin lesions, pharyngitis, tonsillitis, lymphadenopathy – respiratory symptoms potentially developing

Radiologic features

1 Airspace consolidation, occasionally described as 'oval' and resembling a non-cavitary lung abscess
2 Cavitation in ~15%
3 Ipsilateral hilar adenopathy in 25–50%
4 Pleural effusion in 25–50%

Diagnostic criteria

1 4-fold increase in serum antibody levels, the peak occurring 4–8 weeks after the onset of illness
2 Cultures of skin, lymph nodes, sputum or blood (dangerous lab pathogen)
3 Innoculation of mice or guinea pig with culture of necrotic material from liver, spleen or lymph nodes

VARICELLA PNEUMONIA

Varicella-zoster virus can cause pneumonia as a complication of both chickenpox and shingles, the former being more common

- Chickenpox is mainly a mucocutaneous disease, transmitted by respiratory droplets, with an incubation period of 10–21 days

Clinically, it is seen in <1% of children, but complicates approximately 15% of adults with primary varicella infection, and approximately 10% of these patients develop life-threatening pneumonia

- The risk factors for pneumonia include
  - Aging
  - Pregnancy (up to 40% mortality) with greatest risk for pneumonia in the third trimester
  - Immunocompromised patients, e.g. bone marrow or other transplants, children with cancer
  - Steroid treatment
  - Severity of the rash
  - ? Smoking history
- The classic history is that of contact with an infected child in the previous three weeks, followed by the development of fever and non-specific respiratory symptoms one to six days after the vesicular rash (pneumonia has not been reported in the absence of rash)
- Spontaneous resolution is the usual course of disease, although progressive pneumonia can develop from the virus itself or bacterial superinfection
- Systemic complications include myocarditis, nephritis, hepatitis, and adrenal hemorrhage with pregnancy and immunosuppression increasing mortality rates

Labs reveal a variable WBC count without pathognomonic findings

Radiologic features

1 Bilateral patchy airspace consolidation, often nodular in appearance

2 Adenopathy and pleural effusions are uncommon
3 Resolution can take days to months and lags behind clinical improvement
4 Residual widespread nodules may persist with eventual calcification, resulting in multiple calcific nodules 1–2 mm in diameter

Definitive diagnosis of pneumonia can be made by
1 Paired acute and convalescent sera or scrapings from cutaneous lesions for viral culture or immunofluorescent staining

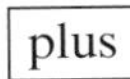

2 Positive PCR on BAL or
3 Positive cultures of BAL or lung tissue

Presumptive diagnosis can be made by a history of exposure, the characteristic skin eruption and radiologic findings

VISCERAL LARVA MIGRANS

Human infection is seen following the ingestion of eggs from dogs (*Toxocara canis*), or less often cats (*Taxocara catis*), which have been in soil for a few weeks, and is therefore mainly a disease of children
Clinically, after ingestion of eggs, larva are carried through the portal vein to the liver and then into the systemic circulation
Pulmonary symptoms include cough, wheezing and shortness of breath, accompanied by peripheral eosinophilia
X-rays reveal non-specific infiltrates while BAL eosinophilia has been described
Serology is the most useful diagnostic test

WHOOPING COUGH

Caused by *Bordetella pertussis*, an encapsulated gram negative coccobacillus that can present in adulthood after vaccination in childhood

Clinically, the incubation period is usually 7–10 days with illness lasting 6–8 weeks and evolving through 3 stages

1 Catarrhal stage of 1–2 weeks with upper respiratory symptoms, cough, fever
2 Paroxysmal stage of 2–4 weeks with the typical paroxysm of cough but absence of fever unless bacterial superinfection is present
   - The distinctive woop is due to sudden inspiration against a closed glottis at the end of a paroxysm
3 Convalescent stage where cough intensity gradually lessens

- Adults present with upper respiratory symptoms and prolonged cough, while the characteristic whoop is less common than in infants and children
- Coughing spasms are less severe and cough less prolonged in vaccinated individuals
- Clinical symptoms relate to the development of bronchitis, bronchiolitis and pneumonia
- Differential diagnosis includes respiratory viral infections, e.g. influenza, adenovirus, RSV, as well as mycoplasma and chlamydia

Radiologic manifestions

1 Segmental pneumonia
2 Atelectasis secondary to mucus plugs
3 Hilar adenopathy – one of few bacterial infections causing lymphadenopathy
4 Bronchiectasis (rare today)

Diagnostic features

1 Lymphocytosis (uncommon in adults)
2 Positive nasopharyngeal cultures are seen in ~50% of adults from the time of exposure to about 2 weeks after symptoms develop
   - Diagnostic yield falls rapidly after two weeks and is rarely positive by week four
3 Fluorescent antibody staining or PCR of nasopharyngeal secretions

4 Positive cultures from symptomatic contacts
5 Serology

Fraser R.S., Muller N.L., Colman N., Paré P.D. (1999) *Diagnosis of Diseases of the Chest* 4th Edn., WB Saunders.

Hoeprich, P., Jordan, M.C., Ronald, A. *Infectious Diseases – A Treatise of Infectious Processes.*: J.B. Lippincott. pp. 349–497.

Heffner, J., Harley, R. (1992) Thoracic actinomycosis. *Semin. Resp. Med.* **13**: 234–240.

Kuzo, R., Goodman, L. (1996) Blastomycosis. *Semin. Roent.* **xxxi**: 45–51.

Miller, G., Brann, N., Einsele, H. *et al.* (1993) Human CMV infection in transplantation. *Nephron* **143**: 343–353.

Morris, D. (1995) Opportunities for diagnosing CMV in pulmonary infections. *Thorax* **50**: 3–5.

Cathomas, G., Morris, P., Pekle, K. *et al.* (1993) Rapid diagnosis of CMV pneumonias in marrow transplant recipients. *Blood* **81**: 1909–1914.

Schluger, N., Rom, W. (1995) The polymerase chain reaction in the diagnosis and evaluation of pulmonary infections. *Am. J. Resp. Cri. Care Med.* **152**: 11–16.

Goodwin, R.A., Loyd, J.E., Des Prez, R.M. (1981) Histoplasmosis in normal host. *Medicine* **60**: 231–266.

Goodwin, R.A., Des Prez, R.M. (1978) Histoplasmosis. *ARRD* **117**: 929–956.

Drutz, D.J., Catanzaro, A. (1978) Coccidioidomycosis. *ARRD* **117**: 559–585.

Goodwin, R.A., Shapiro, J., Thurman, G. *et al.* (1980) Disseminated histoplasmosis: clinical and pathological correlations. *Medicine* **59**: 1–33.

Klein, D.L., *et al.* (1980) Manifestations of aspergillosis. *AJR* **134**: 503–552.

Batra, P., Ritu Sonia Bathra. (1996) Thoracic coccidioidomycosis. *Semin. Roent.* **xxxi**: 28–44.

Conces, D. (1996) Histoplasmosis. *Semin. Roent.* **xxxi**: 14–27.

Binder, R., Faling, J., Pugatch, R. *et al.* (1982) Chronic necrotizing pulmonary aspergillosis: a discrete clinical entity. *Medicine*: 109–124.

Woodring, J., Ciporkin, G. Lee, C. *et al.* (1996) Pulmonary cryptococcosis. *Semin. Roent.* **xxxi**: 67–75.

Sarosi, G. (1991) Community-acquired fungal diseases. *Clinics Chest Medicine* **12**: 337–347.

Murphy, R., Miller, W. (1996) Pulmonary mucormycosis. *Semin. Roent.* **xxxi**: 83–87.
Miller, W. (1996) Aspergillosis: a disease with many faces. *Semin. Roent.* **xxxi**: 52–66.
Bigby, T., Serota, M., Tierney, L. *et al.* (1986) Clinical spectrum of pulmonary mucormycosis. *Chest* **89**: 435–439.
Patz, E.F., Goodman, P.C. (1992) Pulmonary cryptococcosis. *J. Thor. Imaging* **7**: 51–55.
Boyars, M.C. *et al.* (1992) Clinical manifestations of pulmonary fungal infections. *J. Thor. Imaging* **7**: 12–22.
Pluss, J.L., Opal, S. (1986) Pulmonary sporotrichosis: review of treatment and outcome. *Medicine* **65**: 143–153.
Rohwedder, J.J. (1987) Pulmonary sporotrichosis. *Semin. Resp. Med.* **9**: 176–179.
Rolte, M., Strieter, R., Lynch, J. (1992) Nocardiosis. *Semin. Resp. Med.* **13**: 216–233.
Taylor-Robinson, D. (1996) Infection due to species of mycoplasma and ureaplasma: an update. *Clin. Infect. Dis.* **23**: 671–684.
Ortaqvist, A. (1994) Initial investigation and treatment of the patient with severe CAP. *Semin. Resp. Med.* **9**: 166–179.
Bartlett, J.G., Mudy, L. (1995) Community-acquired pneumonia. *NEJM* **333**: 1618–1626.
Torres, A., Serra-Batlles, J., Ferrer, A. *et al.* (1991) Severe community-acquired pneumonia: epidemiology and prognostic features. *ARRD* **144**: 312–318.
Bartlett, J.G. (1993) Anaerobic bacterial infections of the lung and pleural space. *Clin. Infect. Dis.* **16**: S248–S255.
Bartlett, J.G. (1979) Anaerobic bacterial pneumonitis. *ARRD* **119**: 19–23.
Kauppinen, M., Saikku, P. (1995) Pneumonia due to Chlamydia pneumoniae: prevalence, clinical features, diagnosis, and treatment. *Clin. Infect. Dis.* **21**: S244–S252.
Sahn, S.A. (1993) Management of complicated parapneumonic effusions. *ARRD* **148**: 813–817.
Fein, A.M., Feinsilver, S., Niederman, M. *et al.* (1987) 'When the pneumonia doesn't get better'. *Clinics in Chest Medicine* **8**: 529–541.
Murray, H.W. (1975) The proteon manifestation of *Mycoplasma pneumoniae* infection in adults. *Am. J. Med.* **58**: 229–242.
Gogos, C., Bassaris, H., Vagenakis, A. (1992) Varicella pneumonia in adults: a review of pulmonary manifestations, risk factors and treatment. *Respiratory* **59**: 339–343.
Triebwasser, Ussaf, M.C., Harris, R. *et al.* (1967) Varicella pneumonia in adults. *Medicine* **46**: 409–420.

American Thoracic Society (1993) Guidelines for the initial management of adults with CAP: diagnosis, assessment of severity and initial antimicrobial therapy. *ARRD* **148**: 1418–1426.

Lynch, D., Armstrong, J. (1991) A pattern oriented approach to chart radiographs in atypical pneumonia syndromes. *Clinics in Chest Medicine* **12**: 203–222.

Gill, V.J. (1996) Laboratory evaluation of specimens, pp. 586–588. In: Shelhamer, J.H. (Moderator). *The Laboratory Evaluation of Opportunistic Pulmonary Infections. Ann. Int. Med.* **124**: 585–599.

Kuhlman, J. (1996) Pneumocystis infections: the radiologist's perspective. *Radiology* **198**: 623–634.

Naidich, D.P., McGuinness, G. (1991) Pulmonary manifestations of AIDS: CT and radiographic correlations. *Radiol. Clin. North Am.* **29**: 990–1017.

Safrin, S. (1993) *Pneumocystis carinii* pneumonia in patients with the acquired immunodeficiency syndrome. *Semin. Resp. Inf.* **8**: 96–103.

Miller, R.F., Mitchell, S.M. (1995) *Pneumocystis carinii* pneumonia. *Thorax* **50**: 191–200.

Stevens, D. (1995) Coccidioidomycosis. *NEJM* **332**: 1077–1082.

Pachon, J., Prados, M.D., Capote, F. *et al.* (1990) Severe community-acquired pneumonia. Etiology, prognosis and treatment. *ARRD* **142**: 369–373.

Celis, R., Torres, A., Gatell, J. *et al.* (1988) Nosocomial pneumonia. A multivariable analysis of risk and prognosis. *Chest* **93**: 318–324.

Dalhoff, K., Maass, M. (1966) *Chlamydia pneumoniae* in hospitalized patients. *Chest* **110**: 351–356.

McConnell, C., Mueller, C., Marston, B. (1994) Radiographic appearance of *Chlamydia pneumoniae*. Respiratory infections. *Radiology* **192**: 819–826.

Duchin, J., Koster, F., Peters, C.J. *et al.* (1994) Hantavirus pulmonary syndrome: a clinical description of 17 patients with a newly recognized disease. *NEJM* **330**: 949–955.

Feldman, S. (1994) Varicella-zoster virus pneumonitis. *Chest* **106**: 22S–27S.

Bartlett, J., Breiman, R., Mandell, A. *et al.* (1998) Community-acquired pneumonia in adults. Guidelines for management. *Clin. Infect. Dis.* **26**: 811–838.

Fine, M., Auble, T., Yealy, D. *et al.* (1997) A prediction rule to identify low-risk patient with CAP. *NEJM* **336**: 243–250.

Farr, B.M. (1997) Prognosis and decisions in pneumonia. *NEJM* **336**: 288–289.

Moolenaar, R.L., Dalton, C., Lipman, H. *et al.* (1995) Clinical features that differentiate hantavirus pulmonary syndrome from three other acute respiratory illnesses. *Clin. Inf. Dis.* **21**: 643–649.

American Thoracic Society (1995) Hospital acquired pneumonia in adults: diagnosis, assessment of severity, initial antimicrobial therapy and preventive strategies. *Am. J. Resp. Crit. Care Med.* **153**: 1711–1725.

Pluss, G.L., Opal, S.M. (1996) Pulmonary sporotrichosis: review of treatment and outcome. *Medicine* **65**: 143–153.

American Thoracic Society (1995) Hospital-acquired pneumonia in adults: diagnosis, assessment of severity, initial antimicrobial therapy, and preventive strategies. *Am. J. Resp. Crit. Care Med.* **153**: 1711–1725.

Khurshid, A., Barnett, T., Sekosan, M. *et al.* (1999) Disseminated *Pseudallescheria boydii* infection in a nonimmunocompromised host. *Chest* **116**: 572–574.

Sinave, C.P., Hardy, G.J., Fardy, P.W. (1999) The Lemierre syndrome: suppurative thrombophlebitis of the internal jugular vein secondary to oropharyngeal infection. *Medicine* **68**: 85–93.

58 Pneumothorax

Definition: Air in the pleural space. Can be classified as follows

Primary Spontaneous Pneumothorax

Defined as a non-traumatic pneumothorax occurring in patients without obvious pulmonary disease clinically or on chest X-ray, although chest CT usually reveals subapical blebs and bullae (etiology unclear)

Clinical features

- Seen in tall thin individuals, most often between the ages of 20 and 40
- Male/female ratio of about 5:1
- Sporadic or familial
- Risk increases with smoking in a dose-related fashion
- Dyspnea and/or pleuritic chest pain are the most common presenting features (Horner's syndrome rarely described from traction on the sympathetic ganglion)
- Most cases occur at rest with only about 10% on exertion
- Ipsilateral recurrence seen in about 30% of patients within 5 years of the first event, the incidence of recurrence increasing with each repeated event
- Contralateral recurrence seen in about 10% of cases

Radiologically, a pneumothorax is diagnosed by detection of the visceral pleural line which occasionally can be identified only on an expiratory film

- An associated pleural effusion is present in 10–20% of cases, usually serous but bloody in about $\frac{1}{3}$, where it is thought to be due to tearing of adhesions

Secondary Spontaneous Pneumothorax

Defined as a pneumothorax occurring in patients with underlying lung disease, the clinical features often reflecting this

- Patients are usually more symptomatic, with dyspnea resulting from diminished pulmonary reserve
- Recurrence rates exceed those seen in primary pneumothorax, ipsilateral > contralateral
- COPD accounts for about 60% of cases of secondary pneumothorax, etiologies including

Airways disease

- COPD
- Asthma
- Cystic fibrosis
- Bronchopleural fistula

Parenchymal disease

- Bullae, cysts, cavities, pneumatoceles, emphysema
- Interstitial lung diseases, especially those with honeycombing
- Infections, e.g. PCP, necrotizing pneumonia, TB, ecchinococcus, paragonimiasis
- Neoplasms, primary or secondary
- Radiation
- Others

Vascular disease

- Infarcts
- Catamenial
- Vasculitides

Others

- Mitral valve prolapse, gastropleural or colopleural fistulas

Traumatic Pneumothorax

Penetrating injury (direct communication between pleural space and atmosphere)

- Blunt, e.g.
  - Lacerated visceral pleura from a rib fracture
  - Fractured tracheobronchial tree
  - Intrapleural rupture of mediastinal air

- Drug-induced, e.g.
  - Attempted injection into the subclavian or internal jugular veins
  - Drug inhalation and valsalva
- Iatrogenic, e.g.
  - Barotrauma of mechanical ventilation
  - Thoracocentesis, TTNA, pleural or transbronchial biopsy

Radiologically, films are often supine with the visceral pleural line not identified as air accumulates in the anterior cardiophrenic angle and is manifest by

1. Depression of the hemidiaphragm
2. Hyperlucency of the lower chest
3. Double diaphragm sign reflecting the central dome and anterior insertion
4. Deepened lateral costophrenic sulcus
5. Sharp outline of the cardiac apex and adjacent fat when left-sided

Tension Pneumothorax

Hemodynamic emergency which can complicate a spontaneous or traumatic pneumothorax, and characterized by the pleural pressure on the side of the pneumothorax exceeding atmospheric pressure throughout expiration

A one-way valve is created where air enters pleural space in inspiration but cannot exit in expiration, the consequences including

Respiratory

- Altered sensorium with agitation/confusion
- Tachypnea
- Cyanosis
- Contralateral tracheal shift
- Distended ipsilateral hemithorax with little air movement
- Supraclavicular soft tissue mass representing herniated lung

Cardiovascular

- Tachycardia

- Jugular venous distension
- Systemic hypotension (late finding)

Labs

- Hypoxemia, metabolic and respiratory acidosis (late findings)

Radiological findings

1 Air-filled hemithorax with atelectasis of the involved lung
2 Downward displacement of the ipsilateral diaphragm
3 Contralateral shift of the trachea and mediastinum

Fraser R.S., Muller N.L., Colman N., Paré P.D. (1999) *Diagnosis of Diseases of the Chest* 4th Edn., WB Saunders.

Felson, B. (1973) *Chest Roentgenology*.: W.B. Saunders.

Chapman, S., Nakielny, R. (1995) *Aids to Radiological Differential Diagnosis*, 3rd edn.: W.B. Saunders.

Baum, G.L., Crapo, J.D., Celli, B.R., Karlinsky, J.B. (eds) (1997) *Textbook of Pulmonary Diseases*, 6th edn.: Lippincott-Raven.

Fishman, A.P., Elias, J.A., Fishman, J.A., Grippi, M.A., Kaiser, L.R., Senior, R.N. (1998) *Fishman's Pulmonary Diseases and Disorders*, 3rd edn.: McGraw-Hill.

59 Pregnancy-related

Dyspnea

'Normal' physiologic dyspnea of pregnancy reflects elevated progesterone levels which increase minute ventilation, mainly due to an increase in tidal volume with little change in respiratory rate

- The dyspnea or 'awareness of hyperventilation' begins in the first or second trimester, plateaus or improves as term approaches, and may be accompanied by
  - Orthopnea and PND due to an elevated hemidiaphragm
  - Dizziness or syncope when supine, the 'supine hypotensive syndrome' due to IVC compression and associated reduced cardiac output
  - Fatigue due to weight gain or anemia
  - JVD secondary to elevated blood volume
  - Radiologic features of increased lung markings reflecting elevated blood volume and an enlarged cardiac silhouette secondary to a more horizontal heart position

1 **Cardiac pulmonary edema**
   - Rheumatic heart disease and specifically mitral stenosis is the most common cause of heart disease in pregnancy, with failure developing in the 3rd trimester, labor or the early post-partum period
     - Other valvular lesions are less commonly identified
   - Tocolytic pulmonary edema refers to patients on β-agonist therapy who present in edema within 24 hours of treatment and improve rapidly after tocolytic agents are stopped (wedge pressures are variable and unclear whether the pulmonary edema is cardiac or non-cardiac)

- Peripartum cardiomyopathy is an idiopathic dilated cardiomyopathy, usually occurring in the last month of pregnancy or first 6 weeks post-partum, and diagnosed in the absence of an identifiable cause of heart disease
- Pre-eclampsia is manifest by hypertension, edema and proteinuria with seizures defining eclampsia
  - Pulmonary edema is seen in ~ 3% of pre-eclamptics, often in the post-partum period
- Other cardiac diseases including congenital, ischemic or infectious endocarditis

2 **Non-cardiac pulmonary edema**
- 'HELLP' syndrome, a variant of pre-eclampsia, consisting of **H**emolysis, **E**levated **L**iver enzymes and **L**ow **P**latelets, with ARDS, hemorrhage, acute renal failure and hepatic failure as complications
  - Usually presents between 20 and 30 weeks but can be seen post-partum
  - The combination of right upper quadrant pain, shoulder pain and elevated right hemidiaphragm should suggest a subcapsular hepatic hematoma
- Sepsis
- Massive hemorrhage
- Air embolism
- Amniotic fluid embolism
- Overwhelming pneumonia

3 **Pneumonia** both typical as well as atypical
- Decreased cell-mediated immunity can result in increased morbidity and mortality from influenza and varicella-zoster infections
- HIV infections should be ruled out

4 **Septic emboli** to the lungs post-partum from endometritis, infected wound site, pelvic abscess, septic thrombophlebitis

5 **Aspiration** of gastric contents (Mendelsohn's syndrome) post-partum

6 **Venous thromboembolism** reflecting stasis and hypercoagulable state, occurring five times as often compared to non-pregnant females

7 **Asthma** exacerbations are seen in ~⅓ of known asthmatics who are pregnant and is the most common pulmonary disease in pregnancy

8 **Lymphangioleiomyomatosis** (LAM) may have its initial presentation (or exacerbation) in pregnancy

9 **Ruptured hemidiaphragm** manifest as abdominal pains, nausea, vomiting, dyspnea with hypotension developing if bowel strangulation occurs
   - Radiologic features include a domed density resembling an elevated hemidiaphragm, intrathoracic bowel and contralateral mediastinal shift

10 **Pneumomediastinum**

11 **Esophageal rupture and acute mediastinitis**

12 **Pneumothorax**

13 **Urinothorax**

14 Metastatic **choriocarcinoma** usually follows a molar pregnancy and rarely a term pregnancy or abortion
   - Dyspnea can result from tumor emboli, pleural effusions, endobronchial disease or parenchymal metastases
   - Diagnosis is confirmed by finding an elevated HCG level in a non-pregnant patient

15 **Amniotic fluid emboli** result from amniotic fluid unpredictably entering the blood stream via tears in the uterine veins, with particulate materials in the fluid thought responsible for most of the clinical manifestations
   - Most common cause of maternal deaths during labor and the immediate post-partum period
   - Onset is acute, during labor or immediately postpartum and results in ~85% mortality, usually within the first hour, and clinical manifestations include

  - Respiratory – hypoxemia, non-cardiac pulmonary edema, acute pulmonary hypertension, respiratory failure
  - Cardiovascular – hypotension, LV dysfunction, right heart failure secondary to pulmonary hypertension
  - CNS – altered sensorium, seizures
  - Bleeding – uterine or other source secondary to DIC and fibrin depletion
  - Septic picture – infection of amniotic fluid which subsequently embolizes
- Diagnosis is usually made clinically plus ? analysis of blood from a PA catheter demonstrating amniotic fluid debris, although the latter may be present without clinical evidence of disease

16 **Pulmonary air embolism** results from air entering the uterine veins and going to the right heart where its mixing with blood results in fibrin plugs being formed which subsequently occlude the pulmonary circulation
- Clinical manifestations
  - Hypotension
  - Capillary leak pulmonary edema
  - 'Mill wheel' murmur (said to be pathognomonic)
  - Associated systemic air embolism involving the brain, heart or other organs
- Diagnostic criteria
  - High index of suspicion
  - Air in the right heart or pulmonary arteries on chest X-ray
  - Intracerebral air on brain CT

Pleural Effusion in Pregnancy

1 **Transudate**
- Congestive heart failure
- Urinothorax from hydronephrosis

2 **Exudate**
- Ruptured diaphragm
- Pulmonary infarct

- Parapneumonic
- Metastatic choriocarcinoma

3 **Hemothorax**
- Pulmonary infarct
- Metastatic choriocarcinoma

4 **Empyema**
- Parapneumonic

5 **Chyle**
- LAM

Fraser R.S., Muller N.L., Colman N., Paré P.D. (1999) *Diagnosis of Diseases of the Chest* 4th Edn., WB Saunders.

Baum, G.L., Crapo, J.D., Celli, B.R., Karlinsky, J.B. (eds) (1997) *Textbook of Pulmonary Diseases*, 6th edn.: Lippincott-Raven.

Fishman, A.P., Elias, J.A., Fishman, J.A., Grippi, M.A., Kaiser, L.R., Senior, R.N. (1998) *Fishman's Pulmonary Diseases and Disorders*, 3rd edn.: McGraw-Hill.

Lapinsky, L.S., Kruczynski, K., Slutsky, A. (1995) Critical care in the pregnant patient. *Am. J. Resp. Crit. Care Med.* **152**: 427–455.

Broder, S. Paré, P. (1996) Diagnosis and management of pulmonary embolism in pregnancy. *Can. Resp. J.* **3**: 187–192.

Zeldis, S. (1992) Dyspnea during pregnancy. Distinguishing cardiac from pulmonary causes. *Clinics in Chest Medicine* **13**: 567–589.

Demers, C., Ginsbery, J. (1992) Deep vein thrombosis and pulmonary embolism in pregnancy. *Clinics in Chest Medicine* **13**: 645–656.

Masson, R. (1992) Amniotic fluid embolism. *Clinics in Chest Medicine* **13**: 657–665.

Heffner, J., Sahn, S. (1992) Pleural disease in pregnancy. *Clinics in Chest Medicine* **13**: 667–678.

Rodrigues, J., Niederman, M. (1992) Pneumonia complicating pregnancy. *Clinics in Chest Medicine* **13**: 679–691.

60 Pulmonary Edema

ETIOLOGIES

Increased pulmonary venous pressures

1 LV dysfunction:
- **R** – rheumatic/valvular, restrictive myopathy
- **I** – ischemic, infectious, infiltrative
- **C** – congenital, congestive myopathy, cocaine or other drugs
- **H** – hypertrophic myopathy, hypertension, high output states

2 Mitral valve disease

3 Atrial disease
- Myxoma, ball-valve thrombus, cor triatriatum

4 Pulmonary venous disease
- Congenital – stenosis, anomalous pulmonary venous drainage
- Acquired – veno-occlusive disease, fibrosing mediastinitis, *in situ* thrombosis, tumor compression (benign/malignant)

Reduced capillary osmotic pressure
- Hypoalbuminemia secondary to renal disease, liver disease, malabsorption, large volumes of i.v. fluids

Increased capillary permeability
- Causes of ARDS

Neurogenic (combined hydrostatic and increased permeability)

- Head trauma, increased intracranial pressure, post-ictal

Miscellaneous

- Re-expansion
- High altitude
- Post-pneumonectomy
- Severe upper airway obstruction

RADIOLOGIC FEATURES

Interstitium

- Upper lobe redistribution of blood (size and number of upper lobe vessels is similar to those of the lower lobes)
- Loss of sharp definition of bronchovascular markings
- Thickening of interlobular septa (Kerley A + B lines)
- Perihilar and lower zone haziness
- Peribronchial cuffing
- Fibrosis and hemosiderosis from longstanding edema

Airspaces

- Acinar shadows, often confluent medially
- Bilateral and symmetric distribution, spreading from the medulla to the cortex
- Relative sparing of the lung periphery with a 'bat's wing' or 'butterfly' pattern

Pleura

- Thickening of interlobar fissures
- Localization of fluid in fissures, minor > major, resulting in a disappearing or 'phantom' tumor
- Effusions are bilateral > unilateral and when unilateral, usually right-sided

*UNILATERAL EDEMA – ETIOLOGY

1 Prolonged lateral decubitus position
2 Rapid thoracocentesis of fluid or air

3 Bronchial obstruction and a 'drowned lung'
4 Systemic to pulmonary artery shunts with congenital heart disease
5 Unilateral venous obstruction, e.g. veno-occlusive disease, mediastinitis, mediastinal or bronchogenic tumor, left atrial myxoma
6 Reduced or absent perfusion of the contralateral lung, e.g. Swyer-James, hypoplastic pulmonary artery, embolic disease, emphysema, fibrothorax
7 Severe mitral insufficiency with selective involvement of the RUL
   - Often difficult to distinguish from pneumonia

UPPER LOBE FLOW REDISTRIBUTION – DIFFERENTIAL DIAGNOSIS

1 Pulmonary venous hypertension
2 Pulmonary artery hypertension
3 Lower lobe pulmonary emboli
4 Supine position
5 Lower lobe parenchymal disease, e.g. emphysema
6 Left-to-right shunts
7 Hypervolemia

Fraser R.S., Muller N.L., Colman N., Paré P.D. (1999) *Diagnosis of Diseases of the Chest* 4th Edn., WB Saunders.
Felson, B. (1973) *Chest Roentgenology*.: W.B. Saunders.
Chapman, S., Nakielny, R. (1995) *Aids to Radiological Differential Diagnosis*, 3rd edn.: W.B. Saunders.

61 Pulmonary Hypertension

DEFINITION

- Normal systolic pressure <20 mmHg
- Normal diastolic pressure <10 mmHg
- Normal mean PAP 10–18 mmHg
- Pulmonary hypertension defined by mean PAP >25 mmHg

The **gold standard** for diagnosis of pulmonary hypertension is a right heart cath with direct measurement of

1. Pulmonary artery pressure
2. Pulmonary wedge pressure
3. Cardiac output
4. Response of the above to interventions, e.g. drugs, O_2, exercise
5. O_2 sats

Echocardiography (transesophageal > transthoracic) usually makes the initial diagnosis with data on

1. Estimation of pulmonary artery pressure
2. Dimensions, function and hypertrophy of RA, RV, LA, LV
3. Mitral valve stenosis/insufficiency
4. Pulmonary/tricuspid insufficiency
5. Shunts

ETIOLOGIES

1 **Pulmonary venous hypertension** (elevated wedge pressure)

Pulmonary venous obstruction
- Fibrosing mediastinitis/tumor
- Anomalous pulmonary venous drainage
- Congenital stenosis of pulmonary veins
- Veno-occlusive disease (wedge may be normal)
- Pulmonary capillary hemangiomatosis (wedge may be normal)
- *In situ* thrombosis

Left atrial disease
- Left atrial myxoma
- Cor triatriatum
- Ball valve thrombus

Mitral valve disease
- Stenosis/insufficiency

LV dysfunction

2 **Hyperkinetic** (normal wedge pressure)

Atrial
- Atrial septal defect (ASD)
- Anomalous pulmonary venous drainage
- Transposition of the great vessels with ASD

Ventricular
- Ventricular septal defect (VSD)

Aortic
- Patent ductus arteriosus (PDA)
- Aorticopulmonary window
- Truncus arteriosus
- Post-surgical shunts, e.g. Blalock-Taussig (subclavian artery to pulmonary artery)

3 **Obstructive** (normal wedge pressure) with decreased cross-sectional area of the pulmonary vascular tree

Functional, i.e. vasoconstriction

- Cocaine
- Hypoxemia of pulmonary, e.g. COPD, ILD, or extra-pulmonary origin, e.g. OSA altitude, neuromuscular diseases (hypoxemia may only be present at night or on exertion in some patients)

Structural

- Intralumenal, e.g. *in situ* thrombosis, emboli (thromboemboli, talc, fat amniotic fluid, tumor, parasites), myeloid metaplasia, intravascular lymphomatosis
- Intramural, e.g. vasculitis (Takayasu's, Behcet's), collagen vascular diseases (SLE, RA, scleroderma, CREST syndrome), sarcoid, amyloid, pulmonary artery stenosis(es), pulmonary artery sarcoma
- Extramural, e.g. mediastinal fibrosis/tumor

Obliterative

- Emphysema
- Post-lung resection

Combined

- ILD
- HIV, cirrhosis, drugs

4 **Idiopathic** or **primary** (normal wedge pressure)

DIAGNOSTIC WORK-UP

1 **History and physical**

Cardiorespiratory symptoms of dyspnea, anginal chest pains and syncope on exertion may be accompanied by

- History of congenital or acquired cardiac disease
- Evidence of extravascular pulmonary disease involving the airways, parenchyma, pleura, chest wall or mediastinum
- Drug intake by ingestion or illegal injection
- Embolic source, central or peripheral

- Family history of pulmonary hypertension
- Systemic disease which can cause pulmonary artery hypertension, e.g. HIV, liver disease, collagen disease, hematologic disorder
- Physical findings of pulmonary artery hypertension, RV hypertrophy and right heart failure

Cardiac

- RV heave
- Increased P_2
- Right-sided S_3 or S_4
- Pansystolic murmur of TI or diastolic murmur of PI
- Associated findings can include typical systolic murmur of a VSD, fixed split S_2 of ASD, murmurs of MS/MI

Extracardiac

- Prominent 'A' wave with RVH
- Elevated JVP with prominent 'V' waves
- Congestive hepatomegaly (+/− pulsatile)
- Congestive splenomegaly
- Ascites
- Peripheral edema
- Cyanosis

2 **Chest X-ray/CT abnormalities**

X-rays may be normal early in the disease but typical findings are enlargement of the main pulmonary artery and hilar vessels with pruning of the peripheral arterial tree

- With time the above abnormalities increase, in addition to the development of right heart enlargement and calcifications of the pulmonary artery
- The following may provide clues to a specific diagnosis
  - *Airways disease*
    - Hyperinflation with oligemia and bullae, indicating emphysema
  - *Parenchymal disease*
    - Diffuse interstitial disease
    - Conglomerate masses of sarcoid, silicosis, talcosis, CWP

- *Pleural disease*
  - Fibrothoraces
  - Transudative effusions secondary to pulmonary venous hypertension, cirrhosis with ascites and pulmonary hypertension, amyloid infiltration of the heart and pulmonary arteries
  - Exudative effusions secondary to collagen diseases, e.g. RA, SLE, tumor emboli and metastatic pleural disease, thromboemboli with infarction
  - Chylous effusions from LAM
- *Mediastinal disease* with fibrosis, neoplastic compression or obstruction of the pulmonary arterial or venous tree
- *Chest wall disease* in severe kyphoscoliosis or thoracoplasty with secondary hypoxemia and hypercapnia
- *Pleonemia* is seen with left to right shunts and characterized by increased caliber of the pulmonary arteries with visualization of vessels in the peripheral 2 cm of lung where they are not usually seen
  - With increased resistance and shunt reversal, the hypervascularity disappears and oligemia develops
- *Oligemia* is seen with
  - Primary pulmonary hypertension
  - Disorders causing obstruction of the pulmonary arterial tree
  - Hyperkinetic cause with shunt reversal
- Signs of *pulmonary venous hypertension*
  - Increased upper lobe vasculature
  - Kerley B lines
  - Interstitial edema/fibrosis
  - Airspace edema
  - Hemosiderosis
  - Ossifications (mitral stenosis)
  - Pleural effusions

- *Enlarged left atrium/left ventricle*
- *Perihilar mass, pulmonary metastases* or *mediastinal lymphadenopathy* from pulmonary artery sarcoma or metastatic disease with tumor emboli

3 **ABGs**

- Hypoxemia occurs on exertion and may occur at rest in pulmonary hypertension but hypercapnia should suggest
  - Airways disease
    - Upper, e.g. obstructive sleep apnea
    - Lower, e.g. COPD, bronchiolitis
  - Neuro-musculo-skeletal disorders

4 **R/O pulmonary venous hypertension** – elevated wedge pressure

- *Pulmonary venous obstruction* may be secondary to
  - Congenital stenosis of pulmonary veins
  - Bronchogenic carcinoma
  - Sclerosing mediastinitis
  - Pulmonary veno-occlusive disease

  A complication of pulmonary vein obstruction is pulmonary venous infarction, manifest clinically by cough, dyspnea and hemoptysis which may be acute, gradual or paroxysmal in presentation
  - LA and LV pressures are normal
  - Diagnosis made by infusion CT or pulmonary angiography with delayed venous phase when the large veins are involved
- *Left atrial disease* secondary to atrial myxoma, ball-valve thrombus or cor triatriatum
- *Mitral valve disease* – stenosis or insufficiency
- *Left ventricular failure*

5 **R/O shunt** – normal wedge pressure

- Echocardiography with transesophageal echo is able to diagnose some cases of ASD or patent ductus not seen on transthoracic echo
  - Exercise echocardiography can diagnose a subset of

patients with dyspnea on exertion where PAH is found only on exertion
- Cardiovascular MRI may detect and quantify shunts
- Angiogram (cardiac cath)
- Step-up of O_2 sats in the right heart
- Step-down of O_2 sats in the left heart with shunt reversal

6 **R/O pulmonary vascular obstruction** (functional, structural, obliterative) – normal wedge pressure
   - PFTs, COPD being the commonest cause of secondary pulmonary hypertension, PA pressure correlating with the extent of hypoxemia rather than the severity of airways obstruction, e.g. blue bloaters > pink puffers
   - ABGs with O_2 sats measured while awake, asleep, and with exercise
   - Sleep study
   - Spiral CT
   - V/Q scan
   - Cytology of wedged blood
   - Transbroncial biospy, e.g. talc granulomas, tumor emboli
   - Arch aortography, e.g. Takayasu's arteritis
   - Pulmonary angiography/angioscopy to visualize the central and peripheral vessels plus measure pressure gradients
   - Work-up for vasculitis/collagen vascular diseases, e.g. SLE, RA, scleroderma, mixed connective tissue disease, polymyositis
   - LFTs
   - Work-up for an occult neoplasm and resultant tumor emboli, including β-HCG level

CHRONIC THROMBOEMBOLIC PULMONARY HYPERTENSION

Definition: Rare sequela of acute pulmonary emboli, of unknown etiology, usually diagnosed after the development of significant pulmonary hypertension

- An initial acute embolic event may or may not have been diagnosed, followed over months to years by symptoms of increasing dyspnea and progressive pulmonary hypertension (often in the absence of documented recurrent acute embolic episodes)
- Associated clinical features of pulmonary hypertension and right heart failure develop, with flow murmurs described over the lung fields

Diagnostically, echocardiography often initially documents pulmonary artery hypertension, with other investigations

- Chest X-rays range from normal to findings of PAH
- PFTs may be normal or show a reduced DLCO
- PaO_2 varies from normal to low
- V/Q scan findings of segmental or larger perfusion defects (underestimates central obstruction)
- CT demonstration of thromboembolic material in central pulmonary vessels
- *Pulmonary angiography/angioscopy to document the presence, extent and location of disease as well as surgical accessibility

7 After the above investigations, there is a group of patients with **unexplained pulmonary hypertension** who require open lung biopsy for definitive diagnosis
   - Pulmonary veno-occlusive disease
   - Primary pulmonary hypertension
   - Pulmonary capillary hemangiomatosis

PULMONARY VENO-OCCLUSIVE DISEASE (VOD)

Definition: Disease of unknown etiology characterized pathologically by intimal fibrosis of the pulmonary veins and venules with disease also seen in the pulmonary arteries (medial hypertrophy, thrombosis) and lung parenchyma (hemorrhage, fibrosis)

- The pathologic diagnosis can be confused with UIP as well as idiopathic pulmonary hemosiderosis
- VOD can occur in isolation but has been described in association with multiple and diverse disorders

Clinically, the disease should be suspected when patients present with features of

- Undiagnosed pulmonary hypertension and/or
- Atypical pulmonary edema

Hemodynamic abnormalities include elevated pulmonary artery pressures with a normal or elevated wedge pressure

Chest X-ray findings

1 Signs of pulmonary artery hypertension
2 Kerley B lines and interstitial edema
3 Absence of vascular redistribution or an enlarged left atrium

PRIMARY PULMONARY HYPERTENSION (PPH)

Definition: Idiopathic disorder diagnosed only after a negative work-up for left-sided cardiac valvular disease, congenital or acquired myocardial disease, thromboembolic disease, connective tissue disease, clinically important respiratory disease, or other identifiable causes of pulmonary hypertension

- Hemodynamically, there is a normal wedge pressure and an elevated mean pulmonary artery pressure >25 mmHg at rest or >30 mmHg with exercise
- The elevated pulmonary vascular resistance is due to the combination of vasoconstriction, *in situ* thrombosis and wall remodelling, ultimately leading to right ventricular failure
- Biopsy reveals pulmonary arteriopathy with plexiform lesions
- Although a cause and effect relationship is lacking, pulmonary hypertension with similar pathology is seen with

- Familial pulmonary hypertension
- Portal hypertension with cirrhosis
- HIV
- Drugs, including cocaine inhalation, appetite suppressants, e.g. aminorex, amphetamines, fenfluramine and 'bush tea'
- Collagen diseases, e.g. rheumatoid arthritis, systemic lupus, scleroderma, Sjogren's, dermato/polymyositis, mixed connective tissue disease

Clinically, PPH can be sporadic or familial with a mean age of 36 years and a female predominance

- The non-specific symptoms of fatigue, dyspnea, chest pains, syncope and Raynaud's (approximately 10%), result in a mean length of time of two years before the diagnosis is established
- Signs are those of pulmonary hypertension eventually leading to right heart failure
- Oral contraceptives and pregnancy can exacerbate the pulmonary hypertension
- The disease is often progressive with death in a few years, although exceptions are described
- Predictors of survival include
  - Hemodynamic characteristics
  - Exercise tolerance in a 6 minute walk
  - Functional class
  - Anticoagulant therapy
  - Response to vasodilators
- Historically the median survival after diagnosis was 2.5 years but this has improved with recent therapies
- Mortality is usually related to progressive right heart failure or sudden death

Bloods are non-specific with low titer ⊕ ANA in approximately 30% of patients

- Hypoxemia is seen at rest and accentuated with exercise

PFTs vary from normal to an isolated reduction in DCO

Chest X-rays reveal right ventricular enlargement, prominence of the main PA, enlarged hilar arteries tapering rapidly, as well as diffuse oligemia

- X-rays are normal in ~5% of cases

V/Q scans vary from normal to diffuse, patchy, non-segmental perfusion defects with normal ventilation

Pulmonary angiography may be required to document or exclude thromboembolic disease when one or more segmental defects is noted

ECGs reflect right atrial and ventricular enlargement with right-axis deviation, tall peaked P waves, tall anterior R waves, and ST depression +/– T wave inversion anteriorly

Echocardiography can estimate pulmonary artery pressures and rule out congenital, valvular or myocardial disease

- Findings include RV enlargement with paradoxical septal motion as well as RA enlargement with pulmonary and tricuspid regurgitation

Cardiac catheterization reveals an elevated pulmonary artery pressure, increased pulmonary resistance, normal wedge pressure and reduced cardiac output

- In addition to confirmation of the diagnosis, cath excludes other diseases, establishes the severity of disease and prognosis

PULMONARY CAPILLARY HEMANGIOMATOSIS

Definition: Extremely rare disorder characterized by the proliferation of capillary-like channels confined to the lungs ? low grade vascular neoplasm

- Involvement is seen in many structures including the interlobular septae, alveolar walls, pleura, bronchi, pulmonary arteries and veins, the latter thought to be responsible for the pulmonary hypertension

- Clinically, hemoptysis, dyspnea and unexplained pulmonary hypertension are presenting complaints with the diagnosis made on biopsy, the differential including Kaposi's sarcoma and veno-occlusive disease
- Most patients are 20 to 40 years of age and prognosis is poor with patients usually dying within a few years of diagnosis
- Radiologic findings include an interstitial reticulonodular pattern as well as enlarged pulmonary arteries
- Hemodynamically, the pulmonary hypertension is accompanied by normal wedge pressures

Fraser R.S., Muller N.L., Colman N., Paré P.D. (1999) *Diagnosis of Diseases of the Chest* 4th Edn., WB Saunders.

Naidich, D.P., Zerhouni, E.A., Siegelman, S.S. (1998) *Computed Tomography and Magnetic Resonance of the Thorax*, 3rd edn. New York: Raven Press.

Thurlbeck, W., Churg, A. (eds) (1995) *Pathology of the Lung*, 2nd edn.: Thieme Medical Publishers.

Rubin, L. (1997) *Primary pulmonary hypertension. NEJM* **336**: 111–117.

62 Pulmonary-renal Syndromes – Goodpasture's

Definition: Pulmonary-renal syndrome is the combination of glomerulonephritis and diffuse alveolar hemorrhage

- Glomerulonephritis is suspected clinically from an active urine sediment and may be accompanied by a systemic vasculitis, the etiologies including
  - Systemic vasculitis (50%), e.g. Wegener's, Churg-Strauss, microscopic polyarteritis
  - SLE
  - Goodpasture's syndrome (20%)
  - Other causes of glomerulonephritis e.g. post-streptococcal

Goodpasture's Syndrome (GS)

GS, the prototypical pulmonary-renal syndrome, is an antibody-mediated disease due to an anti-glomerular basement membrane (AGBM) antibody that cross-reacts with alveolar basement membrane and glomerular basement membrane

Clinically, it is a disease of unknown etiology with the majority of cases being sporadic

- Ingestion of penicillamine or exposure to volatile hydrocarbon solvents has been implicated in some cases
- Typically seen in young adults with a male predominance of 3–9 times that of females
- Patients generally present with hemoptysis which may be accompanied by dyspnea and hematuria
- The hemoptysis varies from blood-streaked sputum to massive bleeding, although extensive intrapulmonary hemorrhage may occur without overt hemoptysis

- Repeated bleeding can lead to interstitial fibrosis with resultant pulmonary hypertension and cor pulmonale
- Pulmonary manifestations commonly precede renal disease by months but acute oliguric renal failure can develop
- 20–40% of patients will have isolated renal disease while <10% will have only lung involvement
- Extrapulmonary extrarenal disease is rare and should suggest another diagnosis
- The prognosis of untreated disease is poor with death usually from renal failure

Lab findings reveal acute renal failure, an active urine sediment with hematuria, proteinuria and casts, as well as an iron deficiency anemia from alveolar hemorrhage

- Urinalysis is rarely normal with renal disease only documented on biopsy
- Presence of serum AGBM antibodies an the absence of ANCA, ANA and anti-double-stranded DNA antibodies
- Detection of serum AGBM antibody by indirect immunofluorescence can establish the diagnosis rapidly but false negatives can be seen in up to 40% of patients, more sensitive serum assays being an ELISA or radioimmunoassay
- Circulating ANCA is described in up to 30% of patients with GS during the course of their illness reflecting a mixed clinical syndrome

Radiologic features

1. Patchy fluffy airspace disease resembling pulmonary edema or pneumonia
2. Distribution is bilateral more often than unilateral, symmetric or asymmetric
3. Resolution of the above results in an interstitial pattern which can resolve completely in 1–2 weeks
4. Repeated bleeding can result in interstitial fibrosis
5. Renal failure can result in the superimposed findings of uremia (see p. 717)

Diagnostic features

1 Necrotizing glomerulonephritis without vasculitis on light microscopy, as well as linear glomerular staining for immunoglobulin (usually IgG) or complement on immunofluorescence
   - Antibodies may not be detected in lung tissue but only seen on renal biopsy
2 Features of diffuse alveolar hemorrhage (see p. 28)
3 AGBM antibodies in the blood
4 Detection of AGBM antibodies by linear immunofluorescence on lung tissue obtained by transbronchial or open biopsy

Other Pumonary-renal Disorders

Although not classified as pulmonary-renal syndromes, several clinical conditions can present with the combination of

Pulmonary disease	+	Renal disease
• Abnormal x-rays		• ↑ BUN/creatinine
• Pulmonary symptoms		• Abnormal urinalysis
• Abnormal lung function		• Gross or microscopic pathology

Disease **categories** include

A. *Primary renal disease*
- Acute, e.g. renal vein thrombosis → pulmonary emboli
- Chronic, e.g. renal cell carcinoma → lung metastases

B. *Primary pulmonary disease*
- Acute, e.g. Streptococcal pneumonia → glomerulonephritis
- Chronic, e.g. bronchogenic cancer → renal metastases

C. *Concurrent renal and pulmonary disease*
- Acute, e.g. tuberculosis
- Chronic, e.g. sarcoid

Pulmonary disease	**Renal disease**
Granulomatous diseases	
• Sarcoid	• Interstitial nephritis, nephrocalcinosis, renal stones
• Tuberculosis	• Renal tuberculosis
Neoplasms	
• Lymphoma	• Nephrotic syndrome
• Bronchogenic carcinoma	• Renal metastases glomerulonephritis, hypercalcemia, hyperuricemia
• Pulmonary metastases	• From renal cell carcinoma
• Lymphomatoid granulomatosis	• Concurrent renal disease
Infections	
• Acute pneumonia	• Glomerulonephritis or dissemination to kidneys
• Chronic infections	• Amyloidosis of kidneys
Amyloid	• Nephrotic syndrome
Calcinosis	• Secondary to renal failure and secondary hyperparathyroidism
Pulmonary edema	• And pre-renal failure secondary to CHF • Secondary to acute glomerulonephritis or acute renal failure with hypervolemia
Vasculitis/collagen vascular disease	• Glomerulonephritis, arteritis
Alveolar hemorrhage syndromes	• Goodpasture's, others (see p. 708)
Pulmonary emboli	• Secondary to nephrotic syndrome • Paradoxical renal emboli
Tumor emboli	• Secondary to renal cell carcinoma
Septic emboli – right-sided endocarditis	• Secondary glomerulonephritis
Pulmonary effects of uremia	• End-stage kidney disease

Table 62.1

Fraser R.S., Muller N.L., Colman N., Paré P.D. (1999) *Diagnosis of Diseases of the Chest* 4th Edn., WB Saunders.

Baum, G.L., Crapo, J.D., Celli, B.R., Karlinsky, J.B. (eds) (1997) *Textbook of Pulmonary Diseases*, 6th edn.: Lippincott-Raven.

Fishman, A.P., Elias, J.A., Fishman, J.A., Grippi, M.A., Kaiser, L.R., Senior, R.N. (1998) *Fishman's Pulmonary Diseases and Disorders*, 3rd edn.: McGraw-Hill.

Randall Young, K. Jr. (1989) Pulmonary-renal syndromes. *Clinics in Chest Medicine* **10**: 655–675.

Ball, J., Randall Young, K. (1998) Pulmonary manifestations of Goodpasture's syndrome. *Clinics in Chest Medicine* **19**: 777–791.

63 Radiation-induced Lung Disease

Radiation pneumonitis is seen with radiation directed at the lungs, chest wall or mediastinum with the pulmonary response affected by

- Radiation dose
- Volume of lung exposed
- Time course of radiation
- Associated chemotherapy
- Steroid withdrawal

Clinical spectrum includes

1. Radiologic changes from radiation (seen in almost all patients) in the absence of symptoms
2. Non-specific features of cough, dyspnea and fever seen in approximately 10% of cases
3. Rarely a fulminating course with severe hypoxemia, cyanosis and acute cor pulmonale

- Radiation pneumonitis can resolve completely, but usually progresses to a variable degree of fibrosis, which itself can be asymptomatic or present with dyspnea and respiratory failure

Nuclear studies reveal a positive gallium scan as well as reduced perfusion on V/Q scanning

PFTs show a restrictive picture usually beginning about 2 months post-radiation and often normalizing at about 8 months, although changes can be severe and prolonged

Radiologic features of **radiation pneumonitis** are rarely seen immediately following therapy and uncommon for 1–4 weeks, usually appearing at 6–8 weeks and most marked at 3–4 months

1 Loss of sharp definition of the bronchovascular markings which are the earliest and may be the only changes
2 Progression to airspace consolidation and air bronchograms within the radiation ports, with sharp linear borders not conforming to segments or fissures
3 Volume loss with mediastinal shift and diaphragm elevation
4 Pleural effusion or thickening occurring with co-existing radiation pneumonitis and often resolving completely

Uncommonly seen:

5 Obstructive atelectasis when an underlying endobronchial lesion is present
6 Hyperlucent lung ? secondary to obliterative vasculitis
7 Changes outside the radiation port

- The above changes usually peak 3–4 months post-radiotherapy with either complete resolution but more often a gradual merging into radiation fibrosis
- CT changes may antedate chest X-ray abnormalities with 'ground glass' opacities or consolidation being extensive while chest X-rays are still normal

Radiologic features of **radiation fibrosis** are seen by 3–4 months and stabilize at 9–12 months following radiotherapy

1 Volume loss with elevation of the hemidiaphragm, hila or minor fissure and medial retraction of the hilar vessels
2 Airless opacity sharply demarcated from normal lung
3 Bronchiectasis
4 Pleural thickening, calcified pleural plaques or encapsulated pleural fluid

Other changes post-radiation include

5 Thymic cysts
6 Calcified nodes post-radiation for Hodgkin's disease
7 Premature atherosclerosis with calcification of the coronaries, great vessels and congestive cardiomyopathy
8 Malignant mesothelioma
9 Chest wall sarcomas, e.g. fibrosarcoma, osteogenic

sarcoma, developing 5–30 years post-radiotherapy and may mimic recurrent lung cancer

10 BOOP is rarely seen following radiation for breast cancer only, beginning within the radiation field and then extending outwards to the ipsilateral and contralateral lung
11 Radiation esophagitis with dysphagia and aspiration
12 Pericardial effusion/calcifications
13 Bronchopleural fistula

Post-radiation Changes – Differential Diagnosis

1 Recurrent lung tumor manifest by
   - Obliteration of the sharp and linear margins of radiation pneumonitis
   - An enlarging mass developing later than 4 months post-radiation, the time when the radiologic changes have usually peaked
   - Mass lesion with absence of air bronchograms on CT
   - Associated lymphadenopathy
2 Obstructive pneumonitis
3 Second lung cancer following cure of a small cell or non-small cell tumor
4 Superimposed infection, e.g. bacterial, tuberculosis, subacute necrotizing pulmonary aspergillosis
5 Localized pulmonary edema from pulmonary venous obstruction secondary to tumor or mediastinitis
6 Generalized pulmonary edema from radiation myocarditis
7 Malignant mesothelioma developing post-radiotherapy
8 Chest wall sarcoma post-radiotherapy
9 Lymphangitic carcinoma, usually most marked at the lung bases and associated with Kerley B lines
10 Chemotherapy-induced lung disease, typically bilateral with lower lobe predominance
11 Unrelated disease

Fraser R.S., Muller N.L., Colman N., Paré P.D. (1999) *Diagnosis of Diseases of the Chest* 4th Edn., WB Saunders.

Naidich, D.P., Zerhouni, E.A., Siegelman, S.S. (1998) *Computed Tomography and Magnetic Resonance of the Thorax*, 3rd edn. New York: Raven Press.

Moss, A., Gamsu, Genant (1992) Thorax and neck. In: *Computed Tomography of the Body with Magnetic Resonance Imaging.* 2nd edn, vol. 1.: W.B. Saunders.

Movsas, B., Raffin, T., Epstein, A. *et al.* (1997) Pulmonary radiation injury. *Chest* **111**: 1061–1076.

Libshitz, H.I. (1993) Radiation changes in the lung. S*emin. Roent.* **28**: 303–320.

64 Renal Diseases – Pulmonary Manifestations

UREMIA – PULMONARY COMPLICATIONS

Vascular

1 **Thrombo-emboli** in nephrotic syndrome with associated renal vein thrombosis
2 **Hypoxemia** with hemodialysis (etiology unclear)
3 **Hypercapnia** with acute or intermittent peritoneal dialysis due to the large carbohydrate load and increased CO_2 production
4 **Alveolar hemorrhage syndrome** secondary to uremia
5 **Pulmonary edema** can be secondary to
   - Hypervolemia
   - Increased capillary permeability
   - Hypoalbumenia
   - Cardiac dysfunction from anemia, hypertension, AV shunts, uremic cardiomyopathy
   - Occurrence is unpredictable and does not correlate with the degree of azotemia
   - Distribution may be the 'classic' butterfly pattern with bilateral symmetric densities extending from the hila with sparing of the apices and lung periphery, to an asymmetric distribution

Parenchyma

1 **Pulmonary calcinosis** is frequently asymptomatic although it can present with non-specific respiratory symptoms progressing to respiratory failure
   - Described most often in patients on chronic hemodialysis, less often with peritoneal dialysis and uncommonly in chronic renal failure
   - X-rays reveal focal or generalized infiltrates which can mimic pulmonary edema, pneumonia, or tuberculosis when seen in the lung apices
   - PFTs vary from normal to restrictive disease and the diagnosis can be made with
     - Density measurements on CT scan
     - Pyrophosphate bone scan showing pulmonary uptake

2 **Tuberculosis**

3 **Pneumonia**

4 **Bibasilar atelectasis** with peritoneal dialysis

Pleura

1 **Transudative** effusions from CHF, hypervolemia, nephrotic syndrome, peritoneal dialysis

2 **Uremic pleuritis**, an exudative effusion unrelated to the absolute values of the BUN or creatinine
   - Seen in uremia or in patients on dialysis where the presentation varies from dyspnea and pleuritic pain to an asymptomatic finding, pleural +/– pericardial rubs often being heard
   - The effusions are unilateral or bilateral and may be large and bloody and have a lymphocytic predominance
   - They usually resolve spontaneously in weeks but may result in a fibrothorax
   - Uremic effusion is a diagnosis of exclusion with the differential including pulmonary emboli, uremic pericarditis, pneumonia with effusion, tuberculous pleurisy

3 **Urinothorax** where an obstructive uropathy (stones, malignancy, valves, pregnancy) can result in urine extrava-

sation from the urinary tract, with extension into the retroperitoneum and pleural space

- The effusion is a transudate with a fluid creatinine greater than the serum level

Restrictive PFTs
May reflect pulmonary edema, pleural effusions, calcinosis, uremic myopathy or phrenic neuropathy

ACUTE RENAL FAILURE – LUNG DISEASE

Acute Glomurelonephritis

1. **Goodpasture's syndrome**
2. **Systemic lupus erythematosus**
3. **Vasculitis**, e.g. Wegener's granulomatosis, microscopic polyarteritis
4. **Secondary to pneumonia**
5. **Pulmonary emboli** complicating nephrotic syndrome from minimal change, focal segmental, membranous, membranoproliferative or idiopathic rapidly progressive glomerulonephritis
6. **Pulmonary edema** secondary to hypervolemia
7. **Right-sided SBE** resulting in a lung abscess and secondary glomerulonephritis

Acute Interstitial Nephritis

Secondary to **antibiotic** use in pneumonia

Acute Tubular Necrosis

Secondary to systemic **hypotension** from pneumonia with sepsis, tension pneumothorax, massive pulmonary embolus, cardiac failure

RENAL CELL CARCINOMA

Lungs are a common site of metastases via the hematogenous or lymphatic routes

- There are many case reports of spontaneous regression of metastases but seen in <1% of cases

Airways

- Endobronchial metastases

Mediastinum

- Hilar/mediastinal lymphadenopathy including bilateral hilar adenopathy

Pleura

- Malignant effusions
- Pleural nodules or masses

Parenchyma

- *Single or multiple nodules
- Lymphangitic cancer

Vasculature

- Tumor emboli

RENAL TRANSPLANT – PULMONARY COMPLICATIONS

1 **Post-transplant malignancy**
   - *Lymphoma*, usually non-Hodgkin's, with a high incidence of extranodal disease and dissemination
   - *Kaposi's sarcoma* has an incidence 400 times that of the general population
     – Visceral involvement is much more common than lung disease whose radiologic features are similar to those of HIV patients
     – Neoplastic disease can disappear following discontinuation of immunosuppression
- Occult *renal cell carcinoma* is seen in ~6% of chronically dialyzed patients at autopsy

2 **Pneumonia**
   - The time interval post-transplant as well as the degree of immunosuppression will determine the likelihood of specific infections

- Bacterial: acute community-acquired organisms including legionella, mycobacteria, nocardia
- Viral: CMV (most common infection post-transplant)
- Fungal: most often aspergillus but candida, cryptococcus, histoplasma and coccidioides are also described; pneumocystis

3 **Mediastinal lipomatosis** secondary to steroids

Fraser R.S., Muller N.L., Colman N., Paré P.D. (1999) *Diagnosis of Diseases of the Chest* 4th Edn., WB Saunders.
Baum, G.L., Crapo, J.D., Celli, B.R., Karlinsky, J.B. (eds) (1997) *Textbook of Pulmonary Diseases*, 6th edn.: Lippincott-Raven.
Fishman, A.P., Elias, J.A., Fishman, J.A., Grippi, M.A., Kaiser, L.R., Senior, R.N. (1998) *Fishman's Pulmonary Diseases and Disorders*, 3rd edn.: McGraw-Hill.

65 Sarcoid

GENERAL FEATURES

Definition: A systemic disorder of unknown etiology and characterized by non-caseating granulomas

There are no pathognomonic findings and diagnostic criteria include

1 Compatible clinical history, pulmonary or extrapulmonary
2 Compatible chest X-ray
3 Non-caseating granulomas on biopsy (see Biopsy of Granulomas, p. 67)
   - These consist of central mononuclear phagocytes, i.e. epithelioid cells and giant cells (occasionally containing inclusions, e.g. asteroid bodies, Schaumann bodies) and lymphocytes (CD4) as well as a peripheral rim of fibroblasts and lymphocytes (CD8)
   - Evolution of granulomas include coagulative necrosis centrally as well as fibrosis that begins peripherally, with hyalinization in the chronic stage
   - Transbronchial biopsy is recommended first but bronchial mucosal biopsy, nodes (intrathoracic or extrathoracic), skin or other tissue may suffice
4 Exclusion of specific diseases which can give similar findings, e.g. tuberculosis, fungi, beryllium

5 In the absence of tissue confirmation, non-diagnostic but suggestive tests include
   - CD4/CD8 ratio >3.5 on BAL
   - Panda pattern/lambda pattern on total body gallium scan

Epidemiologic features

1 Age at presentation is usually in adults under 40, with a peak at 20–29
   - A second peak is seen in females >50 in Japan and Scandinavian countries

2 Seen in all races with the highest incidence in U.S. blacks, Danes and Swedes
   - Rarely reported from Spain, Portugal, India, South America, Saudi Arabia
   - Whites are often asymptomatic with blacks having more severe disease

3 Several reports of familial clustering with a 19% incidence in black families and 5% in white families in the United States

Clinical presentation varies with racial background, site of organ involvement and frequency of routine screening chest X-rays in the community, the **most common** being

1 Asymptomatic radiologic abnormality, seen in up to 50% of cases

2 Pulmonary symptoms of dyspnea, cough, and chest pains are presenting features in about ⅓ of cases, with the frequency in the four stages being
   - Stage 1 – 5%
   - Stage 2 – 40%
   - Stage 3 – 75%
   - Stage 4 – 100%

3 Systemic complaints of fevers, night sweats, malaise and weight loss are present in about 40% of patients

4 Skin lesions are presenting features in 10–25%

5 Eye lesions are seen in 10–20% of patients initially

Immunologic abnormalities are seen systemically, e.g. cutaneous anergy, circulating immune complexes, as well as intrapulmonary

- Early reaction features activitated T cells (CD4 > CD8) and macrophages, both groups releasing a wide range of cytokines which result in increasing number of inflammatory cells from the peripheral blood and *in situ* proliferation, leading to granuloma formation
- Unclear why the course of lung disease is so variable in different patients

PFTs are difficult to predict from chest X-ray stage although the majority of patients with stage I disease will have normal or mild restrictive disease whereas most patients with stage III or IV disease have the most severe restrictive +/– obstructive abnormalities

- Airways obstruction may be due to endobronchial disease, peribronchial disease, bronchostenosis or bronchiectasis, usually with stage III or IV disease

Patient assessment after the diagnosis is established should include

1. Extent of lung involvement on X-ray and PFTs
2. Indicators of disease 'activity' with a guess as to prognosis
3. Requirement for therapy
4. Presence of extrapulmonary disease, i.e. CBC, calcium, LFTs, renal function/urinalysis, ECG, ophthalmology consult
5. Tuberculin status

CHEST X-RAY STAGING

Stage 0 – **Normal chest X-rays** with extrathoracic disease seen in ~5% of patients

Stage I – **Lymphadenopathy and normal lung parenchyma** seen in ~50% of patients

- Bilateral hilar, paratracheal and tracheobronchial nodes are typical, with unilateral adenopathy in approximately 5% of cases
  - Aortopulmonary nodes are seen in ~50% of cases and subcarinal adenopathy in ~20%
- Nodes can persist for years, enlarge or regress
- Nodes can calcify
- Nodes can compress adjacent structures
  - SVC → SVC syndrome
  - Pulmonary artery compression → oligemia
  - Pulmonary venous obstruction → pulmonary edema
  - Left innominate vein obstruction
  - Tracheal narrowing
  - Bronchial narrowing with atelectasis

Stage II – **Parenchymal disease with adenopathy** is seen in 15–30% of patients

- Distribution of parenchymal disease is typically bilateral symmetric and central but may be
  - Asymmetric
  - Peripheral in distribution simulating eosinophilic pneumonia
  - Predominantly upper lobe simulating post primary tuberculosis
- The pattern of parenchymal disease is usually interstitial and nodular or reticulonodular, less commonly reticular but can be
  - Acinar or airspace consolidation, discrete or confluent; air bronchograms may be present
  - Miliary pattern resembling miliary tuberculosis with nodules usually <3 mm (most often upper-middle lobe)
  - Nodular sarcoid/necrotizing sarcoid granulomatosis with nodules >1 cm and resem-

bling metastases (often accompanied by small nodules)

- Additional findings
  - Pleural effusions rare (approximately 2%)
  - Airways distension, narrowing or obstruction uncommon

Stage III – **Parenchymal disease** is seen in 10–15% of patients

- Changes are similar to those of Stage II without the associated lymphadenopathy

Stage IV – **Pulmonary fibrosis** is seen in <20% of patients

- Upper lobe predominance with associated volume loss
- Parenchymal infiltrates become coarse and coalesce with the findings of fibrosis – honeycombing, traction bronchiectasis, fibrotic 'masses' and linear bands
- Bullae, areas of emphysema and 'cavitary' lesions
- Additional findings include
  - Cardiovascular changes of cor pulmonale and pulmonary hypertension
    - — Seen in a few percent of sarcoid patients
    - — Usually associated with extensive fibrosis
    - — Rarely due to extrinsic compression of the pulmonary arteries or granulomatous inflammation of the vessel walls
  - Pleural thickening (uncommon)
  - Aspergillomas can develop in the cystic spaces (bullae or cystic bronchiectasis) of patients with Stage III and IV disease, usually upper lobe in distribution
    - — Pleural thickening developing adjacent to a cystic space may precede the radiologic appearance of the mycetoma
  - Airways distension, narrowing or obstruction

HRCT

Indications for HRCT include

1. Normal chest X-ray but clinical suspicion of disease
2. Atypical chest X-ray findings
3. Assessment of complications

HRCT features include

1. Airspace consolidation which is often peribronchial with air bronchograms
   - Less commonly there is peripheral consolidation resembling eosinophilic pneumonia
2. 'Ground glass' opacities representing granulomatous inflammation more often than fibrosis
3. Findings of fibrosis
   - Honeycombing/cystic structures
   - Traction bronchiectasis
   - Architectural distortion, i.e. loss of lobular architecture
   - Conglomerate masses
4. Nodular (often spiculated) or reticular densities (representing granulomatous inflammation or fibrosis) distributed in the peribronchovascular interstitium, interlobular septae and the subpleural region along lymphatics
5. Occasional miliary nodules or larger nodules >1 cm in diameter which may cavitate (rare)
6. Lymphadenopathy involving the hila, paratracheal regions and aortopulmonary window in addition to the subcarinal, anterior mediastinal, posterior mediastinal and axillary regions which are often not appreciated on chest X-rays
7. Upper lobe predominance
8. Complicating mycetoma in a bulla, cavity or bronchiectatic cyst

SARCOID *VS.* LYMPHANGITIC CANCER – HRCT

	Sarcoid	Lymphangitic cancer
Lymphadenopathy	+ (± eggshell calcification)	+
Peribronchovascular thickening *Interlobular septal thickening* *Fissural thickening* *Nodules*	+	+
Conglomerate masses	+	–
Pleural effusion	–	+
Distribution	Upper > lower lobes Central > peripheral Bilateral	Lower > upper lobes Central or peripheral Unilateral or bilateral
'Ground glass' opacities	+	–
Findings of fibrosis (*honeycombing, architectural distortion, traction bronchiectasis*)	+	–

Table 65.1

PROGNOSTIC FEATURES

Natural history is variable with spontaneous remissions in ⅔ of patients, usually within the first two years of diagnosis

- Stage I – 80% (persistent adenopathy does not imply 'activity' or need for therapy)
- Stage II – 55%
- Stage III – <30%
- Stage IV – 0%

- Late relapses are seen in about 5% of patients who remitted or stabilized

- A chronic disease course is seen in ~20% of patients but rare in patients whose X-rays normalized from any stage or who have stable Stage I disease
- Significant extrapulmonary disease is seen in about 5% of patients at presentation with sarcoid and increases as the disease evolves
- Overall mortality ranges from 1–5% with most deaths due to pulmonary, cardiac or CNS disease
- Respiratory insufficiency and cor pulmonale may be accompanied by massive hemoptysis from a complicating aspergilloma
- Rare association reported between sarcoid and testicular germ cell tumors

Negative indicators

1 Insidious onset of lung disease with multiple extrapulmonary lesions
2 Radiologic features of fibrosis
3 Blacks worse than caucasians
4 Disease onset after age 40
5 Lack of radiologic improvement after 1–2 years
6 Disease 'activity'
   - Recent development or increasing respiratory symptoms
   - Progressive disease on serial chest X-rays
   - Deterioration on serial PFTs
   - 'Ground glass' opacification on HRCT
   - Serial elevations in serum ACE levels
7 Cardiac disease
8 CNS disease
9 Absence of erythema nodosum
10 Lupus pernio
11 Chronic uveitis
12 Chronic hypercalcemia/nephrocalcinosis

Positive indicators

1 Isolated asymptomatic bilateral hilar lymphadenopathy
2 Acute presentation with Lofgren's syndrome

3 Resolution of radiologic disease
4 Normal PFTs
5 Absence of extrapulmonary disease

Unclear indicators

1 BAL findings re cellular content, enzyme levels
2 Gallium scan
3 Serum ACE levels
4 Nodules, septal thickening, alveolar consolidation on HRCT
5 Human leukocyte antigen (HLA) typing

AIRWAY AND PLEURAL DISEASE

Airways Disease

Nasal disease

- Most often involves the nasal mucosa with epistaxis, nasal discharge
- Nasal septum involvement with ulcers and perforation
- Disease of the nasal bones and cartilage with osteolytic lesions and saddle nose deformity

Sinusitis

Larynageal disease with hoarseness and signs of upper airways obstruction

Endotracheal/endobronchial disease

- Granulomatous inflammation of the airway walls is seen in Stages I, II, III and may be found on endobronchial biopsy in 30–70% of patients
- Lesions can be single or multiple and extend from the trachea to subsegmental bronchi
- The mucosa may be grossly normal initially, with nodules and a cobblestone pattern developing as disease becomes more severe, resulting finally in diffuse bronchial stenosis and occlusion (granulomatous lesions leading to fibrosis and scarring)
- Additional causes of airway narrowing include extrinsic compression from enlarged nodes, airways distension from

pulmonary fibrosis in Stage IV disease as well as independent airway disease e.g. asthma
- Atelectasis can result, with the right middle lobe being most frequently involved
- Clinical manifestations can include recurrent bronchospasm, infections and subsequent bronchiectasis
- Airways involvement, intrinsic or extrinsic, is reflected by an obstructive picture on PFTs

Bronchoscopy
- Non-caseating granulomas may be seen with transbronchial biopsy (TBB), endobronchial biopsy (EBB), or transbronchial needle aspiration (TBNA) of nodes
- Yields with TBB range from 60–95% and are affected by
  - Presence of stage II or III disease
  - Number of biopsies taken
  - Biopsies from areas showing the most changes bronchoscopically
- Recommendation is approximately 5 biopsies from each of two sites in one lung
- Yields from EBB are variable and low with a normal mucosa but up to 90% with endobronchial abnormalities
- The role of TBNA is unclear in the routine evaluation of sarcoid

Pleural Disease
Clinically, seen in approximately 1% of patients with sarcoid and the manifestations include
- **Pleural effusions**
  - More common in stages II and III
  - Exudate biochemically with fluid being unilateral or bilateral
  - Lymphocytic predominance with occasional eosinophilia
  - Fluid may resolve spontaneously, following a course of steroids or progress to pleural thickening and fibrothorax
  - Granulomas can be seen on pleural biopsy

  - No pathognomonic features to the effusion and therefore a diagnosis of exclusion, having ruled out CHF, tuberculosis, fungi, parapneumonic effusion, renal failure
- **Pleural thickening**
  - Seen in stage IV sarcoid
  - Adjacent to an aspergilloma complicating a cystic space
- **Pneumothorax**
  - Seen with advanced fibrocystic disease and caused by the rupture of subpleural blebs
  - Rarely the presenting feature of sarcoid due to necrosis of subpleural granulomas
- **Hemothorax**
  - Rare
- **Chylothorax**
  - Rare

SYSTEMIC DISEASE

Bone, Joint and Muscle Disease

Acute polyarthritis is seen early in the disease with non-specific inflammation clinically

- Peripheral, symmetric disease, most often involving the ankles and knees followed by involvement of joints of the upper extremity
- May be the presenting feature of sarcoid and often seen along with other manifestations of Lofgren's syndrome, e.g. fever, bilateral hilar lymphadenopathy
- Joint X-rays are often normal

Chronic polyarthritis is seen in patients with chronic sarcoid and characterized pathologically by granulomatous inflammation

- Large or small joints are involved with symmetric, asymmetric or rarely monoarticular disease
- Fever and erythema nodosum are uncommon
- X-rays reveal well-defined eccentric erosions, periarticular osteoporosis and articular destruction

Bone disease is seen with chronic sarcoid

- Skeletal involvement can be localized or generalized, usually with osteolytic lesions, the hands most commonly attacked

Skeletal muscle disease is common but usually asymptomatic

- Patients may present with features of acute or chronic myopathy

Calcium Metabolism

The macrophages of sarcoid granulomas convert 25-hydroxyvitamin D to 1,25-dihydroxyvitamin D with increased intestinal calcium absorption resulting in

1 Hypercalcemia, seen in about 10% of patients, ranging from mild to life-threatening
    - Metastatic calcifications may develop in several organs including the lungs
2 Hypercalciuria, seen in up to 50% of patients, and varies from asymptomatic to nephrocalcinosis, nephrolithiasis and renal failure

Cardiovascular Disease

Primary cardiac sarcoid is seen clinically in about 5% of patients but sarcoid granulomas can be found at autopsy in about 20% of cases

- In only about ½ of patients with cardiac sarcoid diagnosed at autopsy is the diagnosis of systemic sarcoid known
- Course of disease is variable and ranges from benign arrythmias to death
- Manifestations are variable, depend upon the location and extent of granulomatous inflammation/fibrosis and include
    - ECG findings of conduction disturbances including bundle branch blocks and complete heart block
    - Ventricular > atrial arrythmias with sudden death due to either
    - CHF or ventricular aneurysm as manifestations of left ventricular disease

- Mitral insufficiency from papillary muscle or left ventricular disease
- Pericarditis with effusion

The **diagnostic gold standard** is percutaneous endomyocardial biopsy demonstrating granulomas but the yield is limited by the patchy distribution of granulomas as well as the common finding of 'non-specific' lymphocytic myocarditis

- Ancillary studies that are suggestive of cardiac involvement include
  - Echocardiogram
  - Cardiopulmonary exercise testing
  - Thallium scan where defects are present at rest but disappear with exercise

Other causes of cardiovascular disease include

- Cor pulmonale secondary to severe lung disease, characterized by parenchymal fibrosis, hypoxemia and pulmonary hypertension (most common abnormality)
- Extrinsic compression of the pulmonary arteries, pulmonary veins, or SVC by enlarged lymph nodes

Digestive Tract

Clinically significant **liver** disease is seen infrequently compared to the finding of granulomas pathologically (up to 90% of patients) and can be manifest as

1. An asymptomatic increase in the liver enzymes bilirubin, alkaline phosphatase and the transaminases
2. Hepatic cirrhosis with complicating portal hypertension and encephalopathy
3. Budd-Chiari syndrome
4. Biliary obstruction from intrahepatic cholestasis or granulomatous involvement of the hepatic duct
5. FUO

Esophageal obstruction and dysphagia from enlarged nodes

Infiltration of the **gastric mucosa** can result in non-specific upper GI symptoms and a gastroscopic appearance of the 'linitis plastica' form of cancer, biopsy revealing noncaseating granulomas

Salivary gland involvement is common with granulomas seen in the minor salivary glands on random biopsy and gallium uptake seen in the major glands, with clinical manifestations including

1 Unilateral or bilateral parotitis
2 Heerfordt's syndrome of fever, facial palsy, anterior uveitis and parotid enlargement

Eye Disease

Eye involvement is seen in about 20% of cases, the manifestations including

Anterior eye involvement in 90% of patients with ophthalmic sarcoid, most often granulomatous uveitis – acute or chronic, as well as conjunctivitis

Posterior eye structures are involved in about 25% of cases, including chorioretinal nodules and optic nerve disease

Granulomatous infiltration of the lacrimal gland, usually bilateral, and often associated with parotid swelling

Bilateral exophthalmos

Hematologic Disease

Symptomatic **splenic** disease is uncommon compared to the finding of granulomas pathologically in up to 70% of patients

- Manifestations can include marked splenomegaly with hypersplenism, abdominal pains and splenic rupture

Lymphopenia is the most common abnormality on a peripheral smear, other findings including anemia, thrombocytopenia and eosinophilia

Lymphadenopathy

Granulomatous infiltration of lymph nodes can result in

1 Grossly normal nodes with only microscopic abnormalities
2 Palpable lymphadenopathy
3 Visible and rarely massive lymphadenopathy

- The involved nodes are rubbery, firm, discrete, mobile and non-tender

- Nodes most commonly involved are the cervical, axillary, epitrochlear and inguinal although any nodal area may be affected
- Compressive symptoms are rare but treatment may be required for cosmetic purposes

Neuroendrocrine Disease

Seen clinically in 5–10% of patients but pathologically in about 15%

- One half of patients with clinical neurosarcoid present initially with neurologic symptoms which may be the sole manifestation of sarcoid (making diagnosis difficult) or occur simultaneously with extra neurologic disease
- All levels of the nervous system may be involved with predilection for the base of the brain, including

Cranial nerve involvement with the following decreasing frequency

1 7th (facial) nerve disease can be unilateral, bilateral or associated with other cranial nerve abnormalities
   - Most common neurologic manifestation of sarcoid with a good prognosis

2 Optic nerve disease with visual disturbances, papillary edema and pupillary abnormalities

3 Nerves 9 and 10 with dysphagia, hoarseness and vocal cord dysfunction

Peripheral nerve involvement including mononeuropathy, mononeuritis multiplex, polyneuropathy, Guillan-Barre

- Clinically, the ulnar and peroneal nerves are most often involved

Aseptic meningitis which may or may not be symptomatic but manifest by increased CSF protein and ACE levels, hypoglycemia and lymphocytic pleocytosis

- Tuberculous and fungal infection must be excluded

Central nervous system lesions – mass-like or infiltrating, with symptoms reflecting the site of disease and resulting increase in intracranial pressure

Hypothalamic-pituitary abnormalities including anterior

pituitary insufficiency with amenorrhea, impotence, adrenal insufficiency, hypothyroidism, diabetes insipidus

- Diagnosis can be made by biopsy of neurologic tissue or compatible neurologic findings on CSF, MRI or CT scan in conjunction with histologic confirmation from other tissue

Skin Disease

Erythema nodosum – non-granulomatous

- Seen in acute sarcoid, commonly in Europeans, Puerto Ricans and Mexicans but rare in U.S. blacks and Japanese
- Acute onset of subcutaneous, erythematous, tender nodules involving the anterior tibial and other extensor surfaces
- Often accompanied by a flu-like illness, bilateral hilar adenopathy and uveitis
- Non-specific for sarcoid with identical lesions seen in other diseases
- Patients presenting with Lofgren's syndrome, i.e. erythema nodosum, fever, polyarthralgias and bilateral hilar adenopathy, have an excellent prognosis with >90% having spontaneous resolution of disease within one year

Granulomatous lupus pernio

- Specific for sarcoid, common in blacks and Puerto Ricans, and characterized by a nodular or plaque-like eruption most often involving the face and neck
- Onset is insidious, the course chronic, with residual scarring being common and spontaneous remissions rare
- Often associated with other manifestations of chronic sarcoid, e.g. pulmonary fibrosis, uveitis, bone cysts

Other granulomatous infiltrations

NECROTIZING SARCOID GRANULOMATOSIS (NSG) – NODULAR SARCOID (NS)

NSG is defined pathologically by a combination of

1 Confluent sarcoid-like granulomas

2 Coagulative necrosis
3 Vasculitis
4 Absence of infection, e.g. histoplasmosis

NS is defined pathologically by masses of granulomas and hyalinized connective tissue in the absence of infection

Clinically, NSG and NS are thought to be variants of sarcoid, but the pathologic and radiologic features are atypical

- Presentation varies from asymptomatic to non-specific pulmonary and systemic symptoms with a female to male ratio of 4:1
- Extrapulmonary disease is generally absent, although liver, eye and neurologic disease are described
- Disease resolves either spontaneously or with steroids in more than 80% of patients

Chest X-ray abnormalities

1 Multiple nodules or ill-defined parenchymal opacities
2 Hilar adenopathy in <50% of cases
3 Cavitation may be present
4 Pleural effusions may be present

Fraser R.S., Muller N.L., Colman N., Paré P.D. (1999) *Diagnosis of Diseases of the Chest* 4th Edn., WB Saunders.

Naidich, D.P., Zerhouni, E.A., Siegelman, S.S. (1998) *Computed Tomography and Magnetic Resonance of the Thorax*, 3rd edn. New York: Raven Press.

Moss, A., Gamsu, Genant (1992) Thorax and neck. In: *Computed Tomography of the Body with Magnetic Resonance Imaging*. 2nd edn, vol. 1.: W.B. Saunders.

Baum, G.L., Crapo, J.D., Celli, B.R., Karlinsky, J.B. (eds) (1997) *Textbook of Pulmonary Diseases*, 6th edn.: Lippincott-Raven.

Fishman, A.P., Elias, J.A., Fishman, J.A., Grippi, M.A., Kaiser, L.R., Senior, R.N. (1998) *Fishman's Pulmonary Diseases and Disorders*, 3rd edn.: McGraw-Hill.

Lynch, J., Kazerooni, E., Gay, S. (1997) Pulmonary sarcoid. *Radiol. Clin.* **18**: 755–785.

Sharma, O.P. (1997) Cardiac and neurologic dysfunction in sarcoidosis. *Clinics in Chest Medicine* **18**: 813–825.

Sharma, O.P. (1997) Neurosarcoidosis: a personal perspective based on a study of 37 patients. *Chest* **112**: 220–228.

Mana, J. (1997) Nuclear imaging. *Clinics in Chest Medicine* **18**: 799–811.

Nishimura, K., Itoh, H., Kitaichi, M. *et al.* (1993) Pulmonary sarcoidosis: correlation of CT and histopathologic findings. *Radiology* **189**: 105–109.

Newman, L., Rose, C., Maier, L. (1997) Sarcoidosis. *NEJM* **336**: 1224–1233.

American Thoracic Society (1999). Statement on sarcoidosis. *Am. J. Resp. Crit. Care Med.* **160**: 736–755.

66 Skin/Nail Disorders – Pulmonary Manifestations

SKIN NODULES – LUNG DISEASE

1 Vasculitis, e.g. Wegener's, Churg-Strauss
2 Erythema nodosum
3 Infections
   - Sporotrichosis
   - Histoplasmosis
   - Blastomycosis
   - Coccidioidomycosis
   - Aspergillosis (disseminated)
   - Bacillary angiomatosis (HIV)
   - Tuberculosis
4 Sarcoid
5 Rheumatoid arthritis
6 Systemic lupus erythematosus
7 Neoplasms
   - Neurofibromatosis
   - Lymphomatoid granulomatosis
   - Metastatic lung cancer
   - Kaposi's sarcoma
   - Lymphoma
   - Melanoma

- Waldenstrom's macroglobulinemia
- Systemic mast cell disease

NEUROFIBROMATOSIS

Airways
- Endotracheal or endobronchial disease

Parenchyma
- Bullae, often apical
- Interstitial fibrosis resembling UIP
- Combination of bullae and interstitial fibrosis
- Primary neurogenic tumors
- Metastatic disease from neurogenic sarcoma

Pleura
- Hemothorax secondary to erosion of intercostal vessels

Chest wall
- Rib notching or destruction
- Extrapleural mass
- Kyphoscoliosis
- Subcutaneous nodules (neurofibromas)

Mediastinum
- Neurofibroma/schwanoma – benign or malignant
- Phaeochromocytoma
- Meningocele/myelomeningocele

NAIL CHANGES – LUNG DISEASE

1. Clubbing/hypertrophic osteoarthropathy
2. Yellow nail syndrome
3. Yellow-brown staining in heavy smokers with COPD
4. Periungual telangiectasia and digital infarcts with scleroderma, SLE, dermatomyositis

YELLOW NAIL SYNDROME

Definition: Rare disorder, initially described in 1964 as the association of yellow nails and lymphedema, the latter reflecting lymphatic aplasia or hypoplasia

- Usually develops in middle age with clinical features including

1. **Nails** (initial finding in ~$\frac{1}{3}$)
   - Yellow-green in color
   - Thick, slowly growing and excessively curved along both axes
   - Easily infected
   - May precede or follow the pleural effusions and spontaneously revert to normal
2. **Lymphedema** (initial finding in ~$\frac{1}{3}$)
   - Involves the lower extremities, breasts, face and upper extremities
3. **Respiratory disease** (initial finding in ~$\frac{1}{3}$)
   - Pleural effusion
     - Etiology unclear ? lymphatic hypoplasia
     - Unilateral or bilateral and may persist for months to years
     - Varies in size from small and asymptomatic to large, recurrent and debilitating
     - Usually exudative with a lymphocytic predominance but may be chylous
     - May precede the nail changes by years
   - Chronic sinusitis
   - Bronchiectasis
   - Recurrent bronchitis and pneumonia
4. **Other**
   - Chylous ascites
   - Chyluria
   - Pericardial effusion
   - Intestinal lymphangectasia
   - Giant cell interstitial infiltrate

TUBEROUS SCLEROSIS

Definition: Autosomal dominant disorder characterized by the classic triad of adenoma sebaceum, mental retardation and seizures

- Pulmonary disease is seen in <1% of patients, with male involvement being rare
- Lung involvement is that seen in LAM with interstitial lung disease, cysts, pneumothoraces and cor pulmonale but chylothorax is less common
- PFTs are also similar to LAM with hyperinflation, airways obstruction and low DCO
- Extrapulmonary disease includes hamartomas of the CNS, retinal phakomas, angiomyolipomas of the kidney, renal and bone cysts, cardiac rhabdomyomas

ERYTHEMA NODOSUM

Inflammatory nodules develop as a hypersensitivity reaction to a variety of disorders affecting the lungs including

1 Sarcoid
2 Drugs, e.g. sulfas or other antibiotics, contraceptives
3 Infections, e.g. tuberculosis, histoplasmosis, coccidioidomycosis, psittacosis, streptococcus, brucellosis, tularemia

- Pulmonary disease can be manifest by
  - Adenopathy, e.g. sarcoid
  - Infiltrates, e.g. drugs
  - Cavitary disease, e.g. coccidioides immitis

MELANOMA

Pulmonary disease is a common manifestation of **metastatic melanoma**, with CT scans able to detect disease not apparent on chest X-ray

- Isolated pulmonary disease is uncommon

- Patients may be asymptomatic or present with non-specific respiratory symptoms

Parenchyma
- Single or multiple nodules
- Miliary pattern
- Lymphangitic spread
- Lung mass
- Patchy air space disease

Pleura
- Malignant pleural effusion

Airways
- Endobronchial metastases

Mediastinum
- Lymphadenopathy

Chest wall
- Bone metastases

Fraser R.S., Muller N.L., Colman N., Paré P.D. (1999) *Diagnosis of Diseases of the Chest* 4th Edn., WB Saunders.

Baum, G.L., Crapo, J.D., Celli, B.R., Karlinsky, J.B. (eds) (1997) *Textbook of Pulmonary Diseases*, 6th edn.: Lippincott-Raven.

Fishman, A.P., Elias, J.A., Fishman, J.A., Grippi, M.A., Kaiser, L.R., Senior, R.N. (1998) *Fishman's Pulmonary Diseases and Disorders*, 3rd edn.: McGraw-Hill.

67 Sleep-related Breathing Disorders

OBSTRUCTIVE SLEEP APNEA AND HYPOPNEA (OSAH)

Definition: Repeated discrete episodes of upper airway obstruction during sleep lasting for 10 sec or greater with cessation (apnea) or reduction (hypopnea) of airflow, resulting in hypoxemia, hypercapnia and/or sleep fragmentation

- Results from the loss of upper airway tone during sleep superimposed upon an anatomically narrowed or excessively collapsable upper airway

Symptoms

'Hallmark symptoms' are those of heavy habitual snoring and excessive daytime sleepiness

Daytime symptoms include

- Excessive sleepiness
- Impaired concentration
- Memory loss
- Irritability, personality change
- Rarely, major depression, frank psychosis

Nocturnal symptoms (patient is typically unaware of apneic events) include

- Heavy snoring
- Witnessed apneas
- Restless sleep

- Nocturnal choking
- Unrefreshing sleep
- Morning headache
- Nocturia, rarely enuresis
- Impotence
- Nocturnal seizures

Factors Predisposing to Upper Airway Collapse/Reduced Airway Size

1 Male gender
   - ? Hormonal modulation of neuromuscular activity in the upper airway

2 Anatomic factors
   - Obesity/fat deposition
   - Endocrine disorders, e.g. hypothyroidism, acromegaly
   - Nasal obstruction
   - Tonsillar hypertrophy
   - Other tumor/obstructing lesion
   - Macroglossia
   - Cranio-facial disproportion (retrognathia, micrognathia)
   - Secretions and airways inflammation, e.g. cigarettes, rhinitis

3 Neuromuscular factors
   - Neuromuscular disease with upper airway involvement
   - Drugs leading to muscle dysfunction: sedatives, alcohol, muscle relaxants
   - Negative pressure ventilation
   - Phrenic pacing

4 Tissue factors
   - Increased tissue compliance (Marfan's, Ehlers-Danlos)

Complications

Neuropsychiatric

1 Daytime sleepiness, impaired concentration/vigilance
   - Impaired work performance, workplace accidents

- Motor vehicle accidents
- Poor financial decisions

2 Mood disturbance
- Social/marital disruption

Cardiovascular

3 Systemic hypertension
- Evidence for an independent association of OSAH with hypertension
- May contribute to poor BP control

4 Arrhythmias
- Bradyarrhythmias, tachyarythmias and heart block are seen with ventricular ectopy if nocturnal hypoxemia is severe
- Isolated nocturnal arrhythmias on Holter may be a clue to OSAH

5 Pulmonary hypertension
- Mild degree is common with moderate to severe levels usually in the context of significant daytime hypoxemia
- Can improve with treatment but often persists

6 Myocardial infarction
- Growing evidence that OSAH is a risk factor with nocturnal ischemia occurring in patients with OSAH and coronary artery disease

7 Stroke
- Increased rate of OSAH (up to 60–70%) in stroke, transient ischemic attacks
- OSAH may predispose to and complicate stroke

8 Congestive heart failure
- OSAH may worsen ventricular function in patients with dilated cardiomyopathy (ischemic, idiopathic, etc.)
- Treatment of OSAH may significantly improve cardiac function

9 Secondary polycythemia
- Unusual and seen in patients with marked awake hypoxemia

Pulmonary

10 Hypoxemia and hypercapnia are seen during wakefulness in 10–20% although ABGs are normal in most OSAH patients
- Due to hypoventilation which usually occurs with underlying lung dysfunction, e.g. COPD, obesity restriction, in subjects with severe nocturnal hypoxemia
- May also be related to pulmonary hypertension in severe cases, which may progress to cor pulmonale
- Chronic awake hypoventilation may progress to overt respiratory failure, with or without an identifiable acute precipitating factor
- OSAH may co-exist with other nocturnal hypoventilation syndromes (obesity, neuromuscular, etc.)

11 Nocturnal asthma
- Snoring and/or OSAH may worsen asthma control in some patients and those with prominent nocturnal wheeze and dyspnea may be improved by treatment of co-existing snoring and/or OSAH

12 Peri-operative airway risk
- OSAH patient should be on treatment prior to major elective surgery
- The upper airway in OSAH is often 'difficult' for anesthetic management with precautions needed during induction
- Post-extubation CPAP should be immediately initiated until patient is fully awake
- Consider effects of post-operative analgesia on the upper airway and assess the need for monitoring

Endocrine/metabolic

13 Sympathetic activation
- Related to nocturnal hypoxemia, arousals from sleep
- Believed to contribute to cardiovascular complications of OSAH

14 Altered salt-water excretion
- Relative nocturnal natriuresis
- Accounts for symptoms of nocturia, enuresis

15 Insulin resistance
- OSAH may independently contribute to insulin resistance in some diabetic patients
- Treatment of OSAH may improve diabetic control in difficult patients

16 Thyroid dysfunction
- Hypothyroidism is an important predisposing factor for OSAH

Diagnostic Work-up

1 History (input of bed partner important) and physical examination including predisposing causes and search for complications (as above)

2 Clinical evaluation alone is not adequate to establish the diagnosis of OSAH and some form of nocturnal respiratory recording is required
- Overnight laboratory polysomnography is the gold standard
- Partial/home nocturnal respiratory recordings may be adequate
  - If there is a 'classic pattern' of oxyhemoglobin desaturation with a strongly suggestive history (may proceed directly to treatment)
  - If the study is negative or equivocal, a complete polysomnogram is required for symptomatic patients

3 Ancillary tests include
- Complete blood count
- Arterial blood gas
- Serum biochemistry
- Specific endocrine testing (acromegaly, thyroid function)
- Pulmonary function testing
- Chest radiograph
- Electrocardiogram
- Holter monitoring

- Fiberoptic nasopharyngoscopy
- Cephalometry
- Upper airway CT or MRI

CENTRAL SLEEP APNEA (CSA)

Definition: Discrete episodes lasting 10 sec or greater of cessation of breathing during sleep due to a loss of central respiratory drive and respiratory effort

- Overall CSA is much less common than OSAH

Hypercapnic CSA

Central causes

- Primary central hypoventilation and apnea
- Previous encephalitis
- Cervical cordotomy
- Multiple sclerosis
- Brainstem lesions

Neuromuscular disease

- Myotonic dystrophy
- Muscular dystrophy
- Myasthenia gravis
- ALS
- Post-polio syndrome
- Dysautonomias
- Acid maltase deficiency

Episodic complete loss of respiratory drive leading to CSA occurs either in the context of overall reduced central respiratory drive and/or impaired ventilation secondary to neuromuscular weakness

- In many of these conditions discrete CSA episodes may be observed in conjunction with sustained nocturnal hypoventilation
- Some underlying conditions may also have associated upper airway dysfunction e.g. neuromuscular, so both CSA and OSAH may be observed
- Patients may present with poor sleep quality, unrefreshing sleep, morning headache, daytime sleepiness, awake hypoxemia, cor pulmonale and progressive respiratory failure

Non-hypercapnic CSA

Group of disorders characterized by periodic breathing in which a mild degree of alveolar hyperventilation appears to contribute to pathogenesis

- There are differences between wakefulness and sleep in the ventilatory sensitivity to CO_2 as well as in the 'apneic threshold', i.e. the PCO_2 below which respiratory rhythm generation ceases
- The apneic threshold is higher during sleep, and in individuals with frequent arousals or sleep-wake transitions, periods of apnea can be induced if baseline CO_2 is reduced slightly, i.e. toward the apneic threshold

1 Cheyne-Stokes respiration (CSR)
   - Characterized by crescendo-decrescendo alteration in tidal volume separated by periods of apnea/hypopnea
   - Thought due to the combination of hyperventilation and a prolonged circulatory time in patients with CHF
   - Observed during sleep in 40–50% of stable severe (NYHA Class 3–4) congestive heart failure patients and potentially reversible if failure improves
   - Symptoms of frequent paroxysmal nocturnal dyspnea, nocturnal angina 2° to hypoxemia and poor quality unrefreshing sleep
   - may be associated with daytime sleepiness as well as other sleep apnea symptoms, although the sleep disorder is often unrecognized clinically
   - May contribute to worsening of cardiac function, which can improve if successfully treated with nasal CPAP
   - CSA is also seen with neurologic disease where cortical injury has occurred

2 High altitude periodic breathing
   - Related to hypoxemia-induced hyperventilation with symptoms of insomnia and nocturnal choking being part of the symptom complex of 'acute mountain sickness'
   - May also occur with chronic high altitude exposure

3 Idiopathic central sleep apnea
   - Clinical presentation may be similar to OSAH
   - Slightly older population with body habitus usually normal while sleep disruption/insomnia are prominent complaints
   - Often associated with mild hyperventilation during both wakefulness and sleep, periodic increases in tidal volume and ventilation during sleep triggering central apneas in the absence of oxyhemoglobin desaturation
   - Does not lead to respiratory failure/cor pulmonale

4 Physiologic periodic breathing associated with sleep-wake state transitions
   - Mild degree of central apnea may be seen at the beginning of the sleep period in normal subjects

NOCTURNAL HYPOVENTILATION

Definition: A sustained reduction in ventilation during sleep, as distinguished from discrete apnea or hypopnea episodes, which is generally more prominent during rapid-eye-movement (REM) sleep than non-REM sleep

- Nocturnal hypoventilation is often not strictly identified on the basis of increased PCO_2 in view of the practical difficulties in measuring this accurately during sleep, but identified on the basis of hypoxemia, usually measured via pulse oximetry
- There are no strict criteria for the extent or duration of hypoxemia which define nocturnal hypoventilation
- Most patients with clinically significant hypoventilation spend a majority of the sleep period with $SaO_2 < 90\%$, particularly during REM

Nocturnal hypoventilation occurs due to sleep-related decrements in respiratory drive, respiratory muscle activity, lung volume and load compensation

- The above lead to abnormal reductions in ventilation in patients with compromised respiratory muscle function and/or who are dependent upon high levels of respiratory drive and muscle activity to maintain adequate ventilation

- Some nocturnal hypoxemia may also be due to changes in ventilation-perfusion matching related to reduced end-expiratory lung volume resulting from inhibition of respiratory muscles during sleep and/or body position effects

Differential Diagnosis

1 **Neuromuscular and chest wall restrictive disorders**

Neuromuscular disorders	Chest wall abnormalities
• Myotonic dystrophy	• Congenital
• Muscular dystrophy	• kyphoscoliosis
• Myasthenia gravis	• Post-surgical (thoracoplasty, chest wall resection)
• ALS	• Post-traumatic
• Post-polio syndrome	
• Acid maltase deficiency	

In neuromuscular patients, FEV_1 is usually <35% predicted when nocturnal hypoventilation occurs

- In scoliosis, nocturnal desaturation is generally observed with curvature >100°
- Nocturnal desaturation may occur well before the development of awake hypoxemia in neuromuscular and chest wall disorders
- Nocturnal respiratory disturbances are believed to be an early step in the progressive development of chronic respiratory insufficiency
- Conversely if these patients are hypoxic awake, they are likely to be more so asleep
- There may be a combination of hypoventilation and CSA or OSA in some patients

2 **Obsesity hypoventilation ('Pickwickian Syndrome')**
Morbid obesity with awake hypoventilation, i.e. hypoxemia and hypercapnia out of keeping with degree of obesity-related restrictive impairment on PFT

- Daytime sleepiness, mental impairment and morning headaches are common while right-sided heart failure may be prominent
- During sleep ABGs worsen with sustained reduction in SaO_2 and increased $PaCO_2$, worst during REM
- There is almost always a contribution of increased upper airway resistance to the hypoventilation and very often these patients also have OSA

3 **COPD**

Severity of nocturnal hypoxemia generally correlates with severity of lung function and presence of daytime hypoxemia

- Not all patients with severe lung dysfunction hypoventilate at night and reliable prevalence figures are unavailable
- Symptoms of sleep disruption, morning headache and daytime fatigue may suggest nocturnal hypoxemia
- OSA may also be present in COPD patients with nocturnal hypoventilation, the likelihood being increased by obesity or heavy alcohol consumption

NOCTURNAL CHOKING AND DYSPNEA

Definition: Respiratory symptoms of choking, suffocation, cough or shortness of breath which occur uniquely or predominantly at night

- May be related primarily to sleep, to assuming the supine position, or both

1 Obstructive sleep apnea
   - Nocturnal choking is an uncommon symptom
   - Typically occurs in very mild cases with rare, sporadic events or in extremely severe, relatively young patients
   - Diagnosis confirmed by a sleep study with symptoms resolved on treatment

2 Congestive heart failure (paroxysmal nocturnal dyspnea – Cheyne-Stokes respiration)

- Typical awakening from sleep within several hours after retiring, with dyspnea or cough improved over approximately 15 minutes in the seated position and may recur throughout the night
- Orthopnea also likely present
- Some 'PND' may be related to arousal during the hyperpneic phase of Cheyne-Stokes breathing in severe CHF patients even when medically stable
- Sleep studies required to evaluate Cheyne-Stokes breathing

3 Nocturnal asthma
   - Typical awakening with dyspnea, wheeze or cough between 3–4 am and relief with bronchodilators
   - May be the first sign of asthma decompensation
   - Look for associations with OSAH, GERD which may worsen asthma
   - Document nocturnal worsening by peak flow measurements

4 Gastro-esophageal reflux with acid aspiration and laryngospasm
   - Awakening with choking sensation and throat 'constriction' resolving in seconds to minutes
   - Associated 'acid taste' often but not always present
   - Other symptoms of reflux may be present, e.g. heartburn, epigastric pain, hoarseness, chronic cough
   - Confirmation with esophageal pH monitoring as well as response to acid-reducing medication

5 Other aspiration episodes
   - Awakening with cough, dyspnea and/or choking sensation
   - Related to aspiration of secretions in patients with upper airway dysfunction, heavy secretions
   - Investigation via swallowing assessment (clinical, cineradiographic)

6 Diaphragm paralysis/paresis
   - 'Nocturnal' symptoms specifically associated with recumbency rather than sleep

- Immediate dyspnea on assuming supine position as well as relief when upright
- If paresis rather than paralysis, symptoms may occur later in the night
- There may be associated nocturnal hypoventilation and central apnea

7 Mediastinal mass
- Symptoms associated with lying flat rather than sleep *per se* with cough or dyspnea on assuming the supine position
- An issue for peri-anesthetic airway management where airway obstruction during induction or post-extubation should be closely monitored

8 Idiopathic
- Nocturnal choking episodes with diagnostic evaluation negative for all of the above
- Conservative management, reassurance and clinical follow-up
- Re-evaluation in 6–12 months if symptoms persist

Fraser R.S., Muller N.L., Colman N., Paré P.D. (1999) *Diagnosis of Diseases of the Chest* 4th Edn., WB Saunders.
Strollo, P., Rogers, R. (1996) Obstructive sleep apnea. *NEJM* **334**: 99–104.
Kryger, M. *et al.* (1995) *Principles and Practice of Sleep Medicine*, 2nd edn. Toronto: W.B. Saunders.
Strollo, P.J., Sanders, M.H. (1998) Sleep Disorders *Clinics in Chest Medicine* Volume 19, number 1.

68 Small Hemithorax

Radiologic Signs

1 Elevated hemidiaphragm
2 Approximation of ribs
3 Mediastinal shift to the ipsilateral side
4 Hyperinflation of opposite lung with herniation along the anterior mediastinum into the involved hemithorax (deep retrosternal airspace is seen on lateral chest X-ray)

Differential Diagnosis

Airways

1 Bronchial obstruction – intralumenal, endobronchial, peribronchial
2 Bronchiolitis, e.g. Swyer-James

Parenchyma

3 Any cause of scarring

Pleura

4 Fibrothorax
5 Mesothelioma

Chest wall

6 Diaphragmatic paralysis

Vasculature – congenital or acquired

7 *Agenesis*
   - Very rare disorder characterized by complete absence of the bronchus on the affected side and often associated with major abnormalities of the heart, kidneys, diaphragm and GI tract

- Patients may be asymptomatic into adulthood and present with an opaque and grossly contracted hemithorax
- Some aeration may be seen due to herniation of the contralateral lung across the midline, the remaining lung being hyperplastic but not hyperlucent
- Differential diagnosis includes atelectasis, post-infectious destruction, old tuberculosis with fibrothorax, prior pneumonectomy
- The complete absence of pulmonary structures is documented on CT scan

8 *Aplasia*
- No vasculature or parenchyma is seen and only a rudimentary bronchus is present

9 Hypoplasia
- Reduced size and number of the airways, parenchyma and vasculature
- May be primary or secondary to various developmental disorders

10 *Proximal interruption* of left or right pulmonary artery
- Hilum is absent, i.e. no pulmonary artery is seen and the lung is supplied by systemic vessels
- Lung is hyperlucent with absent perfusion on V/Q scan but differs from Swyer-James in the absence of gas trapping on expiration as well as normal ventilation
- Left-sided proximal interruption is associated with tetralogy of Fallot and septal defects

11 *Hypogenetic lung syndrome* (scimitar syndrome), is a rare congenital abnormality characterized radiologically by
- Hypoplastic right lung and right pulmonary artery
- Abnormal right bronchial tree
- Anomalous pulmonary vein draining part or all of the right lung, descending in the major fissure in a sweeping curve resembling a scimitar, and entering the IVC below the diaphragm or at its junction with the right atrium

- Partial or complete supply of the lung by a systemic artery, usually from the aorta, resulting in a left to right shunt
- Confirmation of diagnosis by CT with infusion

Clinically, patients are usually symptomatic with

- Dyspnea and fatigue from the shunt
- Possible pulmonary hypertension
- Recurrent respiratory infections
- Hemoptysis

12 *Acquired obstruction* of the pulmonary artery, e.g. pulmonary embolus

Fraser R.S., Muller N.L., Colman N., Paré P.D. (1999) *Diagnosis of Diseases of the Chest* 4th Edn., WB Saunders.

Naidich, D.P., Zerhouni, E.A., Siegelman, S.S. (1998) *Computed Tomography and Magnetic Resonance of the Thorax*, 3rd edn. New York: Raven Press.

Moss, A., Gamsu, Genant (1992) Thorax and neck. In: *Computed Tomography of the Body with Magnetic Resonance Imaging*, 2nd edn, vol. 1.: W.B. Saunders.

69 Systemic Blood Supply to Lung

Congenital

1 **Bronchopulmonary sequestration**
2 **Congenital adenomatoid malformation**
3 **Hypogenetic lung syndrome**
4 **Proximal interruption of a pulmonary artery**
5 **Absence of the main pulmonary artery**
   - Several anatomic variants described
6 **Localized systemic supply of normal lung**
   - A solitary artery arises directly from the aorta (less often one of its branches) and supplies a lower lobe with or without an associated pulmonary artery supply to those segments
   - Normal bronchial tree architecture which excludes a sequestration
   - May present in infancy/childhood with a murmur or heart failure due to a left-to-left shunt, hemoptysis or be asymptomatic
   - Chest X-rays may be normal or reveal increased vascularity in a lower lobe with enlargement or the draining inferior pulmonary vein as well as rib notching
   - CT or pulmonary angiography may detail the pulmonary arteries and veins with definitive diagnosis made on aortography
7 **Systemic-pulmonary vascular fistula**
   - Characterized by a fistula between a normal or anomalous systemic artery and pulmonary artery or vein
   - May present with recurrent hemoptysis, a murmur or be asymptomatic
   - Fistulous connection to a pulmonary artery reveals a step-up in O_2 saturation due to a left-to-right shunt
   - May be primary or secondary, e.g. pulmonic stenosis

Acquired

1 **Aortic aneurysm**

2 **Systemic-pulmonary vascular fistula**
- Post-infectious, e.g. bronchiectasis
- Post-trauma
- Post-surgical

Fraser R.S., Muller N.L., Colman N., Paré P.D. (1999) *Diagnosis of Diseases of the Chest* 4th Edn., WB Saunders.

Naidich, D.P., Zerhouni, E.A., Siegelman, S.S. (1998) *Computed Tomography and Magnetic Resonance of the Thorax*, 2nd edn. New York: Raven Press.

Moss, A., Gamsu, Genant (1992) Thorax and neck. In: *Computed Tomography of the Body with Magnetic Resonance Imaging*, 2nd edn, vol. 1.: W.B. Saunders.

70 Thoracoscopy (Medical)

Indications

1 The most common reason is for diagnosis of an exudative pleural effusion of unknown etiology in spite of the clinical features, laboratory evaluation and thoracentesis
  - Closed biopsy should be done if tuberculosis is suspected but unclear whether it is cost effective with malignancy
    - Exfoliative cytology and needle biopsy are each positive in about 50% of cases of metastatic cancer
      - Biopsy is more likely to be positive with advanced *vs.* localized disease but is negative with tumor exclusively involving the diaphragmatic, visceral or mediastinal pleura
      - Thoracoscopy is diagnostic in 85–100% of cases
    - Mesothelioma results in a positive yield on closed pleural biopsy or cytology in <40% of cases, whereas thoracoscopic yield is near 100%
    - Tuberculous pleurisy is diagnosed in about 80% of cases by closed pleural biopsy, pleural culture and cultures of sputum/gastric washings, whereas thoracoscopic yield is 100%

2 Evaluation of a pleural effusion discovered during the staging of lung cancer
  - Pleural invasion or mediastinal disease can be ruled out to select potentially resectable patients

3 Undiagnosed pleural mass

4 Biopsy of focal or diffuse lung disease (some centers) but requires general anesthesia

5 Talc pleurodesis of malignant effusions or uncommonly non-malignant, e.g. hepatic cirrhosis
6 Talc pleurodesis of spontaneous pneumothorax – often combined with surgical interventions including cautery, bleb resection or pleural abrasion

Contraindications

1 Lack of an accessible pleural space due to adhesions
2 Uncorrected bleeding disorder
3 Unstable cardiac disease
4 Respiratory failure unrelated to the pleural effusion

Complications

1 Mortality <0.1%
2 Persistent air leak from injury to the visceral pleura
3 Hemorrhage in <4% of cases
4 Fevers secondary to
   - Talc pleurodesis
   - Empyema
   - Wound infection
   - Aspiration
5 Dyspnea post-thoracoscopy can be secondary to
   - Failure of the lung to re-expand
     - Air leak (subcutaneous emphysema often present)
     - Blocked or malpositioned chest tube (contralateral mediastinal shift and subcutaneous emphysema may be present)
     - Endobronchial obstruction (ipsilateral mediastinal shift may be present)
   - Re-expansion pulmonary edema associated with rapid drainage of pleural fluid or air
   - Hemothorax from laceration of an intercostal vessel
   - Reaccumulation of the previous pleural effusion
6 Subcutaneous emphysema
7 Seeding of the chest wall along the path of the thoracoscope, most often with mesothelioma
8 Cardiac arrythmia
9 Oxygen desaturation

Harris, R.J., Kavuru, M.S., Mehta, A.C. *et al.* (1995) The impact of thoracoscopy on the management of pleural disease. *Chest* **107**: 845–852.

Harris, R.J., Kavuru, M.S., Rice, T.W. *et al.* (1995) The diagnostic and therapeutic utility of thoracoscopy. *Chest* **108**: 828–841.

Menzies, R., Charbonneau, M. (1991) Thoracoscopy for the diagnosis of pleural disease. *Ann. Int. Med.* **114**: 271–276.

71 Tracheobronchial Disease – Chronic

Patients present with a **several month to year history** of symptoms of **airways disease** including cough, sputum, wheezing, dyspnea, hemoptysis, recurrent respiratory tract infections, ± airways obstruction on spirometry, the **differential diagnosis** including the following

Tracheal Disease

1 **Tracheal bronchus** seen in a few percent of the population and characterized by origin of the RUL bronchus from the trachea
   - Airway clearance is poor with recurrent bronchial infections
   - Diagnosis made on bronchoscopy
2 **Tracheomalacia**, congenital or acquired
3 **Post-intubation injury**
4 **Tracheo-esophageal fistula**
   - Congenital
     – May present in adulthood with life-long cough, worse post-prandial, especially with liquids > solids
     – Infection and neoplasms must be ruled out
   - Acquired
     – *Malignant, e.g. lung, esophagus
     – Post-intubation
     – Infectious, e.g. coccidioidomycosis histo, TB
     – Foreign body

Diagnosis can be made by barium swallow, endoscopy, bronchoscopy +/– installation of methylene blue

Tracheal and/or Bronchial Disease

5 **Tracheobronchomegaly** (Mounier-Kuhn syndrome)
Defined as tracheal dilatation of ≥3 cm measured 2 cm above the aortic arch, enlargement of the right main stem bronchus ≥2.4 cm, or enlargement of the left main stem bronchus ≥2.3 cm
- Etiology is unclear with pathology revealing atrophy of the elastic and muscular tissues in the affected tracheobronchial tree, the dilated, thin-walled trachea and bronchi collapsing on forced expiration
- Syndrome of tracheobronchomegaly and recurrent respiratory tract infections was described by Mounier-Kuhn, the infections due to inefficient cough and clearing of secretions with subsequent lung destruction

Clinical onset is usually in early adulthood, predominantly in men and includes
- Asymptomatic radiologic finding
- Recurrent chest infections leading to bronchiectasis, emphysematous bullae and parenchymal scarring
- Chronic airways obstruction with cor pulmonale and respiratory failure

Radiologic features
- Tracheobronchial dilatations on CT or MRI with collapse demonstrated on cinefluoroscopy or dynamic CT
- Mucosal protrusion between the cartilaginous rings creating 'diverticuli'
- Central bronchiectasis involving the first through fourth-order divisions of bronchi, with a transition to normal airways distally

6 **Relapsing polychondritis**
7 **Intralumenal disease** including a foreign body, broncholith or mucoid impaction
8 **Inhalation injury**
9 **Vasculitis** – Wegener's granulomatosis
10 **Infiltrative disorders** including sarcoid, amyloid, tracheobronchopathia osteochondroplastica, endometriosis

11 **Infections** including tuberculosis, atypical mycobacteria, fungi, nocardia, actinomycosis
12 **Plasma cell granuloma**
13 **Neoplasms**, benign or malignant, primary or secondary
14 **Extrinsic narrowing**, e.g. mediastinal fibrosis

Bronchial Disease

15 **Accessory bronchus** consisting of a blind pouch which enters the bronchus intermedius medially
- May present with recurrent bronchial infections and hemoptysis, the diagnosis made on bronchoscopy

16 **Bronchopulmonary sequestration**
17 **Chronic bronchitis**
18 **Bronchiectasis**
19 **Bronchiolitis**
20 **Asthma**, including allergic bronchopulmonary aspergillosis and bronchocentric granulomatosis
21 **RADS**, i.e. asthma-like syndrome developing in a previously normal person, exposed on a single occasion to a high concentration of a toxic agent
22 **Broncholithiasis**
23 **Foreign body**

Fraser R.S., Muller N.L., Colman N., Paré P.D. (1999) *Diagnosis of Diseases of the Chest* 4th Edn., WB Saunders.

Naidich, D.P., Zerhouni, E.A., Siegelmar, S.S. (1998) *Computed Tomography and Magnetic Resonance of the Thorax*, 3rd edn. New York: Raven Press.

Shin, M.S., Jackson, R.M., Hok, G. (1998) Tracheobronchomegaly: CT diagnosis. *AJR* **150**: 777–779.

72 Transplants – Lung/Heart-lung

SELECTION OF LUNG TRANSPLANT RECIPIENTS

Indications

- Advanced pulmonary or pulmonary vascular disease with limited anticipated survival (<1–2 years)
- Failure of alternative treatment strategies
- Severe functional limitation but still ambulatory
- Age 55 years or less for heart-lung transplantation, 60 or less for bilateral lung transplantation, 65 or less for single lung transplantation

Absolute contraindications (may vary from center to center)

- Severe extrapulmonary organ dysfunction including renal insufficiency, hepatic dysfunction with portal hypertension, left ventricular dysfunction, severe psychiatric disease, suspected non-compliance with therapy, drug or alcohol dependence, severe coronary artery disease (consider heart-lung transplantation)
- Acute critical illness
- Active or recent malignancy with likelihood of recurrence (except for basal cell or squamous cell carcinoma skin)

- Active extrapulmonary infection, including infection with HIV, hepatitis B (surface antigen positive) and hepatitis C with significant liver disease on biopsy
- Recent smoking (<6 months)
- Severe malnutrition (<70% ideal body weight) or obesity (>130% ideal body weight)

Relative contraindications (may vary from center to center)

- Chronic medical conditions which are poorly controlled or associated with end-organ damage
- Multisystem disease (connective tissue disease, etc.)
- Inability to walk with poor rehabilitation potential
- Daily prednisone (or equivalent) dosage >20 mg
- Extensive pleural disease
- Invasive mechanical ventilation
- Airway colonization with pan-resistant bacteria (especially *Burkholderia cepacia*) in patients with cystic fibrosis
- Symptomatic osteoporosis

Five groups of patients are considered for transplant

1. Obstructive disease, e.g. COPD, eosinophilic granuloma
2. Restrictive disease, e.g. IPF (primary or secondary), sarcoid, LAM, drug-induced, others
3. Vascular, e.g. primary or secondary pulmonary hypertension, Eisenmenger's
4. Suppurative, e.g. CF, other causes of bronchiectasis
5. Chronic rejection of a previous lung transplant

TIMING OF REFERRAL FOR LUNG TRANSPLANTATION

Timing of referral should vary according to local anticipated waiting times for transplantation

- Referral of potential candidates is appropriate when they are estimated to have a natural history of less than 1–2 years
- For a given functional level, patients with pulmonary fibrosis should be referred earlier due to poorer anticipated survival awaiting lung transplantation

COPD

- FEV_1 <25% post-bronchodilator
- Clinically significant hypoxemia, hypercapnia, pulmonary hypertension
- Rapid decline in lung function
- Frequent, severe exacerbations

Idiopathic pulmonary fibrosis

- Symptomatic disease, unresponsive to medical therapy
- VC <60–70% predicted
- Resting or exercise hypoxemia

Cystic fibrosis

- FEV_1 <30% predicted
- FEV_1 >30% predicted with rapidly declining lung function, frequent severe exacerbations, progressive weight loss
- Female gender and age <18 years should be considered earlier (associated with poorer prognosis)

Primary pulmonary hypertension

- NYHA class 3 or 4
- Mean pulmonary artery pressure >55 mmHg
- Mean right atrial pressure >15 mmHg
- Cardiac index <2 L/min/m^2
- Failure of medical therapy (epoprostenol, calcium channel blockers) to improve functional class or hemodynamic variables

Eisenmenger's syndrome

- NYHA class 3 or 4 despite optimal medical therapy

MOST COMMON INDICATIONS FOR DIFFERENT TRANSPLANT PROCEDURES

Single lung transplant

- Emphysema (with or without α_1-antitrypsin deficiency)
- Idiopathic pulmonary fibrosis
- Primary pulmonary hypertension
- Congenital heart disease (with cardiac repair)

Bilateral/double lung transplant

- Cystic fibrosis
- Bronchiectasis, septic lung disease
- Emphysema
- Idiopathic pulmonary fibrosis
- Primary pulmonary hypertension

Heart-lung transplantation

- Congenital heart disease, Eisenmenger's syndrome
- Primary pulmonary hypertension
- Cystic fibrosis
- Combined advanced pulmonary and cardiac disease

GUIDELINES FOR DONOR SELECTION

- Age <60 years
- No history of significant lung disease
- Clear lung fields on chest X-ray
- Absence of excessive purulent bronchial secretions
- Adequate oxygenation ($PaO_2 > 300$ mmHg on FiO_2 1.0; $PaO_2/FiO_2 > 250–300$)

SURVIVAL FOLLOWING LUNG TRANSPLANTATION

Actuarial survival

- Outcomes are similar for single and bilateral lung transplant recipients with overall survival of approximately 70% at 1 year, 55% at 3 years and 43% at 5 years
- Survival following heart-lung transplantation is slightly worse than for other lung transplant procedures, with 1 year survival of 60% and 5 year of 40%
- Best overall survival outcomes are seen in recipients with emphysema and cystic fibrosis, with slightly poorer results in recipients with pulmonary fibrosis and pulmonary vascular diseases

Factors predisposing to poor outcome

- Re-transplant
- Donor age >50
- Recipient age >60
- Pre-transplant recipient on mechanical ventilation
- Pre-transplant recipient colonization with pan-resistant *Burkholderia cepacia* (cystic fibrosis patients)
- Donor/recipient cytomegalovirus serologic mismatch

COMPLICATIONS POST-LUNG TRANSPLANTATION

0–30 days

1 **Primary graft failure** (acute reperfusion injury)
2 **Bronchial anastomotic breakdown**
3 **Hemorrhage** – pleural, parenchymal or mediastinal
4 **Cardiac dysfunction**
5 **Infection**
  - Active infection conveyed with the allograft
    - Treatment should be guided by cultures obtained from the donor and recipient at the time of transplant
    - Bacteria are most common, often gram negative although a wide range of organisms is described
    - Broad spectrum antibiotics covering gram negative organisms and staphylococcus are generally given in the perioperative period +/– inhaled anti-pseudomonals in cystic fibrosis
  - Nosocomial bacterial/candida, with the majority of infections in the first month being the same nosocomial infections occurring in non-immunosuppressed surgical patients

6 Acute rejection
  - Rarely fatal but the severity and frequency of episodes of acute rejection appear to be the most important risk factor for the later development of chronic rejection
  - Typically occurs early post-transplant (weeks to months)

- Most common clinical manifestations include low grade fever, dyspnea, cough, weight gain and fall in oxygen saturation
- Chest radiographs may show new interstitial/airspace disease or pleural effusions but may be normal
- Definitive diagnosis is by transbronchial biopsy in association with a compatible clinical picture, a histologic grading system for acute rejection being used – this is based upon the extent and severity of perivascular infiltrates around arterioles and venules, with more severe disease extending into the alveolar septae and associated with parenchymal necrosis, infarction or necrotizing vasculitis
- A presumptive diagnosis (less desirable) can be made by exclusion of infection or heart failure and a rapid response to high dose intravenous steroids

7 **Venous thromboembolism**
8 **Phrenic nerve injury**

30 days to One Year Post-Transplant

1 **Obliterative bronchiolitis (OB)**

- Long-term survival following lung transplant is limited by OB, which is thought to be a manifestation of chronic rejection and affects up to 50% of long-term survivors by 3 years post-transplantation
- The process tends to be insidious in onset with progressive dyspnea on exertion, often with cough and deterioration over time
- May be initiated by a clinical presentation suggesting an upper respiratory tract infection followed by an asthma-like picture with cough, wheezing and dyspnea but a poor response to antibiotics and bronchodilators
- Onset is most commonly 3 months or more following transplantation and highest in the first 2 years but patients remain at risk indefinitely
- Occurs unpredictably and undetectable pre-clinically

- The small airways disease is accompanied by bronchiectasis, colonization with a variety of organisms, e.g. pseudomonas, aspergillus, others, as well as acute infectious exacerbations
- Predisposing factors include the frequency and severity of prior episodes of acute rejection as well as prior CMV infection

Diagnosis

- The early identification of chronic rejection following lung transplantation is problematic due to the lack of a reliable early diagnostic test
- Chest radiograph is usually normal or may show signs of bronchiectasis
- HRCT findings include bronchial dilatation, bronchiectasis, gas trapping and mosaic perfusion, best seen on an expiratory scan (HRCT demonstrates high sensitivity but low specificity for the diagnosis of OB)
- OB tends to be patchy in distribution with transbronchial biopsy diagnosis having a high specificity but low sensitivity
- Pathologic findings are seen in the small cartilagenous airways and include
  - Inhomogenous distribution of peribronchiolar lymphocytic inflammation +/– lymphocytic bronchiolitis

    ↓
  - Loss of the epithelial lining with granulation tissue filling the lumen of the small airways

    ↓
  - Recognizable airways not seen but replaced by scar tissue
  - Other airway diseases include lymphocytic bronchitis, mucus plugs, proximal bronchiectasis and BOOP

Bronchiolitis obliterans syndrome (BOS)

- Due to the low sensitivity of transbronchial biopsy for the detection of OB, the diagnosis of chronic airways rejection is generally based on changes in pulmonary function

Grading of BOS

(International Society for Heart and Lung Transplantation

BOS grade	FEV_1 (% post-transplant baseline)
0	>80%
1	65–79%
2	50–64%
3	<50%

Table 72.1

- The commonly used definition of chronic airways rejection, BOS, is defined as a decline in the FEV_1 of more than 20% from the post-transplant baseline in the absence of acute rejection or active infection
- Once OB is established, long-term survival is reduced
- Variable clinical courses are described, either spontaneously or in response to changes in immunosuppressive therapy including
  - Relentless progression
  - Step-wise falls in lung function
  - Plateau at a lower level of lung function

2 **Infection – 1–6 months post-transplant**

- CMV (see p. 636) is the most frequent and important viral agent post-transplant, reflects recent infection or reactivation, and may be a risk factor for the development of obliterative bronchiolitis
  - Seronegative recipients of seropositive donor organs are at greatest risk for infection
  - The most effective way to prevent infection in CMV seronegative recipients is to avoid seropositive donors and seropositive blood products
  - Alternatively, if either the recipient or a donor is seropositive, treatment with gancyclovir from the time of transplant or when increased viral burden is detected can decrease the incidence and severity of infection

- Disease is variable and includes asymptomatic infection, a flu-like illness, severe pneumonia, other organ dysfunction, e.g. hepatitis, as well as disseminated disease involving the bone marrow, retina, CNS and GI tract
- The diagnosis is definitively made when lung biopsy reveals pneumonia and CMV although BAL showing typical CMV inclusion containing cells is specific but insensitive
- Increased viral burden detected by sequential CMV antigenemia or quantitative PCR can suggest evolving infection
- Viral isolation with pneumonia and absence of other infectious agents is suggestive

- Other agents including herpes viruses (infrequent with current prophylaxis), pneumocystis (rare with prophylaxis), aspergillus, bacteria, e.g. gram negatives, legionella, psudomonas in CF, others
- Immunosuppression levels are gradually reduced as tolerated after 6 months and opportunistic infections are less common, with more of the community-acquired pneumonias seen

3 **Post-transplant lymphoproliferative disorders**

- Seen in ~5% of lung transplant receipients, often within the first year
- Majority are non-Hodgkin's lymphoma of B cell origin and relate to the combination of immunosuppression and Epstein-Barr virus
- Clinically, extranodal disease is most common, usually within the allograft, less commonly involving CNS, liver or other sites

4 **Venous thromboembolism**

5 **Airway complications**, e.g. strictures, bronchomalacia

- Uncommon (<15%) with current surgical techniques
- Can generally be managed with bronchoscopic placement of stents or balloon dilatation

One Year + Post-transplant

1 **Obliterative bronchiolitis**

2 **Infection**

3 **Malignancy**

- Lymphoproliferative disorders as well as non-lymphoid malignancy of the skin, lips, Kaposi's and other tumors

RADIOLOGIC ABNORMALITIES POST-TRANSPLANT

Differential of pulmonary infiltrates

1 Early (hours–weeks)
- Primary graft failure (acute reperfusion injury)
- Infection – bacterial (most common), viral (uncommon), fungal (uncommon)
- Acute rejection

2 Late (months–years)
- Infection – bacterial, viral, fungal
- Post-transplant lymphoproliferative disease
- Bronchiolitis obliterans with organizing pneumonia (distinct from obliterative bronchiolitis)

Differential diagnosis of pulmonary nodules

1 Infection
- Fungal
- Mycobacterial disease

2 Malignancy
- Post-transplant lymphoproliferative disease
- Primary bronchogenic carcinoma
- Metastatic carcinoma

3 Bronchiolitis obliterans with organizing pneumonia (distinct from obliterative bronchiolitis)

King-Biggs, M. (1997) Acute pulmonary allograft rejection. *Clinics in Chest Medicine* **18**: 301–310.

Kelly, K., Hertz, M. (1997) Obliterative bronchiolitis. *Clinics in Chest Medicine* **18**: 319–338.

Trulock, E. (1997) Lung transplantation. State of the art. *Am. J. Resp. Crit. Care Med.* **155**: 789–818.

73 Trauma – Non-surgical

Parenchyma

1 **Lung contusion** is defined as exudation of blood and edema fluid into the lung parenchyma with little tissue disruption
Clinical spectrum varies from asymptomatic to hemoptysis, dyspnea, fever and secondary infection
Radiologic findings can include
   - Asymmetric non-segmental airspace consolidation with the major changes occurring deep to the traumatized areas
     – Air bronchograms often absent due to blood in the airways
   - Abnormalities appear within hours of the injury, improvement beginning in 1–2 days, usually resolving spontaneously in about 5 days
   - Disease progression and evolution into ARDS
   - CT findings of non-segmental peripheral parenchymal opacification can be seen before chest X-ray changes

2 **Pulmonary parenchymal laceration** developing post-trauma can result in single or multiple cystic spaces, i.e. traumatic lung cysts that can remain air-filled, demonstrated an air–fluid level or fill completely with blood, i.e. hematoma
Clinically, patient can be asymptomatic, present with hemoptysis, rarely secondary infection or a broncho-pleural fistula
Radiologic findings
   - Single or multiple cysts, ovoid or elliptical in shape, unilocular or multilocular, in the lung periphery

- Appearance within hours to days of injury developing under the point of maximal injury
- Lesions may be air-filled, blood filled (mass-like), have an air–fluid level or result in an air–meniscus sign
- Often surrounded by pulmonary contusion and may not be visible on chest X-ray until the contusion resolves
- May persist for months following the injury
- An associated hemopneumothorax may be present
- CT is more sensitive than chest X-ray in detection of lacerations

3 **Atelectasis**, either obstructive from blood clots and mucus, secondary to bronchial rupture

4 **Lung torsion** (rarely described) occurs with severe trauma where a lobe or entire lung is twisted 180° with radiologic findings of inappropriate hilar displacement, rapid opacification or changing position on sequential X-rays

5 **ARDS** with potential predisposing factors including lung contusion, sepsis, shock, aspiration, fat emboli, fluid overload and transfusion reactions

Airways

1 **Tracheobronchial rupture** is an uncommon injury which usually follows a crushing injury to the chest

- 80% of cases involve the mainstem bronchi just distal to the carina, with tracheal involvement occurring immediately above the carina, and the diagnosis made on bronchoscopy

Clinical features are non-specific and insensitive including

- Associated pneumothorax not responding to chest tube drainage
- Combined pneumothorax and pneumomediastinum
- Subcutaneous emphysema, cough, dyspnea and hemoptysis

- Chest pains from commonly associated fractures of the first three ribs
- New onset atelectasis
- Little or no signs or symptoms in a small percentage of cases, presenting months to years later with bronchial stenosis, atelectasis and destruction of the distal lung parenchyma

Radiologic findings

- Fractures of the first three ribs
- Pneumothorax
- Pneumomediastinum
- Atelectasis from displacement of the fracture ends and bronchial obstruction

2 **Tracheo-esophageal fistula**

Pleura

1 **Hemothorax** can result from injury to the pleura, diaphragm, chest wall, lung parenchyma or mediastinum, including the heart and great vessels

- Symptoms relate to hypovolemia as well as compressive atelectasis, the latter seen with arterial bleeds while bleeding of pulmonary venous origin is usually self-limited without mass effect
- Associated rib fractures are often present
- Pleural tap may reveal an eosinophilia
- Fluid tends to loculate early, may be accompanied by a pneumothorax and can eventually result in a fibrothorax or post-traumatic empyema

2 **Pneumothorax** may develop due to rib fractures and visceral pleural disruption, tracheobronchial rupture, esophageal rupture or interstitial emphysema, with tension pneumothorax a potential complication

- Iatrogenic causes in trauma patients include central venous access, positive pressure ventilation and insertion of chest tubes
- Diagnosis is made by identification of the visceral

pleural line, seen in the apical or lateral hemithorax when the patient is erect

- When supine, air accumulates in the anterior costophrenic sulcus and is manifest as described on p. 686
- Small pneumothoraces may be missed on chest X-ray and diagnosed only on CT scan

3 **Chylothorax** develops an average of 2 to 10 days post-trauma, the diagnosis being made on thoracocentesis
- More superior injuries to the thoracic duct appear in the left chest with more inferior injuries in the right chest
- A mediastinal collection of chyle can occasionally be diagnosed on CT scan prior to the development of the pleural effusion
- Persistent chylothorax can result in a fibrothorax

4 **Post-traumatic empyema** develops when blood in the pleural space becomes infected, particularly in the presence of an air leak from the lung
- Compressive atelectasis from a hemothorax can result in pneumonia and abscess formation, with extension of infection into the pleura

5 **Bilious effusion** from laceration of the right hemidiaphragm and liver with formation of a biliopleural fistula

6 **Sympathetic effusion** from injury to the spleen, liver or pancreas

Mediastinum

1 **Pneumomediastinum** can develop from esophageal, tracheobronchial or alveolar rupture as well as by air tracking down from the neck following tears in the laryngeal or pharyngeal mucosa, from the retroperitoneum (perforated viscus) or from chest wall wounds
- Manifest radiologically by lucent streaks of air outlining the mediastinal pleura and other mediastinal structures

- Usually best seen in the left superior mediastinum extending down over the heart surface

2 **Mediastinal hemorrhage** manifest as a widened mediastinum, the differential including injury to the thoracic aorta or great vessels
   - Can compress adjacent structures and rarely present with cardiac tamponade

3 **Rupture of the thoracic aorta** or its branches occurs at the site of the ligamentum arteriosum in 95% of cases and immediately above the aortic valve in 5%
   - Morality is ~90% within the first hour, with a few percent of patients developing a chronic traumatic aneurysm
   - Clinically, the diagnosis should be suspected with hypertension of the upper extremities, hypotension in the legs, new onset hoarseness and radiologic signs of (a) mediastinal widening and (b) an abnormal outline of the aortic knob

4 **Esophageal perforation** presents clinically with fever, chills, hematemesis and chest pains from acute mediastinitis, usually accompanied by other significant intrathoracic injuries
   - The latter may proceed to abscess formation and perforation into the pleural cavity or bronchus with fistula formation
   - Physical exam may reveal subcutaneous emphysema and Haman's crunch
   - Pleural fluid characteristics include low pH, high salivary amylase and food particles
   - Diagnosis is established by esophagoscopy and the following radiologic findings which include
     – Widened mediastinum which may contain air
     – Hydrothorax or hydropneumothorax if the mediastinal pleura is ruptured
     – Extravasation of ingested contrast material

5 **Ruptured thoracic duct** with initial accumulation of chyle in the mediastinum and subsequent chylothorax

6 **Cardiac abnormalities**
- Cardiac contusion is most common with other injuries involving the coronary vessels, valves, conducting system, rupture
- Pneumopericardium can follow penetrating or blunt trauma with air in the pericardium mimicking pneumomediastinum
  – Rarely results in cardiac tamponade where a small cardiac silhouette is seen and returns to normal size after insertion of a pericardial drain
- Hemopericardium, the high density pericardial fluid seen on CT scan

Vasculature

1 **Fat emboli** are seen with long bone fractures and present with the clinical triad of respiratory distress, CNS abnormalities and petechiae (see p. 236)
- Chest X-rays vary from normal to bilateral patchy airspace disease which is relatively symmetric, appears 1 to 3 days post-trauma and clears in 7 to 10 days

2 **Thromboembolism**

3 **Air embolism** is seen with a bronchopulmonary venous fistula, air visualized in the left ventricle on echocardiography, with systemic air emboli resulting

4 **Traumatic pulmonary arteriovenous fistula**

Chest Wall

Chest wall damage is the most common injury in blunt and penetrating trauma

1 **Rib fractures** can result in hemothorax, extrapleural hematomas, pneumothorax, hemopneumothorax, flail chest, splenic or hepatic injury and indirectly lead to atelectasis and pneumonia from splinting

- Ribs 1 and 2 are the least injured while ribs 3 through 9 are most commonly injured, often along the posterior axilliary line
- Fractures not initially identified on rib X-rays may appear 3–6 weeks later when callus formation is seen
- Fracture of the uppermost ribs increases the likelihood of serious internal injuries including the great vessels, trachea, etc.
- Fracture of ribs 10 through 12 may suggest injuries to the liver, spleen or diaphragm
- Costochondral separation and resultant pain can be a chronic complication of rib fractures

2 **Flail chest** is defined as a segment of chest wall that moves paradoxically with breathing and is seen where multiple rib fractures occur in two places along the same rib

3 **Sternal fractures** are usually transverse with posterior displacement of the manubrium, best seen on lateral X-ray
   - Pain is the main symptom but associated injuries, particularly myocardial contusion as well as injury to the innominate artery (mediastinal hemorrhage) should be ruled out

4 **Scapular fractures** are often associated with other injuries including rib fractures, lung contusion, pneumothorax, brachial plexus injuries, arterial injuries
   - Scapulothoracic dissociation is best seen on frontal X-ray where the scapula is laterally displaced and often associated with injuries to the brachial plexus or subclavian artery

5 **Subcutanous emphysema** should prompt a search for the origin of air including the larynx, tracheobronchial tree, lung parenchyma, esophagus

6 **Thoracic vertebral fractures** radiologically can result in paraspinal hematomas
   - Associated injuries should be sought to the spinal cord, heart and great vessels, as well as the abdomen

and retroperitoneal areas with lower thoracic spine injuries

7 **Lung herniation** is manifest as a bulge which appears through a chest wall defect during coughing or straining, and is usually benign with strangulation being rare
- CT scan demonstrates lung tissue extending through a rib fracture into the subcutaneous tissues

8 **Diaphragmatic injury** (see Traumatic Hernias, p. 195) can follow blunt or penetrating trauma, e.g. gunshot, stabs
- Left-sided lesions are much commoner than right with visceral herniation being immediate or delayed
- Symptoms relate to respiratory compression from intra-abdominal organs in the chest, abdominal pains secondary to visceral strangulation or associated injuries of the chest/abdomen

Radiologic findings include
- *Visualization of a hollow viscus, stomach or colon, above the hemidiaphragm with compressed bowel at the site of the diaphragmatic tear
- Contralateral mediastinal shift
- Obliteration or distortion of the diaphragmatic outline
- Discontinuity of the diaphragm and the CT collar sign (focal constriction of a herniated viscus) are the most reliable CT features
- MRI features

9 **Splenosis** is a rare complication of combined diaphragmatic and splenic injury, defined as the autotransplantation of splenic tissue
- Often asymptomatic and manifest as solitary or multiple pleural based nodules on chest X-ray and CT
- Should be suspected with a history of trauma and associated findings of rib fractures, bullet fragments or diaphragmatic rupture

Fraser R.S., Muller N.L., Colman N., Paré P.D. (1999) *Diagnosis of Diseases of the Chest* 4th Edn., WB Saunders.

Naidich, D.P., Zerhouni, E.A., Siegelman, S.S. (1998) *Computed Tomography and Magnetic Resonance of the Thorax*, 3rd edn. New York: Raven Press.

Fishman, A.P., Elias, J.A., Fishman, J.A., Grippi, M.A., Kaiser, L.R., Senior, R.N. (1998) *Fishman's Pulmonary Diseases and Disorders*, 3rd edn.: McGraw-Hill.

Pezzella, T., Silva, W., Lancey, R. (1998) Cardiothoracic trauma. *Current Prob. Surg.* **Aug**: 719–770.

Shanmuganathan, K., Mirvis, S. (1999) Imaging diagnosis of nonaortic thoracic injury. (Journal title) **37**: 533–549.

74 Tuberculosis and Non-tuberculous Mycobacteria

Introduction

In most industrialized countries, TB is a disease of subpopulations, the clinical and radiologic manifestations varying with age, country of origin and associated medical conditions

1 Among the elderly born in the pre-antibiotic era, TB is mainly a disease of reactivation with few of the classic symptoms and more often a wasting or 'dwindling' disease
   - Radiologic features may be atypical when associated medical conditions result in immunosuppression
2 In foreign-born and aboriginals, incidence of disease is seen in adolescents and young adults, with symptoms and radiologic features more 'classical'
3 Among the urban poor, alcoholism, HIV infection and drug use contribute to higher rates of disease among

young adults, particularly men, and are often associated with atypical clinical and radiologic manifestations

PRIMARY TB – CLINICAL-RADIOLOGIC PRESENTATIONS

Primary TB, by convention, develops within one year of infection and is traditionally a disease of children, but in North America primary TB may occur in adults of all ages with manifestations as follows

1. **Normal chest X-ray**
   - Asymptomatic patient with a PPD conversion (most common)
2. **Pleural effusion – tuberculous pleurisy**
   Tuberculous infection of the pleural space is generally caused by rupture of a subpleural caseous focus and rarely by hematogenous dissemination
   - Typically seen in adolescents and young adults, occurring 6–9 months following the primary infection
   - In older adults, tuberculous pleural effusions can occur as a manifestation of reactivation disease, presenting more insidiously with minimal fever, no chest pain, dry cough, mild dyspnea and a slowly increasing pleural effusion

   Clinically, tuberculous pleurisy is usually of acute onset with pleuritic chest pains and fever simulating pneumonia
   - Less commonly, the presentation is insidious in onset with fever, weight loss and mild pleuritic chest pain
   - PPD is negative in approximately 25% of cases
   - Sputum smears and cultures are more likely to be positive when an associated pulmonary infiltrate is present
   - Usually self-limited over the short term with clinical and radiologic resolution over several weeks, although approximately 65% of untreated patients will develop pulmonary or extrapulmonary tuberculosis within the subsequent 5 years

Pleural fluid characteristics

- Exudative effusion, usually serous and non-bloody
- pH is normal or slightly low, 7.20–7.40
- Glucose levels are variable and non-diagnostic
- WBC count is variable with an initial neutrophilia being replaced by lymphocytes, the hallmark of disease being >90% lymphocytosis
- Eosinophilia and mesothelial cells are rarely seen
- AFB smears are positive in 5–10% and cultures positive in 25–50% of cases
- The exudative effusion rarely progresses to empyema formation
- Increased adenosine deaminase, an enzyme of T lymphocytes with levels >45 IU/L, although immunosuppressed patients may not demonstrate these values
  - Elevated levels are described with bacterial empyema and rheumatoid arthritis but they do not have the lymphocyte to neutrophil ratio >3, as seen in tuberculosis
- Increased γ interferon levels >140 pg/mL suggest TB
- Positive PCR

Closed **pleural biopsy** for histology, smears and cultures has a high yield (about 80%) but depends upon the adequacy of sampling

Thoracoscopic biopsy has a yield of approximately 95%

Chest X-rays reveal a unilateral pleural effusion, rarely bilateral, which may be accompanied by a parenchymal infiltrate

- Effusion usually resolves completely on treatment but residual pleural thickening or calcification can occur with persistent fluid that is positive for tuberculosis
- Reactivation can later occur with empyema and/or bronchopleural fistula formation

CT scan may demonstrate changes not seen on chest X-ray including

- Parenchymal infiltrate which may cavitate

- Hilar, mediastinal or internal mammary lymphadenopathy
- Unsuspected rib or vertebral body involvement

3 **Airways disease**
- Localized airways obstruction may develop from the compressive effect of enlarged nodes, endobronchial disease or nodes eroding into a bronchus and can result in atelectasis
- Areas most commonly involved are the anterior segment of the RUL and medial segment of the RML with atelectasis persisting until the enlarged lymph nodes regress
- May be preceded by 'obstructive emphysema' radiologically due to a check-valve mechanism
- Symptoms are those of airways obstruction

4 **Mediastinal/hilar enlargement**
- Lymphadenopathy is seen more often in children (up to 95% of cases) than adults (<40%) and is the radiologic hallmark of disease in children
- Hilar and/or mediastinal nodes may be enlarged, unilateral > bilateral, and can calcify
- Right paratracheal or tracheobronchial (hilar) lymph nodes are preferentially involved
- With i.v. contrast, nodes >2 cm in diameter may reveal a characteristic combination of central low density and peripheral rim enhancement (not specific for *M. tuberculosis* but described with *M. avium* complex, histoplasmosis, lymphoma and carcinoma)
- An associated parenchymal infiltrate or atelectasis may be present or adenopathy can be the sole radiologic manifestation of disease in children (but rarely in adults)
- May be symptomatic or asymptomatic
- May resolve completely or become calcified, the combination of parenchymal and nodal calcification being the Ghon complex (also seen in histoplasmosis)
- May extend into the mediastinum with development of

granulomatous mediastinitis and involvement of the trachea, pericardium, esophagus, superior vena cava

5 **Miliary disease** – rare

6 **Parenchymal disease**

- *Airspace consolidation* may present acutely with non-specific respiratory symptoms and a rapid downhill course or the syndrome of 'primary atypical pneumonia'
  - Any lobe may be involved without segmental preference with unifocal parenchymal consolidation or multilobar involvement and patchy bronchopneumonia
  - Consolidation is usually sublobar and subpleural although complete lobar consolidation with bulging fissures is described, usually in association with endobronchial obstruction
  - The parenchymal focus resolves completely in ~$^2/_3$ of cases with residual scarring in ~$^1/_3$, the latter occasionally calcifying
- *Tuberculoma*, a nodular or mass-like opacity, often <3 cm in diameter and thought to be the result of healed primary or post-primary disease
  - Usually upper lobe in location
  - Margins are usually smooth and sharply defined but can be spiculated simulating cancer
  - Occasionally multiple and often associated with 'satellite' lesions
  - Cavitation in ~$^1/_3$ of lesions with calcification in up to $^1/_2$ of cases
  - Usually remains stable but can enlarge over time (as well as reactivate)
  - Associated calcified hilar nodes support the diagnosis
- *Cavitation and endobronchial spread* – rare
- *Fibrosis and parenchymal calcifications* (Ghon focus)
- *Progressive primary disease* whose features are those of post-primary TB

POST-PRIMARY TB – CLINICAL-RADIOLOGIC PRESENTATIONS

10% of newly infected persons will develop clinically apparent TB, 5% within the first few years and the remaining 5% in the remainder of life

- Of the above patients, 85% are pulmonary and 15% are extrapulmonary
- Most cases of post-primary TB reflect reactivation of an antecedent primary infection and uncommonly reinfection of a previously sensitized host
- Reactivation occurs when underlying immune function wanes, e.g. aging, viral infection, chronic disease, immunosuppression
- Reinfection of previously infected and treated patients has been documented with DNA fingerprinting which identifies the genotype of M. Tuberculosis
- The above may be more important in poorer countries where the incidence of TB is high and the chances of repeated exposure and infection greater

1 **Normal chest X-ray**
   - May be seen with early miliary disease, endobronchial or laryngeal tuberculosis

2 **Pleural disease**
   - Pleural effusion
   - Tuberculous empyema
   - Bronchopleural fistula and pneumothorax
   - Pleural thickening and calcification

3 **Airways disease**
   - *Bronchiectasis* usually involves the apical and posterior segments of upper lobes
     – Often asymptomatic although can present with recurrent but usually self-limited hemoptysis without chronic cough and sputum
     – Develops secondary to traction (from fibrosis of the lung parenchyma) proximal bronchostenosis or romete endobronchial TB

- *Endobronchial/endotracheal* tuberculosis occurs secondary to
  - Parenchymal disease with direct implantation of organisms intrabronchially
  - Lymphatic drainage to the peribronchial region with erosion of intrathoracic lymph nodes, the latter visualized on CT scan of the mediastinum or peribronchial regions
  - Hematogenous spread (miliary spread via the bronchial arteries)

Bronchoscopically, mucosal lesions include: granularity from submucosal tubercles (early), exudates with white caseation, ulcerations, cicatricial lesions, polypoid or mass lesions, and extrinsic narrowing from nodes with an eccentric protruding mass
  - The above can result in bronchostenosis and/or atelectasis of a segmental or lobar bronchus, bronchiectasis, as well as tracheal narrowing

- *Bronchostenosis* manifest as
  - Segmental/lobar atelectasis
  - Lobar hyperinflation
  - Mucoid impaction/obstructive pneumonitis
- *Broncholithiasis* from calcification of lymph nodes and their erosion into a bronchus
- *Bronchopleural fistula*
- *Broncho-esophageal or tracheo-esophageal fistula*
- *Laryngeal tuberculosis* seen when patients are heavily smear positive with spread along the respiratory tract to the larynx
  - Symptoms are those of hoarseness and pain in the throat
  - Importance is that contagiousness is dramatically increased

4 **Mediastinal/hilar disease**

- *Lymphadenopathy* uncommon except for HIV-infected individuals
- *Fibrosing/granulomatous mediastinitis* results from extranodal extension of disease where the radiologic features are those of mediastinal widening or a mass

   - Complications can involve the major vessels, esophagus, tracheobronchial tree (see p. 508)
- *Cardiomegaly* from an associated pericardial effusion

5 **Vascular disease**

- *Miliary disease* (see p. 801)
- Local invasion of pulmonary arteries and veins resulting in a *necrotizing granulomatous pulmonary vasculitis*
- *Pulmonary gangrene* from thrombosis of a pulmonary artery
- Development of a *Rasmussen aneurysm*, i.e. a localized dilatation of a pulmonary artery branch contiguous to a tuberculous cavity, rupture of which can result in massive hemoptysis and/or death
- *Chronic pulmonary artery stenosis* from thrombosis/vascular compression (very rare)

6 **Parenchymal disease**

- *Airspace consolidation* of the apico-posterior segments of the upper lobes or superior segments of lower lobes
   - Involvement of other areas of lung usually occurs after the above
   - Volume loss of the affected lobe due to the destructive and fibrotic nature of the disease
   - Progression of the above can result in complete lung opacification and cavitation with 'cavernous' breathing
   - Isolated non-cavitary infiltrates in the lower lobes can be seen in the immunocompromised individuals such as those taking steroids, diabetics or individuals with advanced HIV infection
- *Areas of parenchymal fibrosis and calcification* can follow the airspace consolidation with traction bronchiectasis, volume loss, and marked architectural distortion
   - Upper lobe atelectasis with hilar retraction, tracheal deviation and an 'apical cap' are common
- *Tuberculoma* (see p. 792) can be the site of reactivation where a previously stable lesion develops acute

airspace disease in the surrounding parenchyma, accompanied by new respiratory symptoms

- *Cavitation* is common and seen in ~50% of cases on chest X-ray but more accurately detected on CT, particularly where there is extensive parenchymal destruction from scarring
  - Cavities are multiple more often than single and range in size from a few millimeters to several centimeters, with thick or thin walls
  - A surrounding infiltrate is common but a cavity can occur in isolation
  - Air–fluid levels are often absent
  - Complications of cavitation include
    - *Endobronchial spread
    - Spontaneous pneumothorax
    - Mycetoma formation
- *Acinar shadows* represent small foci of active tuberculosis and are the result of endobronchial spread of disease
  - Confluence of the above results in *acute tuberculous pneumonia* (confluent airspace disease), formerly known as galloping consumption
  - Invariably acid-fast bacilli can be seen on microscopic exam of a direct smear of sputum and mortality is very high without treatment
- *ARDS* complicating miliary tuberculosis
- ? *Scar cancer*

7 **Vertebral or other osteomyelitis/paraspinal abscess**

SIGNS AND SYMPTOMS – PULMONARY/EXTRAPULMONARY

Historically, the first symptom is chronic cough which is initially dry, later becomes productive, slowly worsening in frequency and severity

- Fevers and night sweats are typically next to appear

- Hemoptysis is uncommon initially but develops as disease becomes more advanced
- Anorexia, weight loss and cachexia tend to be present when disease is far advanced

Chest exam is usually normal even with advanced disease
- Classic finding is post-tussive rales, i.e. rales which worsen with coughing
- Bronchial or amphoric breathing with large cavities

Evidence of extrapulmonary disease (coexists with pulmonary disease in about 25% of cases) includes

1 **Lymph nodes** (most frequent form of extrapulmonarpy TB)
   - For unknown reasons there is predilection for this form of disease among individuals from Asia, particularly those from India, Pakistan and surrounding countries, and therefore TB should always be suspected in a young foreign-born adult with lymphadenopathy
   - Most commonly affected are the cervical nodes although almost any lymph node can be affected
   - Presentation is that of a painless discrete swelling initially although sequellae can include painful enlargement, suppuration, sinus tracts and appearance of new nodes during or following Rx
   - Systemic symptoms are usually absent in non-HIV patients and chest X-rays may be normal
   - The diagnosis is best made by needle aspiration with specimens sent for histology and TB culture (smears may he negative)
   - Open biopsy can be performed but may result in a fistula or severe scar formation (excisional Bx occasionally required)

2 **Genito-urinary**
   - Hematogenous spread following primary TB can involve any portion of the GU tract
   - Presentation of urinary tract disease varies from an asymptomatic finding on X-ray to non-specific symptoms and diagnostic work up includes

  - Urinalysis with pyuria, hematuria, negative routine cultures
  - Three early morning urine cultures for TB
  - IVP
  - Biopsy of tissues including testes, epididymis or fallopian tubes
- Genital TB in males most often involves the epididymis but orchitis and prostatitis may develop
- Female involvement occurs more commonly with disease of the fallopian tubes and endometrium resulting in infertility, pelvic pains and menstrual abnormalities

3 **Gastrointestinal**

- Any portion of the GI tract may be involved with the terminal ileum and caecum most common, often simulating Crohn's disease
- Colonic disease can present with bloody diarrhea or a perianal fistula

4 **Spinal TB**

- Spinal TB (Pott's disease) affects the lower thoracic and upper abdominal vertebrae in adults but the upper thoracic spine in children
- Early X-ray changes include narrowing of the disk space and irregularity of the vertebral end plates
- Advanced disease results in collapse of the vertebral bodies with the characteristic gibbus deformity and paravertebral abscess formation
- The accompanying 'cold' abscess may present as a chest wall mass, psoas abscess, or paraplegia due to spinal cord compression
- CT can demonstrate the bony abnormalities, involvement of the spinal canal as well as peripheral rim enhancement and low attenuation center of the associated abscess
- Diagnosis can be made by aspiration of the abscess or bone biopsy

5 **Tuberculous peritonitis**
- Typically presents with ascites and rarely with intestinal obstruction, the classically described 'doughy abdomen' uncommonly seen
- Ascitic fluid will have the same characteristics as pleural fluid but AFB smears and cultures have a low yield
- Peritoneal needle biopsy can be done but laparoscopy has the highest yield, is low risk and can be performed under a local anesthetic

6 **Upper airways disease**
- Usually a complication of advanced cavitary TB with the larynx, pharynx and epiglottis affected
- Suspect this in the presence of hoarseness or dysphagia

7 **Pericardial tuberculosis**
- Presents acutely or subacutely with chest pains, fever +/− friction rub, effusion, tamponade, with local extension resulting in myocarditis, endarteritis of the coronary arteries
- Fluid is exudative, often hemorrhagic, with positive cultures in about 30% of patients but pericardial biopsy has a higher diagnostic yield
- Constrictive pericarditis and calcifications may be sequelae of treated disease

8 **CNS disease**
- Meningitis is the most common CNS complication and is particularly seen with miliary, progressive primary disease and AIDS
  - Diagnosis made by positive smears of CSF (10–20%) or positive cultures (50–80%), in association with a lymphocytosis, low glucose and elevated protein
- Tuberculoma

TUBERCULOUS EMPYEMA

Definition: Grossly purulent fluid in the pleural space that is smear and culture positive for tuberculosis and caused by

1. Progression of a primary tuberculous effusion
2. Reactivation of a remote pleural infection
   - Which was inadequately treated
   - Following therapeutic pneumothorax treatment in the pre-chemotherapy era
   - Following pneumonectomy for tuberculosis

- The fluid has a neutrophil predominance often with WBC $> 100000\,mm^3$, a glucose $< 20\,mg/100\,mL$ and pH < 7.2

Clinically, there is usually a history of remote tuberculosis often having never been adequately treated with drugs

- Patients are often asymptomatic for years due to the empyema being 'walled off', but presentations can include
  - Systemic symptoms of fevers, weight loss, general debility
  - Internal rupture into the tracheobronchial tree with cough and sputum due to a bronchopleural fistula (BPF)
  - External rupture with a chest wall mass and 'empyema necessitas'

Radiologic features

1. An opacified hemithorax with extensive pleural thickening and calcification which may remain stable for 30 years or longer
2. A new air–fluid level in a previous 'fibrothorax', representing the development of a BPF
3. New airspace disease in the opposite lung representing bronchogenic spread from a BPF
4. Thickening of ribs over the empyema due to subperiosteal new bone formation
5. New chest wall mass developing over a 'fibrothorax'
6. CT demonstration of a fluid collection within a calcified 'fibrothorax'
7. In the absence of calcifications, the appearance is that of a non-specific loculated pleural collection

MILIARY DISEASE

Definition: Widespread hematogenous dissemination from an established focus of tuberculosis, either progressive primary disease, or, more often activation of a previously dormant focus

Clinically, hematogenous seeding may occur any time after the primary infection, with the focus of seeding being pulmonary or extrapulmonary

- Miliary spread is usually seen at the extremes of age or in immunocompromised patients, especially HIV-infected
- Onset of disease is insidious with an average of 6 weeks between dissemination and clinical recognition of disease which can include
  - Systemic features of fevers, night sweats and weight loss which may be accompanied by non-specific respiratory symptoms
  - Wasting syndrome resembling metastatic cancer
  - Respiratory failure from ARDS
  - Lymphocytic meningitis
  - Ascites
  - Hepatosplenomegaly and lymphadenopathy
  - Choroid tubercles on fundoscopic exam

PPD may be positive or negative, with anergy in approximately 50% of cases

Hematologic abnormalities include anemia, leucopenia or leucocytosis, thrombocytopenia or thrombocytosis

Radiologic findings

1. 'Classic' bilateral diffuse micronodular pattern with 2–3 mm opacities usually evenly distributed, but asymmetric in ~15% of cases
2. Non-specific interstitial lung disease
3. Coalescent opacities progressing to ARDS
4. CT scan may show 1–2 mm nodules when chest X-rays are normal

5 Nodular thickening of the intralobular septae can resemble lymphangitic cancer
6 Associated abnormalities can include mediastinal lymphadenopathy (90% in children versus 10% in adults), pleural effusion, pneumothorax, parenchymal cavitation, evidence of old tuberculosis
7 Positive gallium scan can be seen with normal chest X-rays
8 Resolution within 2 to 6 months of therapy

Diagnostic Workup

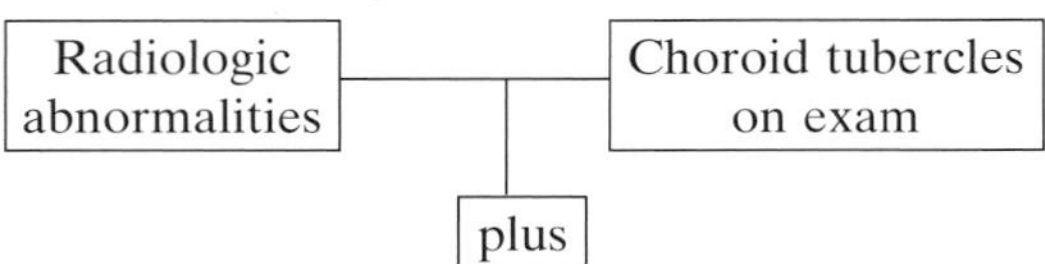

⊕ Sputum or BAL smears (approximately 25%) and cultures (50–75%)

or

Bronchoscopy and transbronchial biopsy (yield 80–90%)

or

⊕ Urine smears (approximately 5%) and cultures (25–50%)

or

⊕ Smears, cultures and histopathology from enlarged superficial nodes, liver or bone marrow

'REMOTE TB' – HEMOPTYSIS

1 TB reactivation, e.g. Rasmussen's aneurysm in a cavitary wall
2 Bronchiectasis
3 Superinfection with atypical mycobacteria
4 Mycetoma in an old tuberculous cavity
5 Broncholithiasis
6 Scar carcinoma
7 Laryngeal TB
8 Tracheobronchial TB

9 Bronchoaortic fistula secondary to active pulmonary TB or tuberculous aortitis

'REMOTE TB' – COMPLICATIONS

1 Reactivation TB in the lungs or at an extrapulmonary site, including miliary disease
2 Development of granulomatous or fibrosing mediastinitis (see p. 508)
3 Colonization and infection with atypical mycobacteria in old tuberculous cavities
4 Subacute necrotizing pulmonary aspergillosis
5 Aspergilloma in an old tuberculous cavity or bronchiectatic cyst
6 Development of 'scar cancer'
7 Hemoptysis (see above)
8 Pneumonia in an area of bronchiectasis
9 Undiagnosed HIV infection
10 Addison's disease and wasting from adrenal destruction

DIAGNOSTIC TESTS FOR ACTIVE TB

1 **Chest X-rays** are readily accessible and results immediately available but not a very reliable test for the diagnosis of TB due to lack of specificity
   - Sensitivity is variable as 10% of individuals with HIV infection and a similar number of recently infected close contacts may have active TB yet normal X-rays

   Radiologic signs suggestive of activity include
   - Unilateral or bilateral airspace consolidation, usually involving the apical-posterior segments of the upper lobes or superior segments of lower lobes
   - Cavitation – thin or thick-walled
   - Endobronchial spread manifest as 5–10 mm acinar nodules
   - Lymphadenopathy involving the mediastinum or hilar areas
   - Miliary pattern

2 **Microbiologic tests – essential for accurate diagnosis**

- Smears of respiratory secretions provide an index of the degree of contagiousness
  - Sputum should be sent for AFB smear and mycobacterial cultures, with early morning specimens preferred as the sputum is more concentrated and there are no food particles which can cause false positive tests
  - 6000–10 000 organisms/mL are needed to see 3 AFB on a slide
  - Microscopic exam of an acid-fast smear will have a sensitivity varying from 20–80%, averaging 55%
  - Multiple specimens have a higher yield than a single specimen
  - Positive smears can reflect non-tuberculous mycobacteria, the frequency being geographic dependent
  - In patients who are ultimately proven to have smear-positive disease
    - A single sputum smear will be positive in 50%
    - At least one of two specimens will be positive in 70%
    - At least one of three will be positive in 80–90%
  - It can take up to 6 specimens to obtain one positive smear result, the most efficient method being to obtain 3 specimens
- Sputum induction using hypertonic (3%) saline should be ordered if sputum is unavailable or the initial specimens are smear negative
  - Optimal yield is obtained using ultrasonic nebulizers that deliver 5 mL/minute of an aerosolized solution for a duration of 15 minutes
  - Sputum induction has a similar yield to broncoscopy and gastric aspiration but is strongly recommended because this method is preferred by patients, has no risk, considerably lower cost and produces less risk of nosocomial transmission
- Bronchoscopy with a yield of 75–80%

- Gastric aspirates can be performed, particularly if expectorated sputum is unavailable e.g. small children, demented elderly patients

3 **Mycobacterial culture** is the gold standard for diagnosis and yield increases with the number of specimens sent, maximum efficiency being three
- 100 organisms/mL are required to grow one colony on culture
- Traditionally, Lowenstein Jensen, Middlebrook agar, or other solid media were used, requiring 6–8 weeks to obtain a result
- Liquid radiometric broth media are presently used which take only 2 weeks
- Cultures have an 80% sensitivity with 20% of patients being culture (and smear)-negative
- 1–2% incidence of false positive cultures is seen secondary to a sputum mix-up or cross contamination in the laboratory

4 **Extrapulmonary TB** can be diagnosed by needle aspirate or biopsy, with specimens sent for histologic examination as well as mycobacterial culture

5 **CT scan** should not be done routinely but can contribute as follows
- Clinical suspicion of TB with equivocal, (e.g. subtle parenchymal infiltrate), or normal chest X-ray, (e.g. miliary disease)
- Detection of cavitation not apparent on chest X-ray
- Detection of lymphadenopathy, the nodes characterized by central areas of low attenuation and peripheral rim enhancement on contrast CT
- Diagnosis of fibrosing mediastinitis
- Detection of endotracheal/endobronchial disease as well as a bronchopleural fistula
- Tuberculous pleurisy where a pleural effusion in association with abnormalities not detected on chest X-ray, e.g. parenchymal infiltrate which may cavitate,

lymphadenopathy, rib or vertebral body involvement, may suggest the diagnosis
- Demonstration of a mycetoma in a tuberculous cavity
- Demonstration of acinar nodules or branching centrilobular opacities, i.e. 'tree in-bud'

6 **Polymerase chain reaction (PCR)** or other nucleic acid amplification tests can give a result in less than four hours
- Better sensitivity than AFB smears but not as sensitive as cultures
- In smear-negative sputum specimens that prove to be culture positive, PCR will be positive in 50–60% while in smear-positive specimens, the sensitivity of PCR is >95%
- Specificity is excellent with very few false positives

Useful applications of PCR include
- A positive AFB smear
- A positive mycobacterial culture
- Confirmation of the presence of *Mycobacterium tuberculosis* in pathologic specimens where caseating granulomas are seen, ZN stain is negative and biopsy specimens were not sent for culture (sensitivity >50%)
- Clinical suspicion of miliary TB with negative sputum smears and positive PCR may avoid an invasive procedure until a therapeutic response is assessed
- Infiltrate in a smoker with negative AFB smears, possible carcinoma but tuberculosis a possibility

7 **Serologic testing** has suboptimal sensitivity and specificity

8 **DNA fingerprinting** is a new technique that can identify individual strains of *M. tuberculosis*, but is a research tool to study the transmission of TB in different settings and has little clinical application at present

TUBERCULIN SKIN TESTING

Tuberculin skin testing is a very poor test for the diagnosis of disease

1 Sensitivity is only 70–80% as 20–30% of those at the time of diagnosis with active disease will have a false negative test
2 Specificity is poor because tuberculin tests are likely to be positive in a high percentage of populations most infected with TB
3 Reasonable to wait 8 weeks from the time of first exposure before evaluating immunocompetent contacts as tuberculin skin test conversion can take 3–7 weeks

Indications

1 Identify new infections in those exposed, e.g. contacts of active cases, workers with occupational exposure
2 Identify latent TB infections in individuals at increased risk of reactivation
   - HIV infection
   - Silicosis
   - Renal failure, especially if dialysis is required
   - Diabetics
   - Patients on immunosuppressive therapy especially prednisone at 20 mg daily or greater
3 Epidemiologic research

Mantoux Technique

- Intradermal injection of 0.1 cc of 5 tuberculin units of ppd on the volar (or palmar) aspect of the forearm
- Readings should be 48–72 hours later
- Transverse diameter of the induration should be measured and recorded in mm with interpretation of a test as positive with the following

5 mm – TB contacts
– HIV positive individuals
– Patients with an abnormal chest X-ray consistent with inactive TB

10 mm – Foreign-born in TB endemic areas
– Patients with other risk factor for true infection, e.g. i.v. drug abuser

- Risk factor for reactivation of disease if infected, e.g. silicosis
- Members of the general population in areas with low rates of tuberculosis where the rates of non-tuberculous mycobacteria are also low, e.g. Northern Europe, Northern USA and Canada

15 mm – Healthy members of the general population in areas of the world where tuberculosis is uncommon but non-tuberculous mycobacteria are common, e.g. Southern USA, some Caribbean islands and Southern European countries

Increased Reaction on Repeat Tuberculin Testing

1 Non-specific increase due to random variation in administration, reading and biologic response resulting in an increase of no more than 5 mm

2 Booster phenomenon where an increased tuberculin reaction of 6 mm or greater is seen when retesting occurs in the absence of a new infection and is due to recall of waned immunity
   - Boosting is a non-specific response to any prior mycobacterial exposure and can be seen with remote TB infection, BCG vaccination, or non-tuberculous mycobacteria
   - Effect is maximal if the interval between tests is 1–3 weeks but the booster effect can be seen up to one year following a first negative test

3 Conversion is defined as the development of new delayed hypersensitivity to mycobacterial antigens following new infection with *M. tuberculosis*, atypical mycobacteria or BCG vaccination
   - The interval from infection to conversion is 8 weeks or less and results in an increase of >6 mm induration

Boosting *vs.* Conversion (Reaction Increase > 6 mm)

1 An increased reaction seen in 1–3 weeks where no exposure occurred is boosting

2 An increased reaction following BCG, close contact with a highly contagious case or following significant exposure during an outbreak is conversion
3 In general the larger the increase in reaction, the more likely it is to be conversion but the best way to distinguish remains the clinical situation
4 If an individual is to have repeated periodic tuberculin testing, e.g. health care workers, then a baseline two-step test should be done upon hiring to exclude the possibility of a booster effect
   - A second tuberculin skin test is done within 3 weeks of an initial negative result, permitting detection of boosting related to BCG vaccination or remote exposure
   - Subsequent tests will be limited to those individuals without boosting, permitting more reliable interpretation of positive results
5 For the low risk (healthy) casual contacts of active cases, it would be preferable to wait until 8 weeks after the end of exposure and perform a single tuberculin skin test *vs.* testing at 4–8 weeks after exposure and repeated 12 weeks after exposure
   - The latter results in falsely diagnosing tuberculin conversion among those who actually manifest the booster phenomenon

ESTIMATION OF CONTAGIOUSNESS

1 Patients with pulmonary parenchymal or laryngeal tuberculosis who generate aerosols of tiny droplets laden with viable TB bacteria
   - The droplets dry rapidly with the smallest ones remaining suspended in air for hours
   - With rare exception extrapulmonary TB is not contagious
2 Cough frequency – more cough translating into greater

contagion, with estimates of as many as 3000 infectious nuclei per cough

3 More extensive pulmonary disease radiologically
4 Smear-positive patients are 4 times more contagious than individuals who are smear-negative, typically those with cavitary or laryngeal tuberculosis, the latter being common in developing countries but rare in North America
   - After starting treatment, patients who were initially smear-negative generally become non-contagious after ~2 weeks of treatment
   - Patients who were smear-positive generally remain contagious as long as the smears and cultures are positive, with only a minority of such patients transiently exhibiting positive sputum smears but negative cultures
   - More than 90% of all smear-positive specimens from initially smear-positive patients will be culture-positive while receiving therapy and are therefore still contagious
   - Among initially smear-positive patients, 50–70% will be culture-positive after 4 weeks of treatment and 5–10% will be culture-positive after 12 weeks of treatment
5 Individuals who are untreated, on ineffective treatment or are non-compliant with their treatment
6 Younger individuals are more contagious
7 Intimacy and duration of contact with the infectious case, especially crowding in poorly ventilated areas

HOW TO CONDUCT A CONTACT INVESTIGATION

'Concentric Circle Approach'

Step 1: Assess the contagiousness of the index case

- Index case is potentially contagious with pulmonary

parenchymal or laryngeal TB not on therapy, particularly when the patient is smear positive and coughing

Step 2: Identify the close contacts

- Defined as persons with daily, or almost daily, contact of several hours
- All persons in the same household are automatically considered close contacts
- Of particular concern are contacts who are very young (0–4 years) or immunocompromised such as HIV-infected

Step 3: Investigation of close contacts

- All close contacts should be tuberculin tested
- Tuberculin reactors should have medical evaluation and a chest X-ray
- Young children are at risk to develop TB meningitis or miliary tuberculosis very rapidly
  - All children under 6 should have medical evaluation even if the tuberculin skin test is negative
  - They should then be treated for latent TB infection for three months even if tuberculin negative
  - Should then be retested and if still negative, treatment stopped
- Close contacts who are immunocompromised should be considered for immediate chemoprophylaxis, after active disease is excluded, even if skin test is negative

Step 4: Reassess contagiousness of index case

- If any among these closest contacts (the 'first circle') have active disease or if the prevalence of TB infection (ppd > 5 mm) is greater than might be expected for that group of individuals, then transmission is considered to have occurred and the index case was contagious

Step 5: Extension of contact investigation

- If transmission has occurred within the 'first circle', the contact investigation is extended to the 'second circle'

- This includes those in regular contact but lasting only a few hours per week, e.g. frequently involves the school, workplace and regular social events such as church or social clubs
- All contacts should be tuberculin tested
- Tuberculin reactors and small children should be managed as per Step 3

Step 6: Assessment of transmission and further extension of contact investigation

- If evidence of transmission is seen in the 'second circle' then the contact investigation should be extended even further
- The 'third circle' includes all persons in contact with the index case, e.g. those with a single exposure for only a few hours and these contacts should be tuberculin tested
- All contacts with a positive tuberculin test (5+ mm) as well as young children or immunocompromised with negative tuberculin tests should have medical evaluation and be managed as per Step 3

TB Contacts in Institutions (see algorithm)

Risk of infection to exposed health care workers and patients varies with

1. Infectivity of the source case
2. Type and extent of contact
3. Delay in isolation and treatment
4. Adequacy of isolation measures
5. Immune status of the contacts

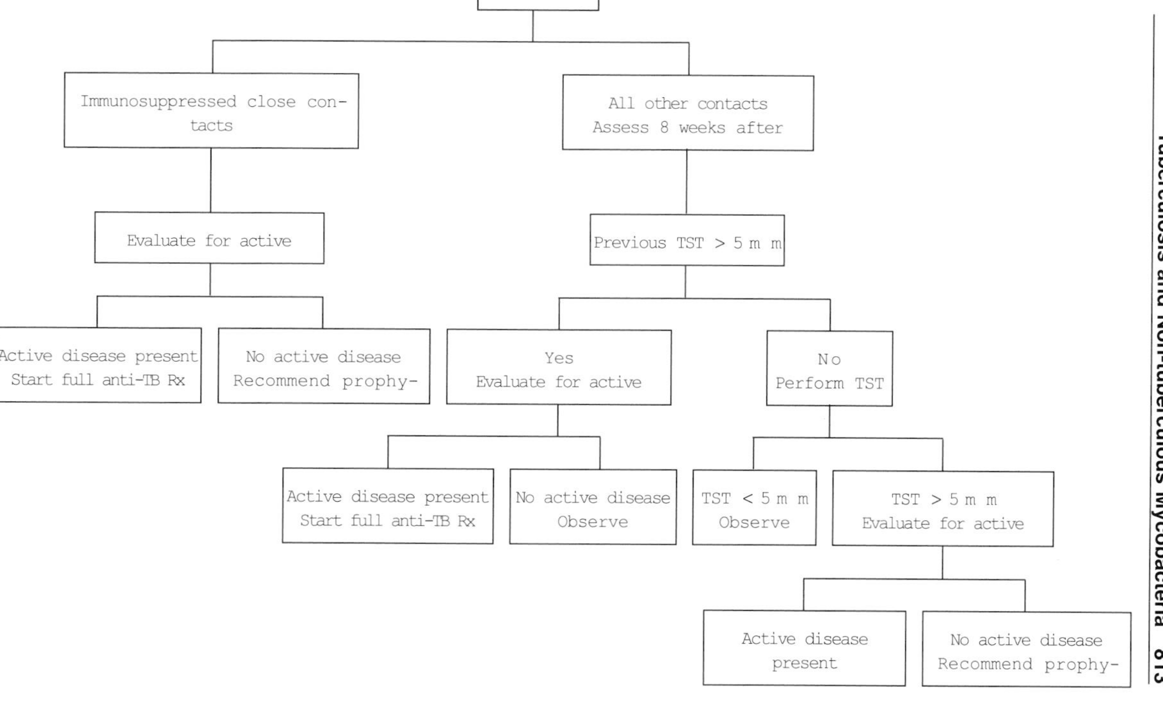

'Tuberculosis: 11. Nosocomial disease' – reprinted from, by permission of the publisher, CMAJ, 1999; **161** (10), pp. 1271–1277

BCG VACCINATION

BCG vaccine is an attenuated strain of *Mycobacterium bovis* developed in 1923 by Calmette and Guérin of the Institut Pasteur in Paris, given to more than 500 million individuals over the past 50 years

Intradermal Route

Used to protect against the development of the disease tuberculosis following infection although it does not prevent acquisition of primary TB infection

- 90% of recipients will develop a positive tuberculin test at 8 weeks following intradermal vaccination with a protective efficacy of
  - 80–90% against TB meningitis or miliary forms in infants
  - 0–80% (in different studies) against pulmonary TB when given to older children or adults
- Tuberculin reactions wane steadily over the next 10 years with
  - 20–50% positive after 5 years
  - 0–25% positive after 10 years or more

Complications of BCG include

1. Superficial scar in most recipients
2. Ulceration can be seen and persist with purulent drainage for 2–3 months
3. Lymphadenopathy/lymphadenitis is common and nodes may suppurate with purulent drainage seen in 1–2%
4. Disseminated BCG

Intravesical Installation

Treatment of bladder cancer by intravesical installation, the most common indication presently in North America

Complications include

1. Granulomatous infection of the testes, epididymis or prostate, pathologically identical to *M. tuberculosis* and usually self-limited

2 Disseminated disease with a miliary pattern on chest X-ray and rare reports of cavitary pulmonary disease

Diagnosis of Disseminated BCG

Rarely follows intravesical installation but seen in immunocompromised patients, usually in immunocompromised infants, with the most common cause being HIV infection due to vertical transmission from HIV positive mothers

- Results in failure to thrive, lethargy, fever and wasting with chest X-rays showing a miliary pattern

Diagnostic features

1 High index of suspicion with the diagnosis considered in anyone who has received BCG by any route in the previous 3–6 months
2 Biopsy of affected organ with caseating granulomas
3 Positive cultures looking for the BCG substrain of *M. bovis*
4 Positive PCR (BCG is part of the *M. tuberculosis* complex)

CULTURE-NEGATIVE ACTIVE TUBERCULOSIS

In recent years approximately 20% of all cases of tuberculosis reported in the United States were culture-negative

- Most common reason for culture-negative disease is extrapulmonary involvement which is diagnosed clinically or radiologically
- Biopsies may be done but cultures are not sent at the time of biopsy
- Culture-negative pulmonary disease is also commonly reported and can occur because
  - Insufficient cultures are done (none or only one)
    - If there is minimal disease, 3 cultures may be required in order to detect one that is positive
  - Disease is so minimal that the number of bacteria present in sputum or respiratory secretions cannot be detected by current laboratory procedures

Diagnosis of culture-negative disease

1 The radiologic pattern should be typical of tuberculosis, i.e. apical-posterior segments of the upper lobes or superior segments of lower lobes
  - Usually non-cavitary since cavitary disease tends to have a high bacillary load and is usually culture-positive (if not smear-positive)

2 Without therapy there should be a slow worsening over 2–3 months

3 No response to usual antibiotics
  - Avoid quinolones if TB is suspected as this may result in a partial response as well as the development of resistance

4 Improvement with anti-TB therapy using 3 to 4 drugs
  - Important if active TB is suspected not to give one drug as this may result in a partial response and contribute to resistance

NON-TUBERCULOUS MYCOBACTERIA (NTM)

Epidemiology

Worldwide in distribution but the incidence and specific species are dependent on geographic locations

- Organisms are present in water, soil, dust as well as fish and other animals
- No evidence of person-to-person transmission by epidemiologic studies, skin testing or DNA fingerprinting, infection acquired by inhalation, aspiration, ingestion (AIDS patients), instrument contamination or traumatic inoculation (skin, joint and soft tissues infections)

Pulmonary disease is caused by

- **M. avium* complex, (MAC includes *M. avium*, *M. intracellulare*, and *M. scrofulaceum*)
  - In the United States, responsible for 80% of all pulmonary NTM disease
  - Overall incidence – 1.1 per 100 000

- **M. kansasei*
  - In the central United States, responsible for approximately 10% of all cases

All others account for 10% of all cases in the United States including

- *M. xenopi*
  - Uncommon in North America but second most common NTM in Western Europe and the most common pathogenic NTM in Southern England
  - Found almost exclusively in hot water, particularly in recirculating hot water systems in large buildings and grows best at 40–47°C
  - Thought to be acquired from inhalation of bioaerosols ? role of showers
  - Joint and disseminated disease are described in immunocompromised patients
- *M. malmoense*
  - Uncommon in North America but rapidly increasing importance in Europe, being the second most common pathogenic NTM in many European countries
  - Commonly associated with underlying pulmonary disease including prior TB, COPD and lung cancer
- *M. szulgai*
  - Rare pathogen (still only case reports) and described to cause progressive pulmonary disease with cavitation as well as joint, skin, lymphatic and disseminated disease
  - Isolation should be considered pathogenic
- *M. simiae*
  - More commonly isolated but rarely a pulmonary pathogen
- *M. bovis/BCG*
  - Very rarely described
  - Transmission from diseased animals to humans reported, therefore seen in veterinarians, abattoir workers
- Rapid growers – *M. chelonae/abscessus/fortuitum*
  - Rarely are pulmonary pathogens

  - Somewhat more common as causes of soft tissue infection

Lymphadenitis due to NTM is seen in young children but rare in adolescents and adults except in HIV infected individuals
- By contrast, 90% of mycobacterial lymphadenitis in adults is caused by *M. tuberculosis*
- *M. avium* is responsible for about 80% of cases with *M. scrofulaceum* causing most of the remainder in the United States but *M. malmoense* increasingly described in northern Europe

Cutaneous disease is most often caused by *M. chelonae/abscessus/fortuitum*, *M. marinum* ('swimming pool or fish tank granuloma'), *M. ulcerans*

Bone and joint infections are seen with a wide range of species while **disseminated disease** is seen in immunocompromised patients with and without AIDS

High Risk Groups

NTM are opportunistic infections that occur in individuals with underlying pulmonary or systemic disease with only about 20% of patients having no documented underlying condition

1. Airways disease
   - COPD
   - Bronchiectasis
2. Pulmonary parenchymal disease
   - Fibrosis secondary to radiation, pneumoconiosis, e.g. silicosis, UIP
   - Bullous disease
   - Lung cancer
   - Remote tuberculosis or mycotic infection
   - Repeated aspiration, particularly the rapid growers
   - Sarcoid
3. Systemic diseases
   - Malignancy, especially hairy cell leukemia
   - Diabetes mellitus
   - Alcoholism
   - Post-gastrectomy
   - Immunosuppression, especially HIV infection

ISOLATION OF NTM – SIGNIFICANCE

Generally when a NTM is isolated from a normally sterile site such as lymph node or other tissue biopsy, there can be little doubt that the NTM is a pathogen

- However NTM are frequently isolated from respiratory secretions in individuals without any evidence of progressive pulmonary disease
- Certain NTM organisms are more, and others less likely, when isolated, to be the cause of progressive pulmonary disease

Usually a pulmonary pathogen when isolated

- *M. kansasei* – 70–80% of the time
- *M. xenopi* – almost all the time
- *M. szulgai* – almost all the time although rarely isolated
- *M. malmoensi* – situation not as well clarified as experience is more limited but appears to be pathogenic 70–80% of the time when isolated
- *M. bovis* – very rarely isolated but when present almost always means there is disease
- *BCG* – very rarely isolated but when it is there is generally pulmonary disease

Sometimes a pulmonary pathogen when isolated

- *M. avium* or avium complex – results vary between series but 20–50% of the time will represent a pathogen
- *M. chelonai/abscessus/fortuitum* – much less data available

Rarely a pulmonary pathogen when isolated

- *M. gordonae* – commonly isolated as colonizer or lab contaminant and may be a contaminant in the hospital water supply or water used in the laboratory – resulting in pseudo-outbreaks
- *M. simiae* – uncommonly isolated; in one series only 10% of isolates were associated with disease
- *M. marinum* – almost never isolated from respiratory secretions; no reports of pulmonary disease
- *M. terrae* – has been described as a contaminant in

clinical specimens and has contaminated hospital water system; no reports of pulmonary disease

ACTIVE INFECTION *VS.* COLONIZATION

Clinical criteria

1 Compatible symptoms with cough and fatigue being most common
2 Exclusion of other pulmonary disease which could be responsible

Radiologic criteria

Progressive pulmonary disease which can take the form of

- Infiltrates +/– nodules
- Nodules
- Cavitary disease
- Multifocal bronchiectasis +/– nodules on HRCT

Positive cultures without radiologic change over years indicates colonization

Bacteriologic criteria

1 Three sputa or bronchial washings over 12 months with
   - Three positive cultures but negative AFB smears
   - Two positive cultures and one positive AFB smear

or

2 One bronchial washing available and
   - Positive culture with 2+, 3+ or 4+ growth
   - Positive culture with 2+, 3+ or 4+ AFB smear

or

3 Tissue diagnosis
   - Lung biopsy growing NTM
   - Granulomatous inflammation and/or AFB on smear with sputum or bronchial washings positive on culture in any numbers
   - Growth from a normally sterile extrapulmonary site

CLINICAL-RADIOLOGIC SYNDROMES (NON-HIV)

1 **Classical**

- In non-HIV infected individuals the course of disease is very slow and typically has been present for years although this may be recognized only in restrospect
- For individual cases, the clinical picture, radiologic features as well as the gross and microscopic pathology are similar to and usually indistinguishable from tuberculosis
- Clinical symptoms include
  - Cough as the most common and earliest feature, initially non-productive with purulent sputum being present in later stages
  - Fever, anorexia and weight loss are late-stage symptoms
  - Shortness of breath may be an important feature when disease is advanced
  - Hemoptysis is rare
  - May present as a wasting syndrome, particularly in the elderly
- Patients often have the traditional predisposing factors
- Most often caused by *M. kansasei* and *M. avium-intracellulare*
- The radiologic features are similar to *M. tuberculosis* with
  - Apical and posterior segmental opacities in the upper lobes
  - Apical pleural thickening
  - Cavitation in about 85% of cases
  - Bronchogenic spread is common with resulting acinar nodules
  - Scarring and volume loss result
  - Disease may be unilateral or bilateral

2 **Non-classical**

- Clinically 80% of cases are seen in females, usually over age 70

- Predisposing conditions are rare
- Constitutional symptoms are uncommon
- Patients may be asymptomatic or present with the insidious onset of non-specific respiratory symptoms
- Radiologic features include
  - Patchy and often bilateral interstitial or alveolar opacities without the apical pattern of reactivation tuberculosis
  - Right middle lobe and lingular disease are most often described
  - Infiltrates are often nodular with associated bronchiectasis

3 **Nodule(s)**

- Patients are usually asymptomatic and sent to surgery for elimination of a neoplastic lesion
- Radiologically there are single or multiple nodules

4 **Aspiration pneumonia**

- Seen in patients at risk for recurrent aspiration, e.g. achalasia with aspirated material, particularly lipid, thought to be an etiologic factor
- The organisms are almost always *M. fortuitum* or *M. chelonae*
- Radiologic features include
  - Confluent bilateral alveolar opacities in 'aspiration segments'
  - A dilated esophagus from achalasia

5 **Disseminated disease**

- Seen in immunocompromised patients on steroids, other immunosuppressives and lymphoproliferative disorders especially hairy cell leukemia
- Blood cultures are often positive
- Systemic symptoms are more prominent than pulmonary
- Radiologic features include
  - Hilar/mediastinal lymphadenopathy
  - Focal or diffuse infiltrates
  - Nodules
  - Cavitation

Differences from Tuberculosis

Radiologic findings

- Pleural effusion, pneumothorax and lymphadenopathy are rare
- Anterior segments of the upper lobes are more commonly involved
- Often less bronchogenic spread but more contiguous spread of disease with focal pleural thickening over the involved areas of lung
- Cavities are often thin-walled, e.g. *M. kansasei*
- *M. avium* may cause multifocal bronchiectasis with clusters of small nodules on HRCT
- Frequent presence of pre-existing airway or parenchymal lung disease
- Lung disease is rare in children and therefore calcified residuals are not seen in adults

Clinical findings

- Hematogenous dissemination after primary infection is rare in normal hosts
- No evidence of person-to-person transmission
- Fevers are uncommon compared to *M. tuberculosis*
- Isolation of organisms in sputum does not necessarily indicate disease
- Whites are more commonly affected than other racial groups
- Symptoms of infection are thought to be due to primary infection and not reactivation
- Underlying chronic lung disease is often present
- Family contacts are not infected

DIAGNOSIS OF SPECIFIC AGENTS

1 Most NTM will grow on solid media (Lowenstein-Jensen) or liquid media (Bactec)
    - Some NTM e.g. *M. avium*, grow more rapidly than *M. tuberculosis* in liquid media and will be isolated in 7–10 days, with rapid growers present within 3–5 days

2 Formerly organisms were identified by their morphology and color of colonies when grown on solid media, hence the old terms photochromogens, scotochromogens, etc.
   - The gold standard presently is high pressure liquid chromatography (HPLC)
3 PCR is a rapid test to distinguish most NTM from *M. tuberculosis*, although *M. bovis* will give a positive PCR result
   - PCR probes are being developed for other species of NTM
4 Skin testing is of little clinical usefulness even though tests have been developed for *M. avium* complex (PPD-B), *M. kansasei* (PPD-Y) and *M. scrofulaceum* (PPD-G)
   - Skin test antigens are not well standardized and cross-reactivity is seen between species

Drug Sensitivity Testing

Limited utility for guiding therapy for NTM because of little data correlating the *in vitro* reactions with an individual patient's response to therapy

Drug sensitivity testing for NTM should be done in referral laboratories only, must be done using solid media and therefore requires 4–6 weeks for results

Many referral laboratories will perform drug sensitivity testing on NTM only if requested by the treating physician and/or there is clinical resistance to first line therapy with failure of standard treatment

M. avium Complex (MAC)

MAC includes *M. avium*, *M. intracellulare* and *M. scrofulaceum*, which are commonly isolated as colonizers in patients with underlying pulmonary disease

- Non-specific respiratory symptoms are accompanied by fever and weight loss in about $^{1}/_{3}$ of patients
- The typical patient does not appear acutely ill and features of chronic diseases, e.g. anemia and hypoalbuminemia, are often absent
- The natural history of lung disease is variable in HIV-

negative patients, varying from indolent to rapidly progressive
- *M. avium* is difficult to treat with mortality increasing in the elderly, immunocompromised and those with underlying disease

Clinical presentations include

1 *Upper lobe cavitary disease simulating *M. tuberculosis* clinically and radiologically
   - Seen in older adults who smoked, frequently with associated alcohol abuse
   - Underlying lung disease is often present including cancer with or without radiotherapy, bronchiectasis, cystic fibrosis, sarcoid
   - Disease is usually progressive if untreated

2 Isolated RML or lingular disease or bilateral nodular/interstitial disease in an upper lobe distribution
   - Multifocal bronchiectasis/nodules are often present on HRCT
   - The above is seen in older white females with no underlying lung disease or previously unrecognized bronchiectasis
   - There is much slower radiologic progression than seen in patients with cavitary disease although progressive disease occurs both radiologically and clinically

3 Solitary lung nodule, with surgical resection usually being curative and further therapy unnecessary

4 Dissemination occurs rarely in the non-AIDS population

5 Lymphadenitis is rare in adults in the absence of HIV infection with children aged 1–5 usually involved, being the most common manifestation of NTM in children
   - Lymph nodes are usually in the head and neck region, unilateral, non-tender, and rarely associated with systemic symptoms
   - They may rapidly enlarge and/or rupture forming a sinus tract with prolonged drainage, the latter occurring as a complication of incision and drainage or incision for surgical biopsy

- Chest X-rays are usually negative and PPD testing is usually negative or weakly positive due to cross-reactivity although some patients may be PPD positive and TB must be ruled out

M. kansasei

Isolated from soil and water with substantial geographic variation, most cases being found in the Midwest and Southwest U.S.

- Pulmonary disease is the most frequent clinical presentation with adult white men being primarily but not solely involved
- Underlying lung disease is often present, particularly old TB or bullous COPD
- Clinical symptoms and chest X-rays resemble tuberculosis
- *M. kansasei* is relatively easily treated with low mortality
- The natural history of untreated disease is progression clinically and radiologically with persistent sputum positivity

Radid Growers – *M. fortuitum, M. chelonae, M. abscessus*

The majority of clinical disease is community-acquired, most often manifest as soft tissue infection, but nosocomial infections are seen

- As a group they are the most common nosocomial NTM, water being the usual source although they have been isolated from soil and house dust
- *M. abscessus* is responsible for about 80% of cases, and *M. fortuitum* about 15%
- MAC is seen concurrently in about 15% of patients with *M. abscessus*

Cutaneous disease can follow penetrating injury with local abscess formation or can occur as a nosocomial infection

- Examples of the latter include post-op wound infection,

e.g. mammoplasty or sternal infection following cardiac surgery, post-injection abscesses or infection of in-dwelling catheters, diagnosis being made by culture of drainage material or tissue

Clinical pulmonary disease

1 Elderly females without underlying pulmonary or systemic disease is most common
   - There is often a prolonged time course from the onset of symptoms to disease diagnosis as chest X-rays are frequently interpreted as chronic scarring
   - X-rays reveal multilobar patchy interstitial or mixed interstitial-airspace infiltrates with upper lobe predominance and cavitation in about 15% of cases
   - HRCT additionally often shows cylindrical bronchiectasis and multiple small nodules similar to that seen in some patients with MAC
2 Pulmonary infection in patients with underlying lung disease, most often old TB but also bronchiectasis, cystic fibrosis, lipoid pneumonia
3 Esophageal disease, e.g. achalasia with chronic vomiting, is seen in about 5% of patients
   - Fever and leucocytosis are accompanied by bilateral alveolar infiltrates on chest X-ray

The presenting features are non-specific respiratory symptoms, often attributed to bronchitis or bronchiectasis, occasionally accompanied by systemic complaints

- The course of disease is usually indolent and slowly progressive but a more fulminent course can occur, especially in those patients with gastro-esophageal disease

Fraser R.S., Muller N.L., Colman N., Paré P.D. (1999) *Diagnosis of Diseases of the Chest* 4th Edn., WB Saunders.

Naidich, D.P., Zerhouni, E.A., Siegelman, S.S. (1998) *Computed Tomography and Magnetic Resonance of the Thorax*, 3rd edn. New York: Raven Press.

Baum, G.L., Crapo, J.D., Celli, B.R., Karlinsky, J.B. (eds) (1997) *Textbook of Pulmonary Diseases*, 6th edn. Lippincott-Raven.

Moore, E. (1993) Atypical mycobacterial infection in the lung: CT appearance. *Radiology* **187**: 777–782.

Miller, W. (1994) Spectrum of pulmonary nontuberculous mycobacterial infection. *Radiology* **191**: 343–350.

Miller, W., Miller, W. (1993) Pulmonary infection with atypical mycobacteria in the normal host. *Semin. Roent.* **xxviii**: 139–149.

Schlugar, N., Rom, W. (1994) Current approaches to the diagnosis and treatment of acute pulmonary tuberculosis. *Am. J. Resp. Crit. Care Med.* **149**: 264–267.

Miller, W. (1994) Tuberculosis in the 1990s. *Radiol. Clin. North Am.* **32**: 649–661.

Miller, W.T., Miller, J.R. (1993) Tuberculosis in the normal host. Radiological findings. *Semin. Roent.* **xxviii**: 109–118.

Kotloff, R. (1993) Infection caused by NTM: clinical aspects. *Semin. Roent.* **xxviii**: 131–138.

Sharma, S.K., Mohan, A., Pande, J.N. *et al.* (1995) Clinical profile, laboratory characteristics and outcome in miliary tuberculosis. *Q. J. Med.* **88**: 29–37.

Hartman, T., Swenson, S., Williams, D. (1993) Mycobacterium avium-intracellulare complex: evaluation with CT. *Radiology* **187**: 23–26.

Barnes, P. (1997) Rapid diagnostic tests for tuberculosis. *Am. J. Resp. Crit. Care Med.* **155**: 1497–1498.

Menzies, D. (1999) Interpretation of repeated tuberculin tests. *Am. J. Resp. Crit. Care Med.* **159**: 15–21.

American Thoracic Society (1990) Diagnosis and treatment of disease caused by nontuberculous mycobacteria. *Am. Rev. Resp. Dis.* **142**: 940–953.

Menzies, D., Tannenbaum, T.N., Fitzgerald, J.M. (1999) Tuberculosis: 10. Prevention. *CMAJ* **161**(6): 717–724.

Schwartzman, K., Menzies, D. (1999) Tuberculosis: 11. Nosocomial disease. *CMAJ* **161**(10): 1271–1277.

Van Rie, A., Warren, R., Richardson, M. *et al.* (1999) Exogenous reinfection as a cause of recurrent tuberculosis after curative treatment. *NEJM* **341**: 1174–1179.

75 Upper Airways Obstruction

Definition: Obstruction of the conducting system from the mouth/nose to the tracheal carina

DIAGNOSTIC WORK-UP

1 **History**
- History of allergic reactions +/– prior episodes
- Recent URI
- Dyspnea, orthopnea, PND with choking on secretions
- Noisy breathing
- Change in voice
- Dysphagia or odynophagia
- Diagnosis of 'asthma' or 'COPD' unresponsive to therapy
- Features of obstructive sleep apnea

2 **Physical**
- Stridor and tachypnea
- Wheezes and rhonchi transmitted from upper airway
- 'Barking' cough
- Drooling
- Hoarseness or muffled voice

- Swollen neck
- Intercostal indrawing

3 **Investigations**

- *PA and lateral chest X-ray*
  - Narrowing of tracheal air column (<10 mm female, <13 mm male in the sagittal or coronal diameter)
  - Loss of the distinct air–tissue border along the wall of the inner trachea
  - Tracheal deviation
  - Signs of chronic obstruction including hyperinflation, pulmonary edema (rare), pulmonary hypertension and cor pulmonale
- *Lateral soft tissues of the neck*
  - Retropharyngeal and retrolaryngeal (pre-vertebral) soft tissue swelling (normal 7 mm at C2 and 21 mm at C5–6)
  - Epiglottic or vallecula swelling
  - Foreign body
  - Hypertrophied tonsils
- *Direct laryngoscopy/bronchoscopy*
- *CT/MRI*
  - Subglottic region and upper trachea are difficult to evaluate endoscopically
- *ABGs*
  - Hypoxemia ± hypercapnia
- *Spirometry and flow–volume curves* with demonstration of fixed or variable obstruction (Fig. 75.1)

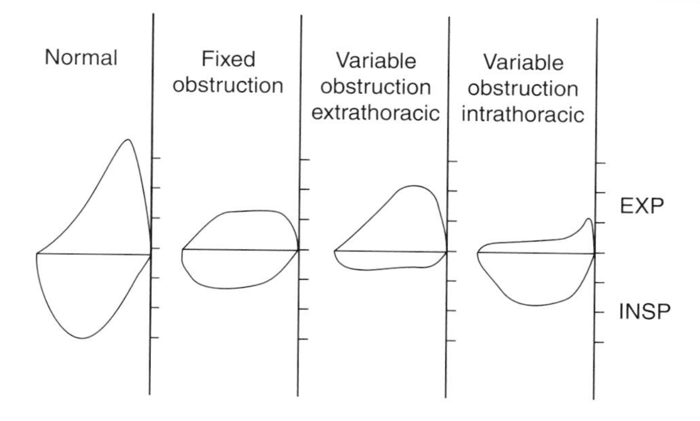

Fig. 75.1 Spirometry and flow volume curves

4 Identify the **likely site** and **potential pathologies**

ACUTE UPPER AIRWAYS OBSTRUCTION

Pharynx

- Airway lumen, e.g. foreign body
- Retropharyngeal space, e.g. abscess, hemorrhage
- Tongue, e.g. edema, fallen back with decreased sensorium
- Floor of mouth, e.g. abscess
- Tonsils, e.g. abscess, tonsillitis
- Pharyngeal wall, e.g. abscess, pharyngitis

Larynx

- Vocal cords, e.g. toxic inhalation, angioedema, trauma
- Subglottis, e.g. trauma
- Airway lumen, e.g. foreign body
- Laryngismus stridoris
- **Epiglottitis**
  - Defined as edema and inflammation of the epiglottis, although other supraglottic structures are frequently involved, including the arytenoids, aryepiglottic folds, pharynx and uvula

- Clinically presents with variable combinations of odynophagia, dyspnea, dysphagia, fever, sore throat, drooling, muffled voice, hoarseness and stridor, complications including
  - Fulminant course with upper airways obstruction and cardiopulmonary arrest
  - Epiglottic or retropharyngeal abscess
  - Systemic complications of bacteremia, pneumonia, meningitis, arthritis

Etiologies
1 *H. influenzae* (most common)
2 *H. parainfluenzae*
3 Streptococcus species
4 *Staph. aureus*
5 Negative cultures

Diagnostic features
1 'Cherry-red' epiglottis by laryngoscopy
2 Thumb sign on lateral neck X-ray
3 CT scan to evaluate the epiglottis and associated supraglottic structures

Larynx and trachea

- Croup (laryngo-tracheitis) is a clinical diagnosis charaterized by
  - URI and low grade fever
  - Barking cough
  - Variable upper airways obstruction
  - Rare in adults with >80% of cases occurring under age 6
  - A viral etiology is typical including respiratory syncitial, parainfluenza, influenza, adenovirus and rhinovirus
  - ENT exam reveals a normal epiglottis and supraglottis with subglottic edema and tracheal narrowing
  - A characteristic but non-specific radiologic feature is the 'steeple sign' with subglottic narrowing on a frontal X-ray
  - Complications include severe upper airways obstruction requiring intubation as well as bacterial tracheitis presenting with bronchoscopic features of edema, purulent exudates and mucosal ulceration of the subglottic trachea

Trachea
- Traumatic edema
- Acute tracheitis
- Wegener's granulomatosis
- Toxic inhalation
- Mediastinal abscess
- Foreign body

SUBACUTE–CHRONIC UPPER AIRWAYS OBSTRUCTION

Pharynx, e.g. tonsillar hypertrophy

Larynx
- Supraglottic, e.g. carcinoma
- Glottic, e.g. bilateral vocal cord paralysis, carcinoma
- Infraglottic, e.g. carcinoma

Trachea – Diffuse or localized tracheal narrowing

TRACHEAL NARROWING

Intralumenal, e.g. foreign body, mucoid pseudotumor

Extrinsic
1. Vascular, e.g. aneurysm, anomalous vessels
2. Neoplastic, e.g. lung, larynx, thyroid, esophagus, mediastinal, lymphomas, others
3. Organomegaly, e.g. goiter
4. Inflammatory, e.g. chronic fibrosing or granulomatous mediastinitis
5. Lymphadenopathy
6. Pulmonary fibrosis, e.g. end-stage sarcoid

Intrinsic
1. Neoplastic, primary or secondary
2. Congenital, e.g. relapsing polychondritis
3. Vasculitis, e.g. Wegener's

4 Infectious, e.g. tuberculous, fungal, bacterial (*Staph. aureus*), viral (parainfluenza)
5 Inhalation injury
6 Inflammatory, e.g. sarcoid, ulcerative colitis
7 Infiltrative, e.g. amyloid
8 Traumatic, e.g. post-intubation or post-tracheostomy
9 Sabre-sheath Trachea
10 Relapsing polychondritis (local or diffuse)
11 Tracheobronchopathia osteochondroplastica
12 Scleroma
13 Inspiratory dilation but expiratory tracheal narrowing – Mounier-Kuhn, tracheomalacia

Sabre-Sheath Trachea

Definition: Excessive coronal narrowing of the intrathoracic trachea with widening of the sagittal tracheal diameter and a ratio of the two diameters, coronal/sagittal, >0.5

- The cervical trachea is spared with an abrupt transition zone at the origin of the intrathoracic trachea at the manubrium
- Clinically it is seen in older male smokers with 95% of patients having COPD and features of airways obstruction, being rarely described in females
- Unclear whether the sabre-sheath trachea is the cause or result of airflow obstruction
- Radiologically, there is narrowing of the intrathoracic trachea in the coronal plane and widening in the sagittal plane
- AP views of the tracheobronchial air column show the diameter of the main stem bronchi to exceed that of the trachea
- On forced expiration, the lateral walls of the trachea collapse inward instead of the posterior tracheal membrane invaginating
- The tracheal cartilages can calcify without the pattern of nodular submucosal calcifications seen in tracheobronchopathia osteochondroplastica
- Other causes of coronal tracheal narrowing, e.g. relapsing

polychondritis, amyloid, etc. do not cause an increased sagittal diameter

Tracheobronchial Papillomatosis

Human papilloma virus infection of the respiratory tract, most commonly presenting with laryngeal disease within the first 3 years of life and rarely beginning in adulthood

- Tracheobronchial or airspace disease develops in ~2% of patients, typically many years after laryngeal involvement
- Clinically, adults have a life-long history of upper airway disease, have often undergone tracheostomy, and present with symptoms of endobronchial disease including cough, hemoptysis, 'asthma', as well as recurrent respiratory infections
- Papillomas can transform into malignancy, most often squamous cell carcinoma

Radiologic findings

1 Tracheal narrowing
2 Bronchial narrowing or obstruction
3 Bronchiectasis
4 Atelectasis
5 Obstructive pneumonitis
6 Abscess formation
7 Multiple lung nodules which can cavitate
8 Carcinoma

Tracheal Neoplasms

Clinically, symptoms relate to the airways, i.e. cough, dyspnea, wheezing, hemoptysis, frequently misdiagnosed as asthma or bronchitis

- Symptoms often delayed until ~50% of the tracheal lumen is obstructed
- Intrathoracic location results in expiratory wheezing and an obstructive picture with a plateau on the expiratory flow–volume curves, whereas a lesion of the extrathoracic trachea is manifest by obstruction of the inspiratory flow volume curves and inspiratory wheezing

- Early lesions are often missed on chest X-ray due to poor appreciation of the tracheal air column

Benign tumors are rare and include chondroma, hamartoma, fibroma, hemangioma, leiomyoma, squamous cell papilloma
- Typically, they are small, well-circumscribed lesions which project into the tracheal lumen but are confined to the tracheal wall
- Calcification may be seen in hamartomas and chondromas

Primary malignant neoplasms are uncommon compared to laryngeal and bronchogenic cancers
- Majority are squamous cell carcinoma and adenoid cystic carcinoma (cylindroma) but other primary tumors include
  - Other cell types of bronchogenic cancer
  - Carcinoid
  - Sarcoma
  - Lymphoma
  - Plasmacytoma
- Squamous and adenoid cystic carcinoma both spread locally into the mediastinum and distally to liver, bone, etc.
- Symptoms are related to local tracheal obstruction, vocal cord involvement in upper tracheal lesions, mediastinal spread, (e.g. SVC syndrome, dysphagia), or distant metastases
- Primary tracheal malignancies should be distinguished from **secondary malignant neoplasms** which occur by direct spread from the thyroid, larynx, esophagus, lung, or hematogenous metastases from breast, melanoma, GU tract, colon

CT scan reveals a soft-tissue density, often sessile and asymmetric with occasional circumferential narrowing of the tracheal lumen
- Direct extension can occur into the mediastinum with displacement, encasement, compression or obstruction of mediastinal structures

Resectability relates to
- Absence of systemic metastases

- Extent of tracheal involvement as submucosal extension may be underestimated
- Extent of extratracheal invasion

Scleroma

Rare chronic granulomatous disease primarily involving the nose and sinuses, caused by *Klebsiella rhinoscleromatis*

- Endemic in Asia, Africa and South America but rare in North America, and characterized by
  - An initial catarrhal stage of purulent rhinorrhea
  - Granulomatous nodules developing along the entire respiratory tract from nose to bronchi with involvement being most severe from top to bottom
  - Enlargement and scarring of granulomas leading to large airways obstruction (seen in <5% of cases)

Relapsing Polychondritis

Rare systemic disease characterized by destruction of cartilage and other connective tissues followed by their replacement with fibrous tissue in multiple anatomic sites

- An inflammatory infiltrate may accompany the fibrosis in clinically active cases as well as a vasculitis of small and large arteries

Clinically, seen in all age groups, peaks between 40–60, sex distribution ranging from equal to 3:1 female/male

- Presenting features can be quite variable with evidence of chondritis frequently seen in several locations, but ear pain is the most frequent initial complaint
- Relapses, remissions and a prolonged course are typical with the natural history of disease being unpredictable

1 *Auricular chondritis is the commonest sign and may result in 'cauliflower-ears', with extension of inflammation to the middle and inner ear
2 *Non-erosive, inflammatory, seronegative polyarthritis involving peripheral joints as well as the costal cartilages is the second most common feature
3 *Nasal chondritis with eventual saddle-nose deformity
4 *Ocular inflammation including conjunctivitis, uveitis, etc.

5 Cardiovascular disease involving the heart and great vessels
6 Systemic symptoms of fevers, night sweats, weight loss
7 *Pulmonary involvement is seen in ~½ of all patients, is the presenting feature in up to ¼, and is responsible for up to 50% of all deaths
   - Cartilagenous destruction extends from the larynx to the bronchial tubes, with its replacement by granulation tissue, fibrosis and calcification
     - Laryngeal disease with hoarseness, stridor, aphasia, cough and tenderness over the upper airway
     - Tracheobronchial involvement with airways obstruction resulting from tracheobronchomalacia, subglottic/tracheal strictures (most common radiologic finding) or inflammatory edema early in the disease
       - Symptoms of the above include cough, wheezing and dyspnea on exertion while airway strictures may be complicated by pneumonia and secondary bronchiectasis
       - Tracheostomy may be required for severe upper airways obstruction although lower airway disease, e.g. mainstem bronchus involvement, may be asymptomatic
       - Disease may be focal or generalized and uncommonly can primarily involve only the bronchial tubes

Diagnostic findings
1 Clinical features as above, most often a history of ear and joint pains
2 Narrowing and/or calcifications of the tracheobronchial tree on chest X-ray or CT with dynamic collapse of airways on cineradiography
3 Calcifications of the pinnae and external auditory meatus on CT scan
4 Airways obstruction ranging from fixed to variable, intrathoracic or extrathoracic
5 Bronchoscopy for visualization of the affected airways with

- Inflammatory or fibrotic narrowing
- Expiratory collapse
- Biopsy of cartilage demonstrating inflammation as well as destruction of cartilage and its replacement with fibrous tissue

Tracheobronchopathia Osteochondroplastica

Rare condition characterized by the presence of multiple osteocartilaginous nodules in the tracheobronchial submucosa projecting into the airway lumen

- Case reports of an association with tracheobronchial amyloid ? end-stage of this disorder in some patients

Clinically, usually seen in patients over age 50 with a male predominance and presentations include

- Asymptomatic finding at autopsy
- Non-specific complaints of dyspnea, cough, wheezing
- Mistaken diagnosis of asthma
- Recurrent respiratory tract infections
- Hemoptysis secondary to mucosal ulcerations

Bronchoscopic features

- 'Beaded' appearance of the tracheobronchial tree due to nodules confined to the cartilagenous areas with sparing of the posterior tracheal membrane
- 'Grating sensation' as the bronchoscope is passed
- Intact mucosa over the nodules
- Distortion and narrowing of the tracheobronchial lumen with lobar narrowing or obstruction

Radiologic features

1. Narrowing and an irregular contour of the tracheal air column, most often involving the lower $\frac{2}{3}$ of the trachea and often extending into the major bronchi
2. Atelectasis or obstructive pneumonitis if bronchial obstruction is complete
3. Pathognomonic CT demonstration of a thickened tracheobronchial wall and calcification of mural nodules

Amyloid

Primary pulmonary amyloid may have several manifestations with tracheobronchial involvement most common

- Disease may be limited to the tracheobronchial tree with focal or diffuse airways narrowing seen on X-ray or CT, reflecting plaques or tumor-like masses (which may calcify)
- Patients may be asymptomatic or present with non-specific respiratory symptoms
- Diagnosis confirmed on bronchoscopy and biopsy of the submucosal mass(es)

Mediastinal Fibrosis

Sequelae of histoplasmosis, tuberculosis or idiopathic, with mediastinal or hilar nodal calcification present on X-ray

- Other mediastinal structures often involved, e.g. pericardium, SVC, esophagus

Tracheomalacia

Defined as a weakness of the tracheal walls with resultant collapsability, etiologies including

1 Williams-Campbell syndrome
2 Secondary to intubation, chronic infection, relapsing polychondritis, tracheostomy, COPD

- Clinically, cough is inefficient with retained secretions, recurrent infections and bronchiectasis
- Patients present with symptoms of airways obstruction
- Radiologically, there is expiratory airways collapse (cine-fluoroscopy, dynamic spiral CT) which can also be seen during fiberoptic bronchoscopy, characterized by greater than 50% narrowing of the anteroposterior tracheal diameter

Post-Intubation or Post-Tracheostomy

1 Tracheal damage is seen at the stoma or at the level of the inflatable cuff
    - The latter compromises blood supply to the mucosa resulting in ischemic necrosis with mucosal ulcerations exposing the cartilaginous rings which are then softened, fragmented, and destroyed from pressure necrosis sequelae of the above including

  - Tracheal stenosis, often circumferential, extending over ~2 cm and due to edema, granulation tissue or mature fibrosis
  - Tracheomalacia with normal inspiratory tracheal diameters but collapse on expiration
  - Tracheal perforation
  - Tracheo-esophageal fistula formation where patients can present immediately post-extubation or many months later
2. Laryngeal edema
3. Vocal cord edema, ulcerations and granuloma formation
   - Usually resolves within 3 months but can present with dyspnea, stridor and hoarseness
4. Laryngospasm from adduction of the vocal cords and spasm of the aryepiglottic folds e.g. post tonsillectomy
5. Bilateral vocal cord paralysis 2° to compression of the anterior branches of the recurrent laryngeal nerves by the endotracheal tube
6. Dislocation of the arytenoids
7. Vocal cord paralysis from trauma, surgery or injury to the recurrent laryngeal nerve

Tuberculous Tracheitis

Rare disease, seen in association with cavitary lung disease

- Tracheal involvement occurs from infected sputum (positive smears), peribronchial lymphatic spread or local extension from mediastinal nodes
- Edematous swelling seen acutely can be followed by scarring and tracheal stenosis

Sarcoid

Upper airway involvement is uncommon and can result from parenchymal fibrosis with distortion and extrinsic narrowing of the airways, compression from mediastinal nodes or endotracheal sarcoid

- Laryngeal involvement, which is very rare without parenchymal or mediastinal involvement, may accompany tracheal disease

Wegener's Granulomatosis

Tracheobronchial involvement can accompany pulmonary parenchymal disease, kidney disease and other organ involvement or may rarely be the only involved site

- The larynx and subglottic region are most often involved with features of upper airway disease, i.e. stridor, wheezing, dyspnea, hemoptysis
- Bronchoscopic findings include ulcerative tracheobronchitis, tracheobronchial stenosis, cobblestone mucosa

Fraser R.S., Muller N.L., Colman N., Paré P.D. (1999) *Diagnosis of Diseases of the Chest* 4th Edn., WB Saunders.

Moss, A., Gamsu, Genant (1992) Thorax and neck. In: *Computed Tomography of the Body with Magnetic Resonance Imaging.* 2nd edn, vol. 1.: W.B. Saunders.

Thurlbeck, W., Churg, A. (eds) (1995) *Pathology of the Lung*, 2nd edn. (Place of publication): Thieme Medical Publishers.

Baum, G.L., Crapo, J.D., Celli, B.R., Karlinsky, J.B. (eds) (1997) *Textbook of Pulmonary Diseases*, 6th edn.: Lippincott-Raven.

Fishman, A.P., Elias, J.A., Fishman, J.A., Grippi, M.A., Kaiser, L.R., Senior, R.N. (1998) *Fishman's Pulmonary Diseases and Disorders*, 3rd edn.: McGraw-Hill.

Frantz, T., Rasgon, B., Queensberry, C. (1994) Acute epiglottitis in adults. *JAMA* **272**: 1358–1360.

Aboussouan, L., Stoller, J. (1994) Diagnosis and management of upper airway obstruction. *Clinics in Chest Medicine* **15**: 35–53.

Gamsu, G., Webb, W.R. (1983) Computed tomography of the trachea and mainstem bronchi. *Semin. Roent.* **18**: 51.

Mayo Smith, M.F. *et al.* (1986) Acute epiglottitis in adults. *NEJM* **314**: 1133–1139.

Shapiro, J., Eavey, R., Baker, S. (1988) Adult supraglottitis: a prospective analysis. *JAMA* **259**: 563–567.

Johnson, J.T. *et al.* (1987) Bacterial tracheitis in adults. *Arch. Otolaryn. Head Neck Surg.* **113**: 204–205.

Stark, P., Norbash, A. (1998) Imaging of the trachea and upper airways in patients with chronic obstructive airway disease. *Radiol. Clin. North Am.* **36**: 91–105.

76 Vasculitis – Pulmonary Manifestations

CLINICAL PRESENTATIONS

Vasculitis involving the respiratory system should be considered with

1. Airways obstruction – upper or lower
2. Undiagnosed pleural effusion
3. Idiopathic pulmonary artery hypertension
4. Parenchymal diseases
    - Hemoptysis, ranging from spotty to diffuse alveolar hemorrhage syndrome
    - Pulmonary-renal syndrome
    - ARDS
    - Lung nodules +/– cavitation
    - Non-resolving or recurrent pulmonary infiltrates
5. Multisystem disease, in association with non-specific respiratory symptoms and variable radiologic abnormalities, including airspace infiltrates, interstitial disease, fleeting infiltrates, nodules
6. Granulomatous lung disease

HISTOPATHOLOGIC CLASSIFICATION

Large Vessel Vasculitis

Lung involvement is rare with isolated case reports in

1 **Temporal arteritis** (Giant cell arteritis)
   - A systemic vasculitis affecting mainly the elderly and the most common form of vasculitis overall
   - Usual presentation is fever, malaise, headache, jaw claudication and visual disturbances
   - Respiratory symptoms are described in a small percentage of patients and include sore throat, cough, hoarseness, and tender cervical structures
   - Granulomatous involvement of the pulmonary vasculature, bronchi and interstitium are described in individual case reports with widely varied radiologic abnormalities, e.g. lung nodules which can cavitate, interstitial opacities, others
   - In-patients with prominent pulmonary disease, both Wegener's and Churg-Strauss, should be excluded

2 **Takayasu's arteritis** (TA) is an uncommon vasculitis affecting the aorta (thoracic +/or abdominal), its major branches, as well as the large and medium sized pulmonary arteries
   - TA primarily affects women, usually Asian and under age 30, with many cases initially diagnosed during pregnancy
   - Clinically, the disease often begins with non-specific constitutional symptoms of fevers, night sweats, weight loss and arthralgias for several weeks to months
   - The classic features subsequently develop including pulseless disease and aortic arch syndrome, renovascular hypertension, claudication of the upper +/or lower extremities, angina, headaches and visual disturbances, the above reflecting ischemia of the affected organs
   - Pulmonary disease is a reflection of the patchy panarteritis and fibrosis of the adventitia, media and intima

responsible for the vascular stenoses, but is often asymptomatic
- Pulmonary artery involvement may be seen in ~50% of patients (CT/MRI) and vascular bruits may be heard over the lung fields
- Pulmonary hypertension is the principal clinical manifestation although massive hemoptysis has been reported
- Pulmonary vascular obstruction can be visualized indirectly on lung scan or directly on pulmonary angiography, spiral CT angiography or MRI, while extensive collaterals can be seen between the bronchial and pulmonary circulations with occlusion, stenosis and post-stenotic dilatation of the pulmonary arteries
- The abnormalities on lung scan may incorrectly suggest the diagnosis of thromboembolic disease
- Chest X-ray abnormalities most often involve the aorta with contour irregularities and calcifications, while CT and MRI further define aortic lesions, e.g. stenotic, dilated, aneurysmal

Medium Vessel Vasculitis

Polyarteritis pathologically only involves arteries, never small vessels, rarely involves the lungs, and then only the bronchial arteries

Small Vessel Vasculitis – ANCA positive or ANCA negative

Defined as vasculitis predominantly involving arterioles, venules and capillaries, i.e. capillaritis
- Lung disease is common in the ANCA positive group which includes
  - Wegener's granulomatosis
  - Microscopic polyangiitis
  - Churg-Strauss (see p. 270)
- The ANCA negative immune complex diseases rarely involve the lungs and include Henoch-Schonlein, drug-induced vasculitis, cryoglobulinemia, others

PULMONARY CAPILLARITIS

Pulmonary capillaritis is a histopathologic diagnosis made on light microscopy and defined by

1 Capillary occlusion by fibrin thrombi
2 Fibrinoid necrosis of the capillary wall
3 Interstitial infiltrate of erythrocytes, hemosiderin, neutrophils
4 Intra-alveolar hemorrhage which can be extensive
5 Absence of an infectious agent identified

- Can be diagnosed by transbronchial or open lung biopsy but may be misdiagnosed as alveolitis
- Pulmonary capillaritis and resultant DAH are usually a manifestation of
  - Underlying systemic vasculitis, e.g. Wegener's, microscopic polyarteritis
  - Collagen vascular disease, e.g. systemic lupus
  - Other systemic disorder, e.g. Behcet's, cryoglobulinemia, Goodpasture's syndrome
- Also described as an isolated disorder, without clinical, serologic or pathologic evidence of a systemic disease

Clinically, the presentation is that of the diffuse alveolar hemorrhage (DAH) syndrome

- Many patients with the DAH syndrome do not have capillaritis, the latter being a constellation of clinical, radiologic, laboratory, pulmonary function and bronchoscopic findings (see p. 28)
- Dyspnea is the most common presenting symptom with hemoptysis, hypoxemia and anemia being quite variable
- Symptoms vary from mild to severe, occasionally resulting in respiratory failure requiring mechanical ventilation
- Chest X-rays reveal diffuse bilateral patchy alveolar infiltrates which prompt the lung biopsy
- The finding of capillaritis should prompt a search for systemic disease with respect to clinical features,

pathologic evidence or serologic abnormalities including anti-GBM antibody, C-ANCA, P-ANCA, anti-DNA antibody, rheumatoid factor

WEGENER'S GRANULOMATOSIS

A multisystem disease, described in all age groups and equally seen in both sexes, pulmonary involvement characterized **pathologically** by the triad of

1 Vasculitis ± capillaritis
2 Parenchymal necrosis
3 Granulomatous inflammation with the exclusion of granulomatous infection by fungi, mycobacteria and helminths

Classic disseminated disease is characterized by the above pathology of the upper and lower respiratory tract, glomerulonephritis and necrotizing vasculitis of systemic organs

Limited or non-renal disease can involve the upper respiratory tract and skin in addition to the lungs, is often insidious in onset with symptoms present for many months before the diagnosis is considered

Clinical Presentations

Pulmonary disease occurs in about 45% of patients at presentation and in ~90% of patients over the course of their disease, including

1 Non-specific respiratory symptoms usually reflecting airway or parenchymal disease
2 Alveolar hemorrhage syndrome which can rapidly progress to respiratory failure
   - Seen in ~5% of cases and may be the presenting feature
   - Diagnosis is established by defining the presence of a diffuse alveolar hemorrhage syndrome which is often accompanied by capillaritis (*vs.* the usual granulomatous inflammation) as well as a positive c-ANCA

3 Upper airways involvement with laryngotracheal disease, particularly subglottic stenosis in ~15% of patients
   - Symptoms vary from hoarseness to stridor and life-threatening upper airways obstruction
4 Lower airways disease with endobronchial abnormalities of ulceration, tracheal/bronchial stenosis, inflammatory lesions without stenosis or hemorrhage
5 Asymptomatic radiologic abnormalities (see below)
6 Airways obstruction on PFTs +/– associated reductions in lung volume when extensive parenchymal disease is present

ENT disease is the most common presenting feature
1 Ears – recurrent otitis media, pains, hearing loss
2 Nose – epistaxis, mucosal swelling, ulcerations, septal perforation, saddle-nose deformation
3 Throat – nasopharyngeal ulcerations
4 Sinuses – sinus pain, purulent discharge

Renal disease manifest as glomerulonephritis is present in ~20% of patients at presentation and in ~80% during the course of disease, often developing within the first 2 years
- An active urine sediment, proteinuria and variable BUN/Cr are seen
- The presence of renal disease on urinalysis or biopsy defines generalized *vs.* limited Wegener's, although disease may change over time with limited evolving into classic Wegener's
- Spontaneous resolution of kidney disease is not seen

Eye disease is seen eventually in ~50% of patients but is often non-specific, although proptosis when present is characteristic

Constitutional symptoms of fevers, weight loss

Other, including cutaneous purpura and nodules, cardiac disease, GI disease, neurologic disease – central or peripheral, arthritis

Radiologic Manifestations

Parenchymal disease

1 Lung nodules, 5 mm–10 cm in diameter, randomly distributed, usually bilateral but occasionally solitary, increasing in number and size with disease progression
   - Cavitation seen in up to 50% with thick-walled cavities becoming thin-walled during treatment
   - Number of nodules as well as associated cavitation are better evaluated on CT

2 Airspace opacities ranging from 'ground glass' to consolidation and representing
   - Granulomatous inflammation
   - Alveolar hemorrhage
   - May be focal or bilateral and diffuse with random distribution

3 Fleeting infiltrates that can resolve before therapy

4 Diffuse reticulonodular disease (rare)

Airways disease

5 Endotracheal disease with subglottic stenosis

6 Endobronchial stenosis and atelectasis

Pleural disease

7 Pleural effusions, due to primary disease, uremia or infection

Mediastinum/hilum

8 Adenopathy (rare)

Secondary pulmonary manifestations

9 Infections, including opportunistic organisms

10 Drug toxicity including direct toxicity as well as drug-induced infections or lymphoma

11 Cardiac failure

12 Renal failure (see effects of uremia p. 717)

Morbidity

1 **Pulmonary**
   - Fibrosis with restrictive PFTs
   - Tracheal stenosis

- Endobronchial stenosis with lobar atelectasis or recurrent post-obstructive pneumonitis
- Obstructive lung disease
- Cyclophosphamide-induced pneumonitis
- Opportunistic infection

2 **ENT** including hearing loss, nasal deformity
3 **Renal failure**
4 **Visual loss**
5 **CNS** infarcts, hemorrhage

When to Suspect Wegener's

Wegener's should be considered in the differential of a wide range of pulmonary disorders including

1. Endotracheal or endobronchial narrowing
2. Lung nodules ± cavitation
3. Pulmonary-renal syndromes
4. Alveolar hemorrhage syndromes
5. Granulomatous lung disease – NYD
6. ANCA ⊕ vasculitis
7. Non-resolving or changing pattern of airspace consolidation
8. Rarely as interstitial lung disease – NYD
9. Pulmonary disease with prominent nasal symptoms
   - R/O cocaine use, SLE, eosinophilic granuloma, lymphoma, Churg-Strauss, sarcoid, fungal infection, scleroma, nasopharyngeal carcinoma
10. Pulmonary disease and a laryngeal mass
    - R/O carcinoma, sarcoid, tuberculosis, histoplasmosis, blastomycosis

Diagnostic Features

1. Compatible clinical presentation with ENT symptoms the most common, followed by pulmonary, renal and eye disease
2. Compatible chest X-rays
3. Focal segmental glomerulonephritis on renal biopsy with little or no immune complex deposition on immunofluorescence or electron microscopy, granules being uncommon

4 ⊕ c-ANCA with anti-proteinase 3 antibodies in ~90% of cases with disseminated disease
   - A minority of patients have ⊕ p-ANCA directed against myeloperoxidase
   - The incidence of a ⊕ ANCA is decreased in limited Wegener's (50% or less) or inactive disease
   - ⊕ c-ANCA is seen in other vasculitides, e.g. polyarteritis, microscopic polyarteritis, Churg-Strauss, polyangiitis overlap syndrome as well as in non-vasculitic disorders, e.g. TB, neoplasms, etc.

5 Pathologic features of vasculitis and granulomatous inflammation involving the upper and/or lower respiratory tract
   - Bronchoscopy can demonstrate areas of stenosis, ulceration or inflammatory pseudotumor and may establish the diagnosis

MICROSCOPIC POLYANGIITIS (MPA)

Small vessel vasculitis of arterioles, capillaries and venules, capillaritis being the most common lesion, and histologically distinguished from

1 Wegener's by the absence of granulomas
2 Henoch-Schonlein or cryoglobulinemia by the absence of immune deposits
3 Polyarteritis nodosa (PAN) which affects only medium sized arteries and has immune complex deposition

Clinically, renal disease is the major feature with rapidly progressive glomerulonephritis and renal impairment, which can deteriorate quickly if untreated

- Other involvement includes cutaneous vasculitis, mononeuritis multiplex and systemic symptoms of fever, myalgias, arthralgias and weight loss
- Pulmonary involvement occurs in ~30% of cases and is usually that of alveolar hemorrhage which can be life-threatening or lead to pulmonary fibrosis

- Upper airway symptoms typical of Wegener's or Churg-Strauss are absent

Labs reveal a positive ANCA in about 80% of cases (p-ANCA > c-ANCA) but negative serology to hepatitis B, unlike PAN

- Urinalysis reveals hematuria and an active sediment
- BAL findings are those of diffuse alveolar hemorrhage

Chest X-rays reflect the alveolar hemorrhage with diffuse alveolar opacities ranging from 'ground glass' opacities to consolidation, while pleural effusions are seen in ~15% of cases

Diagnostic features

1 Compatible clinical picture
2 Histologic evidence of vasculitis involving the lungs or other tissues
3 Positive ANCA (usually p-ANCA) seen in most patients, positive RF in 40%, positive ANA in 20%
4 Crescentic glomerulonephritis

BEHCET'S DISEASE (BD)

Most cases are described from eastern Mediterranean countries and Japan with a male/female predominance

- 5–10% of patients have involvement of the pulmonary vascular tree, reflecting a systemic multifocal vasculitis of arteries (e.g. aortitis), capillaries (e.g. cutanous vasculitis) and veins (e.g. vena cava obstruction)
  - Hemoptysis is the most common pulmonary symptom (~95% of patients), a poor prognostic sign, and can be secondary to pulmonary artery aneurysm rupture, *in situ* thrombosis complicating vasculitis, pulmonary infarction from thromboemboli, contiguous bronchial inflammation with bronchial artery erosion
  - Other non-specific respiratory symptoms can occur, and with hemoptysis usually develop years after systemic disease
  - Pulmonary hypertension
  - Migratory thrombophlebitis of the legs and/or IVC in ~40% of patients

– Hughes-Stovin may be a manifestation of BD, i.e. DVT and multiple pulmonary artery aneurysms

Radiologic features

1 Hilar enlargement reflecting pulmonary artery aneurysms or varix formation
2 Signs of thromboembolic disease with diaphragmatic elevation, line shadows and wedge-shaped peripheral opacities
3 Lobulated opacities or mass lesions reflecting aneurysm formation (single/multiple/unilateral/bilateral)
4 Pulmonary infiltrates with 'stellate' or star-shaped peripheral vessels on CT reflecting vasculitis and aneurysm formation
5 Pleural effusions secondary to pulmonary infarction, vasculitis, hemothorax (rare), chylothorax (rare)
6 Perfusion defects on V/Q scan
7 Pulmonary artery cut-offs or aneurysms on CT or MRI (angiography not recommended due to puncture of inflamed vessels as well as local side-effects)
8 Airspace consolidation or 'ground glass' opacities reflecting pulmonary hemorrhage
9 Mediastinal widening due to brachiocephalic or SVC thrombosis, aortic aneurysm

Diagnosed on the basis of recurrent oral ulcers and two of the following

1 Recurrent genital ulcers
2 Uveitis
3 Typical papulopustular skin lesions
4 Positive pathergy test, i.e. sterile pustules 24–48 hours after cutaneous needle prick

HENOCH-SCHONLEIN PURPURA

Vasculitis syndrome of palpable purpura, arthritis, abdominal pain and glomerulonephritis

- Systemic vasculitis is often diagnosed on skin biopsy which reveals a small vessel vasculitis, most prominent in the postcapillary venules, as well as deposition of IgA-containing immune complexes in skin or renal biopsy
- Described in all age groups but primarily occurs in childhood or adolescence
- Pulmonary disease is rare with vasculitis and alveolar hemorrhage described pathologically
- Clinically there is hemoptysis which can be severe, chest X-rays reflecting the alveolar hemorrhage and manifest as airspace disease

Fraser R.S., Muller N.L., Colman N., Paré P.D. (1999) *Diagnosis of Diseases of the Chest* 4th Edn., WB Saunders.

Thurlbeck W., Churg, A. (eds) (1995) *Pathology of the Lung*, 2nd edn. (Place of publication): Thieme Medical Publishers.

Green, R., Ruoss, S., Kraft, S. *et al.* (1996) Pulmonary capillaritis and alveolar hemorrhage. Update on diagnosis and management. *Chest* **110**: 1305–1316.

Green, R., Ruoss, S. *et al.* (1996) Pulmonary capillaritis and alveolar hemorrhage. *Chest* **110**: 1305–1316.

Leavitt, R.Y., Fauci, A.S. (1986) Pulmonary vasculitis. *ARRD* **134**: 149–166.

Erkan, F., Cavdar, T. (1992) Pulmonary vasculitis in Behcet's disease. *ARRD* **146**: 232–239.

Jennette, J.C., Falk, R. (1997) Small vessel vasculitis. *NEJM* **337**: 1512–1522.

Sullivan, W. *et al.* (1984) A prospective evalaution emphasizing pulmonary involvement in patients with MCTD. *Medicine* **63**: 92–107.

Numan, F., Islak, C., Berkmen J. *et al.* (1994) Behcet's disease: pulmonary arterial involvement in 15 cases. *Radiology* **192**: 465–468.

Raz, I., Okon, E., Chajek-Shanh, T. (1989) Pulmonary manifestations in Behcet's syndrome. *Chest* **95**: 585–589.

Beer, D. (1992) Ancas aweigh. *ARRD* **148**: 1128–1130.

Hoffman, G., Kerr, G., Leavitt, R. *et al.* (1992) Wegener's granulomatosis: an analysis of 158 patients. *AIM* **116**: 488–498.

Fauci, A., Walff, S.M. (1973) Wegener's granulomatosis. *Medicine* **52**: 535–561.

Duna, G., Galpem, C., Hoffman, G. (1995) Wegener's granulomatosis. *Rheum. Dis. Clin. North Am.* **21**: 949–976.

Jemmings. C., King, T., Tuder, R. *et al.* (1997) Diffuse alveolar hemorrhage with underlying isolated pauciimune pulmonary capillaritis. *Am. J. Resp. Crit. Care Med.* **155**: 1101–1109.

Fauci, A. *et al.* (1983) Wegener's granulomatosis: prospective clinical and therapeutic experience with 85 patients for 21 years. *Ann. Intern. Med.* **98**: 76–85.

Sullivan, E., Hoffman, G. (1998) Pulmonary vasculitis. *Clinics in Chest Medicine* **19**: 759–776.

77 Vocal Cord Dysfunction (VCD)

Laryngoscopic diagnosis defined by paradoxical (and/or less often expiratory) closure of the vocal cords in the absence of demonstrable organic disease, the clinical and diagnostic features including

1 **History**

- Most often described in young women but not confined to this group
- Often a psychiatric history including depression, histrionic personality, abuses of a sexual, physical or emotional nature, secondary gain
- Patients are often labelled as asthmatic due to the presentation of intermittent dyspnea and 'noisy breathing', with a history of intubation being not uncommon
- Usually a lack of sputum (unlike asthma)
- Historically there is a lack of subjective response to bronchodilators, although several have often been prescribed including high dose steroids
- Differential diagnosis includes laryngospasm, laryngeal edema, vocal cord paralysis and asthma
- VCD may occur in isolation or co-exist with asthma making diagnosis difficult

2 **Physical**

- In the absence of concurrent asthma, there are inspiratory and expiratory wheezes which originate and are loudest in the neck area, as well as attenuated wheezes over the lung fields thought to be of tracheal origin
- Stridorous sounds are reduced or absent with either nose breathing or panting as well as during sleep

3 **Laryngoscopy**
- There is inspiratory closure of the vocal cords when symptomatic, either spontaneously or after provocation tests, e.g. methacoline, exercise
- Vocal cord closure is seen in fewer patients on both inspiration and expiration or on expiration alone, while about 50% of patients may demonstrate abnormal findings between exacerbations

4 **Labs**
- Severe hypoxemia can develop during acute attacks but chest and sinus X-ray are normal
- There is an absence of eosinophilia (unlike asthma)

5 **PFTs**
- No evidence of expiratory airflow obstruction or bronchodilator responsiveness
- No bronchial hyper-reactivity on challenge testing but VCD can be triggered with methacholine
- There are normal lung volumes and airways resistance when measured plethysmographically
- Flow-volume curve abnormalities include
  - Truncation of the inspiratory limb with decreased inspiratory flows as well as inspiratory fluttering (variable extrathoracic obstruction)
  - $MEF_{50}/MIF_{50} > 1.5$
  - Improved flows with a helium-oxygen mixture
  - Poor reproducibility of the curves

Fraser R.S., Muller N.L., Colman N., Paré P.D. (1999) *Diagnosis of Diseases of the Chest* 4th Edn., WB Saunders.

Fishman, A.P., Elias, J.A., Fishman, J.A., Grippi, M.A., Kaiser, L.R., Senior, R.N. (1998) *Fishman's Pulmonary Diseases and Disorders*, 3rd edn.: McGraw-Hill.

Ramirez, R.J., Leon, I., Rivera, L. (1986) Episodic laryngeal dyskinesia. *Chest* **90**: 716–720.

Newman, K., Mason, U., Schmaling, K. (1995) Clinical feature of vocal cord dysfunction. *Am. J. Resp. Crit. Care Med.* **152**: 1382–1386.

Christopher, K.L. *et al.* (1983) Vocal cord dysfunction presenting as asthma. *NEJM* **308**: 1566.

Subject Index

NOTE: Page numbers in bold refer to principal sections. These may include definition, clinical features, complications, diagnosis and differential diagnosis. vs denotes differential diagnosis